SOCIAL PSYCHIATRY
PRINCIPLES AND CLINICAL PERSPECTIVES

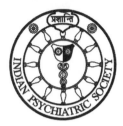

W0009008

Editors

Rakesh K Chadda MD FAMS FRCPsych

Professor and Head
Department of Psychiatry
Chief, National Drug Dependence
Treatment Center
All India Institute of Medical Sciences
New Delhi, India

Vinay Kumar MD

Consultant Psychiatrist
Manoved Mind Hospital and
Research Center
Patna, Bihar, India

Siddharth Sarkar MD DNB

Assistant Professor
Department of Psychiatry and
National Drug Dependence Treatment Center
All India Institute of Medical Sciences
New Delhi, India

Assistant Editors

Rishi Gupta MD DNB

Senior Resident
Department of Psychiatry and
National Drug Dependence Treatment Center
All India Institute of Medical Sciences
New Delhi, India

Nishtha Chawla MD DNB

Senior Resident
Department of Psychiatry and
National Drug Dependence Treatment Center
All India Institute of Medical Sciences
New Delhi, India

Foreword

NN Wig (Late)

JAYPEE BROTHERS MEDICAL PUBLISHERS
The Health Sciences Publisher
New Delhi | London | Panama

Jaypee Brothers Medical Publishers (P) Ltd

Headquarters

Jaypee Brothers Medical Publishers (P) Ltd
4838/24, Ansari Road, Daryaganj
New Delhi 110 002, India
Phone: +91-11-43574357
Fax: +91-11-43574314
Email: jaypee@jaypeebrothers.com

Overseas Offices

J.P. Medical Ltd
83 Victoria Street, London
SW1H 0HW (UK)
Phone: +44 20 3170 8910
Fax: +44 (0)20 3008 6180
Email: info@jpmedpub.com

Jaypee-Highlights Medical Publishers Inc
City of Knowledge, Bld. 235, 2nd Floor, Clayton
Panama City, Panama
Phone: +1 507-301-0496
Fax: +1 507-301-0499
Email: cservice@jphmedical.com

Jaypee Brothers Medical Publishers (P) Ltd
Bhotahity, Kathmandu, Nepal
Phone +977-9741283608
Email: kathmandu@jaypeebrothers.com

Website: www.jaypeebrothers.com
Website: www.jaypeedigital.com

Social Psychiatry: Principles and Clinical Perspectives

First Edition: **2019**

ISBN: 978-93-5270-422-4

Printed at: Paras Offset Pvt. Ltd., New Delhi

Contributors

Vivek Agarwal
Professor
Department of Psychiatry
King George's Medical University
Lucknow, Uttar Pradesh, India
drvivekagarwal06@gmail.com

Shyam Sundar Arumugham
Additional Professor
Department of Psychiatry
National Institute of Mental Health and
Neurosciences
Bengaluru, Karnataka, India
a.shyamsundar@gmail.com

Priti Arun
Professor
Department of Psychiatry
Government Medical College and Hospital
Chandigarh, India
drpritiarun@gmail.com

Ajit Avasthi
Professor and Head
Department of Psychiatry
Postgraduate Institute of Medical
Education and Research
Chandigarh, India
drajitavasthi@yahoo.co.in

Debasish Basu
Professor
Department of Psychiatry
Postgraduate Institute of Medical
Education and Research
Chandigarh, India
db_sm2002@yahoo.com

Prakash Balkrishna Behere
Vice Chancellor and Professor of Psychiatry
Dr DY Patil University
Kolhapur, Maharashtra, India
pbbehere@gmail.com

Aniruddh Prakash Behere
Pediatric Psychiatrist
Helen DeVos Children's Hospital
Spectrum Health, Grand Rapids
Michigan, USA
Clinical Assistant Professor
Michigan State University
Michigan, USA
aniruddhbehere@gmail.com

Rachna Bhargava
Associate Professor
Department of Psychiatry and National Drug
Dependence Treatment Center
All India Institute of Medical Sciences
New Delhi, India
rachnabhargava@gmail.com

Nikita Bhati
PhD Scholar
Department of Psychiatry and
National Drug Dependence Treatment Center
All India Institute of Medical Sciences
New Delhi, India
nikbhati.psych@gmail.com

Ranjan Bhattacharyya
Assistant Professor
Department of Psychiatry
Murshidabad Medical College and Hospital
Murshidabad, West Bengal, India
drrbcal@gmail.com

Manik Changoji Bhise
Associate Professor
Department of Psychiatry
MGM Medical College
Aurangabad, Maharashtra, India
dr.manik.bhise@gmail.com

Dinesh Bhugra
Emeritus Professor of Mental Health and
Cultural Diversity
Institute of Psychiatry
Psychology and Neuroscience, King's College
London, UK
dinesh.bhugra@kcl.ac.uk

Rituparna Biswas
Clinical Psychologist
Vivekananda Institute of Medical Sciences
Kolkata, West Bengal, India
rbiswas92@gmail.com

Rakesh K Chadda
Professor and Head
Department of Psychiatry
Chief, National Drug Dependence Treatment Center
All India Institute of Medical Sciences
New Delhi, India
drrakeshchadda@gmail.com

Subho Chakrabarti
Professor
Department of Psychiatry
Postgraduate Institute of Medical
Education and Research
Chandigarh, India
subhochd@yahoo.com

Suhas Chandran
Resident
Department of Psychiatry
JSS Medical College and Hospital
JSS University
Mysuru, Karnataka, India
suhaschandran90@gmail.com

Damodar Chari
Resident
Department of Psychiatry
Asha Hospital
Hyderabad, Telangana, India

Ishan Chaudhuri
Senior Resident
Department of Psychiatry
Dr DY Patil Medical College
Hospital and Research Center
Pune, Maharashtra, India
ic.bosco@yahoo.co.in

Uday Chaudhuri
Professor
Department of Psychiatry
Vivekananda Institute of Medical Sciences
Kolkata, West Bengal, India
uday.chaudhuri@gmail.com

BS Chavan
Professor and Head
Department of Psychiatry
Government Medical College and Hospital
Chandigarh, India
drchavanbs@gmail.com

Nishtha Chawla
Senior Resident
Department of Psychiatry and
National Drug Dependence Treatment Center
All India Institute of Medical Sciences
New Delhi, India
nishtha.chawla@gmail.com

Anamika Das
Junior Resident
Department of Psychiatry
King George's Medical University
Lucknow, Uttar Pradesh, India
lovembbs@gmail.com

Koushik Sinha Deb
Assistant Professor
Department of Psychiatry
All India Institute of Medical Sciences
New Delhi, India
koushik.sinha.deb@gmail.com

Anju Dhawan
Professor
Department of Psychiatry and National Drug
Dependence Treatment Center
All India Institute of Medical Sciences
New Delhi, India
dranjudhawan@gmail.com

Deeksha Elwadhi
Senior Resident
Department of Psychiatry
Hamdard Institute of Medical Sciences
and Research
New Delhi, India
elwadhideeksha@gmail.com

BN Gangadhar
Senior Professor of Psychiatry
Director and Vice-Chancellor
National Institute of Mental Health
and Neurosciences
Bengaluru, Karnataka, India
kalyanybg@yahoo.com

Rohit Garg
Assistant Professor
Department of Psychiatry
Government Medical College and
Rajindra Hospital
Patiala, Punjab, India
drrohitgarg@hotmail.com

Manju George
Resident
Department of Psychiatry
JSS Medical College and Hospital
JSS University
Mysuru, Karnataka, India
manju9388@gmail.com

Abhishek Ghosh
Assistant Professor
Department of Psychiatry
Postgraduate Institute of
Medical Education and Research
Chandigarh, India
ghoshabhishek12@gmail.com

Subhashini Gopal
Psychologist
Schizophrenia Research Foundation
Chennai, Tamil Nadu, India
subhashini@scarfindia.org

Sandeep Grover
Professor
Department of Psychiatry
Postgraduate Institute of
Medical Education and Research
Chandigarh, India
drsandeepg2002@yahoo.com

Nitin Gupta
Professor
Department of Psychiatry
Government Medical College and Hospital
Chandigarh, India
nitingupta659@yahoo.co.in

Rajiv Gupta
Senior Professor, Director cum CEO
Institute of Mental Health
University of Health Sciences
Rohtak, Haryana, India
rajivguptain2003@yahoo.co.in

Rishi Gupta
Senior Resident
Department of Psychiatry and National Drug
Dependence Treatment Center
All India Institute of Medical Sciences
New Delhi, India
mailrishigupta@gmail.com

Sumeet Gupta
Consultant Psychistrist
Tees, Esk and Wear Valleys
NHS Foundation Trust
Darlington, UK
Sumeet.gupta@nhs.net

Swati Kedia Gupta
Assistant Professor
Amity Institute of Behavioral
Health and Allied Sciences
Amity University
Noida, Uttar Pradesh, India
swati.nakshatra@gmail.com

Gagan Hans
Assistant Professor
Department of Psychiatry
All India Institute of Medical Sciences
New Delhi, India
gaganhans23@gmail.com

Alafia Jeelani
Research Scholar and Junior Consultant
Department of Clinical Psychology
National Institute of Mental
Health and Neurosciences
Bengaluru, Karnataka, India
alafia.jeelani@gmail.com

RC Jiloha
Chairman
Departments of Psychiatry and
Rehabilitation Sciences
Hamdard Institute of Medical
Sciences and Research
New Delhi, India
rcjiloha@hotmail.com

PC Joshi
Professor
Department of Anthropology
University of Delhi
New Delhi, India
pcjoshi@anthro.du.ac.in

Roy Abraham Kallivayalil
Professor
Department of Psychiatry
Pushpagiri Institute of Medical Sciences
Thiruvalla, Kerala, India
roykalli@gmail.com

Gurvinder Kalra
Staff Psychiatrist
Flynn Adult Inpatient Psychiatric Unit
La Trobe Regional Hospital
Mental Health Services
Traralgon, Victoria, Australia
kalragurvinder@gmail.com

Sujit Kumar Kar
Assistant Professor
Department of Psychiatry
King George's Medical University
Lucknow, Uttar Pradesh, India
drsujita@gmail.com

Adarsh Kohli
Professor (Clinical Psychology)
Department of Psychiatry
Postgraduate Institute of Medical
Education and Research
Chandigarh, India
doc_adarsh@hotmail.com

Vijay Krishnan
Former Senior Resident
Department of Psychiatry
All India Institute of Medical Sciences
New Delhi, India
vijayk1984@gmail.com

Krishan Kumar
Assistant Professor
Department of Clinical Psychology
Institute of Mental Health
University of Health Sciences
Rohtak, Haryana, India
keshusony@rediffmail.com

Parmod Kumar
Consultant Psychiatrist
Chandigarh, India

Saurabh Kumar
Senior Research Officer
Department of Psychiatry
All India Institute of Medical Sciences
New Delhi, India
saurabhksingh.singh@gmail.com

Vinay Kumar
Consultant Psychiatrist
Manoved Mind Hospital and Research Center
Patna, Bihar, India
dr.vinaykr@gmail.com

Thenmozhi Lakshmanamoorthy
Assistant Professor
Department of Psychiatry
SRM Medical College and Hospital
and Research Center
Kattankulathur, Tamil Nadu, India
dr.then16@gmail.com

Shreemit Maheshwari
Resident
Department of Psychiatry
JSS Medical College and Hospital
JSS University
Mysuru, Karnataka, India
shreecool_18@yahoo.co.in

Thirunavukarasu Manickam
Professor and Head
Department of Psychiatry
SRM Medical College and Hospital
and Research Center
Kattankulathur, Tamil Nadu, India
arasueshwar@gmail.com

Shivanand Manohar
Assistant Professor
Department of Psychiatry
JSS Medical College and Hospital
JSS University
Mysuru, Karnataka, India
drshivman@gmail.com

Urvakhsh Meherwan Mehta
Assistant Professor
Department of Psychiatry
Wellcome Trust/DBT
India Alliance Early Career Fellow
National Institute of Mental Health and
Neurosciences
Bengaluru, Karnataka, India
Urvakhsh@gmail.com

Girishwar Misra
Vice Chancellor
Mahatma Gandhi Antarrashtriya Hindi
Vishwavidyalaya
Wardha, Maharashtra, India
misragirishwar@hotmail.com

Indiwar Misra
Assistant Professor
Psychology Department
BR Ambedkar College
University of Delhi
New Delhi, India
indiwarmishra@gmail.com

Monica Mongia
Scientist- II
National Drug Dependence Treatment Center
All India Institute of Medical Sciences
New Delhi, India
drmonicamongia2016@gmail.com

R Srinivasa Murthy
Professor of Psychiatry (Retd)
National Institute of Mental
Health and Neurosciences
Bengaluru, Karnataka, India
smurthy030@gmail.com

Ritu Nehra
Professor (Clinical Psychology)
Department of Psychiatry
Postgraduate Institute of
Medical Education and Research
Chandigarh, India
ritu_nehra@rediffmail.com

R Padmavati
Additional Director
Schizophrenia Research Foundation
Chennai, Tamil Nadu, India
padmavati@scarindia.org

Nisha Mani Pandey
Assistant Professor
Department of Geriatric Mental Health
King George's Medical University
Lucknow, Uttar Pradesh, India
nisha15pandey@yahoo.co.in

Pooja Pattanaik
Senior Resident
Department of Psychiatry
Jawaharlal Institute of Postgraduate Medical
Education and Research
Puducherry, India
coolpatnaik10789@gmail.com

Ramandeep Pattanayak
Associate Professor
Department of Psychiatry
All India Institute of Medical Sciences
New Delhi, India
drramandeep@gmail.com

Varghese P Punnoose
Professor
Department of Psychiatry
Government TD Medical College
Alappuzha, Kerala, India
varghese.punnoose@gmail.com

MSVK Raju
Consultant in Psychiatry
Formerly, Professor and Head
Department of Psychiatry
Armed Forces Medical College
Pune, Maharashtra, India
msvkraju@gmail.com

G Prasad Rao
Consultant
Department of Psychiatry
Asha Hospital
Hyderabad, Telangana, India
prasad40@gmail.com

TS Sathyanarayan Rao
Professor
Department of Psychiatry
JSS Medical College and Hospital
JSS University
Mysuru, Karnataka, India
tssrao19@yahoo.com

Ashutosh Ratnam
Senior Resident
Department of Psychiatry
Postgraduate Institute of Medical
Education and Research
Chandigarh, India
ashratnam@yahoo.com

Rajesh Sagar
Professor
Department of Psychiatry
All India Institute of Medical Sciences
New Delhi, India
rsagar29@gmail.com

Swapnajeet Sahoo
Senior Resident
Department of Psychiatry
Postgraduate Institute of Medical
Education and Research
Chandigarh, India
swapnajit.same@gmail.com

Siddharth Sarkar
Assistant Professor
Department of Psychiatry and
National Drug Dependence Center
All India Institute of Medical Sciences
New Delhi, India
sidsarkar22@gmail.com

Pratap Sharan
Professor
Department of Psychiatry
All India Institute of Medical Sciences
New Delhi, India
pratapsharan@gmail.com

Vimal Kumar Sharma
Professor of International Health Development
University of Chester, Chester, UK
Consultant Psychiatrist
Early Intervention Team in Psychosis
Cheshire and

Wirral Partnership NHS Foundation Trust
Chester, UK
Co-Chair, Rural Global Mental Health Section
World Psychiatric Association
v.sharma@chester.ac.uk

Ajeet Sidana
Professor
Department of Psychiatry
Government Medical College and Hospital
Chandigarh, India
ajeetsidana@hotmail.com

Hemendra Singh
Assistant Professor
Department of Psychiatry
Ramaiah Medical College and Hospitals
Bengaluru, Karnataka, India
hemendradoc2010@gmail.com

PK Singh
Professor and Head
Department of Psychiatry
Patna Medical College
Patna, Bihar, India
pkspostline@yahoo.com

Shalini Singh
Senior Resident
National Drug Dependence Treatment Center
All India Institute of Medical Sciences
New Delhi, India
shalin.achra@gmail.com

Baxi Sinha
Consultant Psychiatrist
Tees, Esk and Wear Valleys
NHS Foundation Trust
Stockton, UK
Baxi.sinha@nhs.net

Vinod K Sinha
Ex Director Professor
Central Institute of Psychiatry
Ranchi, Jharkhand, India
vinod_sinhacip@yahoo.co.in

Mamta Sood
Professor
Department of Psychiatry
All India Institute of Medical Sciences
New Delhi, India
soodmamta@gmail.com

Shiva Prakash Srinivasan
Consultant Psychiatrist
Schizophrenia Research Foundation
Chennai, Tamil Nadu, India
drsshivaprakash@gmail.com

Chhitij Srivastava
Assistant Professor
Psychiatry Unit
Moti Lal Nehru Medical College
Allahabad, Uttar Pradesh, India
srivastavachitij@gmail.com

Mona Srivastava
Professor
Department of Psychiatry
Institute of Medical Sciences
Banaras Hindu University
Varanasi, Uttar Pradesh, India
drmonasrivastava@gmail.com

VK Srivastava
Professor
Department of Anthropology
University of Delhi
New Delhi, India
vks1@ymail.com

Abhinav Tandon
Consultant Psychiatrist
Dr AKT Neuropsychiatric Center
Allahabad, Uttar Pradesh, India
abhinavtandon@ymail.com

R Thara
Director
Schizophrenia Research Foundation
Chennai, Tamil Nadu, India
thara@scarfindia.org

Murali Thyloth
Professor and Head
Department of Psychiatry
Ramaiah Medical College and Hospitals
Bengaluru, Karnataka, India
muralithyloth@gmail.com

SC Tiwari
Professor and Head
Department of Geriatric Mental Health
King George's Medical University
Lucknow, Uttar Pradesh, India
sarvada1953@gmail.com

Adarsh Tripathi
Associate Professor
Department of Psychiatry
King George's Medical University
Lucknow, Uttar Pradesh, India
dradarshtripathi@gmail.com

Vijoy K Varma
Formerly Professor and Head
Department of Psychiatry
Postgraduate Institute of Medical
Education and Research
Chandigarh, India
vijoyv@frontier.com

Sriramya Vemulokonda
Research Officer
Asha Hospital
Hyderabad, Telangana, India

Lakshmi Venkatraman
Consultant Psychiatrist
Schizophrenia Research Foundation
Chennai, Tamil Nadu, India
lakmesridhar@yahoo.com

Antonio Ventriglio
Medical Director
Department of Clinical and
Experimental Medicine
University of Foggia
Foggia, Italy
a.ventriglio@liberto.it

KL Vidya
Senior Resident
Central Institute of Psychiatry
Ranchi, Jharkhand, India
dr.vidyakl@gmail.com

Message

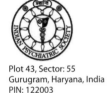

Indian Psychiatric Society

Plot 43, Sector: 55
Gurugram, Haryana, India
PIN: 122003

It gives us immense pleasure to present to you *Social Psychiatry: Principles and Clinical Perspectives*, a landmark book on social psychiatry, published under the aegis of the Indian Psychiatric Society. This book is first of its kind with comprehensiveness of a textbook, and as the title goes, covers not only theoretical aspects but also clinical issues including psychosocial management. It has never been possible to understand and practice psychiatry without taking sociocultural paradigms into consideration. This has become more important and more significant in current period due to good and bad effects of globalization related factors like digitization, urbanization, isolation and migration. This book has been conceptualized well and highlights the various psycho-social issues pertinent to the developing world in general, and Indian society and culture in particular. We hope that this publication will be of great help for all the mental health professionals interested in social psychiatry.

The first and foremost objective of the Indian Psychiatric Society is to promote and advance the subject of Psychiatry, and we are sure that the publication of *Social Psychiatry: Principles and Clinical Perspectives* will further this.

Conceptualizing and editing such a wide range book was a huge task. We appreciate the commitment and hard work put in by the editors. The Indian Psychiatric Society is grateful to all the authors from India and abroad for their valuable academic contribution. We express our sincere thanks to Jaypee Brothers Medical Publishers, an internationally acclaimed medical publisher, for partnering with us, and producing this book so beautifully. We believe that this book would be a source of pertinent information for both students as well as the practicing mental health professionals.

Long live Indian Psychiatric Society

Dr (Brig) MSVK Raju	**Dr Ajit V Bhide**	**Dr Gautam Saha**	**Dr Vinay Kumar**
President	Vice-President	Hon: General Secretary	Chair: Publication Committee

Foreword

Social psychiatry is essence of psychiatric practice, but has often not received due recognition by the psychiatrists in the background of glamorous biological psychiatry. In the modern day world with advancing technologies, changing societal norms and intermingling of cultures, social psychiatry holds even more importance than before. In this background, the book *Social Psychiatry: Principles and Clinical Perspectives* fulfills an important scientific need in the field of psychiatry. The book is a comprehensive compendium of chapters related to social psychiatry. The range of chapters demonstrates that the book intends to capture the entire breadth of topics related to social psychiatry. The social psychiatric aspects of various disorders find due space, and so do the various issues related to social psychiatry. It is enthralling to notice that several issues which are particularly relevant to the Indian cultural context (like rural mental health and farmer suicides) find adequate attention in this book.

India has been an active contributor to the social psychiatry movement in the world. I am pleased to see this book as a yet another important contribution to the cause of social psychiatry at the global scale. This well-crafted book provides perspectives from the practicing and academic psychiatrists who cater to a billion plus individuals of the world. With the contributors being leading experts in the field, including Professors Vijoy K Varma, R Srinivasa Murthy, Dinesh Bhugra, BN Gangadhar and many others, the volume has the potential of an important reference source for those in academic centers as well as those in practice. The readership is intended to be wide and the chapters have been kept at a reasonable level of technicality. Hence, readers from diverse backgrounds are likely to be benefited from this book. I expect that this book would find a unique and crucial position in the narrative of social psychiatry. I would also like to compliment the Indian Psychiatric Society and the Editors of the book for bringing out this important volume to the readership.

NN Wig (Late) MD DPM FRCPsych (Hon) FAMS
Emeritus Professor and Former Head
Department of Psychiatry
Postgraduate Institute of Medical
Education and Research
Chandigarh, India

Preface

The book *Social Psychiatry: Principles and Clinical Perspectives* was conceptualized about a year and half ago by us, Vinay Kumar and Rakesh K Chadda. We had a meeting of a group of interested colleagues during the XXII World Congress of the World Association of Social Psychiatry (WASP 2016) at Hotel the Ashok in December 2016 to discuss the initial proposal. Subsequently the title was finalized. Themes and chapters were finalized over the next 2-3 months. Dr Siddharth Sarkar joined the editorial team in early 2018. We had continued discussions with colleagues and friends for identifying and finalizing the prospective authors as well as the publisher. The Indian Psychiatric Society agreed to publish the book under its banner and Jaypee group was approached and subsequently finalized to publish the book. Here, we would especially like to acknowledge the inputs from Prof Vijoy K Varma, Prof PK Singh, Prof Pratap Sharan, and Prof Nitin Gupta in the initial conceptualization of the book.

This book is divided into 5 sections. Section 1 gives a brief introduction to the discipline of social psychiatry going into its historical development across the world and in India. The section has also a contribution by Prof Dinesh Bhugra, a Past President of the World Psychiatric Association and an international authority in social psychiatry.

Section 2 includes conceptual issues on the relationship between mental health and society. It begins with a chapter on the concept of social psychiatry. It then highlights the family and social context in relation to the mental health of the individual. A chapter is included describing biological underpinnings in social psychiatry. Subsequently, social dimensions of behavior and personality development are discussed, along with the social dimension of spiritual health and psychiatric epidemiology. Psychology of sub-populations of the society are presented, and influence of culture, mythology and religion on mental health are delved upon in two subsequent chapters. The section also presents the social psychiatric aspects of marriage and similar affiliations. The visible and invisible stressors, which have a bearing on psychiatric manifestations, are highlighted in a subsequent chapter.

Section 3 covers the social dimensions of psychiatric disorders. The initial chapter in this section deals with health promotion aspect of evaluating the social well-being and health. Subsequent chapters discern the social psychiatric aspects of individual disorders, including schizophrenia and other psychotic disorders, depressive and bipolar disorders, anxiety disorders, somatoform and dissociative disorders, substance use disorders, psychosexual disorders, personality disorders, and suicide and similar behaviors. Disorders in special populations like childhood and adolescent disorders and psychiatric disorders of the elderly are also covered in this chapter. Physical comorbidity in psychiatry, which is a pertinent concern in the holistic management of patients, is also discussed in this section.

Section 4 expands upon the social interventions that are relevant to the field of social psychiatry. Social support and networking is presented first which highlights the dynamic social networks of the present times. Thereafter, couple therapies, family therapies, and group therapies are discussed. Subsequently, community models of care are presented followed by discussion on the rehabilitation of patients with psychiatric illnesses. Preventive psychiatry, which aims at reducing the incidence and burden of psychiatric disorders is also reviewed in this section. The section concludes by emphasis on cultural interventions for psychiatric disorders.

Section 5, the last section, dwells upon the social issues and mental health. The initial chapter here highlights the stigma of mental illness. Thereafter, migration and mental health are discussed. This is followed by psychiatry in the armed forces, where the application of social psychiatry concepts is an interesting reflection. The legislative aspects of mental health, under which the psychiatry is practiced, is presented next. The social impact of terrorism and extremism, which is very important in today's world, is presented thereafter, followed by discussion on mass media, information technology and mental health. Pertinent issues of farmer suicides in India, rural mental health and urban mental health are discussed subsequently. The section concludes with a discussion on globalization, market economy and mental health.

We hope that the wide range of topics related to the social psychiatry would provide a ready composite reference for the readers. Clinicians, researchers, academicians and policy makers are likely to be benefited from this book. The chapters have been contributed by illustrious experts who are renowned figures in their field. This text is likely to be useful for varied mental health professionals, including psychiatrists, psychologists, mental health nurses, psychiatric social workers, and anyone else who is interested in the field of social psychiatry. This comprehensive compilation would be of interest for both students as well as experts in the field of mental health. We expect that this book provides information and perspective to the readers and contributes to the cause of advancement of social psychiatry.

Social psychiatry has a wide range and multiple interfaces. Due to this reason, we needed experts and academicians not only from the field of psychiatry but also the humanities. We express our sincere thanks to all the authors for their commitment and hard work. We understand that thinking differently and writing on unconventional topics is how much difficult. We are especially grateful to international authors and academic luminaries from humanities for their contribution. Last but not least, leading medical publisher Jaypee Brothers Medical Publishers and its enthusiastic team members deserve all praise for quality production of this book.

Rakesh K Chadda

Vinay Kumar

Siddharth Sarkar

Contents

SECTION

1

Overview

Chapter 1

History of Social Psychiatry

Vijoy K Varma, Rakesh K Chadda

SUMMARY

This chapter is an overview of the history of social psychiatry across the world and is divided into developments in the field in 18th–19th century, genesis of the discipline in early 20th century, developments following the Second World War, formal recognition of the discipline around mid-twentieth century, decline following developments in biological psychiatry, and then re-emergence of social psychiatry. Authors have attempted to cover the global trends, both in the high income as well as the low and middle-income countries. Recognition of mental and substance use disorders as a major contributor to the global burden of disease and failure of biological research to come out with any breakthroughs in treatment have led to a focus on social psychiatry, which was being ignored in recent past. Social psychiatry appears to have a bright future in contemporary psychiatry.

INTRODUCTION

Before going into the history of social psychiatry, it is important to discuss the scope of social psychiatry. In simple words, it could be conceptualized as the subspecialty of psychiatry which deals with the social aspects of the discipline, i.e., role of social factors in genesis, clinical presentation, and treatment of mental disorders (Chadda, 2014). The scope can be further expanded, ranging from the impact of social structures and experiences on onset, course, and outcome of mental disorders to development of appropriate social interventions and service delivery. Julian Leff (2010) describes social psychiatry as a discipline, concerned with the effects of the social environment on the mental health of the individual, and the effects of the mentally ill person on his/her social environment. Social psychiatry has close linkages with the community psychiatry and other social sciences like sociology, social psychology, and social anthropology.

The discipline of social psychiatry has gone through many ups and downs, since the time it was first recognized over 100 years ago, and its importance is being further reinvented from the beginning of the twenty-first century due to the inability of the biological psychiatry to come out with any substantial discoveries after the initial successes.

This chapter is an attempt to trace the history of social psychiatry from beginning to the current period. Authors do not claim to include every aspect of the history since social psychiatry is a vast area.

GENESIS OF THE SPECIALTY

Genesis of social psychiatry can be informally traced back to the late 17th and early 18th century, the period of reforms in the mental asylums like unchaining of the mentally ill, initiated by Vincenzo Chiarugi in Italy, William Tuke in England and Phillippe Pinel in France (Coip, 2009). In the mid-eighteenth century, many developments in psychiatry in Europe and the US were social in nature, important examples being moral treatment and obligation of the state to care for people in need. York Retreat in the UK, established by William Tuke, was one of the most renowned moral treatment asylums in the world. If we talk of South Asia and other continents across the world, persons with mental illness were mostly cared by the families in the community, since formal treatment facilities for mental illness did not exist.

Importance of close linkages between social factors and mental health started getting recognized by the beginning of the twentieth century, following declining standards of care in the mental asylums with the asylums becoming custodial institutions rather than practicing the therapeutic idea of moral treatment. The book *A Mind That Found Itself* published by Clifford Beers in 1908 about the bad treatment he had received as a mental patient in three asylums, brought important developments in social psychiatry in early twentieth century. Beers founded the National Committee for Mental Hygiene, and thus began the mental hygiene movement, which aimed at controlling and preventing mental disorders. This could be termed as one of the initial formal development in social psychiatry (Leff, 2010). Some of the classic epidemiological studies conducted during mid-twentieth century like Midtown Manhattan study (Srole et al., 1962), Stirling County study (Leighton et al., 1963), and social class and mental illness (Hollingshead & Redlich, 1958), are classical examples of social influences on mental disorders, explaining the complexities of the relationship between social class and mental illness. The finding of high prevalence of schizophrenia as reported by Hollingshead and Redlich in the deprived areas of the city of Chicago has been replicated by a number of researchers in similar locations across the world. Social causation hypothesis, which is based on the role of social factors in the causation of schizophrenia, and social drift hypothesis explaining the effect of illness on the social mobility, are based on the above mentioned historical epidemiological works on social class and schizophrenia. It is now well established that social adversities are associated with higher risk to develop mental illnesses. Contribution of sociological factors in personality development was later well stated in the personality theories by Erik Erikson, Harry Stack Sullivan and Karen Horney, given around the mid-twentieth century (Chadda, 2014).

Consequences of the Second World War had a great impact on the mental health scenario in Europe and the US. It is important to mention here that the psychiatric textbooks before the Second World War did not make any mention of social factors in mental illness. The Royal Medico-Psychological Association (which was to later become the Royal College of Psychiatrists) of the UK started a section on psychotherapy and social psychiatry in 1946. In the earlier period, the section focused on the study of social organizations, a conceptual framework which had come from the experiences of military psychiatrists from the Second World War. Two of the proponents of this movement, Maxwell Jones and Tom Main, worked on group therapy, which later evolved into the concept of "therapeutic community" (Leff, 2010).

The World Health Organization (WHO) in its definition of health, way back in 1948, included mental and social wellbeing as integral components of health along with the physical one. Later, George Engel (Engel, 1980) proposed the biopsychosocial model of disease, which emphasizes the contributions of biological, psychological and sociological factors in genesis and management of mental as well as medical illnesses. These developments were indicative of the recognition of the discipline of social psychiatry in the scientific mind in that period.

The initial historical phase of mental health reforms brought by a number of visionary psychiatrists in the mental hospitals before the psychopharmacology revolution, which led to a number of improvements in the condition of the hospitals as well as the inmates, are important examples of the role of social interventions in mental illness. Recognition of the deleterious effects of long-term institutionalization on the wellbeing of the inmates, the positive effects of therapeutic community, and the deinstitutionalization movement are examples of the continuing existence of social psychiatry in that period of time.

INITIAL PROGRESS IN SOCIAL PSYCHIATRY

Social psychiatry had humble beginnings and progress across the world. In the UK, Sir Aubrey Lewis was the first psychiatrist to start research in social psychiatry, also credited with the founding of the Institute of Psychiatry in London. Role of social characteristics of mental hospitals on course and symptomatology of schizophrenia was recognized by the pioneering work by Wing and Brown that under-stimulating conditions lead to more defect symptoms (negative symptoms) and over-stimulating conditions lead to more florid psychotic symptoms (Leff, 2010). The concept of stressful life events and their role in genesis and relapse of different mental disorders including schizophrenia and depression was also recognized around this period (Brown et al., 1987).

A parallel movement of reforms in the mental health was started by the creation of the National Institute of Mental Health (NIMH) in the US in 1948. The coming years saw deinstitutionalization movement, the discovery of chlorpromazine and other antipsychotics and growth of community psychiatry. During this period, there was a lot of focus on social psychiatry in the US. Over the period, the NIMH played a significant role in shifting the focus of care from mental hospitals to the community settings. This was further facilitated by a release of a grant of 2.9 billion dollars by President Kennedy from the federal budget and passing of the Community Mental Health Centre Act by the Senate in 1963. These developments facilitated the community mental health movement in the US and were founded on the principles of social psychiatry. However, with a very large number of patients especially those with chronic schizophrenia or psychosis being discharged from the mental hospitals, it was not possible to provide high-quality care in the community, since the facilities available were not commensurate with the need. A substantial proportion of these patients required long-term rehabilitation, but the community services were not prepared for it. There was also considerable opposition from the lay public which held stigmatizing attitude for the discharged patients. Financial support was not of the magnitude to provide support for all these requirements. This led to the problem of homelessness amongst many patients discharged from the mental hospitals, and some would get readmitted to the mental hospitals while many would end up in the prisons over petty crimes, the trans-institutionalization. A similar phenomenon was observed across different European countries (Coip, 2009; Leff, 2010; Haack & Kumbier, 2012).

One important development occurred in psychiatry in India around this period, when Vidya Sagar started involving families in the care of persons with mental illness in tents outside the premises of the mental hospital at Amritsar. This was the time when families were considered rather toxic in the Western world and responsible for mental illnesses in their wards. Vidya Sagar set an example of family therapy to the Western world (Kapur, 2004; Chadda, 2012). The topic is discussed in more detail in the chapter on the history of social psychiatry in India. India and other countries in the non-Western world, fortunately, did not face the problem of deinstitutionalization, since there were never so many mental hospitals with patients incarcerated in them, and most patients were being looked after by the families and the community (Chadda, 2001).

In the UK, the Royal College of Psychiatrists set up Social and Community Psychiatry Group in 1973, just two years after its establishment, confirming the significance social psychiatry carried. The annual meeting of the College in 1973 included a session on "prospects of social and community psychiatry." The Group took over a number of activities including the development of community psychiatry services, liaison with general practitioners and promoting educational and scientific interests in social psychiatry. The Group was given the status of Section by the College in 1981 (Leff, 2010).

WHO had also important contributions to make in the field of social psychiatry in this period, by its International Pilot Study of Schizophrenia (IPSS) and the study on Determinants of Outcome of Severe Mental Disorder (DOSMeD). IPSS reported wide differences in course and outcome of schizophrenia across different countries in the world, with the developing countries showing better outcome as compared to the developed countries. Role of expressed emotions in relapse in schizophrenia, and its varied distribution across different cultures, as found in the DOSMeD study, were major findings from research in the field of social psychiatry (Leff et al., 1987; Wig et al., 1987; Kulhara et al., 2015).

DECLINE IN INTEREST IN SOCIAL PSYCHIATRY SINCE 1980s

In the last quarter of the twentieth century, there has been a significant improvement in our understanding of the structure and functioning of brain with advances in structural and functional imaging. Our understanding of the etiogenesis of most of mental disorders has also become better. But the exact etiology of most mental disorders remains unknown, though it comes under the broad umbrella of biopsychosocial paradigm. This period was also associated with the introduction of a large number of new medications for mental disorders including a range of antidepressants, antipsychotics, and use of anticonvulsants as mood stabilizers, and a declining interest in psychological, psychoanalytic and social therapies amongst the psychiatrists.

Though a reappraisal of the developments in biological psychiatry in the last 3 decades though confirms considerable progress in fundamental research in genetics and neuroscience related to psychiatry, there have been no breakthrough discoveries in our understanding of the exact etiology or in therapeutics. There have not been any new antipsychotics, antidepressants or mood stabilizers that could be labeled as more effective than the earlier ones (Saraga & Stiefel, 2011). The extensive continued funding for the biological research and declaration of 1990-2000 as the Decade of Brain in the US has led to the improved understanding of human brain and genome, and of the etiogenesis of mental disorders, but no novel biological treatments for psychiatric disorders have come up.

There was a marked decline in funding social psychiatry research received from the 1980s onwards, and most funding went to the biological research in psychiatry. But despite the fund crunch, there have been studies during this period proving the effectiveness of psychosocial treatments for schizophrenia and depression. In fact, family intervention for schizophrenia, cognitive behavior therapy for schizophrenia, and similarly for depression and anxiety disorders stands at a strong ground in the contemporary psychiatry (Priebe et al., 2013).

RE-EMERGENCE OF SOCIAL PSYCHIATRY IN THE 21ST CENTURY

Mental disorders are known to have a neurobiological, psychological and social dimension. The biological research in the last few decades has been able to identify changes in brain functioning in most of the mental disorders, but biology alone can not explain the genesis and clinical presentation of mental disorders. It is generally conceptualized that neurobiological changes in the mental disorders are expressed in form of psychological symptoms, experienced in a social context. The neurobiological findings in an individual patient are considered as the explanation for the illness and symptomatology, which is often expressed in interpersonal context with sociocultural factors affecting the clinical presentation. Similarly, modifications in the neurobiological processes in response to various treatments also explain how and why interventions work. This is also true for psychological, behavioral and cognitive interventions (Priebe et al., 2013).

The Global Burden of Disease, 1990 (GBD 1990) study published in the early nineties was a historical development, which brought focus on mental disorders and the social psychiatry (Murray & Lopez, 1996). GBD 1990 showed that mental and neurological disorders accounted for 10.5% of the total disability-adjusted life years (DALYs). Historically, mental disorders were never considered a health priority across the world, especially when compared with communicable diseases and non-communicable diseases such as cancer or cardiovascular disease, because of focus of the health planning on mortality statistics. The World Development Report in 1993, brought by the World Bank, brought global attention towards the relative burden associated with disease morbidity, rather than mortality alone. Mental, neurological and substance use disorders were identified as major contributors to the global burden of disease. The disease burden was reassessed in 2000, and the estimates showed neuropsychiatric disorders (mental, neurological and substance use disorders) to be responsible for more than a quarter of all non-fatal burden, measured in years lived with disability (YLD). Depression was identified as the most disabling disorder worldwide measured in YLDs, and the fourth leading cause of overall burden measured in DALYs. Depression was associated with the largest amount of disability, accounting for almost 12% of the YLDs. There was an increase in the contribution of mental and neurological disorders to the global burden to 12.3% in 2000 (World Health Organization, 2001). The Global Burden of Diseases, Injuries and Risk Factors Study 2010 (GBD 2010) re-estimated the burden in 2010 (Murray et al., 2012). In the GBD 2010, mental and substance use disorders were separated from neurological disorders in burden assessment. The group accounted for 183·9 million DALYs (95% UI 153·5 million–

216·7 million), or 7·4% (6·2–8·6) of total disease burden in 2010. Global burden caused by the mental and substance use disorders was estimated to be more than that caused by HIV/AIDS and tuberculosis, and diabetes, urogenital, blood, and endocrine diseases, as separate groups. This finding is of great significance.

Dealing with the burden and disability associated with mental disorders is a huge task, which needs changes in the mental health policies, strengthening manpower resources, and targeting barriers to mental health care. The task is especially difficult in the low resource countries. Psychiatric services are though relatively well developed in the Western world, the non-Western countries in Asia, Africa, and South America suffer a gross deficiency in the mental health resources (World Health Organization, 2014). Most of the low and middle-income countries (LAMIC) have a gross deficiency of mental health manpower. According to the Mental Health Atlas (2005), the total number of mental health care workers in 58 countries from the LAMIC group was 362,000, representing 22.3 workers per 100,000 in low income countries and 26.7 per 100,000 in the middle income countries, comprising 6% psychiatrists, 54% nurses and 41% psychosocial care providers, putting the shortage of mental health workers at 1.18 million in the 144 LAMIC countries (Kakuma et al., 2011). A number of alternatives have been suggested to tackle the problem of limited mental health resources especially in the LAMIC. Key Strategies for meeting the challenges could include transforming health systems and policy responses, building human resource capacity, improving treatment and expanding access to care, prevention and implementation of the early interventions, and identifying the root causes, risks, and protective factors (Collins et al., 2011).

It has often been observed that there is a long delay in seeking treatment for mental disorders with reasons often being psychosocial in nature. Duration of untreated psychosis has emerged as an important outcome variable affecting the outcome in psychosis, emphasizing the need for early detection and beginning of treatment (Penttilä et al., 2014). Factors leading to delay in seeking treatment include ignorance, myths, and misconceptions about mental disorders and social stigma, and hence need social interventions. Non-adherence to treatment and not seeking help for mental disorders are other important factors identified to be associated with disability and burden associated with mental disorders and needs active interventions at the hands of social psychiatrists. There has also been a trend towards increasing suicide rates across some countries, which needs to be studied by the social psychiatrists. All these issues necessitate the need for a social paradigm in psychiatry, with social interventions being an important alternative strategy in psychiatric practice. The social paradigm has often been neglected, though the social interventions could be of great help in reducing barriers to seeking treatment, improving adherence, facilitating community rehabilitation and reducing disease-related burden and disability (Chadda, 2016).

SOCIAL CLASS, INEQUALITIES, AND MENTAL HEALTH

It is well known that there is a close association between social class and mental illness. There is also some evidence that social inequalities are associated with an increase in mental morbidity. Unfortunately, there has been increasing social inequalities in the society as well as increasing economic inequality between resourceful and poor countries across the world (Murali & Oyebode, 2004). There has also been a rapid increase in the gap in per capita income between the industrialized and developing world. The developing countries, which comprise 80% of the world's population, contribute to only 21% of the global gross national product. The differences in economic and health status within countries have also been found to be as great as or even greater than those between the rich and poor countries (Pickett & Wilkinson, 2010). Poverty is associated with high levels of common mental health disorders such as anxiety and depression. Similarly, the underprivileged areas are associated with higher rates of hospital admissions, outpatient visits and suicide. Poor financial status has been identified as a predictor of depressive symptoms independent of socioeconomic status, ethnic group and marital status (Heneghan et al., 1998). The New Haven Study of the 1950s and its follow up was one of the earliest studies to report a direct relationship between poverty and high rates of emotional and mental problems. The study had also shown that the different social classes accessed different types of treatment facilities (Hollingshead & Redlich, 1958; Kim et al., 2017).

Unemployment, another social variable, has been reported to be associated with increased prevalence of a number of mental disorders including depression, anxiety, phobias, psychosis and alcohol and substance use disorders (Meltzer et al., 1995). Unemployment has been identified to be one of the strongest predictors of suicide, even after adjusting for other socioeconomic variables (Lewis & Sloggett, 1998). Population-based studies from Netherlands (Bijl et al., 1998) and Ethiopia (Kebede & Alem, 1999) have reported the association of mood disorders with a range of social factors like unemployment, education, and under-achievement. Differences in educational attainment have also been identified as important factors contributing to social inequalities in psychiatric disorder in the world (Patel & Kleinman, 2003). A study from Brazil has shown an independent association of poor educational attainment and low income with increased prevalence of common mental disorders (Ludermir & Lewis, 2001). Thus, a range of social factors like education, income and occupational status which contribute to the socioeconomic status and also social inequalities independently as well as together can act as risk factors for mental illness.

ROLE OF THE WORLD ASSOCIATION OF SOCIAL PSYCHIATRY

The World Association of Social Psychiatry (WASP) has made substantial contributions to the social psychiatry movement across the world over the last 50 years. Joshua Bierer had the unique contribution of initiating the social psychiatry movement starting from the 1950s, and brought together the interested persons to London in the first international congress of social psychiatry in 1964. The meeting was a precursor to the founding of the WASP. Bierer was one of the earliest advocates in the UK for the closure of the custodial mental hospitals and played a leading role in designing and running community-based psychiatric services and psychosocial day hospital programs. Bierer was also the founder editor of the International Journal of Social Psychiatry. Second international congress of social psychiatry was organized in 1969, and the International Association of Social Psychiatry was formally launched with Joshua Bierer as Founder President and Jules Masserman as President. The name of the association was changed to the World Association of Social Psychiatry (WASP) in the international congress at Opatija, Croatia (Leff, 2010; Craig, 2016).

The WASP (earlier under the umbrella of International Association of Social Psychiatry) has the distinction of propagating the cause of social psychiatry across the world by holding regular world congresses every 3 years in different countries across the world. A distinction lies in having its congresses both in the developed as well as the underdeveloped world. India has the unique distinction of organizing the WASP congresses thrice in 1992, 2001 and 2016.

WASP has the objectives of studying the nature of man, the culture, prevention and treatment of man's vicissitudes and behavioral disorders, promoting national and international collaborations among professionals and societies in fields related to social psychiatry, making the knowledge and practice of social psychiatry available to other sciences and to the public, and advancing the physical, social and philosophic wellbeing of the mankind (Craig, 2016). WASP has a number of special sections and task forces, some of which focus on the promotion of personal recovery, family support, and intervention, fighting stigma and migration. Thus, the WASP has played an important role in propagating the cause of the social psychiatry.

INITIATIVES TO BE TAKEN BY SOCIAL PSYCHIATRY

Social psychiatry needs to take a number of initiatives in future in promoting mental health, spreading awareness in the community about the mental disorders, early access to treatment, acting at barriers to pathways to the mental health delivery systems, and identifying and acting at the risk factors for mental disorders. Early interventions need to include educating patients and families, as well as making the society at large aware of the harmful consequences of mental illness. An understanding of the role of social factors in precipitation and perpetuation of mental illnesses is essential in developing a plan for such initiatives. It may not be possible for psychiatrists to reduce social inequalities, but they need to be aware of various psychosocial factors affecting mental health and help-seeking and take initiatives at sensitizing policymakers and others who matter about these aspects (Bhugra & Till, 2013).

Unfortunately, the medical education and also the education in psychiatry has become more biologically focused than a few decades ago. The medical, as well as mental health professionals, often lose sight of the psychosocial factors while interacting with their patients. Role of psychological and social factors in causation, course, outcome, and treatment of various psychiatric disorders is often ignored. This is not a healthy trend, and if this continues, main contributions of psychiatrists will be diagnostic assessment and psychopharmacological treatment, leaving psychotherapy to psychologists and psychosocial care to social workers and care managers? Here, social psychiatry has a crucial role to play, and the social psychiatrists need to sensitize the profession about the need and relevance of social psychiatry as an integral part of the discipline. Same is true for other branches of medicine.

Patients with mental and emotional disorders constitute a substantial part of the clinical practice in primary health care settings. Thus, the primary care physicians also need to be sensitized to this fact and equipped with necessary skills to identify and manage the common psychiatric problems in their routine clinical practice. Future psychiatrists should also be prepared to provide this kind of education and support. The profession needs to be flexible and respond to the changing needs, and be ready to take responsibility towards the society. However, the social psychiatrists also need to be cautious and resist attempts of the society to delegate all responsibility to psychiatry, especially the issues involving cultural sensitivities and values.

It is important to mention here that the role of social factors can't be ignored in mental health despite all the biological advances. Biology can never replace the social factors. Since the psychiatrist works in a social situation and communication is an important part of the psychiatric assessment and psychiatric illnesses mostly manifest in interpersonal situations, social psychiatry will always remain an integral part of psychiatry. The psychiatrist needs to be familiar with various psychosocial risk and protective factors so as to take appropriate steps at mental health promotion and prevention.

A number of recommendations of the World Health Report of 2001, which was devoted to mental health, include social approaches such as providing treatment of mental disorders in primary care, bringing the services at doorsteps, mental health education to the community, involving consumers, families and the community in mental health care, developing human resources, developing linkages with other sectors like education, labor, social welfare, and monitoring community mental health services (World Health Organization, 2001).

CONCLUSION

Social psychiatry is an integral part of psychiatry since mental disorders manifest in interpersonal and social context, and hence for understanding and managing mental disorders, it is not possible to ignore it. The discipline may not be as popular as biological psychiatry due to the glamour attached to the latter but has existed all the time. There have been ups and downs in the importance social psychiatry has received by the psychiatrist and other mental health professionals over the period. Mental health reforms in the mental hospitals are one of the earliest examples of social interventions. Deinstitutionalization, therapeutic community, the concept of day hospital, psychosocial rehabilitation and other psychosocial methods of interventions are some important examples of social psychiatry initiatives in the twentieth century. The relevance of social psychiatry re-emerged in the last 2 decades especially on recognition of mental disorders as a major contributor to the global burden of disease and disease-related disability and absence of any major successes in biological psychiatry after initial hopes.

REFERENCES

Bhugra D, Till A. Public mental health is about social psychiatry. Int J Soc Psychiatry. 2013;59(2):105-6.

Bijl RV, Ravelli A, Van Zessen G. Prevalence of psychiatric disorder in the general population: results of the Netherlands Mental Health Survey and Incidence Study (NEMESIS). Soc Psychiatry Psychiatr Epidemiol. 1998; 33(12):587-95.

Brown GW, Bifulco A, Harris TO. Life events, vulnerability and onset of depression: some refinements. Br J Psychiatry. 1987;150(J):30-42.

Chadda RK. Psychiatric patient in the community: challenges and solutions. J Ment Health Behav. 2001;6:7-15.

Chadda RK. Six decades of community psychiatry in India Int Psychiatry. 2012;9:45-7.

Chadda RK. What social psychiatry has to offer in contemporary psychiatric practice? Ind J Soc Psychiatry. 2014;30:7-13.

Chadda RK. Global burden of mental disorders: meeting the challenge. Ann Nat Acad Med Sci (India). 2016;52:39-55.

Coip R. History of psychiatry. In: Sadock B, Sadock V, Ruiz P (Eds). Comprehensive Textbook of Psychiatry, 9th edition. Philedelphia: Wolters Kluwer/Lippincott/Williams & Wilkins; 2009. Pp. 4474-509.

Collins PY, Patel V, Joestl SS, et al. Grand challenges in global mental health. Nature 2011;472:27-30.

Craig TK. World Association of Social Psychiatry: a brief history (1963-2016). In: Souvenir of the XXII World Congress of Social Psychiatry, New Delhi. 2016.

Engel GL. The clinical application of the biopsychosocial model. Am J Psychiatry. 1980;137(5):535-44.

Haack K, Kumbier E. History of social psychiatry. Curr Opin Psychiatr. 2012;25(6):492-6.

Heneghan AM, Silver EJ, Bauman LJ, et al. Depressive symptoms in inner-city mothers of young children: who is at risk? Pediatrics. 1998;102(6):1394-400.

Hollingshead AB, Redlich FC. Social class and mental illness: a community study. New York: John Wiley; 1958.

Kakuma R, Minas H, Ginneken N Van, et al. Human resources for mental health care: current situation and strategies for action. Lancet. 2011;378(9803):1654-63.

Kapur R. The story of community mental health in india. In: Agarwal S, Goel D, Salhan R, Ichhpujani R, Shrivastava S (Eds). Mental health: An Indian perspective (1946–2003). New Delhi: Directorate General of Health Services, Ministry of Health and Family Welfare, Government of India/Elsevier; 2004. Pp. 92-100.

Kebede D, Alem A. Major mental disorders in Addis Ababa, Ethiopia. I. Schizophrenia, schizoaffective and cognitive disorders. Acta Psychiatrica Scandinavica. 1999;397:11-7.

Kim HS, Hollingshead S, Wohl MJA. Who spends money to play for free? identifying who makes micro-transactions on social casino games (and why). J Gambling Studies. 2017;33(2):525-38.

Kulhara P, Grover S, Kate N. Schizophrenia: Indian research I. Epidemiology, clinical features, neurobiology and psychosocial aspects. In: Malhotra S, Chakrabarti S (Eds). Developments in Psychiatry in India. New Delhi: Springer (India); 2015. Pp. 139-72.

Leff J. The historical development of social psychiatry. In: Morgan C, Bhugra D (Eds). Principles of Social Psychiatry. London: Wiley-Blackwell; 2010. Pp. 3-11.

Leff J, Wig NN, Ghosh A, et al. Expressed emotion and schizophrenia in North India. III. Influence of relatives' expressed emotion on the course of schizophrenia in Chandigarh. Br J Psychiatry. 1987;151:166-73.

Leighton DC, Harding JS, Macklin DB, et al. Psychiatric findings of the Srirling County study. Am J Psychiatry. 1963;119:1021-6.

Lewis G, Sloggett A. Suicide, deprivation, and unemployment: record linkage study. BMJ (Clinical Research Ed.). 1998;317(7168):1283-6.

Ludermir AB, Lewis G. Links between social class and common mental disorders in northeast Brazil. Soc Psychiatry Psychiatr Epidemiol. 2001;36(3):101-7.

Meltzer H, Gill B, Petticrew M, et al. OPCS surveys of psychiatric morbidity in Great Britain London: HMSO; 1995.

Murali V, Oyebode F. Poverty, social inequality and mental health. Adv Psychiatr Treat. 2004;10(3):216-24.

Murray CJL, Lopez AD. The global burden of disease: a comprehensive assessment of mortality and disability from diseases, injuries, and risk factors in 1990 and projected to 2020. Cambridge, MA: Harvard School of Public Health on Behalf of the World Health Organization and the World Bank; 1996.

Murray CJL, Vos T, Lozano R, et al. Disability-adjusted life years DALYs for 291 diseases and injuries in 21 regions, 1990–2010: a systematic analysis for the Global Burden of Disease Study 2010. Lancet. 2012;(380):2197-223.

Patel V, Kleinman A. Poverty and common mental disorders in developing countries. Bull World Health Organ. 2003;81(8):609-15.

Penttilä M, Jääskeläinen E, Hirvonen N, et al. Duration of untreated psychosis as predictor of long-term outcome in schizophrenia: systematic review and meta-analysis. Br J Psychiatry. 2014;205(2): 88-94.

Pickett KE, Wilkinson RG. Inequality: an underacknowledged source of mental illness and distress. Br J Psychiatry. 2010;197(6):426-8.

Priebe S, Tom B, Craig TKJ. The future of academic psychiatry may be social. Br J Psychiatry. 2013;202(5):319-20.

Saraga M, Stiefel F. Psychiatry and the scientific fallacy. Acta Psychiatr Scand. 2011;124(1):70-2.

Srole L, Langner T, Michael S, et al. Mental health in the metropolis: the midtown manhatten study. New York: McGraw-Hill; 1962.

Wig NN, Menon DK, Bedi H, et al. Expressed emotion and schizophrenia in north India I. Cross-cultural transfer of ratings of relatives' expressed emotion. Br J Psychiatry. 1987;151:156-73.

World Health Organization. Mental health: new understandings, new hope. Geneva: World Health Organization; 2001.

World Health Organization. Mental health atlas 2014. Geneva: Department of Mental Health and Substance Abuse/World Health Organization; 2014.

Chapter 2

Social Psychiatry and Contemporary Society

Antonio Ventriglio, Gurvinder Kalra, Dinesh Bhugra

SUMMARY

Social factors form the basis of many psychiatric disorders in that they can not only cause mental illness and distress but can also lead to perpetuation and help seeking. Social psychiatry is that branch of psychiatry which deals with the effects of social environment on the mental health of the individual. It is important to understand that human beings are social animals. Interactions with others lie at the heart of social living and in understanding of psychiatry and its responsibilities in particular. Families are an inherent part of social functioning and these familial and social reactions can lead to difficulties in human functioning both directly and indirectly. It is well recognized that social and environmental factors do influence the presentation and precipitation of psychiatric disorders. Social factors do affect cognitions, behaviors and mood which form the basis of psychiatric disorders. Of course, biological and genetic factors influence psychiatric disorders but in turn these are also affected by social determinants.

INTRODUCTION

Social factors can influence the causation, perpetuation, and responses to stress and psychiatry. Social psychiatry deals with the effects that social environment can have on the mental health of the individual. It must be recognized that basically, human beings are social animals. Interactions with others lie at the heart of social living. Consequently, these familial and social relationships can cause difficulties in human functioning both directly and indirectly. It is inevitable that social and environmental factors will contribute to psychiatric disorders. There may be major problems in our understanding of psychiatric disorders, especially when these are related to diagnoses. One standard way of looking at mental illness is how these abnormalities influence thoughts, actions, and behaviors which constitute types of psychiatric disorders. These are strongly affected by biological and genetic factors. Genetic vulnerability to many psychiatric disorders can lead to abnormal or pathological responses to stress and other social determinants such as unemployment, poverty, overcrowding, lack of green spaces, urbanization, and industrialization, in addition to others. Social determinants thus can contribute to psychiatric disorders. There are social class differences in both understanding and explanations of psychiatric disorders which not surprisingly influence pathways into care. The Society also affects pathways as it is the policymakers who on behalf of the society determine what resources are to be provided for healthcare. It is clear that the field of social medicine includes social and cultural aspects and perspectives of health and medicine and determinants. In spite of the breaking of the genetic code, social determinants continue to play a major role in the genesis and perpetuation of medical disorders. Even the genetic code is under the influence of social and external environmental factors. The roots of disease are still social. All of the diseases, whether it is infectious, genetic, metabolic, traumatic, malignant or degenerative, has social components in the larger perspective or a narrower one.

SOCIAL PERSPECTIVES

McHugh and Slavney offer four different perspectives to psychiatry equally applicable to other branches of medicine (McHugh & Slavney, 1998). These four standard methods for explaining mental disorders implicit in current psychiatric clinical practice include disease, dimensional, behavioral and life story perspectives. These authors argue that the disease perspective is focused on the clinical entity, pathological condition, and etiology whereas a dimensional perspective is applicable to the logic of quantitative gradation and individual variation. Such a perspective relies on normal variation which can be based on attributes such as intelligence or personality trait thus relying on not only a range but also a quantitative spectrum. Therein lies the abnormality which can be identified. Behavioral perspective focuses on goal-directed and goal-driven features of human life and identifies abnormalities in some features such as sexual functioning, eating disorders, etc. Life story perspectives rely on disturbing experiences such as loss leading to grief as well as the developmental aspects of the individual. Psychiatry thus carries within the discipline a social perspective; the notion of cultural and social roles which may be affected and indeed related to social stratification and social class which may be linked to social structures, socio-economic realities and last but not the least socio-political realities.

CULTURES

Hofstede (2001) defines various aspects of cultures which include socio-centric or ego-centric aspects (also described as collectivist and individualist factors respectively); masculine and feminine; how distant individuals in a particular culture feel from the center of power; how cultures avoid uncertainty; and what the long-term orientation of the culture is (Hofstede, 2001). The latter three aspects may well apply better to the cultures of big organizations as that's where Hofstede had carried out his work. The type of society whether it is ego-centric or socio-centric may work at bigger level but does not mean that every individual in that culture will either be same as the larger society. Ego-centricity or individualism refers to society where the ties between individuals are loose, and everyone is expected to look after himself/herself and their immediate or nuclear family whereas socio-centrism or collectivism means that people from birth onwards are integrated into strong cohesive in- groups which throughout their lifetime continue to protect them in exchange for unquestioning loyalty. Whereas individualism represents I-ness, I-consciousness, autonomy, emotional independence, individual initiative, right to privacy, pleasure-seeking, financial security, and need for specific friendship, collectivism represents we-ness, we-consciousness, collective identity, emotional interdependence, group solidarity, sharing duties and obligations, need for stable and predetermined friendships and group decisions (Hofstede, 1980, 1984). The individual identity in ego-centric individuals is about one-self whereas the identity in socio-centric societies and individuals is based on kinship and "tribal" loyalty. Ego-centric individuals are often seen as rational individuals with personal choices who are discreet, autonomous, self-sufficient and respectful of the rights of others. Hofstede (2001) sees them as their role confined by achievement and they believe in equality, equity, non-interference, and detachability. Individuals in socio-centric characteristics are bound by the common good, and social harmony and others are put first before themselves. They see justice and institutions as an extension of the family and follow paternalism and legal moralism. Socio-centric individuals share material as well as non-material resources; they appear to be more susceptible to social influences and self-presentation and face-work; sharing of outcomes, and; feeling involved in others' lives. Ego-centric societies have been shown to be having higher rates of crime, suicide, divorce, child abuse, emotional stress and physical and mental illness and higher levels of Gross National Product. It is entirely possible that egocentric individuals in individualistic cultures will disregard the needs of communities, families or workgroups, and socio-centric individuals will feel concerned about their communities and in- groups. Egocentric individuals in collectivist societies are also more likely to yield to group norms less than socio-centric persons in individualistic cultures whereas people from individualistic cultures are good at entering and leaving new social groups thereby making migration easy and also settling down after such an event. Ego-centric individuals have great skills in forming new in-groups and superficially appear more sociable. Thus it makes sense that egocentric individuals from collectivist societies will settle down better in individualistic societies and on the other hand, socio-centric individuals from collectivist societies, if socially isolated or alienated, will have difficulty in setting down in individualistic societies. Similarly, masculine societies (mostly Latin American societies) allow men to dominate. Feminine societies such as Scandinavian countries believe in gender equality, and child-rearing is a shared activity. Thus different societal and cultural attitudes will influence the social and cognitive development of the child.

UNDERSTANDING OF DISEASE AND ILLNESS AND SOCIAL FACTORS

Diseases are literally disease, and physicians diagnose and treat diseases (Eisenberg, 1977). Patients suffer "illnesses" which are *experiences* of disvalued changes in states of being and in social functioning (Eisenberg, 1977). Sickness, on the other hand, is defined by the society. The disease is often at the heart of the illness experience, but not always. Patients are interested in getting rid of the illness whereas physicians are interested in "curing" disease. Secondly, illness is constituted of social functioning, and focusing on disease will simply ignore this social functioning. Hysteria often has no underlying brain pathology and does not fit into the disease model and is thus an illness. Indigenous healers (and perhaps doctors too) are more responsive to the extra-biological aspects of illness, which were perhaps easier to manipulate. Therefore, any interaction between the patient and their proximal social contacts (family, peers and friends) and distal social contacts (society at large) is part of the clinical assessment and management. Domains of social and cultural aspects, patients' beliefs, practice and experiences and culture of the medicine itself which is affected by health care and health systems and social determinants of disease need to be brought together. All of these are social. As society changes as a result of globalization and urbanization, social factors change, and their emergence can lead to the development of new forms of stress and distress. For example, increasing use of social media such as Twitter, Instagram, etc. has led to increased stress, but we are nowhere near full understanding of the issues related to this and individual users' mental state.

Background: Psychiatry has always been a specialty of medicine, and to the end of the 19th century the term alienism was used to explain the specialty. There is little doubt that society through its political, religious and community leaders (who may all be self-selected) defines and identifies deviance which may be based on statistical variation only. As types of treatments were very limited, patients with psychiatric illness (defined and identified as aliens) were often confined to asylums-institutions which were meant to keep people with mental illness generally hidden away from public eye. This also meant that paradoxically this contributed to stigma and affected further resourcing of services. Although there were some very high profiled psychiatrists and clinicians who were politically and socially well-tuned and tried to change the delivery of services, the purpose of treatment was often punitive in order to make them behave in a way which was seen as being acceptable to the society they were serving. Although there has quite rightly been an emphasis on treatment, inevitably control and seclusion became the norm. Attempts to understand the causation of mental illness had been largely social initially, and as the knowledge of biology and anatomy and human physiology increased, genetic and biological aspects came into their own. Furthermore, a better understanding of psyche perhaps influenced by psychoanalysis contributed to the development of a biopsychosocial model of etiology as well as management. However, often clinician struggle to ascertain which of the three components is of larger importance. Spirituality in many countries and cultures as in India can play a further role in contributing to both stress and alleviation of symptoms. Often the emphasis has been on biological and psychological etiological management only, but not on social consequences of the illness (Ventriglio & Bhugra, 2015). All psychiatry is social as it is based on a number of reasons as discussed below.

First and foremost, human beings are born into cultures and not with cultures. Culture and social milieu play a major role in shaping individual's world-view and cognitive and social development. That is where we all learn to communicate and manage social interactions which go on to define human living. The brain, with its structures and functions, is affected by social factors and causes certain ways of functioning or dysfunction. There is increasing evidence that social determinants of health play a major role in the genesis of both physical and mental illness (Marmot, 2005, 2014). These social determinants include urban factors like poverty, unemployment, overcrowding and a lack of green spaces, among others. The clinical practice of psychiatry (as well as of medicine) is in the social context where society determines the funding, structures, policies, and environment within which clinical and therapeutic encounters take place.

Health should not be seen as a simple absence of disease (Constitution of the World Health Organization, 2006) as has been defined by the WHO (Huber et al., 2011). With increased longevity and people living with complex co-morbidities and also having episodes of health and wellbeing after managing periods of illness such as bipolar illness, it becomes difficult to marry concepts of disease and illness. Therefore, the social domain of illness is about one's ability to manage one's life and social functioning which allows the individuals to lead fulfilling lives and meet their potential and obligations with a degree of independence. Health, therefore, becomes a dynamic balance between opportunities and limitations both of which are strongly influenced by social and environmental conditions. Thus social domain takes on a major role in our understanding of mental health and the practice of clinical psychiatry. We believe that social domain is much more pertinent and can be seen as a crucial aetiological factor too as demonstrated by Brown and Harris's seminal work (Brown & Harris, 1978) on life events and depression. It may be that more organic conditions such as dementia have more clearly identifiable biological substrate, but even their onset can be influenced by social factors, loneliness and lack of support.

Bhugra et al. (2012) describe the psychiatry's contract with society as an implicit agreement as to what is expected of psychiatrists by the society and in return what psychiatrists expect from society (Bhugra et al., 2012). Thus, psychiatrists suggest that they need appropriate resources; an absence of stigma; managing both public mental health and clinical services. There is no doubt that psychiatry must be allowed to get their views across to a wide range of audiences and fight for the good mental health of both the population and service users; as well as educating all stakeholders. As part of their contract, psychiatrists need to explain better what it does, and the judgments psychiatrists make in applying its practices, such as the use of compulsion and psychiatric medication. On the other side, the society needs to ensure adequate resources for services, change policies related to social inequalities and social disparities. Both sides need to be open and honest in their interactions with each other and focus on developing good relationships and communication. Interestingly often this contract is within the medical framework. It is acknowledged that any relationship between psychiatry, society, and management of mental illness has always been complex and mutually ambivalent. As mentioned, the contract often ignores what exactly the role of the psychiatrist is, and how public mental health is often side-lined with a simple acknowledgment or ignored completely. As discussed above, there is a disparity between the patient and the psychiatrist as the former are more interested in illness whereas the latter are interested in disease (Eisenberg, 1977). Under these circumstances, the focus on managing psychiatrically ill patients is narrowed further to medication only to make them comply. In addition in countries such as India where human resources are not adequate, poly-pharmacy in the context of time-limited consultations contribute further complexity to therapeutic interactions. Inevitably this leads to the role of social conditions causing psychiatric disorders being ignored, and advocacy for patients is not as strong and vocal as it could/should be. Virchow (1986) maintained that illness (of any kind) was an indictment of the political system and that politics was nothing other than medicine on a large scale (Virchow, 1986). The idea that medicine is social is not new or even recent , but it keeps being ignored when it is argued by influential people that changes in brain structure are needed to demonstrate the existence of a psychiatric diagnosis (Insel & Lieberman, 2013). At the other extreme is the serious danger of medicalizing normal human emotions such as grief into pathological grief, shyness into social phobia, etc.

In many parts of the world at the undergraduate level, preventive and social medicine forms a major part of training. However, within such curriculum, there is quite rightly a major focus on infectious diseases and occupational health, and often no emphasis is placed whatsoever on mental health aspects of infections or employment. The social medicine model is much more applicable to psychiatry, as such an approach leads to a clearer understanding of what is seen as behaviorally normal and what is construed as deviant. Psychiatrists as managers of society's concerns and expectations can lead to more re-training options (Ventriglio & Bhugra, 2015).

As mentioned above, the life story perspective described by McHugh and Slavney (1998) provides an unusual way of looking at mental disorders. Life story perspective aims to provide a framework for developmental aspects of the individual as well as getting a perspective based on narrative. The development of individuals does not stop in adolescence or youth, and this is a view which needs further exploration and understanding. It is apparent that such a perspective will carry with it social and cultural values and domains. As Eisenberg (1977) states it is the patients who determine not only the importance of the distress and when and where to seek help from, they also determine what the status of their social functioning is, wherein the broader framework of this functioning is set by society at large. This is one way of social control of what is perceived as social deviance which is clearly defined by the society. Many previously commonly diagnosed disorders such as catatonia, hebephrenia, hysteria or conversion disorders have disappeared in the West, at least over the past few decades whereas conditions such as internet addiction and *hikikomori* have emerged. It may reflect changes in psychiatric conditions in response to changes in societies. For example, conversion disorders are rarely seen among white British people in comparison with Indian patients. Whether this means that these disorders are genuinely more common or whether these have transmogrified into something else is important to ascertain. Another example will be introjection of distress by men and using alcohol to deal with it whereas women may use self-harm as a strategy to deal with stress. Similarly, the rise of post-traumatic stress disorder in many countries begs the question whether symptoms have altered in response to social expectations and the role individuals are expected to play in the social system.

Porter pointed out that the 19th-century social reformers in the West were keen to increase the political role of medicine which may have led to introducing this to the undergraduate training of medical students (Porter, 2002, 2006). An additional factor has been a gradual shift from social behavior to lifestyle medicine in the last century as countries have progressed and in many cultures-in-transition such as India. Stonington and Holmes (2006) point out that the way healthcare systems and healthcare models are funded and designed is affected by the social systems (Stonington & Holmes, 2006). Social medicine includes social and cultural studies of health and medicine and social determinants of health and illness (Holtz et al., 2006). These frameworks play a major role in mental healthcare systems. Variations in rates of psychiatric disorders across countries and societies and even within the same society according to gender, race, and ethnicity, social and economic status are recognized. Psychiatry at this stage of its history stands at a similar turning point as medicine did 150 years ago in that our understanding of mental illness is getting better with more understanding about structures and functions of brain and psychopharmacogenomics. It has been shown that attachment patterns in childhood influence brain structures which will, in turn, affect brain functioning and this confirms the notion that social factors are important. Malekpour pointed out that infants upon birth are far more competent, social, responsive and more able to make sense of their environments than previously imagined (Malekpour, 2007). The social interaction starts to build individual identity (Fraiberg, 1959) and attachment patterns modify underlying brain structures. Schore goes on to observe that right brain maturation in its regulatory capacities is experience-dependent and points out that secure attachments in childhood lead to the development of efficient right brain regulatory functions and good infant mental health (Schore, 1994). Perhaps cross-cultural studies looking at child-rearing patterns and linking these with structural brain changes may help understand further the link between the society, social factors, and human functioning. There have been recent suggestions that genetic mutations themselves may be influenced by stressors to push individuals into psychiatric disorders. This has been described as the two hit theory (Maric & Svrakic, 2012). These authors postulate that genetic defects by themselves and per se may not lead to illness but under the influence of other factors may create the second hit leading to expression of pathological mutation. Epigenetics is a relatively new field which deals with our understanding of how environmental influences modulate gene activity.

Stress vulnerability response psychosis models have existed for quite some time, but epigenetics focuses on vulnerability at micro-levels. Kirkbride et al, (2012) postulated that maternal pre-natal nutrition could influence the risk of schizophrenia in the offspring following epigenetic effects (Kirkbride et al., 2012). These factors related perhaps to infections, malnutrition and other dietary factors may well play a role in explaining some of the variations in rates of schizophrenia.

We welcome that DSM-5 (American Psychiatric Association, 2013) has included cultural factors and cultural formulation, but we recommend that socio-cultural dimensions of individual experiences and distress are incorporated in the diagnostic and management frameworks in a clearer way than they have been so far. Patient narratives, life history, and developmental perspective allow us to explore social factors in the context of etiology and biological vulnerabilities on the one hand and their influence on therapeutic engagement and outcomes on the other.

THERAPEUTIC INTERACTION

The practice of psychiatry is much more strongly related to social milieu perhaps more so than many medical specialties. Social environment and social determinants, therefore, need to be applied more rigorously to psychiatric diagnostic framework and management capabilities. The key components of therapeutic encounter in psychiatry belong to the patient and doctor interaction which is strongly influenced by patient perspectives and expectations. Patients' and carers' beliefs, explanatory models, past experiences, the culture of the healthcare system and the profession itself within which psychiatry is practiced are some of the key aspects of patient engagement. Patients' understanding of their own distress and explanatory models which make sense to them (Kleinman, 1980) are part of the social model, and clinicians' emphasis on biological models needs to shift somewhat towards social causation, precipitation, and perpetuation of psychiatric distress. Bhugra (2014) reflects that social causation of psychiatric illness and their role in management must take higher priority than before (Bhugra, 2014). As Ventriglio and Bhugra (2015) highlight that in psychiatric practice, although lip service is paid to social factors, often these are excluded on the basis that biological factors make psychiatry more scientific and thus less liable to accusations of being soft. The emphasis on psychiatry as an art specialty and also as natural science should enable the profession to shed its defensive nature.

A shift in these attitudes may be related to bringing about a change in the way we train medical undergraduates and postgraduates leading to a better understanding and this may be possible through using medical humanities as part of teaching (Ventriglio & Bhugra, 2015) focusing on social factors and the relationship between society and medicine (in particular psychiatry) which will enable a shift from the cult of technology to more humane and humanistic medicine.

CONCLUSION

Psychiatry as a medical specialty needs to speak for its patients and their needs, to take its role and responsibility in public mental health more seriously and vigorously. Furthermore, the task of being an advocate seems to be disappearing in many cultures. Such advocacy is essential not only to improve the care and funding of psychiatric services, but this will also encourage patients to advocate for psychiatry. Most of the advocacy has to be on social factors related to social determinants of mental illness. These social determinants of health apply not only to mental illness but also to physical illnesses. And the two of them influence each other. Increasing social inequalities means that rates of many psychiatric disorders are growing and early interventions must, therefore, focus on public mental health agenda.

REFERENCES

American Psychiatric Association. DSM-5. Washington, DC: American Psychiatric Association Publishing; 2013.

Bhugra D. All medicine is social. J Royal Soc Med. 2014;107(5):183-6.

Bhugra D, Malik A, Ikkos G. Psychiatry's Contract with Society. Oxford: OUP; 2012.

Brown G, Harris T. Social Origins of Depression: A Study of Psychiatric Disorders in Women. New York: The Free Press; 1978.

Eisenberg L. Disease and illness. Culture Med Psychiatry. 1977;1(1):9-23.

Fraiberg S. The Magic Years. New York: Charles Scribner Sons; 1959.

Hofstede G. Culture and organizations. Int Studies Manage Organ. 1980;10(4):15-41.

Hofstede G. Culture's Consequences: International Differences in Work-Related Values. London: Sage; 1984.

Hofstede G. Culture's Consequences. Sherman Oaks: Sage; 2001.

Holtz TH, Holmes S, Stonington S, et al. Health is still social: contemporary examples in the age of the genome. PLoS Med. 2006;3(10):419.

Huber M, Knottnerus JA, Green L, et al. How should we define health? BMJ. 2011;343(2):d4163.

Insel T, Lieberman J. DSM-5 and RDoC: Shared Interests. Washington: National Institute of Mental Health; 2013.

Kirkbride JB, Susser E, Kundakovic M, et al. Prenatal nutrition, epigenetics and schizophrenia risk: can we test causal effects? Epigenomics. 2012;4(3):303-15.

Kleinman A. Patients and Their Healers in the Context of Their Cultures. Berkeley, CA: University of California Press; 1980.

Malekpour M. Effects of attachment on early and later development. Br J Develop Disab. 2007;53(105): 81-95.

Maric NP, Svrakic DM. Why schizophrenia genetics needs epigenetics: a review. Psychiatr Danub. 2012;24(1):2-18.

Marmot M. The Health Gap. London: Bloomsbury; 2005.

Marmot M. Social determinants of health inequalities. Lancet. 2014;365:1099-104.

McHugh P, Slavney P. The Perspectives of Psychiatry. Baltimore, MD: Johns Hopkins University Press; 1998.

Porter D. From social structure to social behaviour in Britain after the second world war. Contempor Br History. 2002;16(3):58-80.

Porter D. How did social medicine evolve, and where is it heading? PLoS Med. 2006;3(10):e399.

Schore AN. Affect Regulation and the Origin of the Self. Mahwah, NJ: Lawrence Erlbaum Associates; 1994.

Stonington S, Holmes: Social medicine in the 21st century. PLos Med. 2006;3(10):e445.

Ventriglio A, Bhugra D. Social justice for the mentally ill. Int J Soc Psychiatry. 2015;61:213-4.

Virchow R. Report on the typhus epidemic in Upper Silesia. In: Rather LJ (Ed). Public Health Reports. Seagemore Beach, MA: Science History Publications; 1986. Pp. 307-19.

World Health Organization. Constitution of the World Health Organization. Geneva: WHO; 2006

Chapter 3

Social Psychiatry: World Scenario

Roy Abraham Kallivayalil, Varghese P Punnoose

SUMMARY

Social psychiatry pays attention to the interaction of man and his social environment, and the effect of this interaction on mental health, rather than just focusing on disease itself. This itself is not a new paradigm, as traditional systems of medicine have, since ages, emphasized the significance of the community and its beliefs in causing or mitigating illness. Social psychiatry builds on this paradigm by bridging the gap between the biological and psychological models of mental illness, providing the "missing link" of the effect of social stimuli on the overall genesis of disease. The World Association of Social Psychiatry (WASP), amongst other goals, aims to promote a greater understanding of social interactions and their effects on psychiatric disorders. The efforts made under the purview of social psychiatry have borne fruit. For example, the mental health legislation of several countries across the world has seen significant reforms fueled by the understanding that social psychiatry provides. Though promising, the emphasis on social psychiatry needs to increase in order for its full potential to be realized.

INTRODUCTION

"Medicalization of life leads to iatrogenic labeling of the ages of man. When this happens, life turns from a succession of different stages of health into a series of periods, each requiring different therapies"—Ivan Illich (1975).

In the practice of medicine and psychiatry today, we have extreme attention to disease. Super-specialization, fragmentation and commercialization of medicine are encouraged either by default or design. There is little attention to the person and his environment, social situation or life stresses. Positive aspects of health like adaptive functioning, resilience, support systems, and quality of life are often not studied. In contrast, social psychiatry involves all stake holders, engaging interactively with persons and families, health professionals, planners, industry, social advocates, and those in the fields of literature, art and films. Imparting academic training with knowledge, skills, and attitudes relevant to the culture and social context are fostered.

A social psychiatry paradigm goes beyond the impact of poverty, wars, social inequality and unemployment on mental health. It encompasses the social nature of human life. Mental disorders are expressed in social interactions and neurobiological phenomena are ultimately meaningless unless they are linked to the real lives of people in their social reality. A social paradigm requires research to study what happens between people rather than what is wrong with an individual, wholly detached from a social context. It will not ignore neurobiological and psychological dimensions, but will link them to social phenomena in the patient's life and in treatment.

WHAT IS SOCIAL PSYCHIATRY?

"Social psychiatry is that branch of psychiatry which is concerned with the effects of the social environment on the mental health of the individual, and with the effects of the mentally ill person on his or her social environment"—Julian Leff (2010). Leff argues that experiences in the past are represented in the subject's memory and operate in the present to trigger psychiatric illnesses, and sometimes precipitate these and at other times produce relapse.

The current concept in psychiatric practice gives emphasis on individual biological susceptibility. What is important will be to study those conditions which make this susceptibility to manifest as disease. There has been an increase in the number of diagnostic categories and subcategories. Components of human experience are disentangled to find individual biological correlates. Our discourse should never miss the theme that humans are basically social animals. Labeling a behavior as eccentricity or mental illness needs consideration of social and cultural factors. What is more important is how individuals relate to each other within the social frame work of a society. This has got fundamental etiological and therapeutic significance.

Psychiatric disorders have been traditionally conceptualized as sociomedical in nature. In the last quarter of 20th century, thanks to the advances in neurosciences, there emerged a tendency to view them as just medical disorders. However, rapid social changes, changes in family structure and dynamics, and increasing pace and complexity of modern life have made a social paradigm in psychiatry increasingly relevant throughout the world in the recent decades. Evidences of social determinants of mental health are convincing. Unfortunately, in the current psychiatric training, the social context, in which mental disorders emerge and perpetuate itself, is neglected. Psychiatric training should reorient itself to give contextual factors their rightful due in the assessment of individual patient. In the social paradigm, treatments of mental illness should primarily be conceptualized as social interactions. Systemic approach for interventions in families and communities, value-based approaches for integrating people with mental disorders in society, interventions to tackle social isolation and stigma, and to improve network of patients with mental illness would make the management of psychiatric disorders more meaningful (Priebe, 2016). So, it is very clear that psychiatry of 21st century requires close collaboration with humanities and social sciences to achieve this meaningfulness.

HISTORICAL PERSPECTIVES

In the non-western cultures, social factors as determinants of mental illness were inherent in their belief systems. So, the traditional systems of medicine in such cultures incorporated religious beliefs and community (social and family) networks in addressing the care of mentally ill. The post-renaissance period witnessed the emergence of empiricism and reductionism in the field of medicine just as in other branches of science. Microbial theories of the pathogenesis of infections and their successful treatment with antibiotics served as the scientific model of understanding diseases. However, this simple "agent-host" model was not enough to explain non-communicable diseases. Soon, there was a realization that "environment" was the missing link between the agent and host. Public health and social medicine built their theories on how the environment interacts with the agent and host, and tried to explain the epidemiology and pathogenesis of medical illnesses. Similarly, in psychiatry, the western medicine was trying to explain mental illness as either due to biological (coarse brain disease—organic) or psychological (individual unconscious factors or learning) factors in a dichotomous fashion. It was soon realized that this dichotomy is not able to capture the complexity of mental illnesses. It was being increasingly recognized that social and cultural factors play an important part in the genesis, expression, and outcome of mental illnesses. Initially, several humane approaches to mental illnesses and later on research evidence from epidemiological studies in schizophrenia across the world gave support to the importance of social factors as determinants of outcome in major mental illnesses. It was in this background that from 1950s onwards (post-World War II) social psychiatry has established itself as an integral part of psychiatric practice and research.

WORLD ASSOCIATION OF SOCIAL PSYCHIATRY

Joshua Bierer organized the First International Congress of Social Psychiatry at London in 1964. Professionals interested in greater understanding of human behavior resolved to make greater efforts in this direction. The Second International Congress of Social Psychiatry was also organized in London in 1969. Joshua Bierer became the first President (1964–1968), followed by Jules H Masserman, USA (1968–1974). Vladimir Hudolin organized the Third International Congress in 1970 at Zagreb, Yugosalvia and served as President from 1974–1978. Constitution of WASP was revised and adopted during Hudolin's tenure. He was succeeded by the following: 1978–1983 George Vassiliou, Greece; 1983–1988 John L Carleton, USA; 1988–1992 A Guilherme Ferreira, Portugal; 1992–1996 Jorge A Costa e Silva, Brazil; 1996–2001 Eliot Sorel, USA; 2001–2004 Shridhar Sharma, India; 2004–2007 Tsutomu Sakuta, Japan; 2007–2010 Julio Arboleda-Flores, Canada; 2010–2013 Driss Moussaoui, Morocco; 2013–2016 Tom KJ Craig, UK; and 2016–2019 Roy Abraham Kallivayalil, India. From the sixth Congress, the International Association for Social Psychiatry was renamed as the World Association of Social Psychiatry (WASP).

WASP aims to promote greater understanding of the interactions between individuals and their physical and human environment (including their society and culture), and the impact of these interactions on the clinical expression, treatment of mental and behavioral problems and disorders, and their prevention. Other aims and objectives include promotion of mental health through education of health workers, policy makers and decision makers and the community at large; promotion of national and international collaboration among professionals and societies in social psychiatry and related disciplines; promotion of research that can facilitate the understanding of the interaction between social factors, psychological functioning and mental health or illness, creating partnerships with professionals of other scientific disciplines, international agencies, and non-governmental organizations working in fields related to social psychiatry, and organizing relevant international congresses and scientific meetings. The WASP organizes a World Congress of Social Psychiatry every 3 years. It also organizes ad hoc, international, regional and local congresses and cosponsored conferences and meetings that facilitate the achievements of its goals. In summary, the WASP aims to study the nature of man and his cultures and the prevention and treatment of his vicissitudes and behavioral disorders, promoting national and international collaboration among professionals and societies in fields related to social psychiatry, making the knowledge and practice of social psychiatry available to other sciences and to the public, and advancing the physical, social, and philosophic well-being of mankind.

In its five decades of existence, the WASP has tried to bring the social and cultural aspects in the etiology and management of mental illnesses to focus in training and planning service delivery with varying degrees of success. It has supported research in areas like cross-cultural studies, expressed emotions and rehabilitation, and led advocacy in areas like stigma reduction. The WASP has been actively collaborating with other stakeholders like the World Psychiatric Association and the World Federation of Mental Health.

HAS SOCIAL PSYCHIATRY LIVED UP TO EXPECTATIONS?

Concepts from social psychiatry have served as preludes and catalysts for reforms and modern legislation in several countries (Haack & Kumbier, 2012). Social psychiatry has given impetus to movements like recovery approach in schizophrenia and person-centered psychiatry in the recent years. Though these are gratifying achievements, it has to be admitted that it has taken a back seat in the recent decades both in the training and in the management decisions.

The case of schizophrenia exemplifies how clinical psychiatry failed to translate potential research findings from social psychiatry to practice. Several cross-cultural studies have demonstrated how social and cultural factors can be crucial in determining the outcome. The WHO led International Pilot Study of Schizophrenia and the subsequent 10 nation study indicated that social and family network support can be protective, a factor which is independent of pharmacological compliance. However, this evidence-based reality has not found its due place in the management plan of the individual as well as that of the population.

Another social aspect of schizophrenia, which has not got its due attention, is the increasing urbanization across the globe in recent times. In 1950, only a third of the population lived in cities. It is estimated that by 2050, 70% of the world's population will be living in urban environments. Some researchers estimate that up to 30% of the risk of schizophrenia is attributable to urban upbringing (van Os J, 2004). Researchers in the newly established field of neurourbanism have suggested the possible brain-based mechanisms of this increased risk (Adli et al., 2017).

Time and again, research has shown that the most effective suicide prevention strategies include identification and treatment of depression in primary care by the basic doctors and restricting the access to lethal methods. The natural practical implication of these findings would be to improve the quality of psychiatry training in general curriculum and legal measures to restrict access to insecticides and guns. But professionals have failed to convince the policy makers even in their fraternity to implement these steps.

It is very unfortunate that social dimensions are not adequately emphasized in the curriculum and training at both undergraduate and postgraduate levels in most teaching institutions. The evaluation systems in examination focus too much on criteria-based diagnosis and evidence-based management, and places little emphasis on the sociocultural context in which the illness develops and the impairments and handicap they produce in social living. The professionals in training generally fail to comprehend the balanced biopsychosocial model of mental illnesses. Management of the individual patient and service delivery plan for the population are also biased by the swinging of pendulum too much to the biological side.

WHAT SOCIAL PSYCHIATRY HAS TO OFFER IN A CHANGING WORLD?

Future mental healthcare needs to consider the changing technological, economic, social, and political context (Kumar, 1995; Bauman, 2000). Recently a project to explore the potential future of the social approach to mental healthcare was done by a group of experts. This group considered several existing "instabilities" in the present scenario and the "drives" which are predominantly external and socially driven. The instabilities identified include the dominant academic status of biological research, scarce funding for social research in mental health, inadequate involvement of family members or informal carers, less collaboration with other agencies like general healthcare, social services and local authorities, need for stronger theories and methods on the effects of social factors on mental health, need to develop effective and more affordable social interventions, gap between knowledge and clinical practice and mental health policies, human resource deficiency in mental healthcare professionals, challenges in keeping up with changes in cultural norms, practical difficulties in implementing a multidisciplinary approach, and paucity of effective preventive strategies. The driving forces for change identified are increasing social inequalities and injustice, ageing population, reduced social role of families, digitalized world, increasing loneliness and social isolation, increasing private participation in mental healthcare, increasing urbanization, globalization, mass migration, increasing individualism, and influence of United Nation Convention on the Rights of People with Disabilities across the globe.

The nature of support and treatment, societies might provide to help the people with mental illness and what role professional services might play in the next 20 years was explored by Giacco et al. (2017). Four possible scenarios were identified:
1. Patient-controlled service
2. Care targeted on social context
3. Emergence of virtual mental health
4. Care that will be regulated on the basis of social disadvantage.

Though these predictions are based on expert opinions from mental health professionals from Europe, it is possible that the scenario will not be much different in non-western world as well.

Patient-controlled services and provision of mental healthcare by artificial intelligence may appear quite challenging for the professionals, but the new age psychiatrists need to be trained for this changing scenario. Mental healthcare is likely to emerge (and desirably so) as a part of a holistic service for people who experience social disadvantage. Social disadvantage cutoffs would be defined according to various dimensions including poverty, social isolation, homelessness, unemployment, marginalization, discrimination, and other more specific aspects such as forced migration. The distinction between physical, psychological, and social distress and care would not be clear.

CONCLUSION

Social psychiatry is at a turning point of its history, and the 21st century will probably belong to it, as the 19th was the one of clinical descriptions and classification, and the 20th was one of psychotherapy and of biological treatments of mental disorders. Social psychiatry is destined to have greater relevance and a brighter future in the coming years. There is a fresh interest in understanding social factors in the etiology of mental illness and a growth in evidence-based psychosocial interventions that are both effective and practical across cultures. Simultaneously, growth in the fields of science, technology, and economics has led to rapid changes in social values. Social psychiatry cannot exist independently of the biological sciences and socioeconomic and ethical issues. Thus, social psychiatry continues to explore the fabric of social environment using it to update our knowledge on human relationships.

We live in a world where the social environment is rapidly evolving, faster than ever in the 2 million years history of *homo sapiens*. Mental health is closely related to social changes. Mental illnesses have reflected the social environment of the times. Mental illnesses cannot be disconnected from their social context. We need to evolve a system of understanding and managing mental disorders, suited to the current age. Ideally, the service provision should be in collaboration and participation by the patient and should be inclusive of the most disadvantaged sections. The profession needs to prepare itself for the challenges of virtual era of care giving. More research is needed to evolve socially based prevention as well as effective social intervention strategies. The policy on management of the individual and that of the population should incorporate evidence from social psychiatry research.

REFERENCES

Adli M, Berger M, Brakemeier EL, et al. Neurourbanism: towards a new discipline. Lancet Psychiatry. 2017;4(3):183-5.

Bauman Z. Liquid Modernity. Cambridge, Polity Press, 2000.

Giacco D, Amering M, Bird V, et al. Scenarios for the future of mental health care: a social perspective. Lancet Psychiatry. 2017;4:256-70.

Haack K, Kumbier E. History of social psychiatry. Curr Opin Psychiatry. 2012;25(6):492-6.

Illich I. Limits to Medicine: Medical Nemesis. London, Marion Boyars, 1975.

Kumar K. From Post-industrial to Post-modern Society. New Theories of the Contemporary World. Chichester, Wiley, 1995.

Leff J. The historical development of social psychiatry, in Principles of Social Psychiatry. In: Morgan C, Bhugra D. (Eds.) Hoboken NJ, Wiley, 2010. pp.1-11

Priebe S. A social paradigm in psychiatry–themes and perspectives. Epidemiol Psychiatr Sci. 2016;25(6):521-7.

Van Os J. Does the urban environment cause psychosis? Br J Psychiatry. 2004;184:287-88.

Chapter 4

History of Social Psychiatry in India

Rakesh K Chadda

SUMMARY

Social psychiatry has informally existed in India for many centuries since persons with mental illness were always being cared for in the community. Some of the age-old practices of the ancient India like Yoga and meditation have been formally recognized as standard nonpharmacological interventions in the modern psychiatry. A formal beginning of social psychiatry in India can be traced back to Dr Vidya Sagar's experiments of involving families in the management of persons with mental illness at Amritsar in the 1950s. Subsequently, the introduction of community outreach programs around the country initially as individual initiatives and later under the National Mental Health Programme (NMHP) of India, community awareness activities under the program, and integration of psychiatry in general hospitals have been other historical developments in social psychiatry in India. Other important developments in social psychiatry included initiatives from the judicial sector in form of initiatives in mental health and enactment of laws aiming at welfare of persons with mental illness. The Indian Association for Social Psychiatry (IASP), which was established in 1984, has also played an important role in the growth of social psychiatry in India.

INTRODUCTION

Social psychiatry has informally existed in India since the time mental illness has. Persons with mental health problems were always looked after in the community by the families, temples, *dargahs* and other similar places. This existed in the absence of formal mental health care systems. A person with mental illness was generally accepted in the community, and social stigma was never as high as in the last few decades. The society could manage its persons with mental illness even in the absence of adequate formal facilities to take care of them. India could manage its mentally ill population within the community even in the absence of mental hospitals in the pre-colonial period, and with a limited number of inpatient beds in the later period (Chadda, 2012; Chadda & Deb, 2013).

Coming to the current situation, India has a substantial deficit of the mental health care resources. The average national deficit of psychiatrists is estimated as 77%. More than one-third of the population of India has more than 90% deficit of psychiatrists. Figures for non-medical mental health professionals like psychologists, psychiatric social workers, and psychiatric nurses are further lower (Thirunavukarasu & Thirunavukarasu, 2010). Thus, there is a large "unmet need" in the community. In the Indian society, psychological distress is not generally considered as something requiring medical treatment, and the modern medical care is considered as having only a limited expertise in the area (Murthy, 2010). The National Mental Health Survey (NMHS) of India of 2016 has estimated treatment gap for various mental disorders as ranging from 70.4–86.3% (Gururaj et al., 2016).

Mental health has always been a challenging issue in India and neighboring countries, and the mental health professionals have developed a number of strategies to meet this challenge. India has to its credit many unique contributions in social psychiatry, which include recognizing the role of family in care of persons with mental illness, integration of psychiatry in general hospitals, community mental health programs, judicial interventions at improving mental health care, protection of rights of the persons with mental illness, and application of the ancient Indian concepts in mental health care.

This chapter is an attempt to summarize the developments in social psychiatry in India and might have missed some of the issues. The subsequent chapters in the book have focused on those issues in detail.

BEGINNINGS OF SOCIAL PSYCHIATRY IN INDIA

A formal beginning of social psychiatry in India can be traced back to 1950s when Dr Vidya Sagar started involving families in the care of persons with mental illness outside the main premises of the mental hospital at Amritsar since it was not feasible to accommodate all the patients in the overcrowded hospital. Dr Sagar made somewhat novel arrangements for the family members to stay with their patients in tents, which were left by the army following the World War 2 on the ground outside the hospital. He and his team provided treatment and group sessions for the patients and the families. This approach helped the family caregivers in learning basic caring skills for their wards. The experiment went a long way in reducing the hostility in the minds of the patients about their family members as they were not being abandoned. The patients following improvement would go back to their homes and the community with a message that mental illness could be treated, reducing the associated stigma (Sagar, 1973; Kapur, 2004). This experiment becomes more significant in the background that 1950s were the period when familial pathology and parental upbringing was considered a major etiological factor in then psychiatry, contributing to the development of mental illness rather than having a role in therapeutics. Going further, it was followed by setting up of family units at other places in India like Vellore and Bangalore (Kapur, 2004; Chadda, 2012).

COMMUNITY PSYCHIATRY MOVEMENT IN INDIA

Community psychiatry movement in India can be traced to the early 1960s when psychiatry units had started opening up in the general hospitals on a large scale and services were also being expanded in some of the mental hospitals, which had started formal training in psychiatry. The time period was parallel to the deinstitutionalization movement in the West following the introduction of chlorpromazine and identification of the institutional syndrome, an after effect of long-term institutionalization. Mental hospitals around the world, especially in the USA and Europe, were being downsized also in response to the human rights initiatives and development of the community psychiatry units. During this period, some dynamic psychiatrists in India also took initiatives to expand the mental health services to the community.

The first such service was started by Dr Satyanand in the form of a weekly community mental health service in 1964 at the Comprehensive Rural Hospital, established at Ballabhgarh near Delhi as community outreach center of the All India Institute of Medical Sciences (AIIMS), New Delhi. Another rural clinic came into being in 1967 at Mandar near Ranchi in Eastern India (Chadda, 2012), started by the then Hospital for Mental Diseases (now Central Institute of Psychiatry), Ranchi. These initiatives were followed by two major developments in the 1970s, which were to change the course of community psychiatry scene in the country. These included the establishment of the community psychiatry services at Raipur Rani in the state of Haryana in Northern India (Wig et al., 1981) and at Sakalwada in Karnataka state in Southern India (Isaac et al., 1982). Both of these projects included outreach clinics at the primary health centers, orientation programs for medical officers and health workers. The experience became the forerunner of the NMHP of India.

Both Raipur Rani and Sakalwada can be called important milestones in the history of social psychiatry in India. Raipur Rani program, which was funded by the World Health Organization (WHO), also gave estimates of the prevalence of mental illness in the rural areas. The project developed methods for identifying mentally ill in the community and studying the community attitudes. Training manuals were developed for doctors, multipurpose health workers, and community health volunteers as a part of the program. Sakalwada program, which was run by the National Institute of Mental Health and Neurosciences (NIMHANS), Bangalore, included many more activities besides the community outreach mental health services, comprising of development of training manuals for doctors and health workers, training programs for primary care physicians, school mental health program, home visits by nurses, and organization of mental health camps (Isaac et al., 1982; Kapur, 2004; Chadda, 2012).

The two programs were followed by the development of similar kind of services by psychiatry departments of many medical colleges in different parts of the country. The NMHS, 2016 has estimated 450 mobile mental units and 249 de-addiction centers providing mental health services in the 12 states of India studied (Gururaj et al., 2016). The total figure for India is likely to be more than double this figure.

ALTERNATIVES TO THE CONVENTIONAL MODELS OF CARE

Alternative and traditional healing practice is an important resource which is used by a large section of the population especially those with mental illnesses in India. A study of the late 1960s from South India had reported nearly 75% of the patients with severe mental illnesses taking treatment from the traditional folk healers. Another study conducted around 30 years later in Delhi in North India found that about 30% of the patients attending a tertiary care neuropsychiatric hospital chose a religious faith healer as the first contact for help (Chadda et al., 2001). Interestingly, more than half of the patients with mental health problems visiting the modern psychiatric facilities consult alternative practitioners at some time during the course of their illness (Mishra et al., 2011). In the recent past, a new group of alternative help resource is becoming popular in India for mental health problems and chronic physical illnesses. This includes folk-healing, spiritual and religious counseling and various kinds of meditation practices (Chadda & Deb, 2013).

Community camp approach is another unique method used for the mental health delivery in India and neighboring countries, where there are not enough services available (Ranganathan, 1994; Chavan & Arun, 1999; Raj et al., 2005). Such an approach has been used in India for a number of decades but has the limitation of maintaining continuity of care, an essential component of mental health services. Such an approach, when used, should incorporate continuity of care. Conducting once a week or once a month clinic at distant places could be a good option. Such a practice has also been used under District Mental Health Programme (DMHP) at a few places and also being used by many private psychiatrists.

CONTRIBUTIONS OF THE GENERAL HOSPITAL PSYCHIATRIC UNITS

The first general hospital psychiatric unit (GHPU) was established in Kolkata by Dr GS Bose in 1933 under the aegis of the Calcutta chapter of the Indian Association for Mental Hygiene at the then Carmichael Medical College (now known as RG Kar Medical College). Interestingly, the college provided only a room and some furnishings, and the rest of money came from the association and Dr Bose. Most of the staff worked on an honorary basis, and the clinic functioned for 2 hours twice-weekly. This was a novel experiment to make mental health services available in the community settings outside the precincts of the high walls of the mental hospitals. After a few years, in 1938, Dr KK Masani started psychiatric services at JJ Hospital (Banerjee, 2001). This was followed by a once-a-week psychiatry clinic in the outpatient department of Patna Medical College Hospital in 1939, under the guidance of Dr Ghoshal (Choudary, 2010) and another service by Dr NS Vahia at KEM Hospital in the early 1940s in Mumbai (Apte, 2010). Starting of these psychiatric units in the general hospitals was an attempt at expanding mental health services, integrating mental health in general health and recognizing the psychological morbidity in the medico-surgical patients.

Just before independence, the Health Survey and Development Committee constituted by the Government of India in 1946 (Bhore Committee, 1946) emphasized the need for training in the social aspects of medicine to boost India's meager mental health resources. Mental health resources at the time of independence comprised of 19 mental hospitals with 10,181 beds and a few GHPUs. The Bhore Committee recommended that psychiatry departments be set up in every general hospital to review and enhance the existing curriculum and training in psychiatry for medical students. Psychiatric services were started in the late 1950s at AIIMS and Irwin Hospital, New Delhi, King George Medical College, Lucknow and Medical College, Amritsar. This was followed by the staring of GHPUs at the Postgraduate Institute of Medical Education and Research (PGIMER) Chandigarh in 1962 and many other medical colleges in Odisha, Tamil Nadu, Punjab, Assam, Gujarat, and other states across the country. GHPUs in India have played an important role in integrating psychiatry in general health services, bringing out psychiatric services outside the high walls of the mental hospitals, reducing stigma and making psychiatric service easily accessible and approachable. GHPUs are also the predominant training center for post-graduation in psychiatry in India.

The GHPUs have led to remarkable mental health service development in mental health services in India, have brought psychiatry to mainstream medicine, and improved its acceptability as a medical discipline in the society. Unlike in the West, GHPUs of India are unique in the sense that the family members stay with their patient during the period of hospitalization. This feature of the GHPUs helps in facilitating improvement in the patient, and also prepares the family member to take care of the patient following discharge in the community. Family conflicts, expressed emotions, and related issues can be dealt with during the hospitalization itself, and family therapy can also be initiated, if required. This feature also helps in acceptability of the patient by family the following discharge from the hospital, akin to the model used by Dr Vidya Sagar (Wig & Avasthi, 2004).

CONTRIBUTIONS FROM THE ANCIENT INDIA

Ancient Indian scriptures are a great source of knowledge on mental health promotion and psychosocial management of mental disorders. *Yoga* is one of the most important contributions of the ancient Indian literature. Indian religious texts like *Gita, Vedas, and Upanishads* are also important resources for lessons on relieving the stress-related disorders, anxiety, and depression and improving mental health. This section briefs on some of these contributions.

Gita, the most popular of the old Indian texts, is a compilation of teachings of Lord Krishna, delivered by him to Arjuna, the warrior prince, in the battlefields of Kurukshetra during the war of Mahabharata. Though in its original form, it is a religious text, in which several verses deal with devotion and interactions with the Divine, it has a broader and more secular dimension. The principles of Gita can be applied in a variety of non-religious areas like administration, management, and leadership. Its lessons include the basic principles of psychotherapy and the art of living. The text is relevant to a number of problems of human life, and many of the teachings have the potential of application in the therapeutic practice. As an example, when Arjuna finds himself confused and in a moral dilemma about going to war with his evil cousins, Lord Krishna counsels him about his duties as a warrior and as a prince to ensure the triumph of truth and freedom, and well-being of the common people. Such a message has therapeutic implications in clinical practice (Bhatia et al., 2013).

Teachings in Gita include a practical, self-contained guide to life, describing emotions and cognitive deviations, and how to gain mastery over the vacillating mind and the consequences of failure. The influence of Gita extends much beyond India and the Hindu religion. Many senior psychiatrists have advocated the use of teachings of Gita in understanding and management of psychic distress and mental disorders (Rao, 1980; Murthy, 2010). Thus, Gita could easily be called an important contribution of the ancient India toward social psychiatry.

Vedas, another important ancient Indian text of knowledge, have given detailed descriptions about the preservation of willpower, emotions, inspiration, and consciousness, which can be considered the principles of positive mental health. There are also descriptions of emotional states like grief, envy, pleasure, hostility, attachment, laziness, and their resolution in the Vedas (Avasthi et al., 2013). *Upanishads*, another ancient Indian text, give descriptions of the basics of psychological functioning including theories of perception, thought, consciousness, and memory (Murthy, 2010).

Ayurveda, the ancient Indian text of medicine, is another excellent resource devoted to medical knowledge. It is also one of the formal systems of medicine in use in modern India. Ayurveda describes life or *Ayu* as a combination of *Shareera* (body), *Indriya* (senses), *Satva* (psyche) and *Atma* (soul). The mind gives directions to the senses, and controls the self, reasoning and deliberation. *Ayurveda* conceptualizes that the human actions are decided by three kinds of desires including the desire for self-preservation, wealth, and a happy future. *Ayurveda* has also given description of psychotherapies using the principle of guilt emanating from the *karmic* deeds, which are to be treated using culturally determined observances like religious rituals and dietary restrictions (Murthy, 2010; Avasthi et al., 2013; Behere et al., 2013). The concept of *karma* or duty can be used in rehabilitation. The role model of teacher-disciple (*Guru-Chela* paradigm) has been used by the Indian psychiatrists in psychotherapy (Neki, 1973).

Examples from ancient Indian epics like Ramayana have also been used in psychotherapy. Coming from a text held in great reverence in India, such examples have a tremendous influence on the Indian psyche. One of such examples is Hanuman Complex, described by Wig (Wig, 2004). Hanuman, a character in Ramayana and also considered a God, was a wise and brave person but had lost awareness of his ability to fly and some other extraordinary powers. While on a mission to search for Queen Sita, who was kidnapped by Ravana, Hanuman was made aware of his full power being reminded by Jambavanta. This example has been used by the Indian psychiatrists in psychotherapy. An Indian patient, who has lost confidence and feels unable to meet life's challenges, is explained that the power to change his life rests within him, giving examples of Lord Hanuman, who is held with great reverence in India. The patient is told that he has only temporarily lost his ability and strength due to his illness, and has to come out of this thought process, and realize his potentials. Thus the concepts described in the ancient Indian texts have great relevance in the modern psychiatry, especially in understanding the psychosocial causation and management of mental disorders.

Similarly, teachings borrowed from Buddhism, Jainism, Sikhism, and some other religions which had origins in India, have a potential use in mental health promotion and also indirectly in the non-pharmacological management of mental disorders.

YOGA AND MEDITATION

Yoga and meditation are two important contributions of the ancient India to the world and have been well recognized in management of anxiety, depression and psychosomatic disorders, and also as a method of stress management. Both yoga and meditation are also an integral component of mental health promotion. These concepts are deeply rooted in the Indian psyche and have been used as techniques for anxiety and stress management.

Yoga had its origin in India several thousand years ago. The word "Yoga" means union, i.e. union of personal consciousness with the cosmic. Basic tenets of Yoga include growth, development, and evolution of mind with a spiritual way of life. The ultimate goal of yoga is to control one's own body, bodily senses, and the seemingly endless internal desires and vicissitudes of the mind. Yoga offers a worldview, a healthy lifestyle, and a series of techniques which bring about changes in human awareness and help in realizing the human potential (Khalsa, 2013).

Swami Vivekanand, a famous Indian saint has described Yoga as *"a means of compressing one's evolution into a single life or a few months or even a few hours of one's bodily existence."* Maharishi Patanjali, also called the "father of Yoga", has compiled and refined various aspects of Yoga in a systematic manner in form of "Yoga Sutras" (aphorisms). Patanjali's Yoga advocates the eightfold path of Yoga, also known as "Ashtanga Yoga", which is said to lead to an all-round development of personality. There are many systems of Yoga, propagated by different experts, but the ultimate aim of all the systems remains the same, which is to bring about an altered state of consciousness, also termed the cosmic consciousness, a state of illumination, or *samadhi*. The practice of Yoga facilitates certain changes within the person, which bring about qualitative and quantitative changes in awareness. Regular practice of Yoga helps in reducing stress and brings about relaxation, and also reduces the decline in physical health (Dwivedi et al., 2016).

Many Indian psychiatrists have studied the beneficial effects of yoga in anxiety disorders, depression, dissociation, psychosomatic disorders and schizophrenia (Vahia & Doongaji, 1973; Gangadhar et al., 2013; Paikkatt et al., 2015).

Meditation is another gift of the ancient India to the world and has a strong association with the Indian ethos and society. Though it might have some religious connotations, meditation has been associated with many religions which had an origin in India including Hinduism, Sikhism, and Buddhism. Starting from the early twentieth century, different techniques of meditation have been promoted by many scholars and got popularized. Some of these include transcendental meditation, vipassana meditation, *dhyana* yoga, primordial sound meditation, Sudarshan Kriya, and so on (Chadda & Deb, 2013). The basic aim of meditation is to bring a state of self-concentration accompanied by body and mind relaxation. It is an important anxiety management technique and helpful in management of functional somatic symptoms, mild depression, and a range of psychosomatic disorders.

INDIAN ADAPTATION OF PSYCHOTHERAPY

Psychotherapy is an important treatment modality, which had its origins in the West. The models of psychotherapy as practiced in the West are not applicable in the Indian setting since most such models are based on the concepts of autonomy and independence, which are often considered alien to the Indian society. Manickam (2010) has reviewed the contributions of many Indian psychiatrists toward an Indian adaptation of psychotherapy (Manickam, 2010). Many Indian psychiatrists including D Satyanand, NC Surya, JS Neki, Vijoy Varma, and C Shamsundar have written about Indian adaptation of psychotherapy.

Use of religious concepts has been a focus in psychotherapy in India. Use of concepts borrowed from the ancient Indian literature in psychotherapy has been discussed in a previous section. Many Indian psychiatrists have attempted to integrate indigenous Indian concepts in psychotherapy. Satyanand has researched on use of the religious symbol of Lord Shiva in psychoanalysis in India (Satyanand, 1961). Surya and Jayaram (1968) have discussed the use of the legend of Savitri in psychotherapy with the Indian patients (Surya & Jayaram, 1968). Erna Hoch, a Swiss psychiatrist, who practiced in India for a long time, has deliberated on the informal psychotherapy carried out by the religious leaders like Pirs and Fakirs, and discussed the scope of the indigenous concepts involved in their practices as "therapy" which worked with the population having faith in them (Hoch, 1979). Concepts of Karma and Dharma, as described in the Indian religious texts have also been used in psychotherapy (Avasthi et al., 2013). Neki has used the concept of Sahaja (Neki, 1977), borrowed from Sikhism, a state of positive mental health, achieved by illumination, equipoise, spontaneity, freedom, and harmony.

Neki (1973), who has written extensively on the use of Indian concepts in psychotherapy, gave the concept of *Guru-Chela* relationship as a model of Eastern psychotherapy in India. In this model, the therapist takes the role of *Guru*, the teacher and the patient takes the role of *Chela*, the disciple. The method is a contrast to the Western models in which both the therapist and the patient are at an equal pedestal. Another important difference from the West is that in India patients often come to treatment accompanied by family members, and the issue of privacy and confidentiality may not exist in many circumstances. These terms do not even exist in Indian socio-cultural context and languages (Neki, 1977). A strict application of confidentiality and privacy in Indian patients may sometimes affect family dynamics adversely. Neki has recommended family therapy or at least a few sessions with the family members to help the progress of psychotherapy.

Long back, Surya (Surya & Jayaram, 1968) pointed out that the Indian patients are more dependent unlike the Western patients, where independence is encouraged in the society. Thus, the patients look for a more active role from the psychiatrist in psychotherapy (Surya & Jayaram, 1968). Varma (Varma, 1982) has also opined about the inapplicability of the Western models of psychotherapy in India. This could be due to a number of reasons like poor psychological sophistication in a large section of population, dependence on the therapist and the elders, family members often coming with the patient in the therapy sessions, social distance between the patient and the therapist, popular concepts of rebirth and fatalism, and guilt attributed to misdeeds in past life. In the Eastern model, the therapist often takes a more active role than the conventional Western models.

Some of the concepts as discussed above may not be as relevant currently as in the past due to globalization, increasing levels of education, and advances in information technology, but are used to a varying degree by the Indian psychiatrists in clinical practice.

CONTRIBUTIONS BY THE INDIAN ASSOCIATION FOR SOCIAL PSYCHIATRY

The IASP has made significant contributions to the growth of social psychiatry in India. IASP started in 1984 with objectives of studying the nature of man and his cultures, prevention and treatment of his vicissitudes and behavior disorders, promoting national and international collaboration among professionals and societies in fields related to social psychiatry, making the knowledge and practice of social psychiatry available to professionals in mental health and other sciences, and to the public by such methods as scientific meetings and publications, and to advance the physical, social, psychological and philosophic well-being of mankind by such methods as promotion of research and deliberations into it. The association had a very dynamic and able giant leadership of stalwarts like Professor A. Venkoba Rao, Professor V.K. Varma, Professor SM Channabasavanna, Professor Shridhar Sharma, Professor BB Sethi, and Dr MAM Khan. IASP also started its own publication, the Indian Journal of Social Psychiatry in 1986, which is now in its 4th decade of publication. IASP holds its national conferences every year and has also hosted the World Congress of Social Psychiatry in India in 1992 and 2016. India had also hosted the 2001 World Association of Social Psychiatry (WASP) Congress under the leadership of Professor Shridhar Sharma, the then President of the WASP. The current president of the WASP is also an Indian, Professor Roy Abraham Kallivayalil.

SOCIAL PSYCHIATRY INITIATIVES AT THE LEVEL OF THE STATE

Following independence from the British, a gradual expansion in mental health services took place in India as a part of general health services. Starting from the 1980s, a number of reforms were initiated, along with the NMHP of India, launched in 1982 (Nizamie & Goyal, 2010). Certain developments occurred as a part of initiatives by the voluntary sector and a few as judicial initiatives (discussed in the next section). Recently in 2014, India declared its Mental Health Policy (MHP) (National Mental Health Policy of India, 2014). NMHP and MHP are important initiatives by the Government of India promoting many of the public health components of social psychiatry.

The NMHP of India had the objectives of ensuring availability and accessibility of minimum mental health care for all the population in the foreseeable future, especially to the most vulnerable and underprivileged sections; encouraging the application of mental health knowledge in general healthcare and in social development; promoting community participation in the mental health service development and to stimulate efforts toward self-help in the community (Nizamie & Goyal, 2010). Though the program was started with great hopes, it could not make much progress in the initial years due to various reasons (Kapur, 2004).

The focus in DMHP has been on early detection and treatment, training of manpower and raising public awareness about the mental disorders. Mental health services were developed at the district level and also at peripheries to make them easily accessible to the community. Training component has included imparting short-term training to the medical officers in diagnosis and treatment of common mental illnesses, and training of the health workers in identifying persons with mental illness and raising community awareness. Public awareness programs are undertaken periodically in the form of information, education, and communication (IEC) activities. Till date, the program has covered about one-third of the districts across the country (R. S. Murthy, 2010).

One of the important features of the NMHP of India was the integration of mental health in general health, which was achieved by setting up of mental health services in the primary care settings, and training the primary care physicians and health workers in the delivery of mental health services. The NMHP also aims at making mental health services accessible to all, especially those in need of it, and includes community participation in the development and expansion of mental health care services (Kapur, 2004; Nizamie & Goyal, 2010; Chadda, 2012).

The MHP of India, which was launched on 10th October 2014 on the occasion of the World Mental Health Day is an important development in the history of social psychiatry in India. The policy aims at providing universal access to mental health care, increasing access to and utilization of comprehensive mental health services, and reducing prevalence and impact of risk factors associated with mental health problems. The policy has the vision to promote mental health, prevent mental illness, enable recovery from mental illness, promote destigmatization and integration of the persons with mental illness, and ensure socioeconomic inclusion of persons with mental illness by providing accessible, affordable and quality health and social care to all persons throughout their lifespan. It emphasizes on the principles of equity, justice, integrated care, evidence-based quality care, and following a participatory and rights-based approach in all training and teaching programs. (National Mental Health Policy of India, 2014).

There have also been some more noticeable developments in social psychiatry related to the welfare of the persons with mental illness in form of policy perspective. Mental illness was included for the first time in the list of illnesses eligible for disability benefits in the Rights of Persons with Disabilities Act, 1995. Subsequently, a number of benefits for the disabled were introduced in many states of India, including disability pension and reservation in jobs for the disabled. However, due to procedural difficulties, inadequate resources for implementation and lack of awareness in the general population, the Act could not achieve the expected results, especially for the persons with mental illness. The Act has been revised and improved to make it more facilitatory. The new Rights of Persons with Disabilities Act, 2016 has a broadened definition of mental illness for the purpose of availing the disability benefits. These reforms can be considered the beginnings, and the steps are likely to bring some relief to the disabled persons and their caregivers.

Persons with mental illness in India do not have access to medical insurance unlike most of the developed world. Various insurance companies offering health insurance have put mental illness under "general exclusions" (suicide, self-inflicted injury or illness, mental disorder, anxiety, stress or depression, use of alcohol or drugs are the categories excluded). Mental Health Care Act (MHCA), 2017 attempts to rectify this deficiency. The MHCA has included a section stating that the Insurance Regulatory Development Authority established under the Insurance Regulatory Development Authority Act, 1999 shall endeavor to ensure that all insurers make provisions for medical insurance for treatment of mental illness on the same basis as is available for treatment of physical illness (Mental Health Care Act, 2017).

INITIATIVES FROM THE JUDICIARY TOWARD IMPROVEMENT OF MENTAL HEALTH CARE

Indian judicial system and the National Human Rights Commission (NHRC) of India, have taken a number of initiatives toward the improvement of the mental health care facilities especially the mental hospitals as well as toward protection of the rights of persons with mental illness. The judiciary and the NHRC took cognizance following reports of failure of the state to take adequate measures in this direction.

In the 1980s, reports had started appearing in the media about the persons with mental illness being kept in prisons and overstaying in mental hospitals by many years following improvement. There were also reports of cases of normal persons being admitted to mental hospitals after being declared as mentally ill, and under trials with mental illness being kept in jails for long periods without trial in some of the states. It also came to notice that some prisoners who were insane at the time of initial trial but improved subsequently, continued to be in the jail even up to 20–30 years due to inaction on the part of the state authorities. In some states like West Bengal, non-criminal mentally ill persons were being kept in jails. There were a set of public interest litigations (PILs) filed in the Supreme Court of India about these practices and also cases were filed against the state government in the High Courts (Sharma & Chadda, 1996; Channabasavanna & Murthy, 2004; Dhanda et al., 2004; Murthy & Nagaraja, 2008).

These instances led to interventions from the Supreme Court of India. Enquiries revealed lack of effective mental health services in jails for the mentally ill prisoners. The Court in its judgment said that the practice of keeping non-criminal mentally ill persons in prisons was unconstitutional and directed the state governments to get all such persons to be examined by psychiatrists and sent to the nearest place of treatment. Further, a number of historical judgments from the Supreme Court of India were instrumental in many reforms in a number of state mental hospitals including those at Shahdara, Agra, Ranchi, and Gwalior. A number of these hospitals have been developed as postgraduate training centers in various mental health disciplines.

Erwadi tragedy of August 2001, in which 26 patients with mental illness, kept in chains in a thatched shed in a dargah in Tamil Nadu (a state in South India), were charred to death in a fire, can be called a black spot in the Indian Psychiatry. But the event brought a lot of social awakening and judicial initiatives. The Supreme Court of India took *suo moto* notice of the event in response to a PIL and issued legal notices to the state of Tamil Nadu and the Union of India. The Court also directed the Union of India to conduct a countrywide survey to map all the mental health facilities, an estimate of all kinds of mental health resources, and the state of care provided in mental health care services. The Court also directed the governments of the states to open mental hospitals, if they did not have one (Murthy & Nagaraja, 2008).

The NHRC of India also keeps a watch of human rights violations of the mentally ill persons and takes suitable action. NHRC has also conducted periodic surveys of various mental hospitals of India since the late 1990s and has made recommendations to the Central and State Governments to take reformatory steps (Channabasavanna & Murthy, 2004; Murthy & Sekar, 2008).

Another important mental health reformatory step which occurred on judicial interventions was the decriminalization of suicide attempt, which had been a great disgrace in the Indian law till recently. The process to decriminalize was initiated by a judgment from the Delhi High Court way back in 1994, but it took more than 20 years of efforts from different sectors to bring a change in the law.

CONCLUSION

India has many significant contributions to social psychiatry, which include application of ancient Indian concepts in mental health promotion and management of mental health problems, community care of persons with mental illness, involvement of families in management of persons with mental illness, community mental health programs, involvement of judiciary in mental health reforms, and also in promoting social psychiatry as a subspecialty of psychiatry.

REFERENCES

Apte JS. Dr NS Vahia (1916–2007). Indian J Psychiatry. 2010;52:205-8.
Avasthi A, Kate N, Grover S. Indianization of psychiatry utilizing indian mental concepts. Indian J Psychiatry. 2013;55(Suppl 2):S136-44.

Banerjee G. First psychiatric clinic in a general hospital in india. Mental Health Rev. 2001;52-5.

Behere P, Das A, Yadav R, et al. Ayurvedic concepts related to psychotherapy. Indian J Psychiatry. 2013;55(6):310.

Bhatia SC, Madabushi J, Kolli V, et al. The Bhagawad Gita and contemporary psychotherapies. Indian J Psychiatry. 2013;55(Suppl.):S315-21.

Bhore J. Health Survey and Development Committee. Government of India, 1946.

Chadda R. Six decades of community psychiatry in india. Int Psychiatry. 2012;9:45-7.

Chadda R, Agarwal V, Singh MC, et al. Help seeking behaviour of psychiatric patients before seeking care at a mental hospital. Int J Soc Psychiatry. 2001;47(4):71-8.

Chadda R, Deb KS. Indian family systems, collectivistic society and psychotherapy. Indian J Psychiatry. 2013;55(6):299.

Channabasavanna SM, Murthy P. The National Human Rights Commission Report 1999: a defining moment. In: Agarwal SP, Goel DS, Salhan RN, Ichhpujani RL, Shrivastava S (Eds). Mental Health: An Indian Perspective (1946–2003). New Delhi: Directorate General of Health Services, Ministry of Health and Family Welfare, Government of India/Elsevier; 2004. pp. 108-12.

Chavan BS, Arun P. Treatment of alcohol and drug abuse in camp setting. Indian J Psychiatry. 1999;41(2):140-4.

Choudary S. Lt Colonel Jal E Dhunjibhoy (1911–1980). Indian J Psychiatry. 2010;52(6):52-141.

Dhanda A, Goel DS, Chadda RK. Law and mental health: common concerns and varied perspectives. In: Agarwal SP, Goel DS, Salhan RN, Ichhpujani RL, Shrivastava S (Eds). Mental Health: An Indian Perspective (1946–2003). New Delhi: Directorate General of Health Services, Ministry of Health and Family Welfare, Government of India/Elsevier; 2004. pp. 170-85.

Dwivedi D, Kumari S, Nagendra HR. Effect of yoga practices in reducing counterproductive work behavior and its predictors. Indian J Psychiatry. 2016;58(2):216-9.

Gangadhar BN, Naveen GH, Rao MG, et al. Positive antidepressant effects of generic yoga in depressive out-patients: a comparative study. Indian Journal of Psychiatry 2013; 55(Suppl-3):369–73

Gururaj G, Varghese M, Benegal V, et al: National Mental Health Survey of India 2015–16. NIMHANS: Bengaluru, 2016.

Hoch E. Process in instant cure. In: Kapur M, Murthy VN, Sathyawathi K, Kapur RL (Eds). Psychotherapeutic Processes. Bangalore: NIMHANS. 1979. pp. 45-69.

Isaac MK, Kapur RL, Chandrashekar CR, et al. Mental health delivery through rural primary care-development and evaluation of a training programme. Indian J Psychiatry. 1982;24(2):131-8.

Kapur RL. The story of community mental health in India. In: Agarwal S, Goel D, Salhan R, Ichhpujani R, Shrivastava S (Eds). Mental Health: An Indian Perspective (1946–2003). New Delhi: Directorate General of Health Services, Ministry of Health and Family Welfare, Government of India/Elsevier; 2004. pp. 92-100.

Khalsa SBS. Yoga for psychiatry and mental health: an ancient practice with modern relevance. Indian J Psychiatry. 2013; 55(Suppl 3):334-6.

Manickam LSS. Psychotherapy in India. Indian J Psychiatry. 2010;52(Suppl 1):S366-70.

Mental Health Care Act: Ministry of Law & Justice, Government of India, 2017.

Mishra N, Nagpal S, Chadda RK, et al. Help-seeking behavior of patients with mental health problems visiting a tertiary care center in north India. Indian J Psychiatry. 2011;53(3):234-8.

Murthy P, Nagaraja D. Judicial interventions and NHRC initiatives in mental health care. In: Nagaraja D, Murthy P (Eds). Mental Health Care and Human Rights. New Delhi: National Human Rights Commission; 2008. pp. 69-84.

Murthy P, Sekar K. A decade after the NHRC quality assurance initiative: current status of government psychiatric hospitals in India. In: Nagaraja D, Murthy P (Eds). Mental Health Care and Human Rights. New Delhi: National Human Rights Commission; 2008. pp. 101-42.

Murthy RS. From local to global-contributions of Indian psychiatry to international psychiatry. Indian J Psychiatry. 2010;52(Suppl 1):S30-7.

National Mental Health Policy of India. Ministry of Health and Family Welfare, Government of India, 2014.

Neki JS. Guru-chela relationship: the possibility of a therapeutic paradigm. Am J Orthopsychiatry. 1973;43(5):755-66.

Neki JS. Psychotherapy in India. Indian J Psychiatry. 1977;19(2):1-10.

Nizamie S, Goyal N. National Mental Health Programme of India a reappraisal. In: Indian Journal of Social Psychiatry. New Delhi: Ministry of Health and Family Welfare, Government of India; 2010.

Paikkatt B, Singh A, Singh P, et al. Efficacy of yoga therapy for the management of psychopathology of patients having chronic schizophrenia. Indian J Psychiatry. 2015;57(4):355.

Raj L, Chavan BS, Bala C. Community "de-addiction" camps: a follow-up study. Indian J Psychiatry. 2005;47:44-7.

Ranganathan S. The Manjakkudi experience: a camp approach towards treating alcoholics. Addiction. 1994;89(9):1071-5.

Sagar V. Challenge of our times. Indian J Psychiatry. 1973;15:95-103.

Satyanand D. A comparative study of scientific and religious psychotherapy with a special study of the role of the commonest shivite symbolic model in total psychoanalysis. Indian J Psychiatry. 1961;3:261-73.

Sharma SD, Chadda RK. Mental Hospitals in India: Current Status and Role in Mental Health Care Delhi: Institute of Human Behaviour & Allied Sciences; 1996.

Surya NC, Jayaram SS. Some basic considerations in the practice of psychotherapy in the Indian setting. Indian J Psychiatry. 1968;4:153-6.

Thirunavukarasu M, Thirunavukarasu P. Training and national deficit of psychiatrists in India—a critical analysis. Indian J Psychiatry. 2010;52:83-8.

Vahia N, Doongaji D. Further experience with the therapy based upon concepts of Patanjali in the treatment of psychiatric disorders. Indian J Psychiatry. 1973;15:32-7.

Varma VK. Present state of psychotherapy in India. Indian J Psychiatry. 1982;24(3):209-26.

Wig NN. Hanuman complex and its resolution: an illustration of psychotherapy from Indian mythology. Indian J Psychiatry. 2004;46:25-8.

Wig NN, Avasthi A. Origin and growth of general hospital psychiatry. In: Agarwal SP, Goel DS, Salhan RN, Ichhpujani RL, Shrivastava S (Eds). Mental Health: An Indian Perspective (1946–2003). New Delhi: Directorate General of Health Services, Ministry of Health and Family Welfare, Government of India/Elsevier; 2004. pp. 101-7.

Wig NN, Murthy RS, Harding TW. A model for rural psychiatric services-Raipur Rani experience. Indian J Psychiatry. 1981;23(4):275-90.

Basics of Social Psychiatry

Chapter 5

Concept of Social Psychiatry

Rakesh K Chadda, Nishtha Chawla, Siddharth Sarkar

SUMMARY

Social psychiatry is a subspecialty of psychiatry which studies social factors affecting psychiatric morbidity, and vice versa. Its domain includes psychosocial issues affecting mental health and social approaches to psychiatric care. Historically, social psychiatry has important contributions to understanding the etiopathogenesis and management of psychiatric disorders. Today, with the adoption of biopsychosocial approaches for explanation and management of psychiatric disorders, social psychiatry holds a strategically important position in contemporary psychiatry, though it has not received its due recognition. It is a known fact that many patients with severe mental illnesses continue to remain nonfunctional despite adequate control of their symptoms with psychotropic medications. This is where psychosocial approaches play an important role, if not more, in integrating the person back into the society. In this chapter, authors have attempted to explain the concept and evolution of social psychiatry. Authors touch upon the interplay between social factors and mental health and its role in treatment of mental disorder. A brief discussion has been made on how the clinical presentation of psychiatric disorders varies with social factors like culture and ethnicity, and what role does the society play in treatment of psychiatric illnesses. Finally, the chapter discusses briefly about what society harnesses for prevention of mental illness.

DEFINITION AND EVOLUTION OF SOCIAL PSYCHIATRY

The relationship between psychiatry and social sciences has been identified since ages. With the advances in science and medicine, social aspects of health, especially its role in outcome, are often ignored by the modern medicine except the public health professionals. The branch of medical sociology originated with the efforts of social scientists, who studied various aspects of human life. Over the period, the concept of social sciences has got incorporated into the branch of psychiatry like no other branch (Krupinski, 1992).

Social psychiatry is a subspeciality of psychiatry which deals with social factors associated with psychiatric morbidity, social effects of mental illness, psychosocial issues, and social approaches to psychiatric care. Its domain includes studying social factors affecting psychiatric illness and psychiatric illness affecting the social factors (Krupinski, 1992). Various authors have tried to define social psychiatry and link psychiatric illnesses to social factors. It has been conceptualized by different authors in varying ways.

Differences in Perspectives on Social Psychiatry

According to Ruesch (1961), social psychiatry has existed, since training started in psychiatry in medical schools. In a comprehensive review, Ruesch (1965) described psychiatry as developing in three distinct directions: psychological, biological, and social. The psychological development included studies of thinking, feeling or dreaming, and understanding a person's total experience. The biological psychiatry, getting impetus from developments in electronics, biochemistry, and pharmacology, progressed beyond the studies of central nervous system to the study of organism as whole as in studies of sleep, food, and sensory deprivation. Social psychiatry, the third development, focused on the structure of community, the significance of the group for the individual and the mechanics of communication. Arthur, who has written extensively on social psychiatry, with a book on social psychiatry to his credit, describes social psychiatry as the study of the role of social phenomena in genesis and manifestations of mental and physical illness, and application of social factors in treatment of mental and emotional disturbances (Arthur, 1971, 1973). Social psychiatry may not look into the cause of illness per se, but describes the pattern of behavior and distress, and how much disturbance it causes to the person and to others (Leighton, 1966).

Ciompi (1994) defines social psychiatry as "the domain of psychiatry which tries to understand and treat psychiatric disturbances in close relation with their social environment". The focus of social psychiatry remains in the community which includes community itself and institutions like daycare centers, halfway homes, rehabilitation centers and therapeutic communities. The specific institutions are meant for those patients who are suffering from moderate to less severe psychiatric illness and for whom continuous hospitalization is not indicated. These patients, however, have a continued need for clinical care and attention of the psychiatrist as they are the lost resources of the community which are recoverable (Ciompi, 1994). To further expand upon it, a broader concept of social psychiatry would include social environment and effects of environment on mental condition, social treatments and social epidemiology.

Social environment of an individual which impacts the mental health as well as the presentation of mental illness, may be as extensive as the whole society, but can be narrowed down to as less as a dyadic relationship like a patient of depression and his/her spouse or a patient of schizophrenia and his/her elderly parents, or for that matter patient and the therapist. All of these are examples of different social relationships affecting the psychiatric illness (Brown et al., 1986). Social breakdown syndrome is an example of malfunctioning environment leading to a pathological condition, characterized by hostility, withdrawal or both. The syndrome is postulated to occur as a result of prolonged hospitalization, seen in background of psychiatric illnesses like schizophrenia, depression, etc. The condition is often associated with severe deterioration, and is largely resistant to therapy, but improves with change in the social environment (Wing & Brown, 1970).

Going back to the early history of psychiatry, moral treatment in psychiatry, initiated by Pinel and his contemporaries, was a form of social treatment, and was used as a measure to prevent social breakdown syndrome. Occupational therapy is also a form of social treatment. The overall purpose of any kind of social treatment has been to reintegrate the person into the "society". As psychiatrists entered more into the dynamics of mental disorder, feeling capable of dealing with patients not only in the hospital but also in the community, social psychiatry showed important developments during mid -20th century, with its concept becoming crystallized with the apparent success of social treatments (Krapf, 1960). Many of these treatments remain relevant in the current context.

According to many authors, psychiatric epidemiology makes a major contribution to social psychiatry. It includes not only measuring the prevalence and incidence but also the differential distribution of mental disorders across different populations/situations and looks into the reason for the same (Pepper & Redlich, 1962; Ransom & Arthur, 1973). Ransom & Arthur (1973) suggested social factors as playing an important role in determining the differential distribution across social classes and variations in treatment provided to different classes. They also included the concept of community psychiatry, sociotherapy, and transcultural psychiatry under the broad rubric of social psychiatry.

Since the science of sociology, social psychiatry, and anthropology share some common features, a number of definitions of social psychiatry are extrapolated from the definitions provided by anthropologists and sociologists. Kirmayer and colleagues opine that the anthropological model for explanation of psychiatric illness emphasizes the cultural shaping of an individual to play an important role in their efforts to give a meaning to their symptoms (Kirmayer et al., 1994).

Rutz (2006) expands the domain of social psychiatry to include raising awareness about various dynamic and regressive mechanisms in the background of development of psychopathology in an individual or groups, and expanding on to the society. Thus, the function of social psychiatry includes analysing effects of societal changes, political decisions, and policy implementations on public and mental health.

Despite the differences in the views of different authors, there is a consensus that social psychiatry deals with the social factors affecting the onset, course, and outcome of the illness, social effects of psychiatric illnesses and social approaches to prevention, treatment, and rehabilitation of psychiatrically ill patients (Dunham, 1959; Caplan, 1964; Leff, 2010; Chadda, 2013).

From Psychobiological to Biopsychosocial Approach

While the historical evolution of social psychiatry as an essential branch of psychiatry, especially in the post-world war II era, is discussed in a separate chapter, this section briefly talks about the introduction of psychobiological approach by Adolf Meyer which later evolved into a biopsychosocial model by George Engel.

Adolf Meyer made a significant contribution toward the formation of "new psychiatry". In the era where all illnesses were explained with the help of "medical model", Meyer emphasized on the importance of including subjective experiences and social behavior of a person suffering from mental illness. He stated with confidence in one of his orations in a congress in 1913, *"Psychiatry deals with the social organ of man"*. He implied that the branch of medicine should deal not only with pathology and treatment of the body organs but with the adaptation of individual as a whole with the society. He conceptualized "social adaptation" as a biological function. Although Meyer's conceptualization faced criticism, it eventually contributed to the development of clinical skills in "new psychiatry" for the 20th century psychiatrists (Lamb, 2015).

Further evolution in the concept of explaining psychiatric illnesses came when certain authors tried to explain their origin through the model of "biopsychosocial" approach. While George Engel (1977) is often credited for the concept, the term "biopsychosocial" was actually coined two decades earlier by Roy Grinker (1954), a psychiatrist and neurologist, in his efforts to emphasize on the biological roots to psychiatric illnesses in the era of Freudian ideology. Engel applied the psychosocial approach into the branch of medicine as a whole, and focused upon the behavioral, social, and psychological dimensions of medical illness (Engel, 1977; Ghaemi, 2009).

Today, we live in the era of biopsychosocial approach to psychiatric illness. However, recent research has stressed more upon biological psychiatry. Hence, the field of social psychiatry has received less attention. Nonetheless, social psychiatry is an important contributor to the understanding of etiology of mental illnesses and effective management of psychiatric disorders.

MODELS OF SOCIAL PSYCHIATRY

Models of social psychiatry draw on patients' personal and social resources in their treatment. They are, hence, often termed as "resource-oriented therapeutic model". The purpose of these models is to ameliorate a patient's dysfunction and improve quality of life. Priebe and colleagues (2014) explain various models for therapy, based on social psychiatry, working on building relationships with the family, friends, their peers or other patients as well as the therapist. Some of the models proposed by the group are discussed as below:

Befriending model: In this model, the volunteers discuss various recreational and social activities with the patient like a friend, using friendship as the resource.

Client-centered therapy model: The therapist provides empathy and unconditional regard to the patient in order to enhance patient's self-efficacy and determination, thus helping improve his functioning and social integration. The patient himself acts as the resource which is encouraged by a supportive therapist.

Positive psychotherapy: Positive psychotherapy encourages inculcation of positive cognitions, behavior and emotions in an individual in contrast to ameliorating agony or correcting cognitions, thus differing in basic concept from the cognitive behavior therapy. It helps achieve positive mental health and not merely treat mental illnesses. A patient is made self-sufficient and self-efficacious by encouraging positive change in him/her.

Self-help groups: Patients with similar problems come together to share their experiences, e.g. alcoholics anonymous. This enables them to understand that they are not the sole sufferers and helps them to get the confidence and second-hand experience to reintegrate with the society.

Systematic family therapy: Family is one of the most invaluable resources that an individual can harbor. Mobilizing family resources through a systematic therapy helps the patient positively.

Therapeutic community: Therapeutic community is an effort to build a community within an institution, where the patients and the staff members work together to maintain the institution. In this way, the resources of the patients are used by the patients for themselves.

Marriage
Mental Health Spiritual health
Depression Culture Mass media
Epidemiology Farmer suicides Elderly
Globalization   Comorbidity

Social psychiatry
Legislation   Group therapy   Stigma
Rehabilitation Positive mental health
Migration   Child and adolescent
Psychopathology
Social support Biopsychosocial
Family

Figure 1: Domains of Social Psychiatry.

The models as discussed above are based on few important themes like building up of social relationships, sharing of experiences with peers and other patients, enabling them to understand their own strengths, and encouraging decision-making abilities and involvement in various recreational activities which will help in their stimulation, inculcating positive and self-correcting behaviors and emotions (Priebe et al., 2014). **Figure 1** summarizes the domains of social psychiatry.

INTERACTION OF SOCIETY WITH PSYCHIATRIC ILLNESS AND TREATMENT

While the association between mental illness and society is two-way, the impact may also be in both positive as well as negative direction. For example, families getting involved in their patients' treatment may be a reason for improved compliance as well as better stimulation and support, but if the expressed emotions outweigh the support, it may prove detrimental. On the other side, caregivers may feel self-efficacious and responsible in seeking treatment for their wards, but may also become a victim of caregiver burnout and become burdened ignoring their own health and needs. In this section, we briefly describe some of the factors which have been shown to have significant impact on the genesis of mental illness, its clinical presentation and treatment, and effect on the society **(Flowchart 1).**

Flowchart 1: Interaction of society, mental illness and its treatment.

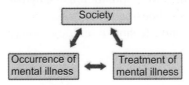

How Does Society Affect Occurrence of Psychiatric Illness?

In contrast to the declining trend in the prevalence and mortality associated with communicable diseases, the prevalence and mortality of noncommunicable diseases is seen to be on the rise, with mental disorders being associated with increasing disability and burden. The increasing burden due to mental disorders has taken place despite having achieved many advances in effective treatments. Multiple factors contribute to this difference between the need and actual treatment provision and barriers to treatment (Kessler et al., 2005; Murphy et al., 2000).

Stigma

If an individual seeks treatment, he/she gets labeled with a psychiatric diagnosis for life. Stigma is faced by the patients of psychiatric illness in all spheres of life like marriage, employment, job, housing, etc. (Wig, 1997). Mass media also plays a significant role by portraying psychiatric illness as well as psychiatric treatment in a negative light (Andrade et al., 2010). The National Mental Health Programme (NMHP) of India was formulated to make mental health care accessible to people, integrated into the primary health care and general health care, which would eventually help in allaying the stigma associated with mental illness. However, many challenges are ahead of it before it gets implemented fully in India.

Social Class

Similar to what is seen in physical illnesses, an inverse relationship exists between socioeconomic status and psychiatric illness. Two kinds of hypothesis are based on social class theories: social causation hypothesis and social drift hypothesis. Social causation hypothesis states that the incidence and prevalence of psychiatric illnesses are more in lower socioeconomic strata because of various social adversities, e.g. poverty, unemployment, homelessness, and single motherhood. Social drift hypothesis, on the other hand, states that psychiatric illnesses have genetic predisposition irrespective of the original socioeconomic class, and those who become mentally ill, are unable to maintain in their social status, get marginalized, thus drifting down to lower strata of the society (Cooper, 2005; Wadsworth & Achenbach, 2005). The phenomenon is discussed in more detail in one of the preceding chapters.

Migration

Migration is associated with increased risk to develop schizophrenia, depression, anxiety disorders, and other psychiatric illnesses. One of the most important hypotheses postulated is the losses experienced by the migrant population leading to significant stress, which in turn leads to the development of psychiatric illness (Das-Munshi et al., 2012). Various contributing factors have been studied in migrant population like language barrier, legal status concerns, culture shock, racial difficulties, housing difficulties, and isolation. These factors lead to a feeling of lowered self-esteem and a feeling of self-dejection (van Os et al., 2010).

Urbanization

Varma and colleagues (1997) showed that the outcome of non-affective psychoses is favorable in rural as compared to urban area (Varma et al., 1997). Urbanization has been linked to various psychiatric conditions ranging from common psychiatric illnesses like substance use disorders, depression, and psychosis to other deviances like delinquency, vandalism, family disintegration, and alienation. Causes could include overcrowding, unemployment, air pollution, social alienation, increased crime, low vitamin D levels, ethnic differences, deprivations, and migration (Kelly et al., 2010; Padhy et al., 2014).

Role of Families and Expressed Emotions

While mental illness causes caregiver burden, caregivers also impact the course and outcome of the illness through various means, e.g. "expressed emotions". While family members have different ways of coping with the burden of caregiving, they also show different reactions to their wards' illness (Chadda et al., 2007; Chadda, 2014; Wig et al., 1987). This has primarily been studied in the context of schizophrenia. There has been a change in perception of relationship between families and psychiatric illness over the last 1 century. In the first half of 20th century, family pathology and upbringing was considered to play an important role in development for mental illness. Experiments of Dr Vidya Sagar in Amritsar in India involving families in care of persons with mental illness brought out the positive role of families in mental health care. In many countries, especially in Asia and Africa, families play an important role in taking care of their wards with mental illness (Bergner et al., 2008). This is especially more so in collectivistic societies like India where family plays an integral role in treatment process (Chadda & Deb, 2013).

Culture

Culture is defined as *"that complex whole which includes knowledge, belief, art, law, morals, customs and any other capabilities and habits acquired by man as a member of society"* (Bhugra & Gupta, 2010). Culture, thus, plays an important influence in the genesis of psychopathology. It may determine the form of psychopathology (e.g. culture bound syndromes), as well the content of psychopathology (changing content of delusions with development of science and fiction). It also influences the frequency of occurrence of disorders (e.g. anorexia nervosa being more common in societies where thinness is idealized) (Tseng, 2007). Ethnicity and culture determine an individual's response to treatment apart from the relationship between the therapist and the patient. The perceived efficacy may vary with dietary habits, smoking, expectations, and a person's belief in a complementary system of medication (Ng et al., 2008).

Positive Impact of Society on Mental Health

Society, though, responsible for the prevailing stigma to mental disorders, also plays an extremely useful role in the treatment of a patient with psychiatric illness. Resources in form of family, peers, and friends play an important role in reintegration of the individual into the society. The society contributes to the stresses related to migration and urbanisation, which affect mental health. At the same time, it is also responsible for creating formal and informal support systems of mental health in the community.

How Do Social Factors Affect Clinical Presentation in Psychiatric Illness?

Psychiatry studies human behavior which is more complex than different organ systems, and lacks any stable biomarker. The grading of symptoms is based on self-report by the patient. The diagnosis is not aided with the help of various signs and investigations. For example, diagnosis of schizophrenia is made when a person explicitly reports hearing "voices" or harbors false and often implausible beliefs. Even if a person behaves in a bizarre way or appears talking and smiling to himself/herself, a diagnosis of schizophrenia can not be confirmed. So, psychiatric diagnoses are constrained in a lot of subjectivity.

A prominent disorder with which multiple patients present especially in the non-Western countries is the somatization disorder, where multiple somatic complaints are presented with no findings on physical investigation. While the symptoms are associated with substantial amount of distress, these respond poorly to pharmacological treatment. Various studies in the literature have shown that somatic symptoms are exaggerated in Asians as compared to Caucasians, and the severity of the symptoms is proportional to the severity of distress (Saint Arnault & Kim, 2008). However, majority of patients are unable to acknowledge any relationship between their physical symptoms and their stress (Simon et al., 1999). Somatic symptoms also accompany depression very commonly, important ones being: gastric upset, abdominal complaints, aches and pains, weakness and palpitations. It has been postulated that such somatic symptoms may be a result of intrapsychic conflict condensing into somatic symptoms, or a way of expression of individual's discontent with the society (Kirmayer & Young, 1998).

DSM-5 has introduced a new term called the "cultural concept of distress", which refers to differences in the way individuals in certain groups understand, perceive and express their problems, symptoms, troubling thoughts, and difficult emotions (American Psychiatric Association, 2013). According to DSM-5, "all forms of distress are locally shaped, including the DSM disorders". The similar concept is proposed by some authors in defining the term, "idioms of distress" which are the culture specific expressions of suffering (Saint Arnault & Kim, 2008).

How Do Mental Illnesses Affect the Society?

Mental illness impacts the society by taking away its individuals' most productive years of life. Social epidemiology includes not only measuring the prevalence of various disorders across different societies (e.g. developed and developing countries or different ethnic groups) but also measuring the costs of psychiatric illnesses, both financial burden, and societal cost. Societal costs include burden of individuals with psychiatric illnesses on the society by failure to attain higher education, unemployment, early marriages, early separations due to marital instability, single motherhood, and various other social and economic difficulties (Kessler et al., 1998).

As expected, the illness with early age of onset which runs a chronic course has the maximum cost to the individual, his/her family as well as the society, as the individual loses the most productive years of one's life. It is, however, difficult to establish a causal association between the two with the findings available in the current literature, and hence difficult to conclude that early treatment of the psychiatric disorders will prove to be beneficial in this regard (Kessler et al., 2007). Some studies have been carried out in the western countries to measure the short-term cost incurred in the treatment of psychiatric illness, for example, money spent on medications, and loss of work by the individuals, which could have translated into earning. Studies have shown considerable cost being spent on common mental illnesses like anxiety disorders and depression (Greenberg & Birnbaum, 2005). As compared to physical illnesses, the amount of money spent on treatment, the amount of disability and the loss of work were found to be higher for mental disorders (Ormel et al., 2008).

How Do Social Factors Interact with the Treatment and Outcome of Mental Illness?

Social factors also play an important role in outcome of mental illness. Since etiology of mental disorders is multifactorial, treatment also has to take into consideration of the biopsychosocial factors. In addition, societal attitudes, illness behaviour, belief systems, choice of treatment and pathways to care have an important influence on treatment seeking and outcome of illness. Current research has started to focus on effects of non-pharmacological, psychosocial interventions in psychiatric disorders (Avasthi, 2016). A large number of patients with psychiatric illness and their family members seek non-psychiatric help before they consult a psychiatrist (Chadda et al., 2001). Studies have been done to find out what affects their choice of treatment.

Pathways to Care

Unlike a patient of fever being seen by general physician, or a patient having blurred vision being seen by an ophthalmologist, a patient with psychiatric illness is seen by a variety of persons ranging from general physicians, neurologists, psychologists, alternative medicine practitioners, psychiatrists, traditional faith healers, local religious leaders, and lay counselors (Andrews et al., 2001). The choice depends on the belief of the person about the illness, accessibility, availability, the prevailing belief in the surrounding environment, recommendation by some relative or friend, and the type of health system of the nation. Often they are referred later to a psychiatrist (Chadda et al., 2001; Mishra et al, 2011).

A study done in a tertiary institute in India showed that the psychiatrists were the most common first point of contact for the patients visiting the centre, with psychiatric care not being very expensive. However, around one-third patients did seek help from faith healers during the course of their illness and more than 80% sought treatment from non-psychiatric physicians at some point in time. The most common reason for bringing patients to tertiary center for treatment was lack of satisfactory response from previous treatment followed by being recommended by someone (Mishra et al., 2011).

In view of high percentage of patients with psychiatric illness seeking treatment from non-psychiatric professionals, it calls for integration of psychiatric care into general health care which has also been emphasized in the NMHP of India (Wig & Murthy, 2015).

Principles of Psychosocial Interventions

Psychosocial care needs a dedicated team approach. The multidisciplinary team consists of psychiatrist, psychologist, social worker, occupational therapist, and community psychiatric nurse. Patient and preferably family members also form a part of the treatment team and are given the opportunity to decide their treatment. Another important principle in social approaches to the treatment of psychiatric illnesses is limited reliance on medications. Certain authors postulate that high doses of antipsychotic medications, despite controlling psychotic symptoms, hamper the overall functioning of individuals because of their side effects. Optimal dosage of antipsychotics combined with family-centered approaches to treatment has shown similar outcomes as compared to treatment focusing only on medications like antipsychotics and hospitalization (Ciompi et al., 1992; Lehtinen, 2000).

Social approaches to treatment emphasize on providing social skills training in community settings where the patient is eventually expected to apply his/her skills. It has been seen that community-based settings result in better outcomes as patient has normalized surroundings, and stays in touch with his/her family (Liberman et al., 2002). It has also been stressed upon to reduce coercive treatment like seclusion and physical restraint for the patients with psychiatric illness. Coercive treatments not only make the experience frightening for the patient but also increases stigma in the society (Wadeson & Carpenter, 1976).

Social Factors and Course of Illness

Majority of the studies determining the course of illness have been done on schizophrenia or psychosis which was classically described by Kraepelin as a chronic illness with a downhill natural course. The current literature, however, differs from overtly pessimistic Kraepelinian view and suggests that the course of schizophrenia can be variable depending upon family environment, social support, psychosocial treatment, and life events of an individual (Strauss & Carpenter, 1974; Vaughn & Leff, 1976). Stress diathesis model plays an important role in onset as well as recurrence of the psychotic disorder, suggesting that stress leads to initiation of illness and further relapses in vulnerable individuals. However, limited amounts of stress leads to mobilization of the individual to function better rather than causing him/her to decompensate (Breier & Strauss, 1983). Following the stress vulnerability model, the interactive developmental model was proposed which postulates that development of humans occurs over time, i.e. vulnerability changes over time, and interaction occurs between developing humans and environment (Kessler, 1994; Strauss & Carpenter, 1974).

WHO's ten country study on determinants of outcome of severe mental disorders showed a better course of schizophrenia in developing countries as compared to developed countries, hypothesizing a role of genetics as well as environmental differences (Jablensky et al., 1992). The course of psychiatric disorders is hypothesized to vary according to the genetic make-up as well as environmental conditions. Social factors have been suggested to have a considerable role in determining the outcome in these studies. Family and cultural attributes may thus matter significantly in the manner in which psychiatric illnesses progresses and recovery ensues.

HARNESSING SOCIAL FACTORS IN PREVENTION OF PSYCHIATRIC ILLNESS

Apart from treatment of those with psychiatric illness, the focus has also been upon preventive strategies for psychiatric disorders. With the advent of crisis intervention, removing or at least reducing social risk factors, and reintegrating the mentally ill into the society, social psychiatry is now becoming synonymous with preventive psychiatry (Uchtenhagen, 2008).

Certain countries in Europe, especially the East European states belonging to the former Soviet Union and the Central Europe have undergone many dramatic changes in recent past related to identity, lifespan planning and predictability in life. This kind of societal stress has been identified to lead to a societal "community syndrome", characterised by depression, alcohol use disorder, aggression, risk-taking behaviour, and suicidality. Vulnerable individuals at the time of stress find difficulty in coping, become hopeless and helpless, and are aggressive toward self or others. Majority find difficulty verbalising their distress, often self-stigmatising their own condition (Rutz, 2006).

Various interventions are employed like providing social support, improving individual's coping abilities, detection and management of prodrome or psychosis in early stages in ultra -high-risk population for psychosis, providing social skills training to intellectually disabled population, developing problem solving strategies and skills for working population or adolescents undergoing stressful life situations, deploying self-help groups which help in enhancing one's social networks, nidotherapy (modifying environment), and working on developing natural support systems (Avasthi, 2016). The World Health Report (2001) has provided guidelines on steps to be taken to prevent occurrence of psychiatric illness like educating public, raising awareness, reducing stigma, reintegration of mentally ill into humanized services, and promoting community-based treatment (World Health Organization, 2001).

Suicide is another important concern which has always been a focus of psychiatric management and research, and has received attention from social psychiatry as well. Different strategies have been suggested as well as adopted in different places irrespective of the cultural background for prevention of suicide, for example, suicide crisis interventions in educational institutions, prohibition of sale of toxic agents (including medication which carry risk with overdose), identification and training of gatekeepers, and restriction on publicity about suicides. Many of them are based on the social level which highlights the importance of social psychiatry in addressing the issue of suicides in the community.

CONCLUSION

Social psychiatry is an important branch of psychiatry which is lately becoming the focus of researchers. Psychiatric disorders are a result of interaction between mind and the environment. There are innumerable social factors which affect mental health, and it is required to study each one of them to design better treatment interventions. One also can't discount the need for designing culturally sensitive instruments to have better comparisons of the prevalence of psychiatric disorders across different cultures and regions. One needs to emphasize on psychosocial intervention in clinical practice in order to achieve better outcomes for the patient as well as the society. Preventive psychiatry is another upcoming field of interest which adopts the principles from social psychiatry.

REFERENCES

Andrade C, Shah N, Venkatesh BK. The depiction of electroconvulsive therapy in Hindi cinema. J ECT. 2010;26:16-22.

Andrews G, Issakidis C, Carter G. Shortfall in mental health service utilisation. Br J Psychiatry. 2001;179:417-25.

American Psychiatric Association. Diagnostic and Statistical Manual of Mental Disorders (DSM-5). Arlington: American Psychiatric Association; 2013.

Arthur RJ. An Introduction to Social Psychiatry. London: Penguin Books; 1971.

Arthur RJ. Social psychiatry: An overview. Am J Psychiatry. 1973;130:841-9.

Avasthi A. Are Social theories still relevant in current psychiatric practice? Indian J Soc Psychiatry. 2016;32:3-9.

Bergner E, Leiner AS, Carter T, et al. The period of untreated psychosis before treatment initiation: A qualitative study of family members' perspectives. Compr Psychiatry. 2008;49:530-6.

Bhugra D, Gupta S. Culture and its influence on diagnosis and management. In: Morgan C, Bhugra D (Eds). Principles of Social Psychiatry. London: John Wiley & Sons; 2010. pp. 117-32.

Breier A, Strauss JS. Self-control in psychotic disorders. Arch Gen Psychiatry. 1983;40:1141

Brown GW, Andrews B, Harris T, et al. Social support, self-esteem and depression. Psychol Med. 1986;16:813-31.

Caplan G. Principles of Preventive Psychiatry. England: Oxford;1964.

Chadda RK. Caring for the family caregivers of persons with mental illness. Indian J Psychiatry. 2014;56:221-7.

Chadda RK, Agarwal V, Singh MC, et al. Help seeking behaviour of psychiatric patients before seeking care at a mental hospital. Int J Soc Psychiatry. 2001;47:71-8.

Chadda RK, Deb KS. Indian family systems, collectivistic society and psychotherapy. Indian J Psychiatry. 2013;55:299-309.

Chadda RK, Singh TB, Ganguly KK. Caregiver burden and coping: a prospective study of relationship between burden and coping in caregivers of patients with schizophrenia and bipolar affective disorder. Soc Psychiatry Psychiatr Epidemiol. 2007;42:923-30.

Ciompi L. Social psychiatry today–what is it? Attempt at a clarification. Schweiz Arch Neurol Psychiatr. 1994;145:7-16.

Ciompi L, Dauwalder HP, Maier C, et al. The pilot project "Soteria Berne": Clinical experiences and results. Br J Psychiatry. 1992;161:145-53.

Cooper B. Schizophrenia, social class and immigrant status: the epidemiological evidence. Epidemiol Psychiatr Soc. 2005;14:137-44.

Das-Munshi J, Leavey G, Stansfeld SA, et al. Migration, social mobility and common mental disorders: critical review of the literature and meta-analysis. Ethn Health. 2012;17:17-53.

Dunham H. Sociological Theory and Mental Disorder. Wayne: State University; 1959.

Engel L. The need for a new medical model: a challenge for biomedicine. Science. 1977;196:129-36.

Ghaemi SN. The rise and fall of biopsychosocial model. Br J Psychiatry. 2009;195:3-4.

Gordon RS. An operational classification of disease prevention. Public Health Rep. 1983;98:107-9.

Greenberg PE, Birnbaum HG. The economic burden of depression in the US: societal and patient perspectives. Expert Opin Pharmacother. 2005;6:369-76.

Gururaj G, Varghese M, Benegal V, et al. National Mental Health Survey of India, 2015-16: Summary. Bengaluru: National Institute of Mental Health and Neuro Sciences; 2016.

Jablensky A, Sartorius N, Ernberg G, et al. Schizophrenia: manifestations, incidence and course in different cultures A World Health Organization Ten-Country Study. Psychological Medicine. Monograph Suppl. 1992;20:1.

Kelly BD, O'Callaghan E, Waddington JL, et al. Schizophrenia and the city: A review of literature and prospective study of psychosis and urbanicity in Ireland. Schizophrenia Res. 2010;116(1):75-89.

Kessler R. Lifetime and 12-month prevalence of DSM-III-R psychiatric disorders in the United States. Arch Gen Psychiatry. 1994;51(1):8-19.

Kessler R, Aguilar-Gaxiola S, Alonso J, et al. The global burden of mental disorders: an update from the WHO World Mental Health (WMH) surveys. Epidemiologia E Psichiatria Sociale. 2011;18(1): 23-33.

Kessler R, Amminger GP, Aguilar-Gaxiola S, et al. Age of onset of mental disorders: a review of recent literature. Curr Opin Psychiatr. 2007;20(4):359-64.

Kessler R, Demler O, Frank RG, et al. Prevalence and treatment of mental disorders: 1990 to 2003. N Engl J Med. 2005;352(24):2515-23.

Kessler R, Walters EE, Forthofer MS. The social consequences of psychiatric disorders, III: Probability of marital stability. Am J Psychiatry. 1998;155(8):1092-6.

Kirmayer LJ, Young A. Culture and Somatization: Clinical, epidemiological and ethnographic perspectives. Psychosomat Med. 1998;60(4):420-30.

Kirmayer LJ, Young A, Robbins JM. Symptom attribution in cultural perspective. Canadian J Psychiatry. 1994;39(10):584-95.

Krapf EE. Concept of social psychiatry. Int J Soc Psychiatry. 1960;6(1-2):6-8.

Krupinski J. Social psychiatry and sociology of mental health: A view on their past and future relevance. Aust N Z J Psychiatry. 1992;26(1):91-7.

Lamb S. Social Skills: Adolf Meyer's revision of clinical skill for the New Psychiatry of the twentieth century. Med History. 2015;59(30);443-64.

Lehtinen V. Two-year outcome in first-episode psychosis treated according to an integrated model. Is immediate neuroleptisation always needed? Eur Psychiatry. 2000;15(5):312-20.

Leighton AH. Social psychiatry and the concept of cause. Am J Psychiatry. 1966;122(8):929-30.

Liberman RP, Glynn S, Blair KE, et al. In vivo amplified skills training: Promoting generalization of independent living skills for clients with schizophrenia. Psychiatry. 2002;65(2):137-55.

Mishra N, Nagpal S, Chadda RK, et al. Help-seeking behaviour of patients with mental health problems visiting a tertiary care center in North India. Indian J Psychiatry. 2011;53(3):234-8.

Murphy JM, Laird NM, Monson RR, et al. A 40-year perspective on the prevalence of depression: The Stirling County Study. Arch Gen Psychiatry. 2000;57(3):209-15.

Ng C, Lin K, Singh B, et al. Ethno-psychopharmacology: advances in current practice. Cambridge: Cambridge University Press; 2008.

Ormel J, Petukhova M, Chatterji S, et al. Disability and treatment of specific mental and physical disorders across the world. Br J Psychiatry. 2008;192(5):368-75.

Padhy S, Sarkar S, Davuluri T, et al. Urban living and psychosis–an overview. Asian J Psychiatry. 2014;12:17-22.

Pepper M, Redlich FC. Social psychiatry. Am J Psychiatry. 1962;118:609-12.

Priebe S, Omer S, Giacco D, et al. Resource-oriented therapeutic models in psychiatry: conceptual overview. Br J Psychiatry. 2014;204:256-61.

Ransom J, Arthur MC. Social Psychiatry: An overview. Am J Psychiatry. 1973;130(8):841-9.

Ruesch J. Research and training in social psychiatry. Am Int J Soc Psychiatry. 1961;7:87-96.

Ruesch J. Social Psychiatry: an overview. Arch Gen Psychiatry. 1965;12(5):501-9.

Rutz W. Social psychiatry and public mental health: present situation and future objectives. Time for rethinking and renaissance? Acta Psychiatr Scand. 2006;113:95-100.

Saint Arnault D, Kim O. Is there an Asian idiom of distress? Somatic symptoms in female Japanese and Korean students. Arch Psychiatr Nurs. 2008;22(1):27-38.

Simon GE, VonKorff M, Piccinelli M, et al. An international study of the relation between somatic symptoms and depression. N Engl J Med. 1999;341(18):1329-35.

Sirey J, Bruce ML, Alexopoulos GS, et al. Perceived stigma as a predictor of treatment discontinuation in young and older outpatients with depression. American J Psychiatry. 2001;158(3):479-81.

Strauss JS, Carpenter WT. Characteristic symptoms and outcome in schizophrenia. Arch Gen Psychiatr. 1974;30(4):429.

Tseng W. Culture and psychopathology. In: Bhugra D,Bhui K (Eds). Textbook of Cultural Psychiatry. Cambridge: Cambridge University Press; 2007. pp. 95-112.

Uchtenhagen AA. Which future for social psychiatry? Int Rev Psychiatry. 2008;20(6):535-9.

Van Os J, Kenis G, Rutten BPF. The environment and schizophrenia. Nature. 2010;468(7321):203-12.

Varma VK, Brown AS, Wig NN, et al. Effects of level of socio-economic development on course of non-affective psychosis. Br J Psychiatry. 1997;171:256-9.

Vaughn CE, Leff JP. The influence of family and social factors on the course of psychiatric illness. A comparison of schizophrenic and depressed neurotic patients. Br J Psychiatry. 1976;129(2):125-37.

Wadeson H, Carpenter W. Impact of the seclusion room experience. J Nerv Ment Dis. 1976;163:318-28.

Wadsworth ME, Achenbach TM. Explaining the link between low socioeconomic status and psychopathology: Testing two mechanisms of the social causation Hypothesis. J Consult Clin Psychol. 2005;73(6):1146-53.

Wig NN. Stigma against mental illness. Indian J Psychiatry. 1997;39(3):187-9.

Wig NN, Menon DK, Bedi H, et al. Expressed emotion and schizophrenia in north India. I. Cross-cultural transfer of ratings of relatives' expressed emotion. Br J Psychiatry. 1987;151:156-60.

Wig NN, Murthy RS. The birth of national mental health program for India. Indian J Psychiatry. 2015; 57(3): 315-19.

Wing JK, Brown JW. Institutionalism and schizophrenia: a comparative study of three mental hospitals: 1960–1968. London: Cambridge University; 1970.

World Health Organization. The World Health Report 2001: Mental Health: New Understanding, New Hope. Geneva: WHO; 2001.

Chapter 6

The Individual, the Family and the Society in Relation to Psychiatry

Ajit Avasthi, Abhishek Ghosh, Ashutosh Ratnam

SUMMARY

Mental illnesses are diseases of isolation, cordoning off the individual from the very social life which defines us as human beings. Society and its executive unit, the family can similarly contribute to the genesis, perpetuation and remedy of mental illness. Much has changed in our conceptualizations of this interaction—the "schizophrenia-generating" models of yore have been discarded and family system methodology was devised. The family is today recognized as a system in homeostasis, coming around and reacting to a change in one part (i.e. the illness of one member) in ways which either add to or ameliorate the problem. High expressed emotions can worsen a mental health crisis, the family can deal with the "burden" of caring for a mentally-ill member with varying degrees of failure/success, and corrective recalibrations like family intervention can serve therapeutic roles. Inherent qualitative properties of a family unit can further arm it with specific advantages in such circumstances, e.g. the Indian joint family structure has been accorded much credit for consistently better outcomes, Indian patients with schizophrenia have had. Similarly, the role society had in making and managing of mental illness also required a complete overhaul of earlier understandings and the formulation of a biopsychosocial model. The methodological study of social makeup produced one paramount consistent finding—that low social class is associated with higher incidences of mental illness. Less consistent results emerged when attempts to define society in qualitative terms (social capital) have been made, but it reinforces how social factors (perhaps more than in any other branch of medicine) merit an important place in any discussion on mental illness. Finally, psychological symptoms or disorders and their outcome at the individual level are determined by the tripartite interactions between family, society, and the individual.

INTRODUCTION

Among the most telling and cruel blows a mental illness deals with, is isolation. Uprooting the individual from the consensual realities and social interactions, that normally define human lives, is perhaps the core handicap psychiatric conditions produce. The corollary also holds good—social institutions like the family and the society at large can either aggravate or ameliorate potential damage. In this chapter, we summarize present understandings of the inter-relationships between the individual afflicted with a mental illness, the family he lives in, and the society he is a part of.

THE EMERGENT ROLE OF THE FAMILY IN MENTAL ILLNESS

George Murdock (1965), an American anthropologist, has defined family as a *"social group characterized by common residence, economic cooperation, and reproduction. It includes adults of both sexes, at least two of whom maintain a socially approved sexual relationship, and one or more children, own or adopted, of the sexually cohabiting adults."* He came to this description after studying the workings and constructs of 250 societies of all kinds (hunting-gathering, pastoral, agrarian and industrialized) and finding that all of these societies possessed some form of lineal social unit that met the definition he would frame, making the family the most universal and enduring form of social organization.

Studies of the family in the context of psychiatric disorders have an unflattering history. Parents were formerly blamed for the origin of schizophrenia in their offspring owing to substandard parenting, "double-bind messages" or "schizophrenogenic" mothering. Such early theories of psychosocial etiology were almost entirely concocted from cross-sectional observations of families in which someone already suffered from a major mental illness. Firstly, the pre-existing deficiency was a blurring of the line between correlation (e.g. the family of a patient with schizophrenia had disordered communication mechanisms) and causation (e.g. these disordered communication mechanisms cause schizophrenia) (Miklowitz, 2004). Secondly, they ignored the possibility of these communication dysfunctions being a manifestation of the substantial disease burden of schizophrenia on the involved caretakers (Dixon et al., 2001; Hatfield et al., 1987). Thirdly, these family communication dysfunctions did not seem to have any diagnostic specificity.

Neither do current understandings of this impact see the family as the primary instrument causing a patient's illness, nor do they allow the patient to function as a "scapegoat" for all of the family's covert dysfunctions. Today, the "family systems" approach has come to the fore, with interest now focusing on (a) how the family unit reacts to and organizes itself to contend with episodes of an individual member's psychiatric illness, and (b) how the family's reactions safeguard against or add to the risk of future recurrences (Miklowitz, 2004).

The family systems theory works with certain basic premises:
1. The family is a system which comprises a set of hierarchies, subsystems, and boundaries,
2. This system is predisposed to maintain equilibrium, i.e. *family homeostasis,* and
3. A change in any one family member affects all other members of the family, (an extension of the attribute of family homeostasis) (Fingerman & Bermann, 2000; Mehta et al., 2009).

The concept of *family homeostasis* is borrowed from the physiological principle of homeostasis put forward by Claude Bernard and Cannon (Bernard, 1974; Cannon, 1932). It envisions the family as "an error-activated system which responds to inputs that are not in accordance with its baseline or rules" and understands "homeostasis" as a "system that uses unique processes of compensation to keep the system relatively stable" (Jackson, 1965). This means that destabilizing changes (minor and transient to severe and chronic) to one part of the family system (e.g. the mental health of a member) will cause adaptive responses in other parts. While the family will try to return to its earlier state of equilibrium, in case this proves impossible, it will form a new equilibrium state through homeostatic mechanisms (Goodell & Hanson, 1999). These mechanisms can be both remedial or pathoplastic, and include (among others) scapegoating, formation of defensive alliances or coalitions, release of tension by repetitive fighting, and "resignation" or compromise (Messer, 1971). The family can, therefore, have a role in the causation, maintenance, and therapy of a major mental illness. One prototypical example is Wegscheider-Cruse's concept of survival roles adopted by members of the dysfunctional family of a chemically dependent individual (Wegscheider-Cruse & Cruse, 2012). Each takes up a unique pathoplastic role (*chief enabler, family hero, family scapegoat, lost child and family mascot*) to precariously maintain the superficially cohesive mould of the family unit.

Family Pathology as a Risk Factor for Mental Illness

When studying causality, it is useful to consider the family as a dynamic environment and see the nature of the psychosocial and biological interactions between its members at different points in the development. The family, thus, plays defining roles in the development of psychopathology through the following mechanisms:

(A) Faulty Parent-Child Relationships

Emerging evidence suggests that the two broad dimensions of dysfunctional parenting occurring in families with later emergent psychopathology are: (i) parental negativity, and (ii) ineffective disciplining practices characterized by harshness, disruptiveness, and inconsistency (Berg-Nielsen et al., 2002).

Expanding from these broad determinants, certain specific parent–child relationship patterns frequently emerge in families that engender children with emotional disturbances (Beltran, 2008).

These include:

i. **Rejection :** Rejection takes many forms like physical neglect, denying love and affection, demonstrating disinterest in the activities and achievements of the child, failing to devote time to the child and showing a lack of respect for the rights and feelings of the child as a person. Such parental rejection fosters low self-esteem, feelings of insecurity and inadequacy, an impaired development of conscience and general intellect, an increased propensity for aggression, and an inability to give and receive love (Sears et al., 1957; Hurley, 1965)

ii. **Overprotection and restrictiveness:** Parental overprotection restricts the child's exposure to opportunities for growth, reality testing and competency development. Such children tend to become overanxious and harbor unreasonable levels of fear (Spokas & Heimberg 2009). A rigid enforcement of roles and standards deprives the child of the autonomy required to grow into a unique individual. While such an approach may foster uniform, socially condoned behavior, it is associated with high levels of dependency, repressed hostility, and a dulling of intellectual striving that is consistent with a vulnerable, anxious profile. A specific association has also emerged between overprotective parenting and both obsessive symptoms in depression and overt obsessive compulsive disorder (Yoshida et al., 2005)

iii. **Over-permissiveness and over-indulgence:** A freehand doling out of reward squanders the opportunity to learn the importance of desirable standards of behavior. Children of overly indulgent parents exhibit a pathological degree of egocentricity and are characteristically spoiled, selfish, inconsiderate and demanding. High permissiveness and low discipline levels correlate positively with antisocial, aggressive, and exploitative behavior (Johnson & Kelley, 2011). This may serve as an explanatory pathway for associations that have emerged between overpermissive parenting and subsequent adolescent anxiety and depressive symptoms (Oyserman et al., 2002)

iv. **Unrealistic demands***:* When a child is given unrealistically high standards to live up to, failure is often the only realistic outcome. These serial exposures to defeat then engender pain, frustration, and an eroded self-worth (Koplewicz & Klass, 2016). Such children manifest both significantly lower self-worth and lower objectively measured achievement (Lieblich, 1971).

(B) Maladaptive Family Structures

The family also functions as the first and most important environment for a growing child—a source of safety, emotional warmth, and social knowhow. In this regard, when considered as a whole, certain kinds of family environments, both by what they offer to and deprive the child of, have been seen to confer a vulnerability for psychopathology (Beltran, 2008).

i. **The inadequate family:** Characterized by an actual want of the basic physical and psychological resources required to meet the demands of an ordinary life, which can be produced both by an actual resource deficit or by a large family size

ii. **The disturbed family:** Characterized by (a) *ongoing* parental conflict and engagement to maintain a fragile dyad equilibrium, leaving the child deprived of love and nurturing, (b) exposing the child to such flawed and emotion-fraught *parental models*, and (c) an *inclusion of the child* into the ongoing parental conflict

iii. **The antisocial family:** Characterized by parental behavior violating the acceptable societal standards, which the child proceeds to model, leaving him incompatible with the prevailing community norms and socially maladjusted

iv. **The disrupted family:** Characterized by their being *incomplete*, as a consequence of death, divorce, estrangement, or some other event like a major illness. Less than the broken state of the home, the parental conflict, which caused the disruption, is considered pathogenic

v. **The discordant family:** Characterized by one or both of the parents harboring a deep-rooted dissatisfaction with the family makeup. This usually manifests itself in passive aggressive actions and communications which rob the family environment of any real warmth and cohesion

vi. **Historically important pathological family structures:** For reasons stated above (Dixon et al., 2001; Hatfield et al., 1987), the following celebrated models of "schizophrenia-inducing" family patterns currently have only historical importance:

a. **Pseudomutuality and pseudohostility**: Wynne and colleagues (1958) believed that families with schizophrenia dealt with both positive and negative emotions in an unreal and false manner. Pseudomutuality means the family projects a false appearance of having mutually rewarding and supportive relationships without actually having any, to defend members against the risk of separation and protect them from the feelings of emptiness that their inherently unrewarding relationships produce. Pseudohostility means the family clings together and maintains some form of unity by engaging in superficial bickering and dissent, masking a deeper need for intimacy that the family has difficulty dealing with directly. This conceals and diverts attention from underlying chronic conflicts and potentially destructive alignments within the family unit.

b. **Marital schism and skew:** Marital schism means the family is in a state of *disequilibrium* due to repeated threats of parental separation (Lidz et al., 1957). Parents tend to denigrate each other's roles and even attempt to collude with children to exclude their partner. Marital skew means the family is in a state of *equilibrium* which is distorted and maintained at the expense of a decaying parental dyad relationship. One parent plays the submissive role while the other is dominant, thus making the marriage a precarious but relatively stable fit.

c. **Double-bind relationship:** Double-bind occurs when a person receives two or more contradicting messages (e.g. superficial *verbal communications* contradicting *behavioral and covert, abstract communication*) from one or more family members with whom a vital relationship exists (Bateson et al., 1956). As the child is not permitted to directly discuss the dilemma (doing so would potentially jeopardize love or approval within the relationship), it is never ascertained which message should be followed through, meaning that however he may respond, one directive will always remain disobeyed, leaving him in a double bind.

d. **Schizophrenogenic mothers:** The term schizophrenic mother was coined by Fromm-Reichmann (1948) to describe mothers with a distinct set of psychological flaws ("rejecting, impervious to the feelings of others, rigid in their moralism concerning sex and having a significant fear of intimacy"). These traits rendered the domestic environment and the process of parenting so toxic that a child would develop schizophrenic behaviors and thought processes to make sense of and survive in the home.

Maintaining Role of the Family in Mental Illness

Much like other psychosocial variables, family relationship variables also play pivotal roles in the course of major psychiatric disorders. Of these, *expressed emotion* (EE) has the most support.

Expressed Emotion (EE)

The development of EE by George Brown is an example of the methodical formulation of a construct based on actual clinical findings—the successful advent of chlorpromazine in the 1950s saw large number of erstwhile "long-stay" institutionalized patients being discharged back into the community after inpatient stabilization on the medication. The developmental narrative of the EE concept took off as (Kanter et al., 1987):

1. The *observation* that certain patients with schizophrenia consistently tended to relapse more often than others, thereby providing the *research question* "Why are certain schizophrenia patients repeatedly relapsing after hospital discharge?" (Vaughn, 1989)

2. A systematic *observation* and *reporting* of the relationships between the patient and his family by Brown et al., (1958)

3. An experimental *testing of potential explanations* of the event (Brown et al., 1962). Links emerged between a relapse outcome and the home environment the patient returned to— three-quarters of patients from highly critical living conditions relapsed and returned for admission to the hospital, compared to one-third of the remaining patients
4. The *designing of a new instrument* to measure the variable (s) of interest (Brown and Rutter 1966), i.e. the Camberwell Family Interview (CFI), named after London's Camberwell district, the site of the original research
5. The *identification of specific factors* associated with post-discharge relapse (Brown et al., 1962). After hundreds of ratings using the CFI, significant and independent relationships emerged between relapse and three determinants: *hostility, emotional over-involvement, and relative's critical comments.*

In assessing EE, five measures are considered:
- **Hostility:** A negative attitude leveled toward the patient because the family believes his/her illness is "controllable" (as the "symptoms" are behaviors) and that the patient is making a deliberate choice not to get better
- **Emotional over-involvement:** Emotional over-involvement represents a cluster of feelings and behaviors of a family member toward the patient encompassing
  - Demonstrations of over-protectiveness or self-sacrifice
  - Excessive emotion imbuement when delivering praise or blame
  - Using exaggerated statements of attitude and preconceptions
- **Critical comments:** The critical attitudes of EE combine aspects of hostility and emotional over-involvement. Here, family members appreciate that both internal and external factors contribute to the mental illness and subsequent behavior disruptions, yet criticism takes place
- **Positive remarks:** Positive remarks or regard comprise statements demonstrating an appreciation or support for a patient's behavior and a verbal/nonverbal reinforcement of his actions
- **Emotional warmth:** Warmth is a defining characteristic of the low EE family. It is demonstrated by an appreciable kindness, concern, and empathy when the caregiver talks about the patient. It is estimated using vocal qualities, with smiling being a common accompaniment.

There is substantial research evidence to show that patients with schizophrenia who live in close contact with high-EE relatives are more than twice as likely to suffer a relapse in the 9–12 months following a hospitalization than those living with low-EE relatives, e.g. a meta-analysis demonstrated that the expected 9–12 month relapse rate for schizophrenia patients living with low-EE families was 35%, compared to a figure of 65% for high EE families (Butzlaff & Hooley, 1998). The high EE-relapse association stands good in the contexts of other diagnoses as well, such as bipolar disorder, unipolar depression, and eating disorders (Hooley & Gotlib, 2000; Miklowitz et al., 1988).

Family Resilience and Treatment

i. **Family intervention:** Considering the role the family environment has in the genesis and perpetuation of psychiatric illness, it can take on a therapeutic role by adopting corrective family dynamic recalibrations or remedial optimizations, such as (Sethi, 1989):

- A sensitivity toward and an ability to fulfill the physical, spiritual, and emotional needs of its members
- Effective communication and flexibility in the performance of family roles
- Balancing security and encouragement with a family member's individuality and autonomy, and a readiness to accept help when required with a capacity for and pride in self-help
- Facilitating formation of constructive relationships within and outside the family
- The ability to turn a crisis or potentially injurious experience into an opportunity for growth
- A collective regard for family unity, loyalty and inter-family cooperation

The construct of *family intervention* is an embodiment of the above adaptations (Murthy, 2003). It comprises the following components:

- Building relationships with caregivers founded on empathy and understanding
- Identifying and augmenting the strengths of caregivers and helping them access community resources
- Interventions to conduce treatment adherence—it is important to note that although adherence maximizes when a patient's family members or caregivers are involved, sole and complete dependence on partners/family members for adherence produces comparatively inferior results (van Gent & Zwart, 1991)
- Interventions directed at early identification of relapse and swift control of crisis situations
- Guiding families to:
  - Reduce social and personal disability
  - Temper their expectations from the patient
  - Improve vocational functioning of the patient
- Emotional reinforcement to caregivers and facilitation of self-help groups for mutual support and networking among families

Successful family intervention transcends relapse prevention, and has actual therapeutic benefits like improving quality of life and augmenting recovery rates in patients with schizophrenia, unipolar and bipolar affective disorders, alcoholism, and borderline personality disorder (Miklowitz et al., 2000; Miller et al., 2005; Gunderson et al., 1997; O"Farrell et al., 2004).

ii. **Role of the Family in Rehabilitation:** Rehabilitation endeavors to enable an individual with mental illness to live the most rewarding and meaningful life possible by

1. *Individual-oriented interventions* that directly aim to optimize his existing skill-set and equip him with new competencies, and
2. Interventions aimed at making *augmentative amendments to the environment* to facilitate a better harmonization (Rössler, 2006).

The family is the first and most immediate psychosocial environment, and bringing about positive changes in family dynamics thereby contributes to a major chunk of the rehabilitation work.

The family's role in a specific rehabilitation process takes on additional importance in a resource and infrastructure-scant society like ours. Seemingly simple act like encouraging a patient to participate in domestic work or engage in social occasions, is genuine alignment with the overall vision of rehabilitation.

The Impact of Mental Illness on the Family–Caregiver Burden

Burden of care is often defined as "a psychological state that ensues from the combination of the *physical work*, and the *emotional and social pressure* (such as the economic restrictions) that arise from taking care of a patient" (Dillehay & Sandy, 1990).

The burden borne by the family members can be (Hoenig & Hamilton, 1966):

1. An *objective burden*, comprising tangible evident consequences, such as household disruptions, economic pressures, personal time shortfalls or a caregiver's inability to work or have a normal social life
2. A *subjective burden*, comprising the caregiver's own perceived impact of the care-giving experience. It delineates the overall negative psychological impact on the caregiver and includes negative feelings like loss, depression and anger, all of which culminate in felt distress and suffering.

Associations have emerged between perceived burden, and:

- **Gender**: Higher burden levels are experienced by relatives of male patients with schizophrenia than those of female patients with schizophrenia (Scazufca & Kuipers, 1996). Regarding the gender of the caregiver, the burden of care is shouldered mostly by women, usually mothers, sisters, or wives, e.g. an American community survey of nearly 700 caregivers demonstrated that 82% of the caregivers were women, among whom 90% were the patient's mother (Awad & Voruganti, 2008)
- **Ethnicity**: Non-white ethnic groups (African-Americans and Hispanics) tended to feel less burdened by the care of a relative with schizophrenia. They were also more accepting of the disability, and more optimistic regarding future prospects (Rosenfarb et al., 2006; Jenkins 1997, 1988)
- **Symptom severity (not profile)**: Among diseases, care providers of patients with a diagnosis of schizophrenia have the highest perceived burden, and among them a substantial majority (30–60%) suffer significant distress (Barrowclough, 2004). Symptom severity shows strong and consistent associations with perceived burden (Mors et al., 1992; Provencher & Mueser 1997; Wolthaus et al., 2002). Such consensus is less forthcoming regarding symptom profiles, with stronger perceived burdens associated with both positive (Provencher & Mueser, 1997; Wolthaus et al., 2002) and negative symptoms (Dyck et al., 1999).

Quite understandably, an increased sense of satisfaction with social support networks serves to decrease subjective and objective caregiver burden. Family caregivers experienced fewer burdens when their social support networks were well-knit, and when their spouse also devoted a substantial amount of time caring for the patient (Potasznik & Nelson, 1984). In turn a patient's support system serves as a significant moderating influence on the eventual family burden: patients having an alternate support system generate less caregiver burden than those without a support system (Crotty & Kulys, 1986). The unfortunate reality is that when the interpersonal relationship networks of neurotic and psychotic patients are compared with those of healthy controls, it emerges that psychotic patients not only have social networks with the smallest numbers of people, but that these networks tend to rarely comprise anyone outside of their own family (Pattison et al., 1975).

Indian research on the same domain mirrors these findings showing how significant associations emerge between the overall burden score and the total illness duration, and with the levels of psychopathology and disability. A negative correlation has been reported between perceived social support and total burden score (Jagannathan et al., 2014). The varied dimensions of caregiver burden (tension, worrying, and supervision) had distinct associations with distinct patient and caregiver profiles (e.g. tension with the caregiver being single, the total amount of time per day spent caring for the patient, and the use of negative coping strategies) (Kate et al., 2013).

Family in Indian Context: Focus on the Strengths

The flagship international collaborative studies of the WHO (Jablensky et al., 1992; Mason et al., 1996; Leff et al., 1992) categorically demonstrated that Indian patients with schizophrenia have significantly better outcomes than their Western counterparts. Much of the credit has been accorded to the contribution by the Indian family structure to the life of the individual patient (Kulhara & Chakrabarti, 2001). Certain qualities of the traditional Indian joint family structure have been described, which lend themselves well to explanations of these better outcomes (Ahuja, 1999).

1. The joint family has an *authoritarian* structure, wherein decision-making power lies with a patriarchal head who exercises this discretion with larger collective interests in mind
2. The setup has a *familistic* organization, i.e. the interests of the family as a whole supersede those of the individual, and individuals internalize collective family goals as consistent with their own
3. Statuses and degrees of authority of family members are *clearly defined* based on seniority, age and relationships, mitigating confusion and strife in times of crisis
4. The family operates using an ideal of *joint responsibility*, with the tacit understanding that responsibilities and burdens will be shared by everyone
5. The distinct needs of individual family members get *equal attention.*

These qualities allow for a better distribution of the burden of care, reduce the emotional charge of the home environment, and thereby contribute to the better outcomes that India has consistently demonstrated (Leff et al., 1992). For example, compared to their Danish counterparts, relatives of Indian patients with schizophrenia expressed significantly fewer critical comments (and positive remarks), and demonstrated less over-involvement. Among the same group of Indian relatives though, those living in cities exhibited considerably higher EE measures of all kinds (except over-involvement) than relatives who were village-dwellers (Wig et al., 1987). This aligns well with the finding that compared to the traditional joint family setup, the nuclear family structure shows higher associations with psychiatric disorders (Sethi & Chaturvedi, 1985).

THE EMERGENT ROLE OF SOCIETY IN MENTAL ILLNESS

The importance of ability to align and engage with society as a dimension of mental health was understood early on:

"Mental health could be judged by the degree to which a person could direct himself to his work, love his fellow man and fulfill his social and communal obligations" - Alfred Adler

However, with regards assessing the role of society in the *genesis and perpetuation* of MI, Engel (1980) argued that the prevailing "biomedical" model was inadequate as it did not include the patient's "human attributes" and so could cater neither for the "person as a whole" nor for "data of a psychological or social nature". This was because the reductionism and mind-body dualism on which the biomedical model was based required that such data first be reduced to physic-chemical terms before it could be accorded and acquire meaning. To address these shortcomings, Engel proposed a biopsychosocial model, which maintained that as multiple biological, social and psychological processes contributed to states of health and illness, a similar collective consideration was required concerning etiology and treatment. The model used a *"systems perspective"*, wherein changes to one part of the system set off changes in another part. For example, increases in any kind of disease activity (biological change) would result in increased anxiety and depression (psychological change) which would produce a reduced engagement with family members and friends (social change) (Young et al., 2007).

The effects of social influence would also require an instrument of quantification and measurement similar to the physic-chemical quantifications of biological influences. One of these defining instruments is *social class*. Max Weber conceptualized a three component theory of social stratification, describing social class as an interplay between variables of "class" (economic standing), "status" (social standing) and "power" (the ability to get one's interests met despite resistance from others) (Weber, 1964; Hurst et al., 2016). The division of society based on the above dimensions into strata of high, intermediate, and low social class produced one of the most consistent and well-documented findings in social science—*the correlation of the lower social class with relatively high rates of mental illness*. Save some notable exceptions anorexia (McClelland & Crisp 2001), bipolar probands (Verdoux & Bourgeois, 1995), suicidality in schizophrenia patients (Silverton et al., 2008) and alcoholism, the incidence of all major and common mental disorders is higher in lower social classes.

Understanding the Relationship between Social Class and Mental Illness

There are two potential interpretations that can be drawn from above association—that either mental illness is an outcome of low social class, or low social standing is a consequence of mental illness. The two theories representing this stand are:

Social Causation Theory (Hollingshead & Redlich, 1958)
The concept states that mental illnesses are *caused* by a state of social deprivation and its inherent adversities and stresses. Such circumstances are likelier to be encountered by people of lower social standing. Though the theory holds good for certain conditions like alcohol abuse and depression, support has not been forthcoming for other conditions like bipolar disorder or schizophrenia (Goldberg, 1988).

Social Selection Theory/Social Drift Theory (Wender et al., 1973)
The concept states mental illnesses are over-represented in lower social classes as individuals with a predisposition to mental illness are left with an impaired social mobility—they tend to

either drift down toward the bottom of the social setup or (if that is where they start out from) fail to rise out of it.

Empirical support for this theory came from Faris and Dunham's Chicago Study (Faris & Dunham 1939) – itself an exercise to test Park and Burgess "concentric zone model of urbanization". This model stated that *social disorganization* (isolation and poor fraternity) was at its worst at the epicenter of an urban community. Outer social zones were the most organized, integrated and stable. Faris and Dunham discovered that the least socially organized inner urban zones had the highest incidence of schizophrenia, a finding they contended was due to the downward drift in economic status and social class that set in after the disease process began.

The Protective Power of a Cohesive Society: Social Capital

Social capital was described by the American political scientist Robert Putnam as: *"features of social life—networks, norms, and trust—that enable participants to act together more effectively to pursue shared objectives"* (Putnam, 1996).

Social capital is a property of groups rather than individuals, distinguishing it from traits of individuals like social networks and social support.

Four largely overlapping theoretical dimensions of the concept have been proposed:

- Collective efficacy
- Social trust/reciprocity
- Participation in voluntary organizations
- Social integration for mutual benefit (Lochner et al., 1999).

The concept is divided into:

- **Structural social capital:** The roles, rules, precedents, behaviors, networks and institutions of a group generate a sense of social inclusion by organizing individuals into groups, bridging schisms between societal groupings or vertically integrating groups with differing levels of social power and influence
- **Cognitive social capital:** The values, attitudes and beliefs of a group produce cooperative behavior (Colletta et al., 2000). The construct represents people's perceptions about their existing social relationships (i.e. "what people feel") using estimations like the degree of interpersonal trust, sharing and reciprocity, and is a measurable indicator of *social cohesion* (Fone et al., 2014).

While the social capital concept is an attractive one and should lend itself to amelioration of the effects of adverse circumstance and context on mental illness, identifiable problems exist in the application of the idea:

1. Measuring social capital is an inherently difficult task, as the requisite distinction between the characteristics of people living in an area and the "contextual characteristics" thus produced (i.e. between the constituents and products) is usually lost. Measurements tend to represent an aggregate of individual qualities (Sooman & Macintyre, 1995; Lochner et al., 1999)
2. Continuing with the conventional proxy of a geographical setting (i.e. a neighborhood or community) for a "social context" is difficult, as improved transport and communication allow communities based on "culture" to be geographically dispersed (McKenzie et al., 2002) or even virtual

3. Social capital research largely concerns itself with the "horizontal" links between persons occupying the same rung of a social setup. This ignores how a community's true collective functionality has to take into account the "vertical" power relations and governance interactions between persons at different tiers (McKenzie et al., 2002).

The inconsistency of research results between social capital and mental illness suggest that the effects of social context on mental health are likely to be a complex interplay between social capital, social drift and expressed emotion. For example, on the one hand, when respondents on the British Household Survey were quantified into social capital groupings, both men and women in the low social capital category were twice as likely to meet the cut-off for caseness on the GHQ (score of 3) than those in the group with the highest social capital rating (McCulloch 2001). While in another study, McKenzie et al. (2002) reported higher hospital readmission rates among those psychosis patients who lived in communities with higher perceived safety scores. This was conjectured to be due to a lower community tolerance of deviant behavior.

Deconstructing the Dimensions of Society's Contribution to Mental Illness

The functionalist theory of social inequality views society as a system of institutions which work together to meet a collective need. Society is idealized to work harmoniously and is held together by (and thereby can be assessed in terms of) the determinants of *cohesion, consensus, cooperation, stability, and persistence.* These principles can thus be studied in relation to their impact on mental health (Eitzen & Zinn, 2012).

Social cohesion represents a collective community-level quality encompassing the prevailing levels of trust, the standards of reciprocity and the vitality of authentic social bonds within the local social structure. As already stated, cognitive social capital is often used as a surrogate for social cohesion (Fone et al., 2014). Another approach is that the degree of community acceptance of minorities can serve as a measurable dimension of social cohesion (OECD 2014). A complementary concept is social exclusion. Four areas of social exclusion are identified including consumption, production, political engagement, and social interaction and a lack of participation in any one is deemed independently sufficing to indicate social exclusion (Burchardt et al., 2002). Persons with chronic mental illnesses are among the most excluded groups in all of society. In the UK, less than 25% are actively employed—the lowest employment rate among all groups of disabled persons (Office for National Statistics, 2003).

Social exclusion in any form has universal associations with mental illness. The prototype template for social exclusion is perhaps discrimination on racial or lineal grounds. After the effects of gender, age and socioeconomic status have been controlled for, both personally experiencing interpersonal racism and perceiving a prevalent racism in society at-large have independent contributions to the risks of developing both common mental disorders and psychosis (Karlsen et al., 2005). In this light, the rampancy of discrimination among minority communities is a matter of concern—among a group of 740 black and minority ethnic (BME) people experiencing mental health difficulties, three quarters (73%) of BME people report having experienced some forms of racial discrimination, and 93.2% reported some forms of discrimination because of their mental ill health (Rehman & Owen, 2013). Social exclusion determines access to healthcare services and also the type of services received. Despite the higher levels of ill health and disability among ethnic minority groups, these groups have poorer access to health services (NHS, 2003). On one hand, people of colored and minority ethnic origin with psychosis showed increased rates of hospitalization and involuntary detention. When people from these groups declare that they need help, they tend to face difficulties obtaining any form of psychiatric treatment (Sproston & Nazroo, 2002). Furthermore, the dearth of competent interpretation services means patients who do not speak English might get access to treatment, but may still end up receiving a different standard of care. In Australia, persons born outside the country are likelier to incur an involuntary mental health-related admission than those born within Australia (Stolk et al., 2008). In Ireland, compared to their proportion in the population, colored adults are over-represented in mental health inpatient units, and children and adolescents from this group are under-represented in their mental health service usage.

The quintessential experience of social destabilization is migration. The most well-known and best studied association of migration is with schizophrenia. Several studies in the 1980s and 1990s showed that compared to the native white population in countries like the UK and Holland, the rates of schizophrenia were higher among all migrant groups, with the highest rates being among Caribbean immigrants (Bhugra 2000; Selten & Sijben, 1994). Other mental illnesses that show similar elevated trends are anxiety and depressive disorders, eating disorders, post-traumatic stress disorder (PTSD), and suicidal ideation.

Several hypotheses have been put forward to attempt to explain why the experience of migration is associated with such elevated rates of schizophrenia (Cochrane & Bal, 1987):

1. **Sending countries have higher rates of schizophrenia:** This theory was debunked by the Determinants of Outcome in Severe Mental Disorders (DOSMeD) study (Jablensky et al., 1992) and studies from Jamaica (Hickling & Rodgers-Johnson 1995), Trinidad (Bhugra et al., 1996) and Barbados (Mahy et al., 1999), showing similar rates of schizophrenia in countries migrants originated from

2. **Schizophrenia predisposes people to migrate:** This theory was debunked as:
   a. Higher rates of schizophrenia are found in second, rather than first generation migrants (Bhugra et al., 1997) making it less likely that the illness process had predisposed them to move
   b. Patients with schizophrenia would probably not be able to undertake and complete the physical ordeal of migration and negotiate immigration procedures (Bhugra & Jones, 2001)
   c. If this theory held good, elevated, and largely equal incidence rates would be present in all ethnic migrant groups, which is not the case

3. **Stress of migration can cause schizophrenia:** The facts that prevented the relatively easy acceptance of this attractive theory were:
   a. Differing rates of common mental disorders among different countries
   b. Rates of schizophrenia tend to substantially elevate more than 10–12 years after migration (Ødegaard, 1932), making it less likely that the actual process of migration is a direct cause

4. **Migrants are misdiagnosed with schizophrenia:** Migrants had misdiagnosis contributed to the elevated incidence rate among the Caribbean immigrant population, it should also have similarly elevated (mis) diagnosis rates among all immigrant groups considering

similar degrees of language differences. This is not the case. Furthermore, robustly standardized clinical definitions, assessments, and operational criteria are in place, making it unlikely that such large differences are due to misdiagnosis (Bhugra & Jones, 2001)

5. **Migrants present inherently different symptom patterns:** This last hypothesis was not part of Cochrane & Bal (1987) original hypothesis set. There is considerable evidence from DOSMeD that cultural differences exist between inception rates of narrow- and broad-definition schizophrenias (Jablensky et al., 1992). It is likely that differing rates of these two variants of schizophrenia among distinct migrant groups will result in differing import weights for diagnosis and management.

CONCLUSION

The individual represents many things to society—a building block, a fabricator, and a finished product. Similarly, society and its executive epitome, the family, play numerous generative and mediating roles in the mental health of the individual (**Flowchart 1**). The extent of harmony between the three is an estimate of both the quantum of work and the degree of success a psychiatric intervention will need to provide or has been able to achieve. Biological underpinning of mental disorders can not be ignored but with the zeal to identify specific brain substrates and genetic or epigenetic components, the substantial contribution of social factors must not be undermined. Just take an example of schizophrenia which supposedly has very high heritability (up to 70%). Migration and urbanicity, the two strongest social predictors of schizophrenia have weighted relative risk of 2–3, whereas after several billion dollars of investment any specific gene variant was found to have a relative risk of barely 1-1.5 (Tandon et al., 2008). A recent genome wide study which found 128 genes to be significantly associated with schizophrenia has also lamented that only 3.4% variance of schizophrenia could be explained with all these genes together (Schizophrenia Working Group of the Psychiatric Genomics Consortium 2014). Having said this, it must be reiterated that with

Flowchart 1: Tripartite interaction between family-society-individual

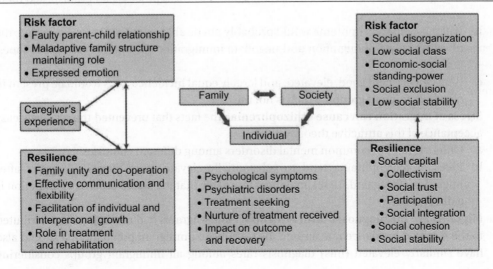

further refinement of methodology and change in the conceptual framework, biological understanding of mental disorders is evolving and improving every day. Competing interests in scientific paradigms commonly lead to either replacement or integration. In replacement, one paradigm perishes from the scientific scene and the other emerges as the sole winner. In integration, two competing paradigms are incorporated into a unified approach. The example of the former could be replacement of Ptolemaic theory with the Copernican models and the example of latter might be retention of Newtonian mechanics even after the invention of the theory of relativity. In our opinion, in current days psychiatry, we need to integrate the older social paradigms with the state of the art biological models, where the biological paradigm might be used for causality and the social models could find significant utility in identification of risk factors, planning optimal intervention, and reintegration of patients. Moreover, strategic studies should also look for the interactions between the two.

There are both risk and protective factors at the levels of family and society. The balance between the two and the interactions with each other determine the effect on the individual. In turn, individuals as a member of the family and larger society interact with them, which not only influence their psychological symptoms or disorders but also determine the outcome.

REFERENCES

Ahuja R. Society in India: Concepts, Theories, and Changing Trends. Jaipur: Rawat Publications; 1999.

Awad AG, Voruganti LNP. The burden of schizophrenia on caregivers: A review. Pharmacoeconomics. 2008;26(2):149-62.

Barrowclough C. In: Sartorius N, Leff J, López-Ibor JJ, and Okasha A (Eds). Families of People with Schizophrenia in Families and Mental Disorders. New Jersey: John Wiley & Sons, Ltd; 2004. pp. 1–24.

Bateson G, Jackson DD, Haley J, et al. Toward a theory of schizophrenia. Behav Sci. 1956;1:251-64.

Beltran J. Abnormal Psychology. Rex Bookstore. 2008.

Berg-Nielsen TS, Vikan A, Dahl AA. Parenting related to child and parental psychopathology: A descriptive review of the literature. Clin Child Psychol Psychiatry. 2002;7 (4):529-52.

Bernard C. Lectures on the Phenomena of Life Common to Animals and Plants. Thomas. 1974.

Bhugra D, Hilwig M, Hossein B, et al. First-contact incidence rates of schizophrenia in Trinidad and one-year follow-up. Br J Psychiatry. 1996;169(5):587-92.

Bhugra D, Leff J, Mallett R, et al. Incidence and outcome of schizophrenia in Whites, African-Caribbeans and Asians in London. Psychol Med. 1997;27(4):791-98.

Bhugra D. Migration and schizophrenia. Acta Psychiatr Scand Suppl. 2000;(407):68-73.

Bhugra D, Jones P. Migration and mental illness. Adv Psychiatr Treat. 2001;7(3):216-22.

Brown GW, Carstairs GM, Topping G. Post-hospital adjustment of chronic mental patients. Lancet. 1958;2(7048): 685-88.

Brown GW, Monck EM, Carstairs GM, et al. Influence of family life on the course of schizophrenic illness. Br J Prev Soc Med. 1962;16 (2):55-68.

Brown GW, Rutter M. The Measurement of family activities and relationships: A methodological study. Hum Relat. 1966;19(3):241-63.

Burchardt T, Le Grand J, Piachaud D. In: Hills J, Le Grand J, Piachaud D (Eds) Degrees of Exclusion: Developing a Dynamic, Multidimensional Measure in Understanding Social Exclusion. Oxford: Oxford University Press; 2002.

Butzlaff RL, Hooley JM. Expressed emotion and psychiatric relapse: A meta-analysis. Arch Gen Psychiatry. 1998;55(6):547-52.

Cannon WB. The Wisdom of the Body. WW Norton & Company; 1932.

Cochrane R, Bal SS. Migration and schizophrenia: An examination of five hypotheses. Soc Psychiatry. 1987;22(4):181-91.

Colletta NJ, Cullen ML. Violent Conflict and the Transformation of Social Capital: Lessons from Cambodia, Rwanda, Guatemala, and Somalia. World Bank Publications; 2000.

Crotty P, Kulys R. Are schizophrenics a burden to their families? Significant others" views. Health Soc Work. 1986 Summer;11(3):173-88.

Dillehay RC, Sandys MR. Caregivers for Alzheimer's patients: What we are learning from research. Int J Aging Hum Dev. 1990;30(4):263-85.

Dixon L, McFarlane WR, Lefley H, et al. Evidence-based practices for services to families of people with psychiatric disabilities. Psychiatr Serv. 2001;52(7):903-10.

Dyck DG, Short R, Vitaliano PP. Predictors of burden and infectious illness in schizophrenia caregivers. Psychosom Med. 1999;61(4):411-9.

Eitzen DS, Zinn MB Globalization: The Transformation of Social Worlds. Wadsworth Cengage Learning. 2012

Engel GL. The clinical application of the biopsychosocial model. Am J Psychiatry. 1980;137(5):535-44.

Faris REL, Dunham HW. Mental Disorders in Urban Areas: An Ecological Study of Schizophrenia and Other Psychoses. University of Chicago Press. 1939.

Fingerman KL, Bermann E. Applications of family systems theory to the study of adulthood. Int J Aging Hum Dev. 2000; 51(1):5-29.

Fone D, White J, Farewell D, et al. Effect of neighbourhood deprivation and social cohesion on mental health inequality: A multilevel population-based longitudinal study. Psychol Med. 2014; 44(11):2449-60.

Fromm-Reichmann F. Notes on the development of treatment of schizophrenics by psychoanalytic psychotherapy. Psychiatry. 1948;11(3):263-73.

Gent EMv, Zwart FM. Psychoeducation of partners of bipolar-manic patients. J Affect Disord. 1991; 21(1):15-8.

Goldberg EM, Morrison SL. Schizophrenia and social class In The Challenge of Epidemiology: Issues and Selected Readings, by Buck, Carol, Pan American Health Org. 1988; pp. 368-83.

Goodell TT, Hanson SMH. Nurse-family interactions in adult critical care: A bowen family systems perspective. J Fam Nurs. 2002; 5(1):72-91.

Gunderson JG, Berkowitz C, Ruiz-Sancho A. Families of borderline patients: A psychoeducational approach. Bull Menninger Clin. 1997;61(4):446-57.

Hatfield AB, Spaniol L, Zipple AM. Expressed emotion: A family perspective. Schizophr Bull. 1987;13(2):221-6.

Hickling FW, Rodgers-Johnson P. The incidence of first contact schizophrenia in Jamaica. Br J Psychiatry. 1995;167(2):193-96.

Hoenig, J, Hamilton MW. The schizophrenic patient in the community and his effect on the household. Int J Soc Psychiatry. 1966;12 (3):165-76.

Hollingshead AB, Redlich FC. Social Class and Mental Illness: Community Study. New Jersey: John Wiley & Sons Inc.; 1958.

Hooley JM, Gotlib IH. A diathesis-stress conceptualization of expressed emotion and clinical outcome. Appl Prev Psychol. 2000;9(3):135-51.

Hurley JR. Parental Acceptance-Rejection and Children's Intelligence. Merrill-Palmer Quarterly. 1965;11(1):19-32.

Hurst CE. Fitz-Gibbon HM, Nurse AM. Social Inequality: Forms, Causes, and Consequences. Routledge. 2016.

Jablensky A, Sartorius N, Ernberg G, et al. Schizophrenia: Manifestations, incidence and course in different cultures. A World Health Organization ten-country study. Psychol Med Monograph Supplement. 1992;20:1-97.

Jackson DD. Family homeostasis and the physician. Calif Med. 1965;103(4):239-42.

Jagannathan A, Thirthalli J, Hamza A, et al. Predictors of family caregiver burden in schizophrenia: Study from an in-patient tertiary care hospital in India. Asian J Psychiatr. 2014;8:94-8.

Jenkins JH. Subjective experience of persistent schizophrenia and depression among US Latinos and Euro-Americans. Br J Psychiatry. 1997;171:20-5.

Jenkins JH. Ethnopsychiatric interpretations of schizophrenic illness: The problem of Nervios within Mexican-American families. Cult Med Psychiatry. 1988;12(3):301-29.

Johnson LE, Kelley HM. Permissive Parenting Style. In: Goldstein S, Naglieri JA (Eds) Encyclopedia of Child Behavior and Development. US: Springer; 2011. pp. 1080.

Kanter J, Lamb HR, Loeper C. Expressed emotion in families: A critical review. Psychiatr Serv. 1987;38(4):374-80.

Karlsen S, James Y, McKenzie K, et al. Racism, psychosis and common mental disorder among ethnic minority groups in England. Psychol Med. 2005;35(12):1795-803.

Kate N, Grover S, Kulhara P, et al. Relationship of caregiver burden with coping strategies, social support, psychological morbidity, and quality of life in the caregivers of schizophrenia. Asian J Psychiatr. 2013;6 (5):380-8

Koplewicz HS, Klass E. Depression in Children and Adolescents. Routledge. 2016.

Kulhara P, Chakrabarti S. Culture and schizophrenia and other psychotic disorders. Psychiatr Clin North Am. 2001;24(3):449-64.

Leff J, Sartorius N, Jablensky A, et al. The International Pilot Study of Schizophrenia: five-year follow-up findings. Psychol Med. 1992; 22(1):131-45.

Leff J, Wig NN, Bedi H, et al. Relatives" expressed emotion and the course of schizophrenia in Chandigarh. A two-year follow-up of a first-contact sample. Br J Psychiatry. 1992;156: 351-56.

Lidz T, Cornelison AR, Fleck S, et al. The intrafamilial environment of schizophrenic patients. II. Marital schism and marital skew. Am J Psychiatry. 1957;114 (3):241-8

Lieblich A. Antecedents of envy reaction. J Pers Assess. 1971;35(1):92-8.

Lochner K, Kawachi I, Kennedy BP. Social capital: A guide to its measurement. Health Place. 1999;5(4):259-70.

Mahy GE, Mallett R, Leff J, Bhugra D: First-contact incidence rate of schizophrenia on Barbados. Br J Psychiatry.1999; 175 (1): 28–33.

Mason P, Harrison G, Glazebrook C, et al. The course of schizophrenia over 13 years. A report from the International Study on Schizophrenia (ISoS) coordinated by the World Health Organization. Br J Psychiatry.1996; 169 (5): 580–86.

McClelland L, Crisp A. Anorexia nervosa and social class. Int J Eat Disord. 200;29(2):150-6..

McCulloch A: Social environments and health: Cross sectional national survey. BMJ. 2001;323(7306): 208-9.

McKenzie K, Whitley R, Weich S: Social capital and mental health. Br J Psychiatry. 2002; 181 (4): 280–83

Mehta A, Robin-Cohen S, Chan LS. Palliative care: A need for a family systems approach. Palliat Support Care. 2009;7(2):235-43.

Messer AA. Mechanisms of family homeostasis. Compr Psychiatry. 1971;12(4):380-8.

Miklowitz DJ. The role of family systems in severe and recurrent psychiatric disorders: A developmental psychopathology view. Dev Psychopathol. 2004;16 (3):667-88.

Miklowitz DJ, Goldstein MJ, Nuechterlein KH, et al. Family factors and the course of bipolar affective disorder. Arch Gen Psychiatry.1988;45 (3):225-31.

Miklowitz DJ, Simoneau TL, George EL, et al. Family-focused treatment of bipolar disorder: 1-year effects of a psychoeducational program in conjunction with pharmacotherapy. Biol Psychiatry. 2000;48(6):582-92.

Miller IW, Keitner GI, Ryan CE, et al. Treatment matching in the posthospital care of depressed patients. Am J Psychiatry. 2005;162(11):2131-8.

Mors O, Sørensen LV, Therkildsen ML. Distress in the relatives of psychiatric patients admitted for the first time. Acta Psychiatr Scand. 1992;85(5):337-44.

Murdock GP. Social Structure. Free Press. 1965.

Murthy RS. Family interventions and empowerment as an approach to enhance mental health resources in developing countries. World Psychiatry. 2003;2(1):35-7.

NHS. Inside Outside. Improving Mental Health Services for Black and Minority Ethnic Communities in England 2003.

O"Farrell TJ, Murphy CM, Stephan SH, et al. Partner violence before and after couples-based alcoholism treatment for male alcoholic patients: The role of treatment involvement and abstinence. J Consult Clin Psychol. 2004;72(2):202-17.

Ødegaard O. Emigration and Insanity: A Study of Mental Disease among Norwegian-Born Population in Minnesota. Levin & Munksgaard. 1932.

OECD. Society at a Glance 2014 OECD Social Indicators: OECD Social Indicators. OECD Publishing, 2014.

Office for National Statistics. Labour Force Survey (LFS). 2003.

Oyserman D, Bybee D, Mowbray C. Influences of maternal mental illness on psychological outcomes for adolescent children. J Adolesc. 2002;25(6):587-602.

Pattison EM, Defrancisco D, Wood P, et al. A psychosocial kinship model for family therapy. Am J Psychiatry. 1975;132(12):1246-51.

Potasznik H, Nelson G. Stress and social support: The burden experienced by the family of a mentally ill person. Am J Community Psychol. 1984;12(5):589-607.

Provencher HL, Mueser KT. positive and negative symptom behaviors and caregiver burden in the relatives of persons with schizophrenia. Schizophr Res. 1997;26 (1):71-80.

Putnam RD. Turning In, Turning Out: The strange disappearance of civic America. Policy Political Science and Politics, 1995;28 (4): 664-83.

Rehman H, Owen D. Mental health survey of ethnic minorities: Research report. London: Ethnos Research and Consultancy. 2013

Rosenfarb IS, Bellack AS, Aziz N. A sociocultural stress, appraisal, and coping model of subjective burden and family attitudes toward patients with schizophrenia. J Abnorm Psychol. 2006;115(1):157-65.

Rössler W. Psychiatric rehabilitation today: An overview. World Psychiatry. 2006;5(3):151-7.

Sears RR, Maccoby EE, Levin H. Patterns of Child Rearing Harper & Row. 1957.

Scazufca M, Kuipers E: Links between expressed emotion and burden of care in relatives of patients with schizophrenia. Br J Psychiatry.1996;168(5):580-87.

Schizophrenia Working Group of the Psychiatric Genomics Consortium: Biological insights from 108 schizophrenia-associated genetic loci. Nature. 2014;511(7510):421-7.

Selten JP, Sijben N: First admission rates for schizophrenia in immigrants to the Netherlands. The Dutch National Register. Soc Psychiatry Psychiatr Epidemiol. 1994;29(2):71-7.

Sethi BB, Chaturvedi PK. A review and role of family studies and mental health. Indian J Soc Psychiatry. 1985;45:216-30.

Sethi BB. Family as a potent therapeutic force. Indian J Psychiatry. 1989;31(1):22-30.

Silverton L, Mednick SA, Holst C, et al. High social class and suicide in persons at risk for schizophrenia. Acta Psychiatr Scand. 2008;117(3):192-7.

Sooman A, Macintyre S. Health and perceptions of the local environment in socially contrasting neighbourhoods in Glasgow. Health Place. 1995;1(1):15-26.

Spokas M, Heimberg RG. Overprotective parenting, social anxiety, and external locus of control: cross-sectional and longitudinal relationships. Cognit Ther Res. 2009;33(6):543.

Sproston K, Nazroo JY. Ethnic Minority Psychiatric Illness Rates in the Community (EMPIRIC): Quantitative report. Department of Health. 2002.

Stolk Y, Minas IH, Klimidis S. Access to mental health services in Victoria: A focus on ethnic communities. Victorian Transcultural Psychiatry Unit; 2008.

Tandon R, Matcheri SK, Nasrallah HA. Schizophrenia, "Just the Facts": What we know in 2008 Part 1: Overview. Schizophrenia Research. 2008;100(1-3):4-19.

van Gent EM, Zwart FM. Psychoeducation of partners of bipolar-manic patients. J Affect Disord. 1991;21(1):15-8.

Vaughn CE. Expressed emotion in family relationships. J Child Psychol Psychiatry. 1989; 30 (1): 13–22.

Verdoux H, Bourgeois M: Social class in unipolar and bipolar probands and relatives. J Affect Disord. 1995; 33 (3): 181–87.

Weber M. Wirtschaft und Gesellschaft: Grundriss der verstehenden Soziologie. Halbbd. 1. Kiepenheuer & Witsch. 1964

Wegscheider-Cruse S, Cruse S. Understanding Codependency, Updated and Expanded: The Science Behind It and How to Break the Cycle. Health Communications, Inc. 2012.

Wender PH, Rosenthal D, Kety SS, et al. Social class and psychopathology in adoptees. A natural experimental method for separating the roles of genetic and experimential factors. Arch Gen Psychiatry.1973;28(3):318-25.

Wig NN, Menon DK, Bedi H, et al. Expressed emotion and schizophrenia in North India. II. Distribution of expressed emotion components among relatives of schizophrenic patients in Aarhus and Chandigarh. Br J Psychiatry.1987;151:160-5.

Wolthaus JED, Dingemans PMAJ, Schene AH, et al. Caregiver burden in recent-onset schizophrenia and spectrum disorders: The influence of symptoms and personality traits. J Nerv Ment Dis. 2002;190(4):241-7.

Wynne LC, Ryckoff IM, Day J, Hirsch SI: Pseudo-mutuality in the family relations of schizophrenics. Psychiatry. 1958; 21(2):205-20.

Yoshida T, Taga C, Matsumoto Y, Fukui K. Paternal overprotection in obsessive-compulsive disorder and depression with obsessive traits. Psychiatry Clin Neurosci. 2005;59(5):533-8.

Young G, Kane AW, Nicholson K. Causality of Psychological Injury: Presenting Evidence in Court. Berlin: Springer Science & Business Media; 2007.

Chapter 7

Concept, Relevance and Management of Social Cognition Impairments in Psychiatry: A Biopsychosocial Approach

Urvakhsh Meherwan Mehta, BN Gangadhar

SUMMARY

Most psychiatric disorders have clinical presentations within a social or interpersonal framework. Apart from subjective distress, the reasons for seeking help include apparent problems in social behavior and the resulting socio-occupational dysfunction. Over the last few decades, scientists from across diverse fields including mental health professionals, anthropologists, evolutionary biologists, neuroscientists and developmental biologists have identified the critical contribution of social cognition to such social behavioral problems. We have now begun to identify a connection between social brain networks, social cognition, and social behaviors in these psychiatric disorders. This chapter focuses on understanding the concepts, dimensions, clinical relevance, assessment and measurements, and management of social cognition impairments in a clinical setting. These sections are guided by a biopsychosocial framework of understanding the connections from the social brain to social behavior through social cognition. Management strategies including cognitive therapies, neuromodulation therapies, novel pharmacotherapies, and traditional life-style practices such as yoga are reviewed and recommendations for clinical practice and future research are discussed.

BACKGROUND: SOCIAL BRAIN TO SOCIAL BEHAVIOR THROUGH SOCIAL COGNITION

Behavioral problems in the social or interpersonal context are common manifestations of a broad range of neuropsychiatric disorders, ranging from developmental (e.g. autism) to degenerative (e.g. frontotemporal dementia) in their origins. The disturbances can broadly be understood as positive phenomena, where patients exhibit undesirable behaviors or negative phenomena, characterized by a lack of desired behavior. Such social behavioral disturbances are related to an underlying deficit or deviation in how the brain processes social information. This ability is also referred to as social cognition, and social neuroscience experiments

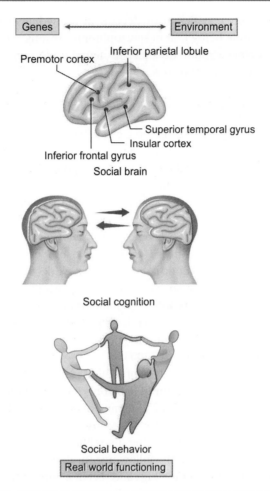

Figure 1: The social chain leading from social brain networks through social cognition to social behavior and functional outcomes.

have demonstrated distinct brain networks underlying these unique higher order cognitive processes.

While a substantial proportion of our social cognition is hard-wired, guided by genetic factors that shape our neuronal networks, the role of social environment (parents, society, and culture) in nurturing its development and expression cannot be underplayed. A common feature across neuropsychiatric disorders is the huge quantum of disability in the domains of personal, family, occupational, and social domains of real world functioning of an individual (Vos et al., 2012). Social cognition impairments and the related social behavioral problems are strong predictors of this commonly observed real world functional disability (Fett et al., 2011). Here, it is important to note that functional disability is a multifactorial construct and there could be other determinants independent of social cognition. Nevertheless, this social chain **(Figure 1)** starting from the social brain shaping social cognition, social behavior, and real-world functioning is often deficient or deviant in individuals with severe psychiatric disorders; a classical example being that of schizophrenia. Through this chapter, we provide a succinct overview of social cognition domains, its neural underpinnings, clinical relevance, and emerging novel management strategies.

CONCEPT AND DOMAINS OF SOCIAL COGNITION

Many of our day-to-day experiences are centered on social cognition like our ability to process socially relevant information within an interpersonal context. These include, but are not restricted to empathy, perspective taking, trust, cooperation, altruism, deception detection, pretense, metaphors, irony, and social blunders or faux pas. Social cognition experiments began in the late 1960s as psychological investigations into the social mind (Heider, 1967), and extended to examining developmental milestones and ontogeny of these processes (Chandler, 1976). At the same time, evolutionary psychology approaches were used to understand the phylogeny of these abilities by identifying comparative processes in social animals like non-human primates (Premack & Woodruff, 1978). The next decade saw its implementation in clinical populations by examining social cognition impairments in children with mental retardation (Blacher, 1982) and adults with traumatic brain injuries (Wais, 1982). However, it was much later that social cognition was seriously examined in disorders such as autism (Dawson & Fernald, 1987) and schizophrenia (Corrigan & Green, 1993), which today are considered as social brain disorders (Burns, 2006a).

Earlier meetings of the National Institute of Mental Health (NIMH)—Measurement and Treatment Research to Improve Cognition in Schizophrenia (MATRICS) initiative (Green et al., 2005, 2008) recommended a set of sub-domains of social cognition to be examined in future studies. Over the last decade, a series of neuroscience-driven experiments have now started to give concerted information regarding neural networks underlying social cognition (Green et al., 2015). We have identified the following four domains of social cognition, based on expert consensus of earlier NIMH meetings and recent evidence from social neuroscience experiments in humans:

1. **Social cue perception:** Social cues are sensory stimuli appearing within a social framework. The perception of these social cues is vital for recognition of identities and emotions in faces and voice, as well as in interpreting gestures and body language (biological motion of head, hands, other body parts, eye contact, lip-reading, etc). This involves initial processing of social information, which later culminates in the precise appraisal of beliefs and intentions in other individuals. The superior temporal sulcus and nearing fusiform face area and fusiform body area are important cortical structures that enable these functions (Allison et al., 2000). The amygdala, an important part of the limbic cortex has a specific role in identifying aversive stimuli that evoke disgust. Factor analytical studies (Mehta et al., 2014b) on social cognition in schizophrenia and healthy individuals also identify a distinct socioemotional processing component that has loadings from scores on tests of social cue detection and facial emotion recognition.

2. **Theory of mind (ToM):** This is a unique cognitive ability present only in higher nonhuman primates and humans. This concept was introduced by primatologists and psychologists Premack and Woodruff in their 1978 article "Does the chimpanzee have a theory of mind?"

as a capacity to impute mental states to oneself and to others. This ability was viewed as a "theory", first, because such states are not overtly observable, and second, because it can be used to make predictions, specifically about the behavior of other individuals (Premack & Woodruff, 1978). Several terminologies have been coined that refer to ToM or to certain aspects of the mental state inferential process. Mental state attributions, mentalizing ability, meta-representations, representational or Machiavellian intelligence, reflexive awareness, folk psychology, taking the intentional stance are few such terminologies (Burns, 2006b, Harrington et al., 2005). The literature identifies the possession of a ToM as manifest in imitation, self-recognition, social relationships, role taking, deception and perspective taking (Heyes, 1998). ToM is defined as the ability to infer intentions, dispositions, and beliefs of others (Green et al., 2008). There are two neural networks that enable our processing of ToM: (a) *the mentalizing network,* which subserves a controlled pretense or simulation-based reflective processing of others' thoughts and is comprised of the medial prefrontal cortex, posterior cingulate cortex, precuneus, and the temporoparietal junctions, and (b) *the mirroring or experience sharing network* comprising of the premotor, inferior frontal, inferior parietal and insular cortices, which helps in a more automatic or a spontaneous embodied simulation driven understanding of others' thoughts. This was also identified as an independent cognitive construct in schizophrenia and healthy subjects using factor analyses (Mehta et al., 2014b). Moreover, experiments in untreated schizophrenia subjects have revealed a significant association between poor ToM performance and reduced mirror neuron system activity (Mehta et al., 2014a).

3. **Emotion regulation:** Our ability to achieve optimal control over our emotions is a dynamic interplay between the generation of emotions and the cognitive appraisal we employ to understand the emotion and respond appropriately (Green et al., 2015). This involves strategies that permit us to generate differing interpretations of emotional stimuli and then regulate how and when we experience and choose to express or respond to these emotions. These complex processes are a function of *emotion generating and experiencing centers* like the amygdala, insula, ventral striatum, thalamus and anterior cingulate, and the *emotion regulation centers* like the dorsolateral prefrontal cortex (maintenance of emotion interpretations in working memory), the ventrolateral prefrontal cortex (selection and inhibition of interpretations) and the dorsomedial prefrontal cortex (self-reflective processes for elaborating the meaning of emotional stimuli).

4. **Attributional styles:** This refers to explanations people generate about possible causes of good and not-so-good events in their lives. It is understood as the ubiquitous tendency to explain the cause of social actions in terms of oneself or others, or the context of the event (Bentall et al., 2009). While individuals experiencing depression tend to have a strong self-blaming bias (attributing negative events to oneself), those with paranoid delusions tend to have a strong self-serving bias (attributing negative events to other people). Transdiagnostic neuroimaging experiments reveal the contribution of brain regions involved in *automatic interpretations* of intentions of others that include the mirroring network (premotor cortex, inferior frontal gyrus and inferior parietal lobule) and those involved in *motivated behaviors* (dorsal striatum, cerebellum and anterior cingulate), which are thought to underlie our attributional biases (Blackwood et al., 2003; Hao et al., 2015; Park et al., 2009; Rose et al., 2014).

CLINICAL RELEVANCE OF SOCIAL COGNITION DEFICITS IN PSYCHIATRY

The last decade has witnessed an exponential increase **(Figure 2)** in the number of published studies on social cognition, especially from clinical and neuroscience perspectives. This is perhaps because of two fairly consistent observations—(a) deficits in social cognition are related to real-world functional disability in patients with severe psychiatric disorders like schizophrenia (Fett et al., 2011) and bipolar disorder (Green, 2006) and (b) these deficits are putative biomarkers for psychiatric disorders (Derntl and Habel, 2011). We will discuss in brief evidence to support these observations, taking schizophrenia as an example.

1. **Relation to functional outcomes:** Schizophrenia, a mental illness caused due to genetic and environmental influences, generally affects individuals during their adolescence or young adulthood. Persons suffering from schizophrenia develop delusions (holding false beliefs, like there is danger to them from others, etc.), hallucinations (e.g. hearing voices when there are none) and disorganized behavior (e.g. wandering aimlessly, talking irrelevantly, etc.). Often, they neglect their self-care, lose aim and motivation in life goals

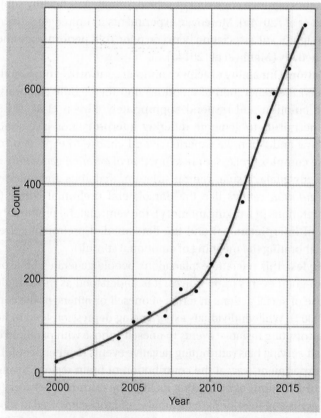

Figure 2: Number of publications with "social cognition" in the title or abstract in PubMed increasing over the years.

(negative symptoms) and lead compromised lives. It is one of the leading causes of disability among young people in the world.

There is a consistent relationship between social cognition deficits and real-world functional ability in patients with schizophrenia. The more the deficits in social cognition, the poorer a person's ability to have a satisfactory day-to-day functioning like personal care, and in meeting family, social, occupational and academic roles. In addition, social cognition deficits may be causally linked to symptoms of schizophrenia (social behaviors). While deficits in social cognition are related to negative symptoms (Mehta et al., 2014c), such as being withdrawn, aloof and apathetic, deviant social cognition (hypermentalizing and externalizing attributional bias) is related to positive symptoms like delusions and poor self-monitoring or insight (Bentall et al., 2009). A host of other factors play a role in determining such complex functional roles in humans. However, social cognition deficits seem to play a significant role in predicting functional abilities directly, as well as indirectly, by mediating the influence of general cognitive dysfunction. A recent meta-analysis on this subject revealed that together general and social cognition influence about 25% of variance in functional outcomes in schizophrenia (Fett et al., 2011). Substantial proportion of this influence was mediated by social cognition deficits rather than neurocognitive deficits, even though both these cognitive functions are strongly related. In our own research, we have used structural equation modeling to study how social cognition could influence functional outcome. We have found that the impact of social cognition on functional outcome is in turn mediated by symptoms such as lack of insight, lack of motivation, and other symptoms of schizophrenia (Bhagyavathi et al., 2015; Mehta et al., 2014c). These observations have resulted in attempts by mental health professionals to train patients using innovative cognitive and social exercises (Eack et al., 2007; Keshavan et al., 2014; Kurtz & Richardson, 2012). However, these strategies show only modest benefits that are difficult to maintain over longer periods of time.

2. **Endophenotype status:** Endophenotypes are subtle manifestations of disorders that lie in between on the path from genes to the disease manifestation, are heritable and are present even in the absence of manifest illness in vulnerable and remitted individuals (Gottesman & Gould, 2003). There is increasing evidence to suggest that social cognition deficits are endophenotype markers for psychiatric disorders, especially schizophrenia. Deficits in all domains of social cognition have been observed even before onset of schizophrenia (Lee et al., 2015). Similar deficits have been demonstrated in even among family members of patients (Eack et al., 2010b), suggesting that these deficits have possible genetic origin. In fact, a recent meta-analysis has demonstrated deficits in facial and voice emotion recognition, and ToM in individuals who are at high-risk for developing schizophrenia (van Donkersgoed et al., 2015). In our investigations in patients who are no longer experiencing hallucinations and delusions, we found extensive deficits across all sub-domains (Mehta et al., 2013). It is important to note that these deficits are, however, not specific to schizophrenia. Nevertheless, they are present in a large magnitude in schizophrenia when compared to other disorders (Yalcin-Siedentopf et al., 2014). These observations suggest that social cognition deficits are putative endophenotypes of schizophrenia and other psychiatric disorders. They possibly have genetic influences and identifying their neural substrates may help us better understand these deficits and treat them.

MANAGEMENT OF SOCIAL COGNITION DEFICITS

From the previous sections, it is apparent that social cognition deficits are clinically relevant predominantly because of their relationship with social behaviors like delusions and negative symptoms, and real world functional outcomes. Hence, treatment strategies are required to focus on first assessing and defining the type of social cognition impairment (deficiency versus deviance) and then using novel biopsychosocial approaches in correcting the deviant processing or training the deficient ability.

1. **Measuring social cognition:** Assessments of social cognition have most often been performed within a research setting to understand its relationship to behaviors and neural underpinnings. There is a broad range of assessment tools to examine social cognition with varying degrees of psychometric properties. Measures of emotion processing vary broadly and include rating of emotions that are displayed in faces (facial emotion recognition) or voices (affective prosody) or rating from brief vignettes of how individuals manage, regulate, or facilitate emotion. The "gold standard" test of comprehending other persons' minds is the ability to understand that others can hold false beliefs that are different from one's own (correct) knowledge (Dennett, 1978). Emotion recognition tests explore two main abilities: the identification (labeling) of an emotion or matching of emotions shown on two faces as being the same or different. The difficulty of the tests can be varied by blending emotions, varying the intensity of emotion, degrading the images or by inverting them (Thatcher effect). Tests of social perception use video-depicted social scenarios. The participants view them and answer questions, which test their ability to observe social cues (Corrigan and Green, 1993). Attributional styles are assessed using hypothetical positive and negative events for which the participants are asked to draw causal inferences and label them as internal personal, external personal or situational (Kinderman & Bentall, 1996).

   Social cognition is under the influence of the sociocultural systems in our immediate milieu. Given the fact that culture has a moderating effect on the contextual expression of social behaviors, and development and processing of social information, it is important to have culture specific tools to examine this complex cognitive ability (Mehta et al., 2011). Within the Indian sociocultural context, ToM, attributional styles and social perception can be measured using the Social Cognition Rating Tools in Indian Setting [SOCRATIS (Mehta & Thirthalli, 2014; Mehta et al., 2011)] and facial emotion recognition can be measured using the Tool for Recognition of Emotions in Neuropsychiatric Disorders [TRENDS (Behere et al., 2008)]. Both these tools have undergone validation in the Indian sociocultural setting and have satisfactory psychometric properties.

2. **Treatment of social cognition impairments:** There is no gold-standard treatment for addressing social cognition impairments in psychiatric disorders yet. Despite initial evidence that atypical antipsychotic drugs improved social cognition (Harvey et al., 2006), subsequent studies have not shown a substantial difference with antipsychotic medications (Kucharska-Pietura & Mortimer, 2013; Sergi et al., 2007). Cognitive processes are certainly more complex than the rather simplistic mechanistic understanding that we have been able to achieve over the last several decades of cognitive neuroscience research. Nevertheless, there have been several attempts over the last two decades to develop novel treatment strategies that can specifically address social cognition impairments. This is

certainly a cutting-edge research area with newer strategies being investigated by the day. The following section is a brief overview of the possible treatment avenues:

a. **Cognitive training:** This is an intervention that uses specifically designed and behaviorally constrained cognitive or socioaffective learning events, delivered in a scalable and reproducible manner, to potentially improve neural system operations (Keshavan et al., 2014). The ultimate target is to correct known neural mechanisms of behavioral impairment to result in clinical change. Social cognitive training is typically delivered in several hour-long sessions every week over a period of few months to a year, in conjunction with general cognitive training and social skills training. It is combined with computer-based cognitive exercises and group-based interactive and communicative strategizing and feedback. Efforts are made to scale up the exercises, maintain motivation to learn, and provide bridging exercises to generalize the gains to real world scenarios. There is evidence that such cognitive training exercises change brain structure (Eack et al., 2010a). Facial emotion recognition and ToM abilities are the most likely to change with modest effect sizes according to a recent review (Kurtz et al., 2016). The effect on negative symptoms is also significant, but not so pronounced on delusions and similar positive symptoms.

b. **Cognitive behavioral therapy for psychosis:** This is a structured, time-bound therapy that establishes links between thoughts, emotions and behaviors, and challenges dysfunctional thoughts. It is mainly used in the treatment of resistant delusions, by correcting the deviant social cognitive processes. The administration of such therapies, as in cognitive training requires skilled manpower and is delivered over several weeks or months. The focus here is to identify key targets in a collaborative manner, and facilitate insight by means of cognitive challenging, logical questioning and behavioral experiments. Principles of formation of delusions based on social cognitive theories of a deviant ToM (hyper-mentalizing) and self-serving or externalizing attributional bias (Abu-Akel, 1999) are also used to understand and then correct the dysfunctional thought pattern. Empirical studies leading to meta-analysis, however, demonstrate minor gains on primary outcomes, such as delusions, but better gains on secondary outcomes like depression and general psychopathology (Hazell et al., 2016, Jauhar et al., 2014). It is therefore important to refine the therapy methods and perhaps examine alternative therapeutic options. This brings us to alternative strategies, which as of today are promising, but have limited evidence. These include non-invasive brain stimulation techniques like transcranial magnetic stimulation (TMS) and transcranial direct current stimulation (tDCS), intranasal oxytocin therapy and traditional life-style practices like yoga.

c. **Intranasal oxytocin:** Emerging evidence on the neurochemical basis of social cognition comes from the study of evolutionarily conserved neuropeptides—oxytocin and vasopressin. These nonapeptides interact with dopaminergic neurons in the nucleus accumbens and ventral tegmental areas to regulate complex social information processing and responses (Young & Wang, 2004). Specifically, oxytocin plays a crucial role in social recognition, social motivation and response to social threat, while vasopressin facilitates social responsiveness and social memory (Skuse & Gallagher, 2009).

A recent study demonstrated reduced plasma vasopressin levels in patients with schizophrenia compared to healthy subjects, and lack of association between plasma oxytocin levels and social cognition performance in patients and their relatives unlike the positive correlation observed in healthy subjects (Rubin et al., 2014). Another study also found lack of association between plasma oxytocin levels and social cognition in schizophrenia patients without delusions (Walss-Bass et al., 2013). This suggests a disruption in the ability of oxytocin to modulate social cognition in patients with schizophrenia. Moreover, intranasal oxytocin has been shown to enhance mirror neuron activity (Perry et al., 2010) in healthy subjects and social cognition ability in patients with schizophrenia (Davis et al., 2014; De Berardis et al., 2013; Gibson et al., 2014). Thus, a dysregulated oxytocin-vasopressin system (Rubin et al., 2014) may mediate social cognition deficits in schizophrenia. In this context, intranasal oxytocin has been examined either as a stand-alone treatment or in combination with social cognition or social skills training in individuals with schizophrenia and autism. While single doses do improve recognition of basic facial emotions in healthy individuals, there are either weak or no definitive improvements on ToM and emotion processing tasks in clinical populations according to recent meta-analyses (Leppanen et al., 2017; Ooi et al., 2017). However, there might be merit in combining intranasal oxytocin with conventional cognitive training sessions to leverage an additive effect of both treatments as has been examined in more recent but limited number of studies (Cacciotti-Saija et al., 2015; Gibson et al., 2014), whose results are promising but not conclusive.

d. **Non-invasive brain stimulation:** Both TMS and tDCS are noninvasive neuromodulatory techniques that utilize magnetic or weak electrical stimulation of focal brain regions to either suppress or activate the underlying cortical structures and their trans-synaptic connections (Hoy & Fitzgerald, 2010). This provides an avenue to modulate brain function by application of the magnetic or weak electrical stimulation based on our current understanding of neural network dysfunction in specific psychiatric disorders. For example, anodal tDCS (facilitating activation) of the right orbitofrontal (ventromedial) prefrontal cortex, when compared to sham stimulation resulted in better facial emotion recognition in a group of healthy individuals (Willis et al., 2015). Similarly, another study demonstrated anodal tDCS to the right dorsolateral prefrontal cortex (DLPFC) and cathodal tDCS to the left DLPFC resulting in faster facial emotion recognition in male healthy volunteers when compared to sham stimulation (Conson et al., 2015). In patients with schizophrenia, a single session of bilateral DLPFC anodal tDCS improved facial emotion processing (Rassovsky et al., 2015). Though these are promising findings, no definitive conclusions can be drawn as the evidence is limited to single session treatments with poor data on durability of effects and their generalizability to social functioning. In the only randomized controlled trial of high frequency TMS (facilitating activation) delivered to the left DLPFC, schizophrenia patients receiving true TMS (10 sessions) showed significant improvements in facial emotion recognition abilities when compared to sham TMS. However, there was no generalizability of these changes on social behavior and symptom outcomes (Wolwer et al., 2014). TMS is now also being used in clinical trials of autism. A clinical trial using deep TMS

(2 weeks) delivered to the bilateral medial prefrontal cortices reported significant gains on social behaviors in adults with autism spectrum disorders when compared to sham TMS (Enticott et al., 2014). A potential site for delivering TMS or tDCS that activates the underlying cortex is the anterior mirror neuron system comprised of the ventral premotor cortex and the inferior frontal gyrus. In a randomized controlled trial of single session, high frequency TMS delivered to the left inferior frontal gyrus, we demonstrated greater mirror neuron system activity in the true group when compared to the sham group of healthy individuals (Mehta et al., 2015). This also replicated our earlier findings of a similar TMS protocol improving mirror neuron system activity in a healthy subject (Mehta et al., 2013). Future studies can examine if repeated sessions of TMS to these regions can improve social cognition in clinical populations. In summary, both TMS and tDCS have been used as novel therapeutic strategies to improve social cognition. The evidence from both these techniques are only preliminary and further refinements are the need of the hour.

e. **Yoga therapy:** Yoga is a multicomponent practice that involves physical postures and exercise, breath regulation techniques, deep relaxation practice and meditation/mindfulness techniques involving attention control (Khalsa, 2013; Rao et al., 2013). While earlier studies have demonstrated the utility of yoga therapy in improving social connectedness (Kinser et al., 2013), depression (Cramer et al., 2013) and negative symptoms of schizophrenia (Duraiswamy et al., 2007; Manjunath et al., 2013), recent studies have examined its effect on specific social cognitive processes. It is likely that yoga therapy improves facial emotion recognition and ToM deficits in schizophrenia. Two studies from the National Institute of Mental Health and Neuro Sciences (NIMHANS), Bengaluru, have demonstrated improvements in emotion recognition ability of patients who received yoga with effect sizes ranging from 0.6 (Behere et al., 2011) to 0.8 (Jayaram et al., 2013). Both these studies employed a randomized controlled design and compared the yoga intervention to physical exercise and/or a treatment-as-usual in a waitlist group. Effects on social cognition in both these studies were observed as early as 1–2 months of yoga therapy. These findings were recently replicated in yet another study that examined other domains of social cognition like social cue detection and ToM. In this study, yoga not only improved all domains of social cognition over a period of 20-sessions delivered over 4–6 weeks, but also improved social behavior (negative symptoms) and real world functional outcomes (Shalini, 2017). Given the effectiveness and feasibility of yoga therapy, this is the most clinically feasible and effective treatment of social cognition deficits in our opinion. Yoga therapy for social cognition deficits is now in the process of being put to regular clinical use at NIMHANS in a graded manner. This is not just for individuals with schizophrenia but also for patients with other neuropsychiatric disorders—adults with autism, social deficits following traumatic brain injury and borderline personality disorder. Possible neurobiological mechanisms through which yoga improves social cognition are discussed in a recent review article (Mehta et al., 2016). In summary, learning and performing coordinated physical postures (asanas) with a teacher facilitates imitation and the process of being imitated. This two-way process can improve social cognition and empathy through reinforcement of the premotor and parietal mirror neuron system (Radhakrishna et al., 2010). Oxytocin may play a role in mediating these processes that further lead to better social connectedness and social outcomes (Aoki & Yamasue, 2015; Jayaram et al., 2013).

CONCLUSION

Most neuropsychiatric disorders have a common impairment in social cognition, which results in abnormal social behaviors. In the more severe disorders, these impairments (deficient or deviant) also predict real world functional outcomes. Social cognition has specific domains based on the underlying neural processes, and a broad range of deficit patterns are expressed across individual neuropsychiatric disorders. Correcting or retraining these impairments requires us to employ a biopsychosocial approach. The management begins with performing detailed assessments within a sociocultural framework using culturally valid rating instruments. It also requires a thorough understanding of the putative neural networks underlying the individual's clinical condition presenting with social cognition impairments. A thorough assessment of social behavior and social functioning is also necessary. Based on the above assessments—cognitive, behavioral, and neurobiological, a comprehensive treatment plan can be planned. Treatment options range from cognitive therapies to brain stimulation and novel pharmacotherapy using oxytocin and traditional yoga therapy. Among the various therapies, the best evidence so far is for yoga therapy and this is now gradually being introduced in routine clinical practice. Given the costs of brain stimulation and oxytocin and the manpower intensive requirements of cognitive therapies, yoga therapy also seems to be a more feasible therapeutic option. A concerted biopsychosocial understanding of how yoga therapy works includes the behavioral processes of imitating others and being imitated by others, which through the possible effects of oxytocin enhances the mirroring networks of the performer's brain resulting in better social cognition. Future investigations will build on these preliminary leads, and continue to explore within a biopsychosocial framework better therapeutic avenues for patients with severe neuropsychiatric disorders. These include refining the current treatment options, innovating to develop more advanced therapies (for example, better pharmacotherapy) and integrating the above treatment options to leverage additive benefits in a rational and scientifically guided manner.

ACKNOWLEDGMENT

Dr Mehta is supported by the Wellcome Trust/DBT India Alliance Early Career Fellowship (Grant No. IA/E/12/1/500755).

REFERENCES

Abu-Akel A. Impaired theory of mind in schizophrenia. Prag Cogn. 1999;7:247-82.

Allison T, Puce A, McCarthy G. Social perception from visual cues: role of the STS region. Trends Cogn Sci. 2000;4(7):267-78.

Aoki Y, Yamasue H. Reply: Does imitation act as an oxytocin nebulizer in autism spectrum disorder? Brain. 2015;138:e361.

Behere RV, Arasappa R, Jagannathan A, et al. Effect of yoga therapy on facial emotion recognition deficits, symptoms and functioning in patients with schizophrenia. Acta Psychiatr Scand. 2011;123:147-53.

Behere RV, Raghunandan V, Venkatasubramanian G, et al. Trends—a tool for recognition of emotions in neuropsychiatric disorders. Indian J Psychol Med. 2008;30:32-8.

Bentall RP, Rowse G, Shryane N, et al. The cognitive and affective structure of paranoid delusions: a trans-diagnostic investigation of patients with schizophrenia spectrum disorders and depression. Arch Gen Psychiatry. 2009;66:236-47.

Bhagyavathi HD, Mehta UM, Thirthalli J, et al. Cascading and combined effects of cognitive deficits and residual symptoms on functional outcome in schizophrenia. A path-analytical approach. Psychiatry Res. 2015;229:264-71.

Blacher J. Assessing social cognition in young mentally retarded and nonretarded children. Am J Ment Defic. 1982;86:473-84.

Blackwood NJ, Bentall RP, ffytche DH, et al. Self-responsibility and the self-serving bias: an fMRI investigation of causal attributions. Neuroimage. 2003;20:1076-85.

Burns J. The social brain hypothesis of schizophrenia. World Psychiatry. 2006a;5:77-81.

Burns JK. Psychosis: a costly by-product of social brain evolution in Homo sapiens. Prog Neuropsycho-pharmacol Biol Psychiatry. 2006b;30:797-814.

Cacciotti-Saija C, Langdon R, Ward PB, et al. A double-blind randomized controlled trial of oxytocin nasal spray and social cognition training for young people with early psychosis. Schizophr Bull. 2015;41:483-93.

Chandler MJ: Social cognition and life-span approaches to the study of child development. Adv Child Dev Behav. 1976;11:225-39.

Conson M, Errico D, Mazzarella E, et al. Transcranial electrical stimulation over dorsolateral prefrontal cortex modulates processing of social cognitive and affective information. PLoS One. 2015;10:e0126448.

Corrigan PW, Green MF. Schizophrenic patients' sensitivity to social cues: the role of abstraction. Am J Psychiatry. 1993;150:589-94.

Cramer H, Lauche R, Langhorst J, et al. Yoga for depression: a systematic review and meta-analysis. Depress Anxiety. 2013;30:1068-83.

Davis MC, Green MF, Lee J, et al. Oxytocin-augmented social cognitive skills training in schizophrenia. Neuropsychopharmacol. 2014;39:2070-77.

Dawson G, Fernald M. Perspective-taking ability and its relationship to the social behavior of autistic children. J Autism Dev Disord. 1987;17:487-98.

De Berardis D, Marini S, Iasevoli F, et al. The role of intranasal oxytocin in the treatment of patients with schizophrenia: a systematic review. CNS Neurol Disord Drug Targets. 2013;12:252-64.

Dennett DC. Brainstorm: Philosophical Essays on Mind and Psychology. Cambridge:MIT Press; 1978.

Derntl B, Habel U. Deficits in social cognition: a marker for psychiatric disorders? Eur Arch Psychiatry Clin Neurosci. 2011;261 (Suppl) 2:S145-9.

Duraiswamy G, Thirthalli J, Nagendra HR, et al. Yoga therapy as an add-on treatment in the management of patients with schizophrenia—a randomized controlled trial. Acta Psychiatr Scand. 2007;116: 226-32.

Eack SM, Hogarty GE, Cho RY, et al. Neuroprotective effects of cognitive enhancement therapy against gray matter loss in early schizophrenia: results from a 2-year randomized controlled trial. Arch Gen Psychiatry. 2010a;67:674-82.

Eack SM, Hogarty GE, Greenwald DP, et al. Cognitive enhancement therapy improves emotional intelli-gence in early course schizophrenia: preliminary effects. Schizophr Res. 2007;89:308-11.

Eack SM, Mermon DE, Montrose DM, et al. Social cognition deficits among individuals at familial high risk for schizophrenia. Schizophr Bull. 2010b;36:1081-8.

Enticott PG, Fitzgibbon BM, Kennedy HA, et al. A double-blind, randomized trial of deep repetitive tran-scranial magnetic stimulation (rTMS) for autism spectrum disorder. Brain Stimul. 2014;7:206-11.

Fett AK, Viechtbauer W, Dominguez MD, et al. The relationship between neurocognition and social cognition with functional outcomes in schizophrenia: a meta-analysis. Neurosci Biobehav Rev. 2011;35:573-88.

Gibson CM, Penn DL, Smedley et al. A pilot six-week randomized controlled trial of oxytocin on social cognition and social skills in schizophrenia. Schizophr Res. 2014;156:261-5.

Gottesman, II, Gould TD. The endophenotype concept in psychiatry: etymology and strategic intentions. Am J Psychiatry. 2003;160:636-45.

Green MF. Cognitive impairment and functional outcome in schizophrenia and bipolar disorder. J Clin Psychiatry. 2006;67:e12.

Green MF, Horan WP, Lee J. Social cognition in schizophrenia. Nat Rev Neurosci. 2015;16:620-31.

Green MF, Olivier B, Crawley JN, et al. Social cognition in schizophrenia: recommendations from the measurement and treatment research to improve cognition in schizophrenia new approaches conference. Schizophr Bull. 2005;31:882-7.

Green MF, Penn DL, Bentall R, et al. Social cognition in schizophrenia: an NIMH workshop on definitions, assessment, and research opportunities. Schizophr Bull. 2008;34:1211-20.

Hao L, Yang J, Wang Y, et al. Neural correlates of causal attribution in negative events of depressed patients: Evidence from an fMRI study. Clin Neurophysiol. 2015;126:1331-7.

Harrington L, Siegert RJ, McClure J. Theory of mind in schizophrenia: a critical review. Cogn Neuropsychiatry. 2005;10:249-86.

Harvey PD, Patterson TL, Potter LS, et al. Improvement in social competence with short-term atypical antipsychotic treatment: a randomized, double-blind comparison of quetiapine versus risperidone for social competence, social cognition, and neuropsychological functioning. Am J Psychiatry. 2006;163:1918-25.

Hazell CM, Hayward M, Cavanagh K, et al. A systematic review and meta-analysis of low intensity CBT for psychosis. Clin Psychol Rev. 2016;45:183-92.

Heider F. On social cognition. Am Psychol. 1967;22:25-31.

Heyes CM. Theory of mind in nonhuman primates. Behav Brain Sci. 1998;21:101-14.

Hoy KE, Fitzgerald PB. Brain stimulation in psychiatry and its effects on cognition. Nat Rev Neurol. 2010;6:267-75.

Jauhar S, McKenna PJ, Radua J, et al. Cognitive-behavioural therapy for the symptoms of schizophrenia: systematic review and meta-analysis with examination of potential bias. Br J Psychiatry. 2014;204:20-9.

Jayaram N, Varambally S, Behere RV, et al. Effect of yoga therapy on plasma oxytocin and facial emotion recognition deficits in patients of schizophrenia. Indian J Psychiatry. 2013;55:S409-13.

Keshavan MS, Vinogradov S, Rumsey J, et al. Cognitive training in mental disorders: update and future directions. Am J Psychiatry. 2014;171:510-22.

Khalsa SB. Yoga for psychiatry and mental health: an ancient practice with modern relevance. Indian J Psychiatry. 2013;55:S334-6.

Kinderman P, Bentall RP. A new measure of causal locus: The internal, personal and situational attributions questionnaire. Pers Individ Dif.. 1996;20:261-4.

Kinser PA, Bourguignon C, Whaley D, et al. Feasibility, acceptability, and effects of gentle Hatha yoga for women with major depression: findings from a randomized controlled mixed-methods study. Arch Psychiatr Nurs. 2013;27:137-47.

Kucharska-Pietura K, Mortimer A. Can antipsychotics improve social cognition in patients with schizophrenia? CNS Drugs. 2013;27:335-43.

Kurtz MM, Gagen E, Rocha NB, et al. Comprehensive treatments for social cognitive deficits in schizophrenia: A critical review and effect-size analysis of controlled studies. Clin Psychol Rev. 2016;43:80-9.

Kurtz MM, Richardson CL. Social cognitive training for schizophrenia: a meta-analytic investigation of controlled research. Schizophr Bull. 2012;38:1092-104.

Lee TY, Hong SB, Shin NY, et al. Social cognitive functioning in prodromal psychosis: A meta-analysis. Schizophr Res. 2015;164:28-34.

Leppanen J, Ng KW, Tchanturia K, et al. Meta-analysis of the effects of intranasal oxytocin on interpretation and expression of emotions. Neurosci Biobehav Rev. 2017;78:125-44.

Manjunath RB, Varambally S, Thirthalli J, et al. Efficacy of yoga as an add-on treatment for in-patients with functional psychotic disorder. Indian J Psychiatry. 2013;55:S374-8.

Mehta UM, Agarwal SM, Kalmady SV, et al. Enhancing putative mirror neuron activity with magnetic stimulation: A single-case functional neuroimaging study. Biol Psychiatry. 2013;74:e1-2.

Mehta UM, Keshavan MS, Gangadhar BN. Bridging the schism of schizophrenia through yoga—review of putative mechanisms. Int Rev Psychiatry. 2016;28:254-64.

Mehta UM, Thirthalli J. External validity of the Social Cognition Rating Tools in Indian Setting. Asian J Psychiatr. 2014;8:106-8.

Mehta UM, Thirthalli J, Basavaraju R, et al. Reduced mirror neuron activity in schizophrenia and its association with theory of mind deficits: evidence from a transcranial magnetic stimulation study. Schizophr Bull. 2014a;40:1083-94.

Mehta UM, Thirthalli J, Bhagyavathi HD, et al. Similar and contrasting dimensions of social cognition in schizophrenia and healthy subjects. Schizophr Res. 2014b;157:70-7.

Mehta UM, Thirthalli J, Gangadhar BN, et al. Need for culture specific tools to assess social cognition in schizophrenia. Schizophr Res. 2011;133:255-6.

Mehta UM, Thirthalli J, Kumar CN, et al. Negative symptoms mediate the influence of theory of mind on functional status in schizophrenia. Soc Psychiatry Psychiatr Epidemiol. 2014c;49:1151-6.

Mehta UM, Thirthalli J, Naveen Kumar C, et al. Schizophrenia patients experience substantial social cognition deficits across multiple domains in remission. Asian J Psychiatry. 2013;6:324-9.

Mehta UM, Thirthalli J, Naveen Kumar C, et al. Validation of Social Cognition Rating Tools in Indian Setting (SOCRATIS): A new test-battery to assess social cognition. Asian J Psychiatry. 2011;4:203-9.

Mehta UM, Waghmare AV, Thirthalli J, et al. Is the human mirror neuron system plastic? Evidence from a transcranial magnetic stimulation study. Asian J Psychiatry. 2015 ;17:71-7.

Ooi YP, Weng SJ, Kossowsky J, et al. Oxytocin and autism spectrum disorders: A systematic review and meta-analysis of randomized controlled trials. Pharmacopsychiatry. 2017;50:5-13.

Park KM, Kim JJ, Ku J, et al. Neural basis of attributional style in schizophrenia. Neurosci Lett. 2009;459: 35-40.

Perry A, Bentin S, Shalev I, et al. Intranasal oxytocin modulates EEG mu/alpha and beta rhythms during perception of biological motion. Psychoneuroendocrinol. 2010;35:1446-53.

Premack DG, Woodruff G. Does the chimpanzee have a theory of mind? Behav Brain Sci. 1978:515-26.

Radhakrishna S, Nagarathna R, Nagendra HR. Integrated approach to yoga therapy and autism spectrum disorders. J Ayurveda Integr Med. 2010;1:120-4.

Rao NP, Varambally S, Gangadhar BN. Yoga school of thought and psychiatry: Therapeutic potential. Indian J Psychiatry. 2013;55:S145-9.

Rassovsky Y, Dunn W, Wynn J, et al. The effect of transcranial direct current stimulation on social cognition in schizophrenia: a preliminary study. Schizophr Res. 2015;165:171-4.

Rose EJ, Hargreaves A, Morris D, et al. Effects of a novel schizophrenia risk variants 7914558 at CNNM2 on brain structure and attributional style. Br J Psychiatry. 2014;204(2):115-21.

Rubin LH, Carter CS, Bishop JR, et al. Reduced levels of vasopressin and reduced behavioral modulation of oxytocin in psychotic disorders. Schizophr Bull. 2014;40:1374-84.

Sergi MJ, Green MF, Widmark C, et al. Social cognition [corrected] and neurocognition: effects of risperidone, olanzapine, and haloperidol. Am J Psychiatry. 2007;164:1585-92.

Shalini N. Effect of add-on yoga therapy on social cognition deficits and mirror neuron activity in patients with schizophrenia—a single blind randomized controlled trial. MD dissertation submitted to the Department of Psychiatry. National Institute of Mental Health & Neurosciences (NIMHANS), Bengaluru; 2017.

Skuse DH, Gallagher L. Dopaminergic-neuropeptide interactions in the social brain. Trends Cogn Sci. 2009;13:27-35.

van Donkersgoed RJ, Wunderink L, Nieboer R, et al. Social Cognition in Individuals at Ultra-High Risk for Psychosis: A Meta-Analysis. PLoS One. 2015;10:e0141075.

Vos T, Flaxman AD, Naghavi M, et al. Years lived with disability (YLDs) for 1160 sequelae of 289 diseases and injuries 1990-2010: a systematic analysis for the Global Burden of Disease Study 2010. Lancet. 2012;380:2163-96.

Wais M. [Disturbances of the social cognition in right-hemisphere brain-damaged patients]. Fortschr Neurol Psychiatr. 1982;50:203-6.

Walss-Bass C, Fernandes JM, Roberts DL, et al. Differential correlations between plasma oxytocin and social cognitive capacity and bias in schizophrenia. Schizophr Res. 2013;147:387-92.

Willis ML, Murphy JM, Ridley NJ, et al. Anodal tDCS targeting the right orbitofrontal cortex enhances facial expression recognition. Soc Cogn Affect Neurosci. 2015;10:1677-83.

Wolwer W, Lowe A, Brinkmeyer J, et al. Repetitive transcranial magnetic stimulation (rTMS) improves facial affect recognition in schizophrenia. Brain Stimul. 2014;7:559-63.

Yalcin-Siedentopf N, Hoertnagl CM, Biedermann F, et al. Facial affect recognition in symptomatically remitted patients with schizophrenia and bipolar disorder. Schizophr Res. 2014;152:440-5.

Young LJ, Wang Z. The neurobiology of pair bonding. Nat Neurosci. 2004;7:1048-54.

Chapter 8

Social Determinants of Behavior

Rajesh Sagar, Rishi Gupta

SUMMARY

An "organism" is a biological system, and "behavior" is any work performed by this system. The sciences of psychiatry and psychology have long tried to make sense of this complex entity in an attempt to better understand it, and treat those cases which exhibit deviant and maladaptive patterns of behavior. In a bid to understand human behavior, as with all other aspects of medical science, the debate of nature versus nurture has emerged. Determinants of behavior may be biological, i.e. a person's genes may determine what his pattern of behavior may be in a specific situation. Alternatively, they may be social. These social determinants of behavior are what this chapter concerns itself with. Social determinants of behavior may broadly be divided into how we perceive and process social influences, how social factors affect us, and how we interact with the society. We begin by elaborating upon attitudes, which are set patterns of perceiving, processing, assessing, and responding to social situations. We touch upon the role of cognitive dissonance, and how it shapes our behavior, and the role of persuasion in molding our attitudes and behavior. We then look at the role of attribution and biases, and how these affect our perception of the social world. We elaborate on the role of stereotypes and prejudices in determining our behavior toward people who are similar and dissimilar to us. Finally, we look at the role of conformity, imitation, obedience, and attraction in human social interactions.

INTRODUCTION

Human behavior has been one of the key subjects of study in the sciences of psychiatry and psychology. Explaining normal and abnormal behavior remains one of their primary goals. More specifically, the science of psychology has concerned itself with determining the origins and determinants of human behavior in all its vastness. In pursuing these goals, the ubiquitous debate of nature versus nurture has emerged, dividing the determinants of behavior into biological and social.

The proponents of biological determinism propose that human behavior arises out of innate traits, established by a person's genetic makeup, and the myriad of physiological processes that comprise the human being. It has long been observed that children exhibit behavior similar to parents, and that personality traits are, at least in part, inherited (Horn et al., 1976). The genetic basis has been established for a range of adaptive and maladaptive human behaviors, including aggression and substance use (Lindzey et al., 1971). Numerous studies have also linked different human behaviors with different neurobiological paradigms, and several behavioral syndromes have been associated with the dysfunction of specific brain areas. Klüver–Bucy syndrome, arising out of a damaged amygdala, is probably the most distinctive example of this proposition (Lilly et al., 1983).

On the flip side of the coin, the proponents of the "nurture" theory of human behavior maintain that most human behavior arises out of socially determined factors, and that a person is what the society makes him to be. It is this view that we shall be elaborating upon in this chapter.

It is difficult to imagine life in isolation. Human beings are inherently social organisms, so-much-so that solitary confinement is one of the most severe forms of punishment mankind has invented. Ever since birth, the baby's life is intricately intertwined with those around him. Since a very young age, children observe their parents and elders and learn to mimic their behaviors. Initially, this mimicking is without understanding, but as abstract thought develops, the process of social learning sets in (Bandura & Walters, 1963), molding the way a child and teenager behaves. On several occasions, the child is instructed by parents as to what is the appropriate and expected behavior in a particular situation, and thus is highlighted the role of obedience. For example, in several subcultures of the Indian society, children are taught to touch their elders' feet or fold their hands to greet "*Namaste*", and this early teaching becomes the basis of one of the hallmarks of a behavior specific to the Indian society. As the child enters teenage, (s)he is subject to yet another strong behavioral driving force, i.e. conformity. They tend to behave as their peers do, whether the behavior is adaptive or maladaptive. Gradually, as they grow older, people develop their own attitudes, prejudices and stereotypes, and these broadly govern their interaction with the society. Eventually, it is a complex interaction of all these processes which determine the behavior of a particular individual.

One way to make sense of these numerous processes is to categorize them into:

1. How we perceive and process social situations (social perception and cognition, comprising of attitudes, stereotypes, prejudices, attribution, biases, and other cognitive processes which help us make sense of the world around us, e.g. counterfactual thinking)?
2. How social factors affect us (e.g. conformity, obedience, imitation, and leadership)?
3. How we interact with the society (e.g. attraction, social transactions, group dynamics, and prosocial behavior)?

Culture and religion too are an integral part of the society. However, we shall refrain from elaborating on these topics, as these have been covered in dedicated chapters elsewhere in the book (see Chapter 12 on Culture, Mythology, and Religion). What follows is an elaboration of some of the major social determinants of human behavior?

ATTITUDES

Most simply put, attitudes are the methods we employ to evaluate and respond to all objects, events and situations in our social world (Kassin et al., 2011). Attitudes have a cognitive, emotional, and a behavioral component. Take for example the attitude of people toward exercise. Someone might think that "exercise is good for general well-being" (cognition). They might feel that they enjoy exercising (emotion). Finally, they might go to a gymnasium every day (behavior). This collective cognitive and emotional evaluation of the concept of exercise, along with the associated behavior, is the "attitude" of one particular person toward exercise.

Attitudes develop through different types of learning, including classical conditioning, operant conditioning, and observational learning. The most important of these is the process of social or observational learning—learning by observing one's social environment.

A common example of the development of a specific attitude by classical conditioning is product advertisements. Advertisers pair their product with an attractive or known celebrity, thus creating a positive affective link between the two. This fact that a positive affect generated during advertising is directly transferred onto the product, regardless of the beliefs related to the product, has long been established (Gresham & Shimp, 1985). It has also been demonstrated that the observer need not even be aware that he is being presented with stimuli for classical conditioning in order for attitudes to be effectively modified. Such presentation of stimuli is called *subliminal conditioning*. In one such study, participants were shown pairs of words for a brief period, and were asked to indicate whether or not there was a dot present above or below the words. In reality, the two words in each pair were a word for drinking water and a word with a positive connotation. The authors noticed that even though the participants did not know that they were being subjected to classical conditioning, after the task they were more likely to request a drink of water than the control group, thus demonstrating the phenomenon of subliminal conditioning (Veltkamp et al., 2011). An even more subtle method exists, called *mere exposure* (Bornstein & D'Agostino, 1992), in which a stimulus is presented for a duration too short for the memory of the stimulus to be formed. It has been shown that even with mere exposure, positive attitudes can be formed.

Operant conditioning too plays an important role in the formation of attitudes. Ever since childhood, expressing the "correct" views leads to verbal and nonverbal positive reinforcement, and indeed it has been shown that at least in the first 10–15 years of their life, children express views similar to those of their parents, following which they do the same for their peers (Oskamp & Schultz, 2005). Finally, attitudes can be formed by observational learning (Bandura & Walters, 1963), that is, we learn merely by seeing others, seen commonly amongst the adolsecents.

It has been demonstrated that attitudes themselves are not the sole determinants of behavior, but are rather subject to social constraints like norms. That is, people do not always behave exactly according to their attitudes, but mold their responses according to what the situation allows. A meta-analysis of 797 studies totaling 1001 effect sizes found that the mean correlation between attitude and behavior fell by ~30% when social pressure and difficulty of behavior were raised to 1 standard deviation above the mean (Wallace et al., 2005). Another aspect which modulates our behavior concerning our attitudes in social situations is pluralistic ignorance (Geisinger, 2005). Pluralistic ignorance is the phenomenon in which people believe that others around them hold a different attitude toward a situation than they do, and thus they curb their default behavior which was to arise out of their own attitude.

The fact that social situations affect behavioral expressions of attitudes is demonstrated well by the Hawthorne effect (a positive social interaction between the clinician and the respondent affects the responses of the respondent) (McCarney et al., 2007), and the Halo effect (the response of the subject is affected by his preconceived notions) (Nisbett & Wilson, 1977).

When people behave in a manner different than what is accorded by their attitudes, the distressful state which is induced is called cognitive dissonance (Festinger, 1962).

COGNITIVE DISSONANCE

A person may not agree with all the ideas of his colleagues, but still praises them when asked to evaluate these ideas. This is a natural human tendency, and is usually done in order to prevent conflict, despite the fact that such an expression of praise itself conflicts with the person's own attitude. This conflict leads to the state of cognitive dissonance. It has been demonstrated that we try to minimize cognitive dissonance (Elliot & Devine, 1994). People may do this via different methods. They may change their behavior, for example, convince themselves that their colleague's idea is not so bad. They may add new information, which might help improve their perception of the situation, or they may trivialize the entire event (Simon et al., 1995). Also, it has been shown that people might engage in the process of self-affirmation (Elliot & Devine, 1994), in which they focus on alternative positive self-attributes, thus negating the distressful state induced by cognitive dissonance.

Another observation which has been made with regards to cognitive dissonance is that peoples' attitudes are more likely to change if the incentive for behaving in a deviant manner is small. If the incentive is large, then the incentive itself is recognized as the reason for the deviant behavior, while if the incentive is small, it is inadequate in itself to nullify cognitive dissonance, and thus, a greater attitude change is brought about to reduce cognitive dissonance.

PERSUASION

Persuasion is the process of changing someone's attitude and eventually the behavior (Hovland et al., 1953). Extensive research has been carried out in the field of persuasion, especially in the context of advertising. It has been shown that when experts deliver the same message, it is more persuasive than when non-experts deliver it. People are more prone to be persuaded if they are not completely paying attention to the process of persuasion, but are distracted in some manner. The messages, which are not recognized as having the goal of changing attitudes, are more likely to do so, rather than those which clearly attempt to do so. Attractive sources are more likely to be successful at persuasion, and rapid delivery of information is better at changing attitudes (Briñol & Petty, 2009). Finally, strong emotions, like fear, induce a much more effective and rapid attitude change (Bourne, 2010).

It has been proposed that there are two primary processes by which social information is processed. The first model is called the *elaboration likelihood model* (Petty et al., 2002). In this model, also called the direct route of information processing, the subject pays full attention to the information that is being presented to him and processes it rationally and systematically. It has been shown that when this route is being employed, the credibility of the arguments which are being provided is the main decisive factor for whether attitude change will take place or not (Bhattacherjee & Sanford, 2006). This method takes more effort and is employed when a greater amount of time is available, or when the topic under evaluation is of greater salience. The *heuristic-systematic model* (Todorov et al., 2002), based on the peripheral route of information processing, utilizes less energy and time, and is employed when the subject is distracted, or the topic does not hold much salience. When this process is employed, the attributes of the presenter hold more significance in changing attitudes, than the actual validity of the arguments.

Thus, we see that attitudes determine the default behaviors we may exhibit in specific situations, how social constraints prevent these behaviors leading to cognitive dissonance, and how the act of persuasion can change someone's attitudes, and eventually, their behavior. Next, we see how the phenomena of attribution, stereotyping, and prejudice affect behavior.

ATTRIBUTION AND BIASES

One of the primary goals of social cognition is to explain others' behavior, so that one may be able to predict their future behavior, and thus respond adequately and appropriately. Attribution is the process by which a person ascribes a reason to someone else's behavior, and thus characterizes and categorizes them. For example, if we see a person shouting at a cashier in a department store, we might ascribe the characteristics of "irritable" and "impatient" to that person. This in turn helps us modulate our behavior with respect to that person in the future, should the need to interact with that person arise.

In "native" psychology, it has been described that humans often attempt to ascribe any observed behavior to either personal or environmental factors (Heider, 1982). If the behavior is attributed to environmental factors, less significance is attached to it than if it is attributed to personal factors. Kelley's attribution theory carries this forward and describes three factors, based upon which it is determined whether to attribute behaviors to internal or external factors (Bonaccorsi & Piccaluga, 1994). These three factors are "consistency," "consensus," and "distinctiveness." "Consistency" of responses is judged over time and situations. "Consensus" is whether other people respond in a similar manner to the same situation. "Distinctiveness" is the property of reacting to similar situations in a different manner by the same person. If all three factors are high, then the behavior is attributed to external factors. For example, in the situation as mentioned earlier, where some person is shouting at the cashier, if that person shouts at most cashiers, if other people too shout at the same cashier, and if that person does not shout at other people in the same store, then it is assumed that there is some external factor motivating this behavior. On the other hand, if consistency is high, but consensus and distinctiveness are low, then the behavior is attributed to personal factors. For example, if that person shouts at most cashiers, other people do not shout at that cashier, and the person shouts at most people in that shop, then it is assumed that this behavior stems from his personal factors. Thus, attribution is an important determinant of human behavior, especially in social situations.

The judgment drawn during the process of attribution is not always accurate though. For example, in the previously mentioned situation, though we ascribe the characteristic "irritable" to the person in question, the case may be that the cashier has actually made some serious mistake and that the person's behavior is justified. This brings us to the concept of *bias*. In the situation mentioned above, we may falsely overestimate the significance of personal factors in the person's behavior, when in reality the source was entirely environmental. This type of bias is called *correspondence bias,* also known as *fundamental attribution error* (Reeder, 2013). It has been shown that this type of bias varies with culture. More individualistic societies like the Western societies tend to attribute behaviors to dispositional traits rather than situational traits, while more collectivistic societies like Asian societies tend to do the reverse, i.e. attribute behaviors to the situation rather than the person (Choi & Nisbett, 1998). Another type of bias which has been observed is the *self-serving bias* (Forsyth, 2008). In this type of bias, humans tend to attribute behaviors with a positive outcome to themselves and behaviors with negative outcomes to situational factors. For example, performing well in one's job is attributed to oneself, while performing poorly is attributed to poor working conditions. It has also been noted that this bias also extends to those, whom we identify as similar to ourselves, for example, our community.

STEREOTYPES, PREJUDICES, AND DISCRIMINATION

Stereotypes are set patterns and schemas of prejudgment, which are heuristically used to assess any given person or event. We often tend to judge the social situations and events by stereotypes. The affective components of these cognitive prejudgments are called prejudices. The behavioral manifestations thereof are called acts of discrimination. Stereotyping, prejudices, and discrimination are parts of strong negative attitudes toward members of specific groups, based only on the fact that they are members of that group (Perkins, 1992). Several different explanations for the origin of such attitudes have been put forth.

The *realistic conflict theory* (Brief et al., 2005) states that due to the paucity of values commodities, resources, and conveniences, that are coveted by most people, there is a natural conflict between them. They thus tend to discriminate against members of other groups inherently. Another source of prejudice is what is sometimes called the ultimate attribution error (Pettigrew, 1979). In this phenomenon, we tend to classify everyone as "us" and "them," and we tend to treat the members of the "us" group more favorably than the "them" group. A third way in which prejudices may develop is through observational learning. Children may see their parents behave in a discriminatory manner toward a particular community, and thus behave similarly.

These attitudes of stereotyping and prejudice are an important behavioral driving force in social situations.

IMITATION AND CONFORMITY

Human beings have a natural inborn tendency to imitate others. A child will imitate his elders by making similar sounds and similar gestures. A teenager will imitate his peers and other influential people by engaging in similar behaviors.

Conformity is the act of adjusting one's beliefs and behavior to better match the society one is present in. In this pursuit, one is guided by *rules* and *social norms* (Cialdini & Goldstein, 2004). These norms may be *descriptive norms* or *injunctive norms*. Descriptive norms are those norms which guide a person about the general manner in which people behave. For example, it is expected that a child will behave in a respectable manner to his elders. In contrast, injunctive norms are specific instructions, as to what is and is not acceptable behavior in a particular situation; for example, signs telling drivers not to honk their horns in the vicinity of a school or a hospital. Norms and rules can be as informal, as a friend telling others the time at which he expects to meet them at his house. Conversely, they may be as formal as the written law of the land, wherein one might invite punishment for deviating from the same.

It has been demonstrated that the pressure to conform to others can even affect one's own judgment. In a classical social experiment, participants were asked to compare the length of three lines with that of a standard and choose which one of the lines was of the same length. When they were asked to perform this exercise alone, they responded with almost perfect accuracy. However, when they were grouped with 7–8 other people, all of whom were trained to point at the wrong line, the accuracy of response of the original respondents went down to 67% (Asch, 1956). This experiment highlighted how we are prone to alter our judgment under the pressure of conformity, even though we are capable of making perfectly valid decisions on our own. Thus, conformity too is an important determinant of human social behavior.

OBEDIENCE

In certain social situations, one person of a higher stature than another may instruct the other to do something, and the second person is obligated to follow that instruction. This is called obedience. Obedience was classically demonstrated in the Milgram experiments (Milgram, 1974). Prof Stanley Milgram of Yale University wanted to find out whether people are willing to inflict harm upon others only as a result of following orders, and if so, to what degree. He designed an experiment, in which participants were invited under the charade of testing for memory. Each experimental setup consisted of the instructor (the authority figure), the "teacher," who was the real subject under study, and the "learner," whom the teacher thought to be another participant, but in reality, was a confederate in the experiment. Through a rigged draw of lots, it was ensured that the participant under study always received the role of "teacher." He was instructed that he was to read out pairs of words, and then was to ask the "learner" to name the second word of a pair, after naming the first word. The "learner," who was strapped in a chair, was to answer by pressing a button. The teacher was told that if the learner's answers are wrong, he has to give the learner an electric shock, in increments of 15 volts, by pressing a button. The teacher was also given a sample gentle shock to demonstrate what the learner would initially feel. The learner, of course, was to receive no shocks but was supposed to emulate being electrocuted by playing back sounds of agony using a tape recorder. The outcome was the final voltage till which the "teachers" would be willing to give the electric shock. If the teacher tried to stop in between, he was given verbal cues like "you must continue," "you cannot stop," and only if he asked to stop despite four verbal cues was the experiment stopped. A pre-experiment poll of students and professors revealed that they thought only ~4% of the participants would be willing to go to the theoretical maximum of 450 volts. However, the results of the experiment revealed that a shocking 67% of the participants gave the "learner" shocks of up to 450 volts. Though most participants protested, most of them continued under the verbal commands of the instructor, who was established as the authority figure. This experiment shows the importance of obedience in the society, and to what lengths of deviant behavior people are willing to go, just because they are following orders. Psychologists have suggested that there may be several reasons for this obedience and conformity. These include social comparison processes, avoiding social disapproval, and the need to be liked and accepted (Hamilton & Biggart, 1985).

INTERPERSONAL ATTRACTION

The extent to which we like or dislike each other is probably one of the strongest motivators of human social behavior. It is important to understand the determinants of this attraction. It has long been known that familiarity, similarity, and proximity play a significant role in the development of attraction. Zajonc described the repeated exposure effect, which states that the more frequently one is exposed to a person, object or idea, the more is one's tendency to evaluate them positively (Zajonc, 1965). Similarly, a recent meta-analysis of 468 effect sizes has demonstrated that similarity between two people has a strong correlation with the interpersonal attraction between them. It has long been demonstrated that interpersonal attraction is stronger when the person is experiencing a positive affect (Izard, 1960). Last, but not the least, is the importance of physical attractiveness. Research findings indeed indicate that there is a strong positive correlation between physical beauty and interpersonal attraction (Luo & Zhang, 2009).

CONCLUSION

There are innumerable social determinants of behavior, the most important of which have been summarized in the text above. Hence, the complex process of human behavior is determined by personal factors, environmental factors, and factors which determine the interaction of these two. Also, not to be discounted are the biological determinants of behavior, which alter each person's behavior is a manner unique to that person. Understanding these factors will help us better devise strategies for intervening in cases of maladaptive behavior, a task central to our science.

REFERENCES

Asch SE. Studies of independence and conformity: I. A minority of one against a unanimous majority. Psychol Med Monogr Suppl. 1956;70(9):1-70.

Bandura A, Walters RH. Social Learning and Personality Development. New York: Holt, Rinehart and Winston; 1963.

Bhattacherjee A, Sanford C. Influence processes for information technology acceptance: An elaboration likelihood model. MIS Quarterly. 2006;30(4):805-25.

Bonaccorsi A, Piccaluga A. A theoretical framework for the evaluation of university-industry relationships. R&D Management. 1994;24(3):229-47.

Bornstein RF, D'Agostino PR. Stimulus recognition and the mere exposure effect. J Pers Soc Psychol. 1992;63(4):545-52.

Bourne A. The Role of Fear in HIV Prevention. Sigma Research. 2010.

Brief AP, Umphress EE, Dietz J, et al. Community matters: Realistic group conflict theory and the impact of diversity. Acad Manage J. 2005;48(5):830-44.

Briñol P, Petty RE. Source factors in persuasion: a self-validation approach. Eur Rev Soc Psychol. 2009; 20:49-96.

Choi I, Nisbett RE. Situational salience and cultural differences in the correspondence bias and actor-observer bias. Pers Soc Psychol Bull. 1998;24(9):949-60.

Cialdini RB, Goldstein NJ. Social influence: compliance and conformity. Annu Rev Psychol. 2004;55: 591-621.

Elliot AJ, Devine PG. On the motivational nature of cognitive dissonance. J Pers Soc Psychol. 1994;67(3):382-94.

Festinger L. A Theory of Cognitive Dissonance. Stanford University Press; 1962.

Forsyth DR. Self-serving bias. International Encyclopedia of the Social Sciences. 2008;7:429.

Geisinger A. Are norms efficient? Pluralistic ignorance, heuristics and the use of norms as private regulation. Alabama Law Review. 2005;57(1):1-30.

Gresham LG, Shimp TA. Attitude toward the advertisement and brand attitudes: A classical conditioning perspective. J Advert. 1985;14(1):10-7.

Hamilton GG, Biggart NW. Why people obey. Sociological Perspectives. 1985;28(1):3-28.

Heider F. The psychology of interpersonal relations. J Psychol. 1982;21:336.

Horn JM, Plomin R, Rosenman R. Heritability of personality traits in adult male twins. Behav Genet. 1976;6(1):17-30.

Hovland CI, Janis IL, Kelly HH. Communication and persuasion: psychological studies of opinion change. Am Sociol Rev. 1953;19(3):315.

Izard CE. Personality similarity, positive affect, and interpersonal attraction 1. J Abnorm Soc Psychol. 1960;61:484-5.

Kassin S, Fein S, Markus HR. Social Psychology. Boston: Cengage Learning; 2011.

Lilly R, Cummings JL, Benson DF, et al. The human Klüver-Bucy syndrome. Neurology. 1983;33(9):1141.

Lindzey G, Loehlin J, Manosevitz M, et al. Behavioral genetics. Annu Rev Psychol. 1971;22(1):39-94.

Luo S, Zhang G. What leads to romantic attraction: similarity, reciprocity, security, or beauty? Evidence from a speed-dating study. J Pers. 2009;77(4):933-63.

McCarney R, Warner J, Iliffe S, et al. The Hawthorne Effect: a randomised, controlled trial. BMC Med Res Methodol. 2007;7(1):30.

Milgram S. Obedience to Authority: An Experimental View. Tavistock; 1974.

Nisbett RE, Wilson TD. The Halo Effect: evidence for unconscious alteration of judgments. J Pers Soc Psychol. 1977;35(4):250-6.

Oskamp S, Schultz WP. Attitudes and Opinions. Psychology Press; 2005.

Perkins HW. Student religiosity and social justice concerns in England and the United States: are they still related? JSSR. 1992;31(3):353-60.

Pettigrew TF. The ultimate attribution error: extending Allport's cognitive analysis of prejudice. Pers Soc Psychol Bull. 1979;5(4):461-76.

Petty RE, Priester JR, Brinol P. Implications of the elaboration likelihood model of persuasion. In: Media Effects: Advances in Theory and Research. Lawrence Erlbaum Associated; 2002;157-970.

Reeder G. Fundamental attribution error/correspondence bias. In: Dunn DS (Ed). Oxford Bibliographies in Psychology. New York: Oxford University Press; 2013. pp. 34-56.

Simon L, Greenberg J, Brehm JW. Trivialization: the forgotten mode of dissonance reduction. J Pers Soc Psychol. 1995;68(2):247-60.

Todorov A, Chaiken S, Henderson M. The heuristic-systematic model of social information processing. In: The Persuasion Handbook: Developments in Theory and Practice. Thousand Oaks: SAGE Publications; 2002. pp. 195-213.

Veltkamp M, Custers R, Aarts H. Motivating consumer behavior by subliminal conditioning in the absence of basic needs. Striking even while the iron is coldJ Consum Psychol. 2011;21(1):49-56.

Wallace DS, Paulson RM, Lord CG. Which Behaviors Do Attitudes Predict? Meta-Analyzing the Effects of Social Pressure and Perceived Difficulty. Review of General Psychology. 2005;9(3):214-27.

Zajonc R. Social facilitation. Science. 1965;149(3681):26974.

Social Determinants of Personality Development

Thirunavukarasu Manickam, Thenmozhi Lakshmanamoorthy

SUMMARY

Personality can be defined as a complex system of psychological elements and processes, whose formation and functioning results from synergistic interaction of multiple subsystems. These subsystems function with different degrees of interdependence as well as independence. The development of such a system cannot be understood simply by a cause-effect model. Multiple biological and psychosocial subsystems are restructured during the course of development of personality. It is an on-going process where there is reciprocal interaction with the environment. It is the interaction with the social world that paves the way for development of personality as an agency. It is not a single act that defines personality of an individual, but the patterns of emotion, cognition, and behavior reveal the underlying personality system. A coherent and complete sense of self is formed by the interaction of individual with his/her sociocultural environment. People form belief systems about their personal qualities and of others from their experiences in the social world and by discussing their experiences with other members of society.

INTRODUCTION

The psychological mechanisms which help the individuals in acquiring competency in the society, in adapting to the environment, and in planning and executing their actions, thus achieving personal meaning in their life, fall under the rubric of social-cognitive theories of personality. These theories elaborate on the reciprocity in the interactions between the personality structures and the sociocultural environment. The influence of social factors or the social determinants of personality development are discussed in this chapter.

CULTURE

Paul H Mussen says, *"Each culture expects, and trains its members to behave in the ways that are acceptable to the group. To a marked degree, the child's cultural group defines the range of experiences and situations, he is likely to encounter and the values and personality characteristics, that will be reinforced and hence learned"* (Kumar, 2009).

"Society is made up of symbols that teach us to understand the world. We use these symbols to develop a sense of self or identity. We then take this identity into the world to interact with other identities to create society"

George Herbert Mead (1934)

Shweder (1991) has defined cultural psychology as a field of psychology which studies the social practices and cultural traditions shaping the human psyche, by regulating its expression and transformation, resulting in the unity of the psyche for the mankind to a lesser extent than what occurs in ethnic divergences in mind, self, and emotion. Shweder opines that based on the resources and the process of extracting meanings from the sociocultural environment one belongs to, the mental life and subjective experiences of that person are changed. There is intermingling between the persons and their culture and it is often difficult to derive independent and dependent variables out of these two.

The development of an individual's personality has marked influences from the culture in which he/she is brought up.

Shweder and Bourne (1984) did a comparative study of the Hindu Indians' and Americans' open-ended descriptions and postulated that the descriptions which Hindu Indians gave were more concrete and context-dependent. On the other hand, Americans gave more abstract and context-free descriptions. The authors, hence described a sociocentric self among the Hindu Indians, i.e. their conception of a person is more holistic and socio-centric. The Americans described it as having more autonomous and abstract conception of the person, called as the egocentric self.

There are various assumptions about the personality conceptions within a culture which may be independence of the self or may have views dependent on each other (Markus & Kitayama, 1998). In the developed countries, independent view of personality is more prevalent. The concept incorporates:

- An individual is an independent and autonomous entity, characterized by a set of qualities, attributes, and processes which are distinct from other individuals
- Behavior is caused by a set of internal processes and attributes
- The distinction between different individuals is a result of differences in their internal attributes and processes. It is the distinctiveness that makes a person unique
- In the interest of maintaining consistency in behavior across different situations and to ensure stability over time, people are encouraged to express their attributes and processes in behavior
- Studying the personality is important because it helps us understand predicting and controlling behavior of a person (Markus & Kitayama, 1998).

Interdependent view of personality is most prevalent in Asian, African, Latin American and a number of Southern European countries. This type of personality incorporates:

- People are interdependent and form a part of encompassing social relationship
- Behavior is a result of being responsive to other organisms with whom a person has interdependence. Behaviors originate from relationships and identification of an individual through his interactions within a given social relationship
- The behavior of an individual varies from situation to situation and time to time, in accordance with the social context.

Collectivism and individualism are broader terms, often used interchangeably with interdependence-independence. The differences between individualism and collectivism have been highlighted by Triandis (1995) as:

- Seeing oneself as an autonomous and independent person in contrast to seeing oneself as a part of the group, connected to it

■ Personal goals taking priority over group goals
■ Personal attributes emphasized in guiding a behavior in contrast to the roles and norms.

Some of the individualistic traits include pleasure-seeking, assertiveness, curiosity, creativity, competitiveness, self-assurance, efficiency, initiative, and directedness. On the other hand, collectivistic traits include respectfulness, attentiveness, empathy, humility, self-control, dependence, dutifulness, cooperativeness, conformity, sacrifice, nurturance, moderation, etc. (Triandis, 1993). An individual in a collectivistic society is perceived more in context of his/her relationships, roles, etc. and less in context of an autonomous person with internal attributes (Markus & Kitayama, 1998; Rhee et al., 1995). In a collectivistic society, an individual's behavior is determined from his/her social roles and norms, unlike individualistic societies, where the behavior is determined by internal dispositions such as personality traits or attitudes (Markus & Kitayama, 1998; Triandis, 1995). The individuals with independent selves are identified primarily by their central attributes, and are motivated to identify, confirm and enhance their positive internal attributes (Heine & Lehman, 1995, 1997; Kitayama et al., 1997).

Tolerance for contraindications is found to be higher in East Asians as compared to Americans (Choi & Nisbett, 2000). In context of motivation, influence plays a different role in collectivistic-individualistic cultures. A study done in European-American children found that the motivation of children was higher if choices were made by children and lower when choices were made by authorities or peers (Iyengar & Lepper, 1999). In contrast to the European-American children, the Asian-American children showed highest level of motivation in response to choice being made for them by trusted authority figures. Lower motivation was seen in the latter group when they were allowed to make personal choice.

Lying is more accepted in collectivistic than individualistic cultures, if it helps the group or saves face. This is also quoted by the famous Tamil poet and philosopher Thiruvalluvar in his work Thirukkural as follows:

"Poimaiyum vaaimai yidaththa puraidheerndha nanmai payakkum enin"

The above phrase denotes that a lie may attain the same value as the truth, if it is said for the good, without any flaw (Diaz, 2000).

According to Trilling (1972), people with strong sense of self, as seen in individualistic culture, are able to determine who they are. They seek authenticity and sincerity. When they are influenced by traditions and obligations, as in collectivistic societies, they reduce the emphasis of authenticity.

FAMILY/PARENTING

While culture gives the norms and values, it is the family which moulds the individual to them. Personality is shaped from the development of "the self". The child develops the sense of self through the process of "socialization". According to Horton & Hunt (1976), the process of internalizing the norms of a group for enabling the emergence of a distinct self, unique to an individual, is called socialization. Self develops by interacting with others, influenced by multiple social factors, and forms the core of personality. An individual's interactions with the world give rise to his/her personality. The concept of "looking glass self' was given by Cooley (1902) emphasizing self to be a product of individual's social interactions with other people. According to Cooley, a person's primary groups like family play the most significant role in formation of personality. The "looking glass self" assures the child, which aspects of the assumed role will bring praise or blame, and which ones are acceptable to others and which ones unacceptable.

The behavioral and personality characteristics of children are influenced by the psychological and emotional environment of the family. Their quality of relationship with their parents determines their adjustment and interactions with each other (Sarmast, 2006).

Personality development is strongly influenced by social learning. Humans have the capacity to learn by observation, thus expanding their knowledge and competencies at a good pace through the information conveyed by various models. Almost all behavioral, cognitive, and affective learning from direct experience can be obtained by observing actions of others and consequences from their actions. Sense of self and personality are strongly influenced by the primary contact like parents because they are one of the first models for learning (Rosenthal & Zimmerman, 1978; Bandura, 1986).

Parenting styles have an important influence on personality development. Parenting styles can be conceptualized as a *"constellation of attitudes toward the child that are communicated to the child and that, taken together, create an emotional climate in which the parent's behaviors are expressed"*(Darling & Steinberg, 1993). Two dimensions in education have also been found to influence/predict child's behavior: responsiveness and demandingness (Baumrind, 1971). Responsiveness includes nutrition, warmth, emotional expressiveness, and reinforcements associated with the child's care. Demandingness refers to the demands and expectations in relation to the child. Baumrind (1971) has described four patterns of parenting, based on these dimensions: authoritative (high on both dimensions), authoritarian (high on demandingness and low on responsiveness), permissive (high on responsiveness and low on demandingness), and neglectful (low on both dimensions). Child's personality is affected differently and distinctly by each style. For example, authoritative parents have children with better social-emotional development and academic performance (Desjardins et al., 2008). Such children also tend to show better organization, and rational orientation (Hill, 1995). Adolescents of such parents are scientifically competent, less neglectful, and have a better psychological development as well as less of physical symptoms (Steinberg et al., 1994). Children of permissive parents have difficulty in self-control, curiosity, and self-confidence, and difficulty in controlling impulses, recognizing values and anti-values (Baumrind, 1971; Bornstein, 2002). Authoritarian style of parenting is often characterized by humiliating children, and giving no explanation about the punishment. This leads to impairment in processing messages from parents, and the children experience constant fear (Hartup & Laursen, 1993). Relationship between authoritarian and openness parenting style is inverse, while between authoritative and openness parenting style is direct. A positive relationship has been observed between three personality traits (viz., agreeableness, extroversion, and openness) and two parenting styles (viz., authoritative and permissive), and a negative relationship with authoritarian parenting style. The personality trait of conscientiousness has a positive relationship with authoritative and authoritarian parenting styles and negative relationship with permissive parenting style (Maddahi et al, 2012).

EDUCATION/SCHOOL

Next to family, school is the place where early learning takes place. Educating is humanizing. Teachers play a significant role in the child's personality development. They organize space and time for children, establishing relationship with them. They also propose, involve and enrich experience for cultural aptitude, thus helping them develop activities with the suitable objects in the environment and culture (Duarte, 1993; Carvalho, 2011). With the increasing complexity of the activities, personality, and intellectual capacity grow and develop further. Bissoli (2005) summarizes this development as:

- **Development** is the result of the subject's activity which involves his/her emotion and cognition simultaneously, giving shape to **reasons** that may or may not be conscious;
- **Reasons** formation is the result of the human necessities which are more and more complex and historically conditioned for the educational work;
- **Personality formation** is directly related to the social situation of the child development and to their living emotional-cognition, which presents as a source of meanings and feelings given by him/her to the human adjectives and to the relations among people.

Knowledge about oneself and the world around plays an important role in contact of humans with reality. Learning is an active process which happens throughout one's life. Through learning, man acquires new behaviors and actions or changes previously acquired ones effectively. Three processes are necessary for cognitive learning, viz. observation, sensory conditioning, and acquiring knowledge. Education as well as intellectual training are required for formation of human personality. Textbooks are not sufficient, and a student learns and gains knowledge from direct observation and perception of reality. Not just cognitive learning, a child also learns from the process of problem learning. In problem learning, the student approaches and analyses the problem, attempts to find ideas for its solution and to verify those ideas. The success of the individual within these three basic phases depends on his independent and creative attitude. Divergent thinking provides unlimited solutions for a problem. Learning experiences have both the intellectual-cognitive elements and the affective-conative elements. Hence, practically two processes are involved in learning, viz. cognitive processes (for intellectual reasons), and affective processes (for emotional satisfaction). As a parallel to intellectual and physical maturity, affective, or emotional maturity occurs over time with practiced forms of emotional activities. An important effect of learning through experience is acquiring invaluable skills which cannot be acquired even if greatest possible emphasis is placed on development of cognitive process. Then comes the productive activity which consists of transformation of reality, and creation of something which has not previously existed. All forms of activity provide education to human will and character. It also helps in development of proper attitude to work, social and private property, and working people. School education and the aspects learnt from it are vital in development of personality in order to have a person's fullest participation in the society (Okon, 1979). A state wide study done in Germany, using a quasi-natural experiment of shortening the high school track as a reform to assess the short-term effect of the reduction of curriculum on students' personality, found that reduction in the curriculum resulted in more extroverted students who were emotionally less stable (Dahmann & Anger, 2014). Thus, an optimum period of schooling is important for personality development.

Findings from the Perry Preschool Project provide an example of the possibility that schooling experiences can change the non-cognitive factors like personality traits (Heckman, 2007; Heckman et al., 2013). The Perry Preschool Project intervention program was initiated to enhance cognitive skills development of the at-risk children. Although little effect was seen on long-term academic or cognitive skills, the intervention participants outperformed non-participants on various important outcomes of life, for example, employment and low criminal behavior. This suggested that the benefits of the interventions were associated with personality factors rather than cognitive abilities. Thus, noncognitive psychological factors, such as personality traits are potentially influenced by educational experiences.

ECONOMIC FACTORS

Whether economic factors such as poverty influence personality development, is debatable. There are a few studies which show that children who grow in low socioeconomic background, exhibit more externalizing and internalizing behaviors, as compared to children grown-up in financially wealthy environment. The role of neighborhood poverty in personality development has been discussed. It has been suggested in literature that neighborhood influences academic and behavioral development in children (Leventhal & Brooks-Gunn, 2000). The best indicators of development have been postulated to be the indicators of neighborhood economic vitality. Successful development is hypothesized to be unlikely in neighborhoods having substantial proportions of families below the poverty line and small proportions of adults having professional occupations.

It has been proposed that economic deprivation in neighborhood raises the chances of maternal depression, and decreases the quality of emotional and intellectual support provided at home (Klebanov et al., 1994). Child's development may be constrained, as depressed mothers may not be responsive to their children's needs (Petterson & Albers, 2001). Similarly, the disadvantaged neighborhoods have weak social control and limited consensus on values. Disadvantaged neighborhood has been associated with antisocial behavior in adolescence, which might be mediated by informal control measured at the level of neighborhood (Sampson & Morenoff, 1997). Maladaptive personalities are more likely to occur in children living in economically disadvantaged neighborhoods, as compared to those living in affluent ones. However, the relation is generally small. Children living in high-poverty neighborhoods, as compared to those living in low-poverty neighborhoods, are more likely to show maladaptive changes in their personality profiles, like decreased resilience, over-control, and increased problem behavior, despite controlling for family-level factors such as maternal education, household income, family size, father's absence, and the home environment (Hart et al., 2008).

Development of antisocial personality or a personality dynamic characterized by an inability for delayed gratification, primary and concrete thinking process, sexual escapades, alcoholism, and a sense of helplessness and hopelessness about the future, is not just a part of belonging to a poor and minority individuals' society. However, demands associated with poverty and racial or ethnic conditions pose a number of challenges to the psychic structure of the poor which are not experienced by the more privileged sections (Javier et al, 1995). The nature, quality, and flavor of the personality structure of these individuals are determined by the way challenges are faced and eventually resolved.

CONCLUSION

Human beings are autonomous, reactive and interactive agents. Human behavior and action is the product of dynamic interplay between personal and situational influences. Personality development studies have shown that longitudinally, the stability of interindividual differences in personality increases with age, which means personality development is a lifelong process. Though genes lay the building blocks, even among genes there is a complex relationship and the final expression of personality is determined by the interplay of genes and various environmental factors. The genetic expression into traits is modified by environmental factors such as the social determinants discussed in this chapter. Personality is not entirely inherited as are genes. The influence of genes on our personality is also dependent upon the social factors, as the context of life unfolds day-by-day. Modifying these social determinants in a constructive manner will definitely help individuals develop personalities to participate efficiently and contribute to the society.

REFERENCES

Bandura A. Social Foundations of Thought and Action: A Social Cognitive Theory. New Jersey: Englewood Cliffs; 1986.

Baumrind D. Current patterns of parental authority. Developmental Psychological Monographs. 1971;4:1-1020.

Bissoli MF. Education and Development of the Child's Personality: Contributions of the Historical-Cultural Theory. Thesis of Doctorate, Marília-SP. State University Paulista; 2005.

Bornstein M. Handbook on Parenting Children and Parenting. Mahwah, New Jersey: Erlbaum Print; 2002.

Carvalho RNS. The Construction of the Curriculum of and in day care: a look at everyday life. Master's Dissertation, Faculty of Education, Manaus, Federal University of Amazonas; 2011.

Choi I, Nisbett RE. Cultural psychology of surprise: holistic theories and recognition of contradiction. J Pers Soc Psychol. 2000;79(6):890-905.

Cooley CH. Human Nature and Social Order. New York: Schocken books; 1902.

Dahmann S, Anger S. The impact of education on personality: Evidence from a German high school reform. Germany: Institute for the Study of Labor; 2014.

Darling N, Steinberg L. Parenting style as context: An integrative model. Psychological Bulletin. 1993;113(3):487-96.

Desjardins J, Zelenski JM, Coplan RJ. An investigation of maternal personality, Parenting styles and subjective well-being. Personality and Individual Differences. 2008; 44:587-97.

Diaz SM. Tirukkural: With English Translation and Explanation. Coimbatore, India: Ramanandha Adigalar Foundation; 2000.

Duarte N. The Individuality for-Itself: Contribution to a Social-historical Theory of the Formation of the Individual. Campinas: Associated Authors; 1993.

Hart D, Atkins R, Matsuba MK. The association of neighbourhood poverty with personality change in childhood. J Pers Soc Psychol. 2008;94(6):1048-61.

Hartup W, Laursen B. Conflict and context in peer relation, In: Hart CA (Ed) in Children on Playgrounds: Research & Perspectives. New York: Suny Press; 1993, pp. 44-84.

Heckman JJ. The economics, technology and neuroscience of human capability formation. Proc Natl Acad Sci U S A. 2007;104(33):13250-5.

Heckman JJ, Pinto R, Savelyev PA. Understanding the mechanisms through which an influential early childhood program boosted adult outcomes. Am Econ Rev. 2013;103(6):2052-86.

Heine SJ, Lehman DR. Cultural variation in unrealistic optimism: Does the West feel more invulnerable than the East? J Pers Soc Psychol. 1995;68:595-607.

Heine SJ, Lehman DR. Culture, dissonance, and self-affirmation. Pers Soc Psychol Bull. 1997;23:389-400.

Hill NE. The relationship between family environment and parenting Style: A preliminary study of African American families. J Black Psychol. 1995;21:408-23.

Horton PB, Hunt CL. Sociology, 4th edition. New York. McGraw Hill; 1976.

Iyengar SS, Lepper MR. Rethinking the value of choice: a cultural perspective on intrinsic motivation. J Pers Soc Psychol. 1999;76:349-66.

Javier RA, Herron WG, Yanos PT. Urban poverty, ethnicity, and personality development. J Soc Distress Homeless. 1995;4(3):219-35.

Kitayama S, Markus HR, Matsumoto H, Norasakkunkit V. Individual and collective processes in the construction of the self: self-enhancement in the United States and self-criticism in Japan. J Pers Soc Psychol. 1997;72(6):1245-67.

Klebanov P, Brooks-Gunn J, Duncan G. Does neighbourhood and family poverty affect mothers parenting, mental health, and social support? J Marriage Fam. 1994;56(2):441-55.

Kumar P. Organisational Behaviour. New Delhi: GenNext Publication; 2009.

Leventhal T, Brooks-Gunn J. The neighbourhoods they live in: The effects of neighbourhood residence on child and adolescent outcomes. Psychol Bull. 2000;126(2):309-37.

Maddahi ME, Javidi N, Samadzadeh M, Amini M. The study of relationship between parenting styles and personality dimensions in sample of college students. Indian Journal of Science & Technology. 2012;5:3332-6.

Markus HR, Kitayama S. The cultural psychology of personality. Journal of Cross-Cultural Psychology. 1998;29:63-87.

Mead GH. Mind, Self, and Society. Chicago: University of Chicago Press; 1934.

Okon W. All-round education and development of the personality. Prospects UNESCO. 1979;3:261-74.

Petterson SM, Albers AB. Effects of poverty and maternal depression on early child development. Child Dev. 2001;72(6):1794-813.

Rhee E, Uleman JS, Lee HK, Roman RJ. Spontaneous self-descriptions and ethnic identities in individualistic and collectivistic cultures. J Pers Soc Psychol. 1995;69(1):142-52.

Rosenthal TL, Zimmerman BJ. Social Learning and Cognition. New York: Academic Press; 1978.

Sampson RJ, Morenoff JD. Ecological perspectives on neighbourhood context of urban poverty: Past and present. In: Duncan GJ, Aber JL (Eds). Neighbourhood Poverty: Policy Implications in Studying Neighbourhoods. New York: Russell Sage Foundation; 1997; 2:1-22.

Sarmast A. Relationship Between Parenting Styles and Stress Coping Styles: Symposium of National Conference in Psychology & Society, Islam. Azad University, Tehran: Salavan Press; 2006.

Shweder RA. Thinking Through Cultures: Expeditions in Cultural Psychology. Cambridge, Harvard University Press, 1991.

Shweder RA, Bourne EJ. Does the concept of the person vary cross culturally. In: Shweder RA, Levine RA (Eds). Cultural Theory: Essays on Mind, Self, and Emotion. Cambridge: Cambridge University Press; 1984. pp. 158-99.

Steinberg I, Lamborn SD, Darling N, et al. Over-time changes in adjustment and competence among adolescents from authoritative, authoritarian, indulgent, and uninvolved families. Child Dev. 1994;65(3):754-70.

Triandis HA. Collectivism and individualism as cultural syndromes. Cross-cultural Research. 1993; 27:155-80.

Triandis HC. Individualism and Collectivism. Boulder: Westview Press; 1995.

Trilling L. Sincerity and Authenticity. London: Oxford University Press; 1972.

Chapter 10

Interpersonal Bonding and Communication

Rachna Bhargava, Swati Kedia Gupta, Nikita Bhati, Pooja Pattanaik

SUMMARY

The need to belong can be construed as an intrinsic, biological phenomenon that begins with the first bond between a mother and an infant. As the individual grows, he/she develops other relationships, which move from being an acquaintance to developing strong and intimate bonds. Development of healthy bonds early in life is strongly correlated with mental health and well-being. Bonding and communication share a strong, reciprocal relationship, wherein bonding develops as a result of communication and there is observable change in quality of communication as the bonds between the two individuals become stronger. However, the era of technology and digitalization has had positive as well as negative effects on both communication and interpersonal bonding. And therefore, it becomes imperative to delineate the interrelationship between these aspects, and strategize ways of developing and maintaining healthy interpersonal relationships.

INTRODUCTION

Attachment and bonding are dynamic terms, which are often used interchangeably. Bonding, attachment, communication and related concepts have been drawing interest of various scientists and non-scientists for decades. These concepts have not just intrigued scientists from mental health disciplines, but many other disciplines, such as pediatrics, anthropology, philosophy, neurobiology, etc. Over the years, various theories have been proposed to understand why and how we develop our bonds (Baxter & Braithwaite, 2008).

The need to belong and to establish and maintain lasting positive and significant interpersonal relationship is a universal phenomenon. However, its intensity as well as expression tends to vary across individuals, societies, and cultures (Bowlby, 1969; Ainsworth, 1989). It is a well-known fact that the Eastern culture is more homogeneous and collectivistic in nature, while the Western culture is more individualistic and heterogeneous (Desai, 2006). Hence, variations across cultures in terms of bonding, interpersonal relationships, and communication patterns have been documented (Triandis, 2001; Karandashev, 2015).

Freud asserted the need for interpersonal belonging, although he emphasized the sexual drive to maintain the same (Freud, 1930), while Maslow ranked the "need to belong" in middle of the motivational hierarchy (Maslow, 1968). Recent theorists have described bonding as the commitment and emotional attachment that a person forms over a course of his/her lifespan with different people like parents, siblings, friends, colleagues, romantic partners, and other members of his/her community (Fisher & Lerner, 2005). Bonding has often been construed as a gradual, continuing, reciprocal process that moves from acquaintanceship to attachment, and ties the individual in a coordinated, constructive social relationship.

ATTACHMENT AND INTERPERSONAL BONDING ACROSS LIFESPAN

Bonding begins as early as life begins. Infants have an innate predisposition to respond to people. Even a few hours old infant prefers to look at human faces and react to mother's voice (Sai, 2005). This stage has often been described as that of "absorption" for both mother and infant, wherein both are mutually preoccupied with each other. Gradually, infants learn to seek attention actively to which the mother instinctively responds leading to "attenuation". As the caregiver consistently meets the infant's needs, the infant develops trust in the availability and responsivity of the caregiver.

Bowlby, a pioneer in giving the concept of attachment, had strongly posited that the attachment figure and emotional bond toward the attachment figure is irreplaceable with anyone else. He asserted that "attachment behavior is held to characterize human beings from cradle to the grave" (Bowlby, 1958).

Positive and enduring bonds that develop during early stage play an important role in the physiological and psychological functioning of both the caregiver and the infants. Studies have often shown that positive and secure attachment in infants makes them more resilient to developing physical illness such as asthma, cardiorespiratory and infectious diseases, and psychological illnesses like depression and anxiety, and also improves their academic performance (Leeb et al., 2011).

At this time, the child tends to explore the environment and the attachment figure serves as the secure base, to which the child can return to. The stress of exploring and the subsequent soothing and encouragement by the attachment figure makes the child feel more confident about him/herself and he/she learns to self-regulate his/her emotions, fears and needs (Howe, 2005). Thus, by the end of the second year, the child develops an attachment relationship within which he/she can communicate effectively, and feel safe (Siegel & Soloman, 2003). This has also been conceptualized as "attachment behavioral system" (in attachment theory) where in an infant's system gets activated under stress, illness, or threats of separation and the "threatened" child re-establishes emotional security with an attachment figure.

During these early years, the child internalizes cognitive and affective representations of the attachment figure, which was termed by Bowlby as internal working model of the caregiver (Ainsworth et al., 1978). These internal working models serve as "template" for further relationship and influence the quality of close relationships, including the therapeutic relationship (Chui & Leung, 2016).

In the third and fourth year, although the attachment figure continues to be the primary source of socialization, the child ventures out even further, socializes with others and forms peer groups. At this stage, the attachment figure shows disapproval or prohibits the child in carrying out certain actions, also known as "misattunement", which may lead to the child experiencing shame or guilt. However, if the caregiver also demonstrates love, acceptance and security, the child comes to understand him/herself as being cared for. Mentalization and affect regulation in this stage sets the ground for development of sense of self and agency (Fonagi et al., 2004).

Peer-bonding develops as the child starts school and can range from acquaintances to friends with whom one spends a considerable time and pursues common interests and activities to few close relationships. These bonds are characterized by varying degree of affection and care felt by the two people in the relationship.

A major shift in the bonding and attachment patterns occurs at the time of adolescence, ushered in by hormonal changes, by physical maturity and development of reproductive capacity (Cooper et al., 2013). This period is also characterized by individuation from parents and increased influence of peers (Hay & Ashman, 2003). A third important change in this period is cognitive development, which leads the adolescents to re-evaluate all their relationship including those with their parents (Furman et al., 2002; Hill et al., 2007), wherein they are less emotionally and behaviorally dependent on them.

Many factors play role in determining the adolescent attachment outcomes during this phase of life. Gender has been one of the key factors and it has often been suggested that girls demonstrate more attachment security with parents as compared to boys (Choi et al., 2012). Another very important factor that determines attachment security is the level of parental support that is demonstrated through guidance, encouragement, and availability (Azam & Hanif, 2011). Features of mature relationship, i.e. approval, companionship and disclosure, are also related to adolescent attachment. Since it is a period of individuation, it is important that parents become more of companions than sole caretakers. A recent study on attachment patterns of 223 adolescents with their parents found that positive relationship experiences like companionship, approval, satisfaction, and support increased attachment security in the sample, whereas negative experiences such as pressure and criticism predicted decrease in attachment security (Ruhl et al., 2015).

Hazan and Shaver (1987), in their seminal work, applied concepts of attachment developed from parent-child studies to romantic relationships. They found that having a secure attachment pattern in childhood predicted stable, consistent, and coherent self-image that further determined secure and positive relationships in adulthood. Fortunately, it has also been demonstrated that individuals are not completely dependent on the early attachment patterns and may be able to develop healthy bonds over their lifespan.

The attachment theory was expanded to include other bonds that develop over a lifetime specifically with romantic partners (Mikulincer & Shaver, 2007). These attachment behaviors also trigger other behavioral systems (e.g. caregiving, sexual behaviors, etc.). The relationship is more reciprocal with both partners relying on each other to fulfill their attachment needs. Sternberg (1986) proposed passion, intimacy and compassion to be the three vital components of pair or sexual bonding. He postulated that passion attracts the two people to each other, intimacy creates emotional and behavioral bonds, and commitment keeps the partners together. In a way, sexual bonds serve evolutionary purpose. Although, pair-bonding is not necessary for reproduction, its presence ensures development of attachment patterns and involvement of both partners as caregivers (Fraley et al., 2005). Moreover, various studies have consistently shown that married individuals show better physical and mental health than those who have never been married, or are widowed or divorced (Robles et al., 2014). Sexual activity is found to release oxytocin and arginine vasopressin, which are the hormones implicated in development of bonding and trust (Lim & Young, 2006). Sexual bonds lay the foundation for more long-lasting relationship, which completes the cycle with childbirth.

ROLE OF COMMUNICATION IN BONDING

Bonding and communication are intrinsically tied with one another. Communication in any form is an important prerequisite for bonds to develop. Berne believed that insight could be better discovered by analyzing social transactions. Berne (1964) mapped interpersonal relationships to three ego-states of the individuals involved: the *parent, adult,* and *child* state. He then investigated communications between individuals based on the current state of each. He called these interpersonal interactions *transactions*. A varying patterns of transactions pop-up repeatedly in everyday life. It has been shown that individuals are more likely to express emotions in close relationships, and intensity of emotional expression depends upon the degree of closeness (Clark & Finkel, 2005; Pietromonaco & Barrett, 2000). On one hand, it can enhance the communication between the individuals, but it can also lead to misunderstandings if the non-verbal cues are misinterpreted. On the other hand, the nature of communication changes as two individuals bond.

Communication patterns have changed fundamentally over the last decade with text messaging and social media (Facebook, Twitter, YouTube, Instagram, etc.) overriding all other means of personal communication. In this era of globalization and digital communication, it is not surprising that bonding and dynamics of interpersonal relationships are also undergoing changes impacted by the way newer communication patterns (communication style and content) have emerged.

Parental Bonding and Communication

Attachment perspective has a significant role to play in demonstrating various aspects of interpersonal communication from children to adults. During early stage of parent-child relationship, the parents transmit their own patterns of relating to children, initially through behavioral-affective interaction patterns, but later also through verbal dialogue about past, future, and hypothetical experiences. Bowlby, in his later writings, emphasized that the child's internal working models of self and attachment figures are established when their parents accept and respond to their children's emotional communication, and allow the internal working models of child be open to change with new experiences (Pietromonaco & Barrett, 2000).

During infancy, communication between caregiver and infant is primarily nonverbal. According to the evolutionary theory, the infant's emotional display serves an important function of letting the caregiver know of his/her internal state. The infant seeks attention by gestures, e.g. asking to be picked up by emotions like smiling and crying. The caregiver responds by cooing to the infant, responding to infant's emotions. The reciprocal interaction at this stage helps in development of attachment between caregiver and infant (Winstona & Chicot, 2016).

As the child grows up and develops speech, verbal as well as nonverbal mode of communication are used. Parents also use verbal as well as nonverbal ways of communication to discipline the child, set boundaries, define acceptable and nonacceptable behaviors, and show love and affection. However, with changing time and evolving technology, a divide is a common observation in households even in Indian setting. If parents are wrapped up in work at home due to technology, children too grow distant with over-involvement in social media sites. Studies have documented "spillover" effect in terms of work of parents blurring the boundaries of work and home. At the same time, issues like the loss of connection and confusion over disciplining the technology-native child has affected family relationships (Chesley, 2005).

Bonding with Friends and Communication

Cushman and his associates postulated that friends and mate relationship development progresses through three-step filtering process. These three filters are: *field of available, field of approachable* and *field of reciprocals (Cushman & Cahn, 1985)*. The "field of available" refers to presence of all individuals present with whom relationship can be formed. The "field of approachable" narrows down to all those, whom the individual finds desirable enough to form a relationship with. And finally the "field of reciprocals" includes those who have reciprocated to the friendly overtures of the individual. They further believed that a particular set of rules, i.e. intimacy/intensity, is the guiding source of these relationships development.

In the process of making friends, one first becomes acquainted with another person where verbal communication is formal, and nonverbal communication and emotional expression are minimal. The acquaintance then may become a casual friend, moving on to become a good and then the closest friend. As the individual moves from acquaintance stage to best friend, the depth and breadth of communication increases, and communication in the last stage is highly personal. Both individuals would freely express their thoughts, emotions and needs, and share common beliefs and interests (Knapp & Daly, 2005).

Lenhart et al. (2010) noted that one of the major reasons for rapid development of internet communication (instant messaging, texting, and social network sites) among college students was to establish and maintain friendships. Valkenburg and Peter (2010) reviewed literature on adolescents' online communication, and found it to be related to different aspects of psychosocial development, including increased self-esteem, opportunity for friendship formation, increased quality of friendships, and sexual self-exploration. The level of anonymity and familiarity between those communicating, the level of compulsion in internet use, and the motivation for using the technology has mediated the communication pattern.

With growing digitalization across the world, more people are resorting to virtual computer-mediated communication. This has triggered considerable interest among researchers to assess the communication and emotional experience of connectedness between friends in digital world. Sherman et al. (2013) assessed emotional connectivity and bonding through information communication media and found that participants reported feeling connected in all conditions [i.e. in-person interaction, video chat, audio chat, and instant messages (IM)]. Greatest bonding was reported during in-person interaction, followed by video chat, audio chat, and IM.

Friendships and relationships at all age levels have expanded but since the communication is "shallow" and one may be left wondering regarding the intensity of bonding, as many times it is possible that the communication may be happening for several years without meeting.

Romantic Relationships and Communication

Intimate relationship development also goes through various stages. From being an acquaintance, one goes to casual dating, moving onto dating steadily, getting engaged to finally getting married. Communication is the key for development of relationship and for moving from one stage to the next. As in friendship, in the initial stages, communication is more formal and there is minimal expression of emotions. As the bonding develops, the length and breadth of common interest areas increases. Also, there is a reciprocal relationship wherein, more the two individuals share in common in terms of interests and needs, more the intimacy increases. As the two individuals become intimate, each one shares and expresses emotions and experiences openly, and tends to speak tenderly. Personal idioms and "personalized communication", i.e. use of secrets and meanings that you would not share with anyone else, is frequently used. Both the individuals actively work toward resolving conflicts amicably, and at the same time, know how to "punish" the person if need be (Knapp & Daly, 2005).

In recent years, role of interpersonal communication in understanding attachment among adult romantic relationships has been of interest (Feeney, 2008). Literature has shown that style of couples' attachment was associated with the quality of daily interaction, nonverbal expression (Rholes, 2001), styles of self-disclosure (Locke, 2008), relational maintenance strategies and supportive communication (Rholes, 2001).

The impact of communication technology like smart phones and social networking sites has been studied in establishing and maintaining sexual and romantic relationships (Jonason et al., 2009), and developing intimate relationships. Bergdall et al. (2012) found calls and text messaging as the widely used communication methods across various relationship phases. Further, the mobile usage was dependent on kind of relationship and the expectations of the partners.

INADEQUATE BONDING, DYSFUNCTIONAL COMMUNICATION AND PSYCHOPATHOLOGY

It is a well-established fact that the lack of communication or negative communication patterns can have long lasting impact on bonding and attachment, for example, conflicts within family, divorce or breaking of friendships leading to various psychological problems, psychopathology and antisocial behavior (Ifeagwazi, 2017). Though the relationship of inadequate communication and attachment with psychopathology has been well studied separately, there is limited research comprehensively assessing the link between communication deviation, attachment issues, and psychological morbidity.

Attachment, Bonding Issues, and Psychological Morbidity

According to attachment theories, when the child interacts with inconsistent, unreliable or insensitive attachment figures, he/she ends up developing insecure attachments, which predispose him/her to break down psychologically at the time of crisis. In such a scenario, child may exhibit one of the two patterns of behavior—he/she may minimize attachment behavior exhibited through passive and withdrawn behavior with little display of emotional distress ("avoidant attachment") or he/she may show demanding and clingy behavior ("anxious attachment"). The former is associated with "inhibitedness" exhibited by restricted expression of emotions, and problems in intimacy; whereas, the latter is associated with "emotional dysregulation", exhibited by emotional lability, identity confusion, anxiety, cognitive distortions, and suspiciousness (Mikulincer & Shaver, 2012).

Over the last decade, various studies that have examined attachment effect on psychopathology have shown insecure attachment to be associated with several mental health issues such as depression, anxiety disorders, suicidal tendencies, and eating disorders (Mikulincer & Shaver, 2012). A great deal of work has also gone to understand the relationship between insecure attachments and personality disorders (Mosquera et al., 2014; Levy et al., 2015). Studies demonstrate that specific type of attachment insecurity differs across personality disorders (Meyer & Pilkonis, 2005). For example, anxious attachment is found to be associated with dependent, histrionic and borderline disorders, and avoidant attachment is associated with schizoid and avoidant disorders (Livesley & Jang, 2007).

A related line of research has been to determine the extent to which difficulties in attachment and bonding affect psychopathology. Recent research has shown that dysfunctional bonding is not directly related to development of psychopathology except separation anxiety disorder. Various other factors such as temperament, intelligence, and life history converge with or amplify the effects of attachment and bonding to further determine vulnerability (Mikulincer & Shaver, 2012).

The significance of secure attachment has been documented in all ages. The ways couples' communicate during conflict also tend to be related to partners' attachment styles. For instance, securely attached individuals are more likely to use constructive conflict resolution strategies (Pistole, 1989), whereas individuals with avoidant or anxious attachment styles were linked to negative conflict tactics (Creasey & Hesson-McInnis, 2001).

Durkheim's (1897) concept of social bonding has been extended by researchers in the area of criminology. Delinquent behavior has been seen as an outcome of weak or absent social bonding of an individual to society. People are reluctant to deviate from social norms because of the fear of negative perception by significant others, losing an important relationship or important future opportunities, and violation of one's moral beliefs. Hirschi has described four factors that comprise of social bond: attachment, commitment, involvement, and belief (Hirschi, 1969).

Communication Problems and Psychological Morbidity

Poor communication is a common feature noted among families with psychosocial adversities. Poor interaction can lead to family problems including severe family conflicts, failure in solving the problems, and lack of intimacy and emotional relations. Interaction is not only talking but is listening to others so that we could understand what they say (Peterson & Green, 2009). Four pathways have been described about maladaptive communication leading to psychiatric illness: social skill deficits, communication deviance (CD), expressed emotions (EE), and lack of social support (Segrin & Givertz, 2015). The greatest evidence of association between CD and development of psychiatric illness exists for schizophrenia spectrum disorder. Two meta-analyses have found a high effect size for association of parental CD with schizophrenia spectrum disorder in the offsprings (De Sousa et al.,2014; Riosko et al., 2014). Studies from the West as well as from India have demonstrated higher caregiver burden in families with EE (Magliano et al., 2006; Nirmala et al., 2011). Impact of EE needs to be understood in sociocultural context. Prognosis of schizophrenia is reported to be better in developing countries such as India. The relationship between EE and psychopathology is understandable in this context as South and East Asian countries such as India and Japan reporting rates of EE as 10–30% compared to European countries and Mexico reporting rates of 40–70%. A landmark multicentric study on schizophrenia carried out by the World Health Organization more than three decades earlier still finds relevance even today. Good prognosis was associated with lower rates of EE (Wig et al., 1987; Satyakam et al., 2013).

Substantial literature also exists regarding the role of adult attachment and communication patterns in mediating depression and marital adjustment (Markman et al., 2010). In teenager-father relationship, avoidance patterns have been reported to cause juvenile delinquency and in teenager-mother relationship the non-constructive approach related to delinquency in teenagers (Van Doorn et al., 2008).

Bonding and Communication Technology

Social media presupposes interactivity, reciprocity, and involvement. At the same time, negative factors also come forth—loss of privacy, over communicativeness, social alienation, and dependency issues. The pattern of continuous and excessive internet/mobile use gradually impacts activities of daily living, mental health, and socio-occupational functioning (Radesky et al., 2016).

As communication technology helps to narrow social distance among young adults, some concerns have also emerged like electronic aggression, defined as aggression using cell phones and internet, including text messages with the intent to embarrass, harass, or threaten a peer (David-Ferdon & Hertz, 2007), sexual behavior, and dating violence (Picard, 2007) which have a detrimental effect on bonding. A qualitative study described these behaviors across relationship stages among adolescents, and found communication technology facilitated and spurred arguments leading to violent incidents through calls, texts, and social networking sites (Draucker & Martsolf, 2010). The constant availability of a partner through the technologies facilitates persistent exposure to this abusive behavior, and makes stopping or avoiding abuse particularly challenging. More research evidence is required to have an in-depth understanding of the changing dynamics in the relationships ever since the technology has become an integral part in the lives of not only adolescents and youth but also in all ages.

MENDING BROKEN BONDS: ROLE OF BONDING AND SPECIFIC COMMUNICATION SKILLS

Lack of attachment securities predisposes the individual to develop psychopathology, and therefore creation and maintenance of attachment security can improve mental health of the individual. In experimental studies, it has been found that activating mental representation of supportive attachment figures (a technique known as "security priming") mitigates cognitive symptoms of post-traumatic stress disorder and improves general mental well-being (Mikulincer et al., 2001).

Therapeutic relationship has been an area of recent evidence-based researches to assess the impact, and understand the processes involved during therapy. Sonkin (2005) proposed that a therapist can fulfill the position of an attachment figure and can be instrumental in changing the attachment style. A multicentric study found that if the therapist is perceived to be sensitive and supportive by the client, there is significant decrease in depressive symptoms, which is maintained over 18-month period (Zuroff & Blatt, 2006). Modifying and understanding interaction patterns based on Berne's transactional analysis has been found to reduce parent child conflicts (Taher & Maryam, 2016).

CONCLUSION

Twenty-first century marks the change in communication patterns in intrapersonal, inter-personal, group and mass communication processes and content. Social rules are being redefined from one culture to another. Virtual relations of youths are overpowering to get youth alienated from the real world leading to weakening interpersonal communication. Intergenerational gap adds to the confusion in parenting, impacting the mental health and interpersonal relationships in family, friends and society in general. There is an urgent need for evidence based researches to understand the complex impact of virtual life and intergenerational cultural dissonance (clash between parent-child over cultural values) on bonding and behavior.

REFERENCES

Ainsworth MD, Blehar MC, Waters E. et al. Patterns of Attachment: A Psychological Study of the Strange Situation. Hillsdale, NJ, Erlbaum; 1978. p.18.

Ainsworth MD. Attachments beyond infancy. Am Psychol. 1989;44:709-16.

Azam A, Hanif R. Impact of parents' marital conflicts on parental attachment and social competence of adolescents. Eur J Dev Psychol. 2011;8:157-70.

Baxter LA, Braithwaite DO. Engaging Theories in Interpersonal Communication: Multiple Perspectives. Thousand Oaks, CA: Sage Publications Inc. 2008.

Bergdall AR, Kraft JM, Andes K, et al. Love and hooking up in the new millennium: Communication technology and relationships among urban African American and Puerto Rican young adults. J Sex Res. 2012;49:570-82.

Berne E. Games People Play–The Basic Hand Book of Transactional Analysis. New York: Ballantine Books; 1964.

Bowlby J. Attachment and loss: Vol. 1. Attachment. Vol. 2. New York: Basic Books, 1969.

Bowlby J. The nature of the child's tie to his mother. Int J Psychoanal. 1958;39:350-73.

Chesley N. Blurring boundaries? Linking technology use, spillover, individual distress, and family satisfaction. J Marriage and Family. 2005;67:1237-48.

Choi S, Hutchison B, Lemberger ME, et al. A longitudinal study of the developmental trajectories of parental attachment and career maturity of South Korean adolescents. Career Development Quarterly. 2012;60:163-77.

Chui WY, Leung MT. Adult attachment internal working model of self and other, self-esteem and romantic relationship satisfaction in Chinese culture: By multilevel–multigroup structural equation modelling. In: Leung MT, Tan L (Eds). Applied Psychology Readings. Singapore: Springer; 2016. pp. 209-28.

Clark MS, Finkel EJ. Willingness to express emotion: The impact of relationship type, communal orientation, and their interaction. Personal Relationships. 2005;12:169-80.

Cooper PJ, Pauletti RE, Tobin DD, et al. Mother-child attachment and gender identity in preadolescence. Sex Roles. 2013;69:618-31.

Creasey G, Hesson-McInnis M. Affective responses, cognitive appraisals, and conflict tactics in late adolescent romantic relationships: Associations with attachment orientations. J Counseling Psychology. 2001;48:85.

Cushman DP, Cahn DD. Communication in Interpersonal Relationships. Albany, NY: State University of New York Press; 1985.

David-Ferdon C, Hertz MF. Electronic media, violence, and adolescents: An emerging public health problem. J Adoles Health. 2007;41:S1-5.

Desai JS. Intergenerational Conflict within Asian American Families: The Role of Acculturation, Ethnic Identity, Individualism, and Collectivism. Chicago, IL: Loyola University of Chicago; 2006.

De Sousa P, Varese F, Sellwood W, et al. Parental communication and psychosis: A meta-analysis. Schizophrenia Bulletin. 2014;40:756-68.

Draucker CB, Martsolf DS. The role of electronic communication technology in adolescent dating violence. J Child Adoles Psychiatr Nursing. 2010;23:133-42.

Durkheim E. Suicide: A Study in Sociology. New York: Free Press; 1897; 1951.

Feeney JA, Noller P, Callan VJ. Attachment and sexuality in close relationships. In: Harvey JH, Wenzel A, Sprecher A (Eds). Handbook of Sexuality in Close Relationships. Mahwah: Lawrence Erlbaum Associates Publishers; 1994. p. 183.

Feeney JA. Adult romantic attachment. In: Cassidy J, Shaver PR (Eds). Handbook of Attachment: Theory, Research, and Clinical Applications, 2nd edition. New York: The Guilford Press, 2008. p. 456.

Fisher CB, Lerner RM. Encyclopedia of Applied. Developmental Science (Vol. 2). Thousand Oaks, CA: Sage Publications Inc; 2005.

Fonagy P, Gergely G, Jurist EL (Eds). Affect Regulation, Mentalization and the Development of the Self. London: Karnac Books; 2004.

Fraley RC, Brumbaugh CC, Marks MJ. The evolution and function of adult attachment: a comparative and phylogenetic analysis. J Pers Soc Psychol. 2005;89:731-46.

Freud S. Civilization and its Discontents (J. Riviere, Trans.). London: Hogarth Press; 1930.

Furman W, Simon VA, Shaffer L, et al. Adolescents' working models and styles for relationships with parents, friends, and romantic partners. Child Dev. 2002;73:241-55.

Hay I, Ashman AF. The development of adolescents' emotional stability and general self-concept: The interplay of parents, peers, and gender. Int J Dis Dev Edu. 2003;50:77-91.

Hazan C, Shaver P. Romantic love conceptualized as an attachment process. J Pers Soc Psychol. 1987;52:511-24.

Hill NE, Bromell L, Tyson DF, et al. Developmental commentary: Ecological perspectives on parental influences during adolescence. J Clin Child Adoles Psychol. 2007;36:367-77.

Hirschi T. Causes of Delinquency. Berkeley CA: University of CA Press; 1969.

Howe D. Child Abuse and Neglect: Attachment, Development and Intervention. London: Palgrave Macmillan; 2005.

Ifeagwazi CM. The Impact of dysfunctional family communication patterns on psychopathology. Int J Comm. 2017;4:7(1).

Jonason PK, Li NP, Cason MJ. The "booty call": A compromise between men's and women's ideal mating strategies. J Sex Res. 2009;46:460-70.

Karandashev V. A cultural perspective on romantic love. Online Readings in Psychology and Culture. 2015;5:1-21.

Knapp ML, Daly JA. Handbook of Interpersonal Communication, 3rd edition. Oakland, USA: SAGE Publication; 2005.

Leeb RT, Lewis T, Zolotor AJ. A review of physical and mental health consequences of child abuse and neglect and implications for practice. Am J Lifestyle Med. 2011;5:454-68.

Lenhart A, Purcell K, Smith A, et al. Social Media and Mobile Internet Use among Teens and Young Adults. Millennials Pew internet & American Life Project; 2010.

Levy KN, Johnson BN, Clouthier TL, et al. An attachment theoretical framework for personality disorders. Canadian Psychology/Psychologie Canadienne. 2015;56:197.

Lim MM, Young LJ. Neuropeptidergic regulation of affiliative behavior and social bonding in animals. Horm Behav. 2006;50:506-17.

Locke KD. Attachment styles and interpersonal approach and avoidance goals in everyday couple interactions. Personal Relationships. 2008;15:359-74.

Magliano L, Fiorillo A, De Rosa C, et al. Family burden and social network in schizophrenia vs. physical diseases: Preliminary results from an Italian national study. Acta Psychiatr Scand. 2006;113:60-3.

Markman HJ, Rhoades GK, Stanley SM, et al. The premarital communication roots of marital distress and divorce: the first five years of marriage. J Fam Psychol. 2010;24:289-98.

Maslow AH. Toward a Psychology of Being. NewYork: Van Reinhold; 1968.

Meyer B, Pilkonis PA. An attachment model of personality disorders. In: Lenzenweger MF, Clarkin JF (Eds). Major Theories of Personality Disorder. New York: Guilford; 2005; 231-81.

Mikulincer M, Hirschberger G, Nachmias O, et al. The affective component of the secure base schema: affective priming with representations of attachment security. J Pers Soc Psychol. 2001;81:305-21.

Mikulincer M, Shaver PR, Horesh N. Attachment bases of emotion regulation and posttraumatic adjustment. In: Snyder DK, Simpson JA, Hughes JN (Eds). Emotion Regulation in Families: Pathways to Dysfunction and Health. Washington: American Psychological Association; 2006. pp. 77-99.

Mikulincer M, Shaver PR. An attachment perspective on psychopathology. World Psychiatry. 2012;11:11-5.

Mikulincer M, Shaver PR. Attachment theory and emotions in close relationships: Exploring the attachment-related dynamics of emotional reactions to relational events. Personal Relationships. 2005;12:149-68.

Mikulincer M, Shaver PR. Boosting attachment security to promote mental health, pro-social values, and inter-group tolerance. Psychology. 2007;18:139-56.

Mosquera D, Gonzalez A, Leeds AM. Early experience, structural dissociation, and emotional dysregulation in borderline personality disorder: the role of insecure and disorganized attachment. Borderline Personality Disorder and Emotion Dysregulation. 2014;1:15.

Nirmala BP, Vranda MN, Reddy S. Expressed emotion and caregiver burden in patients with schizophrenia. Indian J Psychol Med. 2011;33:119.

Peterson R, Green S. Families First-Keys to Successful Family Functioning. Communication. Virginia Cooperative Extension; 2009.

Picard P. Tech abuse in teen relationships study. New York: Liz Claiborne, Inc; 2007.

Pietromonaco PR, Barrett LF. The internal working models concept: What do we really know about the self in relation to others? Rev Gen Psychol. 2000;4:155-75.

Pistole MC. Attachment in adult romantic relationships: Style of conflict resolution and relationship satisfaction. J Soc Pers Relat. 1989;6:505-10.

Radesky JS, Kistin C, Eisenberg S, et al. Parent perspectives on their mobile technology use: The excitement and exhaustion of parenting while connected. J Dev Behav Pediatr. 2016;37:694-701.

Rholes WS, Simpson JA, Campbell L, et al. Adult attachment and the transition to parenthood. J Pers Soc Psychol. 2001;81:421.

Robles TF, Slatcher RB, Trombello JM, et al. Marital quality and health: A meta-analytic review. Psychol Bull. 2014;140:1-80.

Roisko RI, Wahlberg KE, Miettunen JO, et al. Association of parental communication deviance with offspring's psychiatric and thought disorders: A systematic review and meta-analysis. Eur Psychiatr. 2014;29:20-31.

Ruhl H, Dolan EA, Buhrmester D. Adolescent attachment trajectories with mothers and fathers: The importance of parent–child relationship experiences and gender. J Res Adoles. 2015;25:427-42.

Sai FZ. The role of the mother's voice in developing mother's face preference: Evidence for intermodal perception at birth. Inf Child Dev. 2005;14:29-50.

Satyakam M, Rath NM. Expressed emotion in psychiatric disorders. East J Psychiatr. 2013:17.

Segrin C, Givertz M, Swaitkowski P, et al. Over parenting is associated with child problems and a critical family environment. J Child Family Stud. 2015;24:470-9.

Sherman LE, Michikyan M, Greenfield PM. The effects of text, audio, video, and in-person communication on bonding between friends. J Psychosoc Res Cybersp. 2013;7:2-3.

Siegel DJ, Solomon M (Eds). Healing Trauma: Attachment, Mind, Body and Brain. New York: W.W. Norton & Company; 2003.

Sonkin DJ. Attachment theory and psychotherapy. Calif Therap. 2005;17:68-77.

Sternberg RJ. A triangular theory of love. Psychol Rev. 1986;93:119.

Taher TD, Maryam JS. The effect of Eric Berne's transactional analysis on parent-child conflict. Int J Phil Soc Psychol Sci. 2016;2:40-5.

TN, Livesley WJ, Jang KL. Insecure attachment and personality disorder: a twin study of adults. Eur J Pers. 2007;21:191-208.

Triandis HC. Individualism-collectivism and personality. J Pers. 2001;69:907-24.

Valkenburg PM, Peter J. Online communication among adolescents: An integrated model of its attraction, opportunities, and risks. J Adoles Health. 2011;48:121-7.

Van Doorn MD, Branje SJT, Meeus WHJ. Conflict resolution in parent-adolescent relationships and adolescent delinquency. J Early Adoles. 2008;28:503-27.

Wig NN, Menon DK, Bedi H, et al. Expressed emotion and schizophrenia in north India: II. Distribution of expressed emotion components among relatives of schizophrenicpatients in Aarhus and Chandigarh. Br J Psychiatry. 1987;151:160-5.

Winstona R, Chicot R. The importance of early bonding on the long-term mental health and resilience of children. Lond J Prim Care. 2016;8:12-4.

Zuroff DC, Blatt SJ. The therapeutic relationship in the brief treatment of depression: contributions to clinical improvement and enhanced adaptive capacities. J Consult Clin Psychol. 2006;74: 199-206.

Psychology of Subpopulations in the Indian Society

Girishwar Misra, Nisha Mani Pandey, Indiwar Misra

SUMMARY

Subpopulations are the clusters of individuals who are recognized as a particular group of a larger society to which they belong. These groups face substandard life and often have to face a number of challenges in pursuing a life with dignity. Such situations foster negative attitude about self and society. Even sometimes they are not able to identify meaning in life. This chapter identifies some major subgroups of the Indian society and explores how such exclusivity from the general society negatively affects their psychological well-being, and physical and mental health status. Integrated efforts to change the life conditions and extending support would help ameliorating the health problems of these groups.

INTRODUCTION

Subpopulation or subgroup refers to the cluster of individuals who are recognized as a particular group within a larger society. These subpopulations are generally defined on implicit theories of personality which are inferred on the basis of individuals' potential behaviors, emotional reactions, personality attributes, attitudes, and values (Cantor & Mischel, 1979; Kaplan, 1972; Schneider 1973). Such categorizations are commonly based on personality traits and intellectual properties of the individuals belonging to the subgroup. These subgroups are usually perceived to hold certain apparent characteristics which are recognized by personality traits, professional background, and belief systems. Survival of subgroups in the society is essentially knitted with stereotypes about physical features, typical overt behaviors, demographic demarcations as well as imperceptible/abstract features like thoughts, feelings, beliefs, and experiences. Members of a particular subgroup often imbibe such characterizations and generally feel comfortable with it, and designate it as their own subgroup. This chapter briefly outlines the psychology of some subpopulations of the Indian society in the context of shared mentality prevalent in the society. To this end, it highlights four key aspects of life including social processes, mental health, and biological and psychosocial milieu.

Before discussing about psychology of subgroups of the society, a brief description about various subpopulations is in order. India is a home to around 1.21 billion people and is the 2nd most populous country of the world (Census India, 2011). It will be worth mentioning that the population density itself is a big reason in the emergence of marginalized groups; as this adds more and more people in various marginalized subgroups. Further, according to the latest census report of 2011, the population of schedule tribes (STs) and scheduled castes (SCs) in India is 104.55 and 201.38 million, respectively, and; majority of them are illiterate (SCs = 66.07%; STs = 58.95 %). Since long, this subpopulation has been considered as a marginalized group and majority of them remain underprivileged on many counts, i.e. psychosocial, economic, educational, etc. Disability is another reason for marginalization. The recent census (2011) reveals that 26.8 million people are disabled in the country. A group of migrated people in labor class also generate a subgroup which confronts a number of challenges. It is reported that interstate migration is predominated by the labor to balance the supply and demand of work force generated by regional inequality (Ministry of Social Justice and Empowerment, 2004-05). In 2011, for the first time the Indian Census collected details about another group of marginalized people, i.e. transgender, and found that there are 487,803 individuals who belong to this category. According to the Ministry of Social Justice and Empowerment, about 27.5% of total population lives below the poverty line. Of these, the majority belongs to SCs (rural = 36.8%; urban = 39.9%) followed by other backward classes (OBCs) (rural = 26.7%; urban = 31.4%) and others (rural = 16.1%; urban =16.0%) (Planning Commission, 2014).

It will be worth mentioning that the foundation of Indian society has been basically governed by an inflexible occupation-based hierarchical caste and class system. Indeed caste (*Jati*) has been playing a vital role in upbringing, socialization, and choosing an occupation. Upper caste people generally endorse a negative outlook for the lower caste people who were treated as untouchable (*Asprishya*) people in the society. They were not even allowed to mix with general population. A number of reform movements were launched, and gradually the society is now coming out from the spell of caste and class system. However, empowerment still plays a vital role and many of them are impoverished and underprivileged and not getting due psychosocial support of the society, and are demarcated as marginalized group of the population. The Ministry of Social Justice and Empowerment is taking an initiative to bring these people into the mainstream.

Why Psychology of Subgroups of Society?

The subgroups may be referred in a number of ways viz. weaker sections of the society or poorest of the poor having no shelter, disabled or impaired individuals, persons born into particular community (tribes, ethnic group), migrants, or homosexual groups, etc. who face social exclusion/segregation, i.e. marginality. The marginalized subgroups have comparatively less control and poor resources for fulfilling their basic needs. They hardly have the opportunities to fulfil their basic needs, get proper education, and avail healthcare facilities easily. Most of the time, people of such marginal subgroups lack supportive and positive outlook of the general population and therefore, remain isolated and feel somewhat restricted to behave as normal human beings. Sometimes these subgroups have to face marginality from the very beginning of life. At times they are stigmatized. That situation persists and some might attain it due to disability/impairment, changing socio-economic matrices or sexual orientation, etc. The members of such subgroups have specific attitudes, beliefs, thinking, motivation, living practices, etc. Often they do not get a favorable outlook of the society and face disapproval. They have to face a number of problems to fulfil their basic needs, and most of their lives end up in meeting out their basic needs and resolving these problems. Marginalization eliminates the individual from the society as a whole, and their satisfaction from social lives at individual, interpersonal, and societal levels remain very limited.

Let us have an overview of various subgroups of society who are exclusively being treated as marginalized group, and face a number of psychosocial challenges as well as physical or environmental deprivation which render them vulnerable. Most of these subgroups endorse specific local beliefs and attitudes which generally lead to faulty behavioral patterns regarding lifestyle, sanitation, child rearing practices, cooking and eating, interpersonal skills, living and nurturing, and concepts about self and society. Most of these behavioral patterns are generally responsible for generating health related problems. Being a marginalized group of society, they often remain unaware about healthy behavioral patterns as well as the official initiatives related to the basic amenities like sanitation, nutrition, health care and health promotion.

Economically Weaker Section of Society

Globalization is being considered as a sign of development of the society. But capitalism is playing a vital role in generating socio-economic gaps in the society; the poor are facing more deprivation as their basic needs of survival are not being met due to various reasons. The term economically weaker section (EWS) refers to those individuals or households whose level of income is lower than a definite threshold which may be arbitrary across the states. More and more people are becoming homeless and weaker or have to quit parental occupations or systems of social support (Moroney & Chomsky, 2000; Petras & Veltmeyer, 2001; Pilger 2016). People who are economically weak, have comparatively less control over their lives and the resources available to them. Their attitude towards livelihood entirely differs from other sections as majority of their time is spent in satiating their basic needs. Most of the time they remain stressed in managing their bread and butter. Generally, they develop negative attitude towards life due to many reasons related to their survival.

The EWS often have the negative kind of stress which develops uncertainty, refusal, anger, worriedness, and feeling of sadness. Such type of negativity has an adverse effect on one's physical stature. Further, regular stress often leads to many health problems like pains and aches, distresses, rashes, sleeplessness, restlessness, anxiety, ulcers, depression, hypertension, etc. These stresses seize their positive outlook towards life and at times the individual feels troubled and has a hard time to cope. This directly has a negative impact on one's self-efficacy. Studies reveal that self-efficacy is related with various socio-economic domains like income (Gurin et al., 1978); education (Adams et al., 2007); and vocational outcome expectations (Ali et al., 2005). Specific consequences of negative socio-economic conditions are well-established, as self-efficacy is severely reduced following job loss (Pearlin, 1981; Gecas & Seff, 1989), and as a consequence of chronic economic hardship (Popkin, 1990).

Destitute

A person who resides without a shelter and is deprived of any kind of organized and structured care is called as a destitute. Destitute do not have resources and therefore, are unable to meet out their elementary necessities like accommodation, cordiality, diet, water, and health.

According to Census of India (2011) around 1.8 million population of the country are homeless. Destitution has become the term commonly used to refer to the poverty experienced by an asylum seeker and for them who do not have familial, social, emotional, and financial support. A person living without support is unable to understand the meaning of support, and their behavior and attitude towards self, life, and society is found to be entirely different. They often develop physical health problems, emotional or psychiatric problems, face abuse, or indulge in antisocial activities. It is reported that destitute females who reside in institutions, exhibit absence of a normal inhibitory pattern, emotional hunger, emotional superficiality, and absence of normal tension and anxiety (Padmam, 2003). Studies reveal that stress and depression are positively correlated for homeless women (Ayerst, 1999). Further, incidence of depression among destitute women all across the world is higher than among non-destitute women and men (Brown et al., 2002; Kaslow et al., 2000; Kneisl & Trigoboff, 2004; Lilly, 2002; Sharma, 2014). This may be the result of any of the deprivation related to physio-economic and/ experiential factors (Misra & Tripathi, 1980). Destitute often face various negative experiences in life like financial crisis, accommodation issues, loneliness, hatred from others, and are thus more susceptible to develop one or other kind of mental illnesses and need special care and attention.

Persons with Disabilities

In 1980, the World Health Organization defined disability as individual's limitation or restriction of an activity as a result of impairment, whereas impairment denotes loss or abnormality of psychological, physical, or anatomical structure or function at the system or organ level that may or may not be permanent and that may or may not result in disability (World Health Organization, 1980). People who are unable to perform their usual day-to-day activities by self or are dependent on others for most of their activities are referred as persons with disabilities (PWDs). In other words, an individual who lacks physical or mental capacities, is called as PwD. Disability is measured on the basis of severity of impairment. The PwDs are considered as the weakest of the weak as they are dependent on others and are deprived of most of the basic amenities. Due to their physical and mental limits, PwD's participation in educational, social and professional activities are hindered most of the time.

It is reported that PwD have to face a number of challenges. A recent study reveals that adolescents with disability had poorer health and were more exposed to both traditional bullying and cyber harassment (Fridh et al., 2015). This public health issue needs more attention in schools and society in general; disability in India needs to be considered as a social, cultural, and political phenomenon (Ghai, 2015).

A person with physical disability generally has the feeling of insecurity related to his safety and security. PwD often develop a negative attitude about self or life and are often subjected to discriminatory behavior from the society which also inculcates in them a feeling of dejection. This type of attitude or discriminatory behavior of social surroundings may lead to low self-esteem in PwDs. Coping with disability is a big issue in the society. Various disabilities due to mental illnesses have detrimental impact on educational, professional, social, and family functioning of the sufferers.

Migrants

Migrants can be found all across the world, and therefore, studies on migration are a concern of the world. There are various reasons for migration. It is a process through which people move from a permanent place to another, more or less stable place for a significant time period. In India, there is significant migration from rural to urban areas (Mitra & Murayama, 2009). Migration is found to be a significant event of life, and therefore has its debilitating effect on one's life (Ebrahim, 2010; Kessler, 1997). It is reported that around 44–105 million people reside in urban slums (NSSO, 2013). Migrants are more susceptible to develop mental ailments like depression as they repeatedly face many problems for earning their bread and butter. A study from Indonesia reported that migration imposes considerable costs on mental health and encourages higher levels of smoking. The effects differ between women and men. Female migrants tend to internalize the stress experienced in migration and display depressive symptoms, whereas male migrants tend to externalize various stressors by smoking more cigarettes if they already smoke, though they do not start smoking (Lu, 2010). Further, due to migration one has to face acculturation or discrimination, loss of social support and family disruption (NSSO, 2013; Subbaraman et al., 2014).

Tribes or Adivasi

The groups of people like forest dwellers or those living in hills who are often fully dependent on their own land and largely unaware of modern society are called Tribes/Adivasi/Vanvasi. India has the largest tribal population all across the world. According to Census 2011 statistics, 8.6% of total Indian population, i.e. 104 million are tribes. After independence, some policies and programs have been pursued for uplifting the lives of tribes (UNICEF, 2010). It is an established fact that the early developmental stage (1–8 years) of life is significantly important when language, psycho-socio-motor activities as well as socio-emotional development occur. Tribal children are generally disadvantaged and are often excluded despite the fact that various policies and programmes have been pursued for their enrichment (UNICEF, 2010). Tribal life has an adverse impact on overall development of their children. Tribal people have their demarcated remote geographical area, their own culture, beliefs and language, and negligible contact with the society.

Lesbian, Gay, Bisexual, and Transgender

Heterosexuality is the hallmark of normal human relations. In such a situation, lesbians, gays, bisexuals, and transgenders (LGBTs) are not accepted by the society. Earlier LGBTs were designated an abnormal category. However, from the late 60s and early 70s, a debate on LGBTs had continued for their classification as mental disorders, and in 1973, the debate ended up with the removal of homosexuality from the 2nd edition of the *Diagnostic and Statistical Manual of Mental Disorders* (*DSM II*; American Psychiatric Association, 1973). However, in the society the number and proportion of LGBTs are small and therefore, many a times they have to face a number of challenges. In general, the society does not have a positive outlook about LGBTs; at times they are embarrassed, face humiliation from the society and are not treated well. In spite of legislations, they face a number of stressors for their existence and therefore, feel deprived of many social needs. Fear of rejection and discrimination may develop anxiety or stress in this group of individuals.

It will be worth mentioning that all these subgroups are overloaded with so many issues that they hardly dare to think for their betterment, and most of the time their capabilities remain suppressed. Their major part of life is consumed in fulfilling the basic needs. They face a number of social restrictions, and therefore, tend to believe that they do not have meaning in life, are excluded from the society in general, accepted as unusual segment and don't get proper social support. For fulfilling their basic needs, most of the time people of this subgroup remain engaged in serving others. In such a situation, many times they remain neglected and start believing that their life is meant only for assisting others and not anything else. It is also true that if an individual falls in these subgroups; their status and situations hinder them in accessing proper services, income, and belongings, and restrict their liberty, freedom, and growth. Moreover, due to such situations, a possibility to develop detrimental belief and attitude about self and society may occur. Each and every described subgroup of the society need proper support and strength from the society as social supports are needed to improve the life satisfaction among the population aged 45 or more with low social class. By understanding the psychology of these subgroups of society, many of the illnesses can be controlled and prevented. And this can be possible if the attitude, belief and social cognition of the members of the particular subgroups are analyzed critically. It will be worth mentioning that behavior of an individual with convinced mindset may remain unaware about his/her deeds (Ferguson et al., 2005). Problem focused initiatives may be one of the best suited strategies for changing attitude of subgroups by introducing healthy behavioral patterns and eliminating faulty beliefs. For the modification in the intrapsychic configuration of a subgroup, one needs to take the help of those social institutions which already exist in the system. Further, with the help of group leaders or local influential people, the subgroups may be taken in confidence and benefited.

CONCLUSION

Subpopulations need an inclusive approach to the feeling, thoughts, and behaviors of various subgroups of the society. Awareness programs may develop understanding for their own rights. Also they should be productively involved in the social system; and resources to meet their basic needs have to be generated. To help the people of these subgroups to overcome their challenges in constructive ways, participatory approach and action research would be very effective. Further, an interdisciplinary approach by weaving together the personal, relational and social milieu may help overcoming the problems of subgroups. Furthermore, an emphasis on participatory and action oriented work will hold promise for supporting those who are feeling marginalized due to their membership of a particular subgroup that shows resistance to change. Such concerted efforts may help in developing positive attitude and belief which further will be helpful in developing their capabilities and skills in a positive manner and strengthen the psychology of subgroups. However, this needs firm determination at individual and group levels, and also an extensive academic, political, and scientific will and approach.

REFERENCES

Adams J, Martin-Ruiz C, Pearce MS, White M, et al. No association between socioeconomic status and white blood cell telomere length. Aging Cell. 2007;6(1):125-8.

Ali SR, McWhirter EH, Chronister KM. Self-efficacy and vocational outcome expectations for adolescents of lower socioeconomic status: A pilot study. J Career Assess. 2005;13:40(1)-58.

Ayerst SL. Depression and stress in street youth. Adolesc. 1999;34(135):567-75.

Brown VB, Melchior LA, Waite-O'Brien N, Huba GJ. Effects of women-sensitive, long-term residential treatment on psychological functioning of diverse populations of women. J Subst Abuse Treat. 2002;23(2):133-44.

Cantor N, Mischel W. Prototypes in person perception. In ML Berkowitz (Ed), Advances in Experimental Social Psychology. (Vol 12) NY Academic Press. 1979; pp. 3-52.

Census India 2011. Office of the Registrar General & Census Commissioner, Indian Ministry of Home Affairs, Government of India, 2011

Ebrahim S, Kinra S, Bowen L, et al. The effect of rural-to-urban migration on obesity and diabetes in India: a cross-sectional study. PLoS Med. 2010;7(4):e1000268.

Ferguson MJ, Bargh JA, Nayak DA. After-affects: How automatic evaluations influence the interpretation of subsequent, unrelated stimuli. J Exp Soc Psychol. 2005;41(2):182-91.

Fridh M, Lindström M, Rosvall M Subjective health complaints in adolescent victims of cyber harassment: moderation through support from parents/friends - a Swedish population-based study. BMC Public Health. 2015; 15:949.

Gecas V, Seff MA. Social class, occupational conditions, and self-esteem. Sociol Perspect. 1989;32:353-64.

Ghai, Anita. Rethinking Disability in India. New Delhi: Routledge; 2015.

Gurin P, Gurin G, Morrison BM. Personal and ideological aspects of internal and external control. Social Psychol. 1978;41:275-96.

Kaplan HB. Toward a general theory of psychosocial deviance: The case of aggressive behavior. Soc Sci Med. 1972;6(5):593-617.

Kaslow N, Thompson M, Meadows L, et al. Risk factors for suicide attempts among African American women. Depress Anxiety. 2000;12(1):13-20.

Kessler RC. The effects of stressful life events on depression. Annu Rev Psychol. 1997;48(1):191-214.

Kneisl CR, Trigoboff E. Contemporary Psychiatric-Mental Health Nursing. Prentice Hall, New Jersey: Pearson Education; 2004.

Lilly E. Women and depression: Not just—the blues. Alabama Nurse. 2002;29:24.

Lu Y. Mental health and risk behaviours of rural–urban migrants: Longitudinal evidence from Indonesia. Popul Stud (Camb). 2010;64(2):147-63.

Misra G, Tripathi LB. Psychological Consequences of Prolonged Deprivation. Agra, India: National Psychological Corporation. 1980.

Misra G, Tripathi KN. Psychological Dimensions of poverty and deprivation. In: J. Pandey (Ed). Psychology in India Revisited: Developments in the Discipline (Vol.3) Applied Social and Organizational Psychology. New Delhi: Sage Publications; 2004. pp.118-215.

Mitra A, Murayama M. Rural to urban migration: a district-level analysis for India. Int J Migration Health Soc Care. 2009;5(2):35-52.

Moroney M, Chomsky N. Rogue States: The Rule of Force in World Affairs. Cambridge MA: South End Press; 2000.

NSSO: Key Indicators of Urban Slums in India. National Sample Survey 69th Round. July 2012–December 2012. New Delhi: Ministry of Statistics and Programme Implementation; 2013.

Padmam MR. Destitute Women in Kerala. Psychological Resources and Psycho-social Needs. Centre for Development Studies; 2003.

Pearlin LI, Menaghan EG, Lieberman MA, Mullan JT. The stress process. J Health Soc Behav. 1981;22(4): 337-56.

Petras JF, Veltmeyer H. Globalization Unmasked: Imperialism in the 21st Century. New York: Zed Books; 2001.

Pilger J. The New Rulers of the World. New York: Verso Books; 2016.

Planning Commission. Review of Expert Group to Review the Methodology for Estimation of Poverty, Government of India, 2014.

Popkin SJ. Welfare:Views from the bottom. Soc Prob. 1990;37:64-79.

Schneider DJ. Implicit personality theory: A review. Psychol Bull. 1973;79(5):294-309.

Sharma A. Stress and depression in destitute and normal females. Int J Acad Res Psychol. 2014;1:1-6.

Subbaraman R, Nolan L, Shitole T, et al. The psychological toll of slum living in Mumbai, India: A mixed methods study. Soc Sci Med. 2014;119:155-69.

UNICEF. The Status of Tribal Children in India. Published Report; 2010.pp 10-6.

World Health Organization. International classification of impairments, disabilities, and handicaps: a manual of classification relating to the consequences of disease; publ. for trial purposes in accordance with resolution WHA29. 35 for the Twenty-ninth World Health Assembly, May 1976. 1980.

Chapter 12

Culture, Mythology, and Religion

PC Joshi, VK Srivastava

SUMMARY

This chapter looks at the relationship between culture, religion, and mythology, with particular reference to the Indian context. Broadly, it argues that culture, although having its genesis in the discipline of anthropology, is today the overarching concept in the world of scholarship, and one of its institutions is the religion. Myths are the stories which were believed to have been created in the "distant past", the past which does not have a specific and bounded "time period". In spite of their antiquity, myths are evergreen, and seem to be relevant at all points in time. Besides textual and scripture based religion, there exists popular and practiced religion providing meaning to the day-to-day life experiences of the people. Religion in practice blends local history, myths, legends and age-old religious practices, besides syncretizing elements of other religions. Thus, each of the Indian religions has its own set of myths, and also that which it shares with the other religious communities, and they collectively exercise a tremendous impact on the minds of people, eventually having its bearing on mental health and behavioral aspects of human beings.

CONCEPT OF CULTURE

"Culture is uniquely human", so said Bronislaw Malinowski (1944), the renowned anthropologist of the Polish origin. One of the central concerns of the early anthropologists was to distinguish human beings from other animals, although they had all accepted the biologist's conclusion that humans also belong to the Order of Primates of the Animal Kingdom. The anthropological point was that in the long-drawn process of evolution, human beings have lost a number of physical traits, such as the tail, or decimated some of them, like reduction in the size of canine, and alongside, acquired a number of the other characteristics which facilitated the emergence of culture. Since such evolutionary changes did not occur with the other animals they have remained bereft of culture and have to depend solely upon their biological endowments.

One of the biological changes that progressively occurred was in the cranial capacity of human beings, who as a result became "thinking and reflecting beings". Because of the changes that had occurred in their limbs, hands and the positioning of the thumb, the ideas that came in the minds of people could be concretely transformed into material objects. Human beings started fabricating the naturally found resources, and the "world of artifacts", the product of human handiwork, was born. The ideas and the technological skills could be easily transmitted through speech and language to the posterity. For whatever human beings produced in order to survive on the face of the earth, the term that the anthropologists used from the second-half of the nineteenth century, after the masterly work of Edward B Tylor, was "culture" (Voget, 1975). In the last one hundred and seventy-five years, a number of definitions of culture have been given. Each author has emphasized one or the other aspect of culture, however, all these definitions agree on the following points:

- In its fully developed form, culture is confined to human beings. Rudimentary evidences of culture come from the study of the social life of higher primates, particularly chimpanzee, but culture in its true form is distinctly human
- Culture comprises the tangible and intangible aspects. This distinction is principally of analytical significance, for in reality, behind each tangible object is a set of ideas (the intangible/non-material things), which actually leads to its shaping, and the ideas may find their concrete manifestations in material forms. A clarification in this context is offered below
- Human beings have great capacity to think, produce ideas, think about the future, have visions, fictionalize events, invent bodies of ideology and found schools of thought; and not every idea, they have, acquires a material shape. Thus, the relationship between non-material and material aspects of culture should not be seen in a mechanical way, as if each idea will have a material representation. The opposite, however, is true—behind each material entity, there is a corpus of ideas
- Culture is cumulative. Its activities, achievements, codes and procedures of conduct, norms and morality, and changes that occur in each one of them over time are recorded orally as well as in writing, when the latter originated. Human beings reflect upon their past culture, analyzing and learning from it
- Culture is socially transmitted. One of the prime functions of social institutions (be it family, school, peer group, or neighborhood) is to transmit the cultural products to the following generations.

RELIGIOUS SYSTEM: MYTHS, BELIEFS, AND PRACTICES ARE INTEGRAL TO CULTURE

Human beings are "intellect-gifted" and "ideas-generating". They raise questions and remain restless unless they have found satisfactory answers to their queries. Further, they keep on testing critically their already available answers in different situations, for they know that their answers may be time- as well as space-bound, and if the answers deserve to be changed or re-framed, they do so.

One of the many facts that has always deeply concerned men and women in all societies is their periodic encounter with death, near-death experiences, and the experiences of illness and incapacitation of the body which prophesy the imminent and permanent departure of the being. That this is the fate of all living beings (and of the non-living entities) dawns upon the people, creating a puzzling situation: Why are we born to die? How can we become "immortal"? What happens to "us" after death? Who decides the time and place of death? Related with these "fundamental questions", ever bothering, ever engaging, are the questions of inequality and suddenness of the occurrence of events: Why some are born disabled, poor, ugly? Why some remain unsuccessful in life despite the toil they uninterruptedly put in, and why some have silver spoons in their mouths even when they are nasty, cruel, haughty, and unkind? And, why we do not know what may happen the next moment? The uncertainty of life has always been an intellectual enigma, necessitating intense and profound thinking on these questions.

Thus, the subjects of prime concern have been systematizing the meaning in one's living, making the short-lived life "symbolically immortal", answering the questions of life after death and of transmigration of spirit, reincarnation, rebirth as an animal or plant, and of illness, suffering, and pain (Geertz, 1973). These questions and concerns led to the discovery of an entity or a set of entities placed above all living and nonliving things, which affect the course of life. Thus, was discovered the "idea of holy", comprising objects and thoughts that are unblemished, free from imperfections, all powerful, complete, boon-granting and miracles-producing, and above all, superior to all, thus safeguarding the long-term welfare of people who repose their faith in the "holy".

The complex of these thoughts and actions that is concerned with the "fundamental questions" of life and death and the matters of "permanence" and "impermanence", "certainty" and "uncertainty", and "joy" and "pain" is known as "religion" or the "religious system". The following thoughts are generally identified with its understanding:

- Religion is universally found; even in those polities which claim to have wiped out religion and established a society "free" from it, as has been the case with the Communist states, where religion has continued to survive clandestinely at the level of households. It has so happened that whenever the state sanctions on religion relaxed, it returned with full vigor as if it was always there, always intact
- Religion is a way of asserting the hierarchy of power and strength, and to acknowledge the "tininess" and "puniness" of human beings. Political institution may also assert a hierarchy of some sort but what is crucial to religion is the acknowledgement of the "transience" of human existence, suffocated at every nook and corner with sufferings, some bearable, some unbearable
- Religion posits the concrete and the abstract forms of supreme, transcendental, invincible, and omnifarious power, a submission to which is regarded as the greatest human duty. The power is referred to by many local terms, the English equivalent of which is God; that is the reason why in a definition of religion, the concept of God (or moral prescriptions or truths which are believed to be of the same stature as God is) is regarded as its most important component
- Some writers are shy of using the term God in their definitions of religion. Instead, they use words such as "extra-mundane", "spiritual", "unseen order", "holy entities", etc., conveying the same idea as it is conveyed by the concept of God. Scholars, who point out that the world religions like Buddhism and Jainism do not have the concept of God, do say that these religions have "sacred precepts and unassailable truths", which are preternatural, almost equal to the sacredness of God, in which the people repose their faith. Against this backdrop, it was natural that Émile Durkheim (1912) defined religion in terms of the idea of sacredness: Religion comprises a set of beliefs and practices concerned with sacred things, which are set apart and forbidden; and as a property, sacredness is superimposed on objects and ideas. Things are thus sacred not because of their intrinsic qualities but because they are enveloped by sacredness

- An instrumental thought in the minds of people is that the pantheon in which they have faith will grant them their boons, take care of their long-term welfare, relieve them of miseries and woes, and ensure them an eternal place in the "abode" of God. Religion becomes an ally of people. Failures in life do not dampen the faith of people in divinity. On the contrary, they think that they were unsuccessful because they lacked in their devotion to the almighty, or their ritual performances lacked correctness. Deities need to be placated mentally as well as in ritual actions; only then one may hope for divine favor and compassion.

THE SCIENCE OF MYTHOLOGY

It is because of the celebrated contribution of Claude Lévi-Strauss (1963), the French structuralist, that the study of myths acquired not only a respectable but also a scientific status. Scholars before him, and even many of his contemporaries, studied myths that they had collected from different societies as examples of folklore rather than as the "mental product" that could guide us to the understanding of the working of human mind.

For Lévi-Strauss, myths were a significant material (of human creation), for they helped us in grasping how the human mind worked, how it processed information, how different pieces of knowledge were combined, and why there were amazing similarities between the folklore, or kin terms, of different societies, separated by distances of thousands of miles. Similarities between societies could not always be attributed to the processes of diffusion and migration. Perhaps, Lévi-Strauss said, all human beings think in the same way, using the same chunks of information they derived from their external environment. In a nutshell, this logic pointed to the "unity of human mind." That is why it is said that Lévi-Strauss was interested in the study of the Universal Mind, rather than the multiplicity of human societies.

Here, for understanding Lévi-Strauss's method, an analogy from the psychiatrist's work is in order. It is from the episodes of mental imagery (the "mental output"), a person (and his kith and kin) convey to the psychiatrist in their interactions, that the latter infers the behavioral disorders of the sick. In the same way, from the "mental output" of the people, the myths and stories, the kin terms and rules of marriage, the anthropologist endeavors to know the working and the content of the human mind. As a psychiatrist (or a psychiatric social worker) collects the detailed life history of the sick before reaching a diagnosis, in a similar way, the anthropologist meticulously collects the myths, interviewing a myriad of respondents, and also the published reports, for they are a key to discerning the mystery of human mind.

The term "belief" implies accepting the "truthfulness of an idea, thought, event, happening, and entity", despite the skepticism that many others may express on them. Beliefs of people are often unshakeable. They are closely interwoven with the "stories" and "happenings" of the past, for which the term used is myth. Perhaps, Lévi-Strauss gave the finest definition of myth: It is a story of the feats of the characters which is set in a time-frame known as "once upon a time". A myth is independent of the time dimension—the story happened at one time, but people are least interested in knowing the exact time, or least interested in ascertaining its veracity. For them, myths are creditable with truth; the events counted in the myths actually happened and people believe in them. To exemplify: for the people, the great war between the lineage members of the Kuru actually took place, one which is narrated in the epic of

Mahabharata, notwithstanding what the archeological work that BB Lal undertook in the village of Hastinapur (Mathura, Uttar Pradesh) led us to believe. That the kingdom of golden Lanka was situated beyond the coastline of Rameshwaram is an inerrable fact for the believers irrespective of what the archaeological researches of HD Sankalia tell us.

Religion and myths are closely connected. Behind every precept that is followed is a story that legitimizes it. Myths are sometimes intricate, complexly elaborate, and yield several messages that must be adhered. Lévi-Strauss spent more than 50 years analyzing the myths dealing with different aspects of reality (such as food and eating practices, clothing, pottery, and sexuality), showing that they are an essential part of culture. Although myths deal with different institutions of society, they are overwhelmingly represented in religion. Stronger the hold of religion on society, stronger and well-entrenched are the myths.

Let us now look at the Indian religions for the dynamics of culture, religion, and myths.

THE INDIAN SCENE: UNITY IN DIVERSITY

India is a land of multiple religions, sects, creeds, denominations, faiths, and cults. Quite regularly, one hears of the emergence of new "religions", "new religious movements", the cults of god persons and mystics, each claiming a wide following (Madan, 1992). The number of television channels that cater to matters of religion and its mythic world has multiplied, indicating a wide viewership. Instead of declining, as was thought in the late 19th and early 20th centuries, and also by a large number of skeptics throughout the human existence, religion has not disappeared. Its hold on society has definitely decreased and the number of "non-believers" has escalated, but its gripping presence on modern society cannot go unnoticed.

Contemporary India, according to the Census-2011, has six main religious communities, which respectively are Hindu (79.80%), Muslim (14.25%), Christian (2.30%), Sikh (1.72%), Buddhist (0.70%), and Jain (0.37%); the seventh is labeled as the "Others" (0.66%), which also includes "tribal religions"; another 0.24% did not state their religion. Thus, India's "composite religious culture" is a product of the unrelaxing interaction between Indic religions, which were born here, and those which arrived here from different parts of the world at different points of time.

Hinduism is one of the oldest, continuously existing religions, and yet it was named as such only in the nineteenth century. What is now called Hinduism consists of amalgamation, refinement, adaptation, and absorption of multiple traditions and ritualistic practices at various times and from various places. Therefore, unlike other known religions of the world, Hinduism does not have a founder or prophet, a single text, a single path to follow and finally no single authority. The essence of Hinduism lies in its being highly pluralistic, dynamic, adaptive, syncretic, and built up of flexible tenets, something akin to a sponge which has the ability to absorb, adopt, and adapt. A highly ritualistic person is as much a Hindu as is the one who rejects the paraphernalia of rituals, or one who does not believe in the existence of God.

The contrast between the text-based and the practiced Hinduism in various local areas has been understood in the dichotomy of great and little traditions. The great tradition is practiced at the pilgrim centers, like Kashi, Haridwar, Puri, and Rameshwaram. Hinduism in such places is text-dependent, Brahmanical and structured, whereas the little tradition is epitomized in the form of village deities and the cult of the mother goddess. These localized pantheons are non-Brahmanical, non-vegetarian, and unstructured. The appropriation of the little tradition by the great tradition and the percolation of the great tradition to the local communities have inspired the internal transformation of Hinduism. That it is an endless process is a fact known to all.

While Hinduism does not subscribe to a single book, the early Hinduism is equated with the orally transmitted Vedas, namely Rig Veda, Yajur Veda, Sama Veda, and Atharva Veda. The Vedas believed to be revealed to the sages under a meditative state were transmitted orally for centuries, to be finally converted into a textual form. Among the Veda, Atharva Veda consists of prescriptions and methods to treat (and cure) situations arising out of supernatural forces, like ghosts, demons, spirits, etc.

Along with the Vedas, there are supplementary compositions called Brahmanas, Aranyakas and Upanishads. Hindu mythologies are contained in Purana literature, which contains the descriptions of the feats of gods, goddesses, and the other divine forces. The epics of Ramayana and Mahabharata describe the two incarnations of Vishnu, viz. Rama and Krishna, respectively. Both the epics are very lengthy, covering 100,000 and 25,000 verses respectively. These epics are available in multiple versions in India and its neighboring countries. For example, there are nearly 300 versions of Ramayana and likewise the Mahabharata stories also vary from one context to another.

Popular Hinduism assumes multiple forms within which Hindus practice their religion. At the upper layer, there are temples of pan-Indian deities and their associated attendants, such as Vishnu, Shiva, Rama, Krishna, Ganesha, Hanuman, and their regional forms. With these gods are the goddesses like Parvati, Lakshmi, Durga, Saraswati, along with the other forms like Kali. A very well-defined cycle of fasts, festivals, fairs, and rituals is associated with these great deities.

Besides these, there are localized village level deities related to village land, ancestors, local heroes, martyrs and sundry other divine entities found in rivers, streams, waterfalls, ponds, forests, trees, cremation grounds, and other places. Many of these supernatural entities are benevolent but some are considered to be highly malicious, demanding elaborate rituals and sacrifices. These supernatural agencies are propitiated in anthropomorphic to amorphous forms through Brahmanical and non-Brahmanical interventions. At localized level, quite often Hinduism is practiced in a syncretic fashion where boundaries of purity-impurity, auspiciousness and inauspiciousness, and religion and caste are often blurred. At regional level, there exist various cults and fellowships to which many Hindus subscribe. People accept fellowship under Radhaswami, Balaknath, Gorakhnath, and myriad god persons. In present times, the prevalence of such cults is on rise wherein people are given *mantra* (holy litany) or *nam* (name of some divine entity) by the *guru* (preceptor) to be practiced for achieving the desired results.

Hindu pantheon is a very complex and dynamic system with supposedly a number of deities nearing, as it is said proverbially, 330 million. Thus there are gods and goddesses identified with the mainstream and textual Hinduism alongside innumerable localized folk deities. In the early Vedic times, the prominent gods were Rudra, Agni, Indra, Soma, Vayu, Adityas, Varunas, Visvadevas, Brahma, Prajapati, Maruts, Pusan, and Asvin. At present, we have the trinity gods as Brahma, Vishnu and Shiva, with Saraswati, Parvati and Lakshmi as Goddesses along with their incarnations, subordinates, manifestations, and emanations. These include incarnations like Rama, Krishna, Narsimha, Venkateswara, Raghunatha, Vittalnatha, Jagannatha, Dakshinamurty, and Jyotirlinga with attendant gods like Ganesh, Kumara, Nandi, Hanuman, Garuda, besides Kali, Durga, Ambe, Kamakhya, Sati, and Vaishnodevi.

Spirit possession, shamanism, and tantrik traditions are an inseparable component of Hinduism in many parts of India. Spirit possession exists in two forms, namely forceful possession of an innocent human body by an evil force, like ghost, demon and any other malevolent agencies, and voluntary possession by a medium of a benevolent spirit. In the first case, the bad spirit is driven out by means of exorcism while in the latter, the medium who invites the spirit answers questions, suggests ways and gives blessings. Shamans are believed to control supernatural powers by means of special meditative practices, and thus are employed by their clients for various magico-religious assignments.

As a microcosm of the world, India is a home to all kinds of religions. As stated earlier, being a home to world religions, like Hinduism, Jainism, Buddhism, and Sikhism, it is also a place where Islam and Christianity have arrived in their nascent states. The fire-worshipping Parsis have also found India to be the most conducive home for the preservation of their religion. One of the important characteristics of the religions coming from outside has been the exchange of ideas and actions they had with Hinduism. The religions originating in India have a lot in common with Hinduism as these began their respective journeys as reformist religions and protest movements.

The term Jain is derived from the root *ji* meaning "to conquer". The central theme of Jainism therefore is to conquer the senses and *karma* (actions) for achieving liberation from worldly bondage. The followers of Jainism are required to live a life devoid of falsehood, violence, and stealing. They also avoid taking meat, wine, honey, and meal after sunset. Jain mythology is very closely related to Hindu and Buddhist mythology as these were compiled simultaneously. Many of the Hindu divinities find mention in the Jain myths. The Jain mythology gives biographical accounts of tirthankaras (the ford-makers), like Rsabha, Parsva, Malli, Mahavira and others. The Jain concept of cosmology likewise is closely related to Hindu and Buddhist cosmology.

Buddhism is derived from the term Buddha, having its root in *budh* meaning to "wake up" to the worldly realities. Its founder Siddhartha Gautama attained enlightenment under a fig tree in Gaya. Buddhism is a very pragmatic religion. It encourages the disciple to discover the path of truth by contemplation. In the mechanism of three marks of existence, four noble truths, five *skandha*s (concepts), six realms and eightfold path, one can achieve *nirvana* (or liberation), the ultimate goal of human life. Buddhist mythologies are greatly inspired by Hinduism. In Agganna Sutta, the story of creation is depicted. The Jataka tales comprise many stories describing the previous birth of Gautama Buddha in human and animal forms.

The word Sikhism is derived from the word *sikh*, which means the "pupils of the Gurus". Sikhism has emerged as a reformist religion against the dogmatic Hinduism and Islam of medieval India. Guru Nanak, the founder of Sikhism, was against the external practices prevailing in Hinduism and Islam, and so he advocated for the idea of searching of God within one's self. Of the ten Gurus that the Sikhs have, the 5th Guru, Arjan, collected the writings of Gurus along with the other known poet-saints into a book called Adi Granth. After the 10th Guru, the system of Guru was abolished and the Adi Grantha became the major icon of the

Sikhs, who treat the Holy Book as a living entity. There are no separate mythologies of the Sikhs who subscribe to the Hindu mythologies.

Christianity originated in Palestine's region called Judea and was established by Jesus of Nazareth. It has now become the largest religion of the world with nearly one-third of the world population subscribing to it. The term Christianity is derived from the Greek word *christos* which means "anointed", referring to Jesus as the messiah. The Holy Bible, Church and the concept of trinity play an important role in Christianity. There is immense heterogeneity in terms of Church within Christianity which has arisen due to the acceptance of the "message" in different historical and sociocultural contexts by its followers.

In India, Christianity arrived as early as the 4th century with the Syriac Christian trading community which settled in Malabar Coast of Kerala. There have been successive attempts by various missionaries to convert native Indians into Christianity. As a result, at present, nearly 2.30% of Indian population is Christian which includes various scheduled caste and scheduled tribe communities. Regions such as Kerala, Tamil Nadu, Central Indian tribal belt, and North-east India have a good concentration of the Christian population.

Islam means "submission to the will of God." It dates back to 622 CE when its promulgator and founder, Prophet Muhammad migrated from his native city, Mecca, to Madina and established the first Islamic state. The followers of Islam called Muslim must affirm the oneness of God. The Holy Book, the Quran, which was revealed to the Prophet, is to be read and recited as the Word of God. Muslims believe in God's angels and messengers, of whom Prophet Muhammad was the last and the most perfect. Muslims must say daily prayers, observe the yearly month of fasting, give alms, and if circumstances allow, go to Mecca in pilgrimage.

Islam arrived in India in 712 CE. Immigrants were not in large number. They also did not know the local customs and practices. In these circumstances, they had to look for the native support. The local people were also attracted to the egalitarian ideology and practices of Islam—the fact that all humans were believed to be equal before God was a great social fact, by contrast to the highly unequal system of the Hindu. Conversions began. Behind these were the political and ideological factors. However, the converts continued with the cultural and social practices of their pre-conversion days. This gradually helped in the emergence of the composite culture in India.

Parsis are the fire-worshipping Zoroastrians, a very small religious minority of India, now numbering nearly 57,00. The term Parsi is derived from the word "Persian" meaning people hailing from Persia, the present day Iran. Parsis have adopted Indian culture yet they are able to maintain their distinctive religious beliefs and practices. Their religious books are Book of Arda Viraf, Book of Jamasp, Story of Sanjan, etc.

In the Census category of the "Other", the religions practices by the scheduled tribe societies of India have been included, although many of them have been influenced by and converted to Hinduism, Islam, Christianity, and Buddhism. However, in addition, they tend to subscribe to the indigenous spirits, ancestors, legends and totems more or less in a syncretic manner. There are many scheduled tribal families which have not changed their religion, i.e. the Jharkhand tribal people believing in Adi Dharma or Sarna Dharma or the Sanamahi Meities of Manipur. The basic tenets of tribal religions are belief in ancestral spirits, spirits of the nature, totemism, spirit-mediumship, shamanism, sacrifice and witchcraft. Many tribal societies also believe in sorcery and black magic, using this as an explanation of several types of illnesses.

CULTURE AND ILLNESS

From an anthropological perspective, it may be said that culture is the cause and remedy of illnesses. From the ceaseless interaction between religion and mythology results the "world view" of the people. Today, the word "cultural model" is preferred over its earlier usage of "world view". Cultural models determine the classification of conditions as "illnesses"—what may be regarded as illness in one context may not be so in the other. Religious ideas and mythology govern the cultural construction of the cosmos, the kind of beliefs people have about the world around them. If they believe that their universe is populated by malicious, capricious, and bloodthirsty spirits, then there will be a high probability of people suffering from supernatural possessions and afflictions.

The domain of the culture-bound syndromes amply points to the need to understand people's ways of living before they could successfully be treated for psychological ailments and behavioral disorders. Here lies the need to grasp the relationship between culture, religion, and myths, before the profile of a population's health and illness could be meaningfully grasped.

REFERENCES

Durkheim É. The Elementary Form of the Religious Life. Beverly Hills, CA: Sage; 1912.
Geertz C. The Interpretation of Cultures. Selected Essays. New York: Basic Books Inc.; 1973.
Lévi-Strauss C. Structural Anthropology. New York: Basic Books Inc.; 1963.
Madan TN. Religion in India. New Delhi: Oxford University Press; 1992.
Malinowski B. A Scientific Theory of Culture and Other Essays. New York: A Galaxy Press; 1944.
Voget FW. A History of Ethnology. New York: Holt Rinehart and Winston; 1975.

Chapter 13

Social Stressors: Visible and Invisible

PK Singh

SUMMARY

Social stressors are the most common and severe type of stress that people have to face in life, other being physical and psychic. Cumulative stress beyond a critical limit can be pathogenic leading to both physical and mental disorders. Inclusion of these concepts into mainstream medicine is just about a 100-year-old. A social stressor can either be a life event, a chronic strain or a combination of both. It can either be visible or invisible. Starting with various definitions of social stressors and their types as well as sources, this chapter deals with various factors, which determine the severity of stress and how can it be assessed. The impact of social roles, education, culture, mass-media, and social institutions in causing stressors of social type has been discussed at length. Various scales developed for assessment of stress and its severity have also been touched upon in a section. Some light has been thrown upon the health consequences of stressors.

INTRODUCTION

Stress and stressors are now mainstream medical concepts. It was not so about a 100-year-ago. The term "stress", as it is currently used, was coined by Hans Selye in 1936, who defined it as "the non-specific response of the body to any demand for change" (What is Stress?, 2017). It was his monumental work on stress-physiology leading to formulation of the concepts of "General Adaptation Syndrome", that ensured a permanent place for these concepts within the purview of medical sciences. However, even before him some astute and legendary physicians, such as Dr William Harvey in 17th century and Dr William Osler in 19th century, had instinctively felt the link between adverse life events and onset of illness based on their observations (Rodin & Key, 1994; Grayboys, 1984). These concepts have now become integrated into the thinking of not only medical professionals but also of the general masses, the lay and literate both. Concept and techniques of stress-management are now a matter of everyday discussion. Stress can be physical, psychic, or social. All of these produce effect on the organism through similar psychophysical pathways. Stress responses induced within the organism by various kinds of stressors are nonspecific, global, organismic, and almost similar in character. Stressors and stress responses are the two components, which are contained within the broad rubric of the concept of stress. "Stressor" refers to the adverse influence that challenges the system and the "stress-response" refers to system's answer to it to either contain it or undo it.

SOCIAL STRESSOR: DEFINITION

Social stressor is one of the various types of stressors. A stressor is any influence on the organism, external or internal, which obligates it to deploy adaptive responses within its internal and/or external milieu with the goal of maintaining systemic order and thereby ensuring survival of the organism. Stress has also been defined as "a state of imbalance within a person, elicited by an actual or perceived disparity between environmental demands and the person's capacity to cope with these demands" (Sociology of Health and Medicine, 2017). Stress is ubiquitous and universal. Life cannot be imagined or be made devoid of stress. It is integral to and inseparable from the process of living. The only thing that can be regulated, individually and collectively, is the frequency and intensity of stressors that any individual may have to deal with. Capacity to deal with life's stresses has been included as one of the hallmarks of sound mental health by the World Health Organization (WHO, 2014).

Stressors can be physical, psychological, or social in origin. Social stressors, even though inadequately talked and discussed about, are amongst the most important sources of severe stresses. Social dimension of man is the source of his origin, is the source of his survival and the source of his satisfaction in life. It is also the source of his most intense pains and pleasures. By corollary therefore, it is also the source of many of the most important stressors of life. "The most common form of stress encountered by people stems from one's social environment and is perceived as more intense than other types of stressors" (Wood & Bhatnagar, 2015).

Social stressor has been defined by the Encyclopaedia of Behavioral Medicine as "a situation which threatens one's relationship, esteem or belonging within a dyad, group or larger social context" (Juth & Dickerson, 2013). Wikipedia defines social stress as "stress that stems from one's relationship with others and from social environment in general" (Social Stress[a], 2017). Wadman et al (2011) define social stress as "the feelings of discomfort or anxiety that individuals may experience in social situations and the associated tendency to avoid potentially stressful social situations". Ifeld (1977) defined social stressor as "circumstances of daily social roles that are generally considered problematic or undesirable". Broadly speaking, social stressors refer to those social events, influences, interactions, and dispositions that contribute to stress generation.

TYPES OF SOCIAL STRESSOR

Some social stressors are only too obvious to require any special expertise to identify them. They are overtly "visible" and therefore can easily be identified and counted. Whereas there are others which continue to affect the organism surreptitiously in adverse manner despite there being a semblance of calmness at the surface. Many of these social situations are the products of our own making which we have collectively adopted either in the name of modernity and progress or in the name of tradition and culture. These are the sources, which may be referred to as "Invisible Social Stressors". These invisible sources are important because they are universal, and tend to impact the individual continuously; there is generally no escape from them, and they are not available for scrutiny because we are all a party to it. They are often a part of our collective choice. Such invisible stressors are like smoldering under-cover fire, which turns the core elements of the system into ashes.

Whether visible or invisible it is impossible to make a count or a complete list of different types of social stressors that one may come across because there are innumerable ways or permutations and combinations by which social factors and forces can present themselves as stressors to individuals. Therefore, social context and social milieu are very important determinants of what happens inside an individual at psychic and somatic levels. No individual is an island. Every individual has a set of social network through which he receives sustenance, security, esteem, support, and at times stress also. The closer a person is in the social network, greater he has the potential to inflict stress-producing impacts.

Traditionally social stressors have been divided into two groups. The first group includes life events, which are discrete, identifiable, painful adverse life occurrences, which come suddenly and unannounced. The second group comprises the chronic strains, which refer to long-lasting problems of interpersonal or otherwise situational adversity and maladjustment. There is a third situation where adverse life event and chronic strain can both be present together. It is easier to count and measure the life events as has been attempted through many scales, which are useful but address only part of the phenomena of social stressors. The list of stressful life events included in all these scales, as discussed later, gives us a reasonably comprehensive glimpse of many of the commonly experienced major life events by the masses. These life events may be termed as "Visible Social Stressors".

The others type of stressors, which do not produce one-time immediate impact like adverse life events are the ones which produce continuous, generally cumulative, negative effects out of disharmonious relationship with other significant individuals or group. Such stressors are known as chronic strain and are most difficult to be reliably quantified. They are generally invisible and not overtly observable, leading individuals to undergo continuous immeasurable sufferings. For these reasons, they are more strongly linked and correlated with adverse health consequences, both physical and/or mental. Such chronic strains are most often seen at places of most intimate relationships, such as between spouses, between child and parents, in situations of love and sex problems, problems with coworkers, boss and subordinates, with friends and peers, with in-laws, with neighbors, etc. The personal, sociocultural and legislative principles which guide such relationships are generally a matter of personal and societal choice, convictions, and approvals. Therefore, we are collectively responsible for the quantum of stressors originating from such relational paradigms. The degree to which any person is oriented and attuned to self or society determines the outcome of his interpersonal associations and interactions to a large extent. Individuals need society and societies need individuals to sustain and survive. Neither can exist without the other. Therefore, the balance of power available to both, gifted by mother nature and granted by society, has to be equitably proportioned between the self and society for optimal and maximal harmony. The irony of modern times is that this balance is heavily, and may be irrationally tilted toward the individual, leading to many anomalous and stressogenic situations in society, leading to further weakening of social institutions including families as a consequence. Chronic strains have formally been defined as "the relatively enduring problems, conflicts and threats that many people face in their daily lives" (Social Stress, 2017). They can originate from any area of human habitation and activity. As mentioned earlier, it is almost impossible to make a comprehensive list of situations where life can be stressful. Life, in all its shades, can be either fulfilling or stressogenic, depending on the vagaries of circumstances. It can happen within family, at workplace, at school, on the roads or in the market. It can happen within the ambit of dyadic relationship or the framework of group dynamics. Some social stressors may be anticipated, but others may be completely unpredictable. But they all originate from within the very process of living. Chronic strain may be conceptualized to result from the "role strains" at the individual level or "interpersonal strains" at the interactive level (NCI Dictionary of Cancer Terms, 2017).

SOURCES OF SOCIAL STRESS

Social Role: "All the world is a stage and all the men and women are merely players" wrote William Shakespeare in "As You Like It" in 16th century. True to the spirit of this quote, every individual has a role, generally multiple roles to play in this world during his lifetime. Every role is played with a set of rules, rights, and responsibilities to fulfill certain specified expectations and requirements of the society with the ultimate goal of meeting all the necessities for living, loving, and working; also for growing to actualize one's potentials and contribute creatively and comprehensively to the society. Playing a role successfully can be emotionally fulfilling, egosyntonic, and health promoting. However, overplaying it or playing roles in a compromised and distorted manner can be pathogenic. Role related stressful paradigms can be role overload, role conflict, role mismatch, role captivity, or role restructuring.

Role overload: It can be because of cumulative effect of large number of multiple roles being undertaken by a single individual or addition of several responsibilities assigned to any single role. It is typically seen in high end executives or routinely among working housewives who have to stretch themselves to befit both the domestic and the office roles inclusive of nurturance of family members and caregiving of the sick and the elderly. Apart from the consequence of adding up leading to role overload, another consequence of carrying multiple roles is the situation of role conflict wherein the demands of one role may routinely or occasionally interfere with fulfillment of the expectation of another role. This situation of role conflict may often prove to be a great source of stress.

Role mismatch: It is a situation wherein an individual is bestowed upon a role much larger than his innate capacities or a role much below what he can actually perform. When an individual finds himself stuck in a role, which he does not want to remain in, he is in a state of role-captivity. Another stressful situation is when the ascribed or acquired role gets accrued with newer and additional responsibilities over a period of time to trespass individual's capacity to meet it. This is called role restructuring.

Media and market: These have both become ubiquitous, globalized, and overpowering in the modern times. They both also seem to be serving the core interests of each other. Often in this whole process, they both are completely negligent and exploitative of the fundamental interests of the individuals from which they derive their sustenance. They tend to oversubscribe every individual. They also tend to be intrusive to the extent that they breach the barrier between public and private domains of individuals and thus create many anomalous and stressful situations. Media has evolved from its initial position of being a medium of communication to having become the masterly manipulator of minds of people. The kind of control media today exercises over the majority segment of masses, especially the young people, can only be matched by the dogmatic religions of bygone years. Market is also a coparticipant in this process because it needs massive media engagement to pursue its goals of expansion, profit making and gaining business edge over fellow competitors, at times by going to the extent of becoming insensitively predatory. Together they create a fertile ground for genesis of immeasurable amount of invisible stress. They invoke and encourage individuals to a kind of unrestrained and round-the-clock hyper-consumerism, for the mother. Nature has not prepared the human system either at the sensory, motor or material levels. The fall out of this is that individuals are enticed to face and deal with an additional source of avoidable stress. Appearance of a virtual world, the cyberspace of enormous nearly unfathomable dimensions, has added immeasurably to the total quantum of stressors. The real world has now to compete with the virtual world to assert its authenticity and primacy.

Education: Modern education also does not seem to prepare an individual for life in terms of being able to live harmoniously and peacefully with self and others. Education too has become a tool in the hands of market-economy by responding just to their demands and requirements. Human beings are groomed through education to become efficient producers of goods and services assisted by rapidly advancing science and technology to fit into the available slots in the market. Science and technology have made tremendous advancements, more particularly in last few decades. It has definitely made life easier for the masses and thereby has earned their trust. But simultaneously it has also made life much more complex by unleashing a flood of mostly superfluous options and multiplicity; also by making things happen at the "speed of thought" by creating a virtual world which has an edge of superiority over the real world in terms of attraction and appeal. Technology has paradoxically facilitated both loneliness and socialization, former by empowering individual's autonomy through various technologies and the latter by providing a virtual platform through virtual social networking sites. All this is happening at a very rapid speed and on a scale of enormous magnitude. Inability of the human system to adapt or even deal with this speed and scale of change is a significant and perpetual source of strain and stress to every one specially for people who have relatively compromised mental or physical abilities because of age or disease. Rise of science has also led to relative weakening of religion, which has marked inbuilt stress-busting mechanisms.

Value system: Many sacrosanct values of modern times such as equality, liberty, and privacy, have their own trajectories of contributing to stress. Principle of equality, carried too far, leads to loss of hierarchy, further leading to weakening of authority to a level critically below what is required for acculturation, and positive and constructive control even by the well-wishers. Principle of equality at times also leads to premature grant of full autonomy to persons even in the developing and immature phase of life, leading often to detrimental consequences. Principle of privacy at social level is again a double-edged weapon. Protective to some extent, privacy may lead to island like situation, if carried too far, and ultimately to self-annihilation in the end. This further tends to prove that society is the source of sustenance, survival, and satisfaction. Data regarding increasing prevalence of divorce and single parent families to alarming and unhealthy levels indicate that everything is not well with our value systems that are guiding and regulating the everyday and intimate relationships in the modern times in our society. Out of conviction or convenience, society has abdicated its responsibility of exercising some reasonable control over its individual members. The only value modern society seems to be left with is that every individual is his own master and final arbiter regarding all matters related to him. However, this position is not in keeping with his real nature or good for his social health. Spirit of competition, that is fostered, encouraged, and idolized in all relationships, leads to a permanent adversarial disposition in all-important relationships, creating a permanent scope for frequent friction and genesis of stress. Mutually complementary and supplementary relationships, which should form the fundamental principle for all dyadic relationships, generally are not talked about out of considerations of inadvertently undermining the principles of liberty and personal autonomy. We forget in this process that mutually adversarial relationship is mutually subtracting in the sense that they undermine each other, whereas mutually complementary relationship is mutually additive; the former generates stress and the latter generates support. In the former situation, together the partners either will never grow or grow in a tardive manner; whereas in the latter situation, together they will always grow. Even though adversarial alignment is stress producing for both the genders, it has more unfavorable impact on women. The doctrine of freedom has been misconstrued and practiced as freedom to be autocratic and unrestrained regarding anything that one wants to do and acquire at all cost. Freedom has come to mean as freedom to the id, and no freedom to superego and ego. Freedom is demanded as a matter of right without any implied strings of reciprocation with corresponding duties and responsibilities. Rights have become another inviolable word. One can demand anything as a matter of rights without being questioned in anyway or feeling unjustified. The demand for rights may appear justified from an individualistic perspective. However, this demand is implicitly directed toward the society which must receive something in return. This return-gift is in the form of duty that every competent individual must deliver to the society. Widespread satisfactory performance of duty by individuals in society gives birth to the twin offsprings of trust and togetherness, which have definite and positive stress-busting potential. Therefore, a judicious balance between rights and duties has to be accomplished and exercised. If rights and duties were to be arranged vertically in a hierarchical format, duty would find its place in the first slot. If everyone were to perform their designated duties, all in the society would benefit or at least maximum benefit to the maximum people would get delivered. On the other hand, if everyone was to confine themselves to demanding their rights alone, none in the society would benefit because it will lead to scarcity of resource and services in society.

Social institutions: Rampant and nearly universal corruption along with inefficiency and insensitivity of administrative machinery; judiciary which mostly delivers a highly delayed and at times dubious justice; and, legislations which are often incongruent and archaic with multiple loopholes, are everyday sources of unending, mostly invisible social stressors. Failure of these social mechanisms has led to increasing socioeconomic disparities, generating poverty on one hand, and compulsion and attraction for migration on the other. Migration itself is full of potential for stress generation. Apart from the stress of having to adapt to completely new and strange environment, it also creates the compulsion of having to live with either cultural dissonance or multicultural identity. Back home, the consequence of migration is altered demography of villages, with reduced potential for handling stress, because young and active members are not at home. No one is spared as everyone has to interface with these social institutions at many stages of their life. Interaction with these social institutions too is an integral part of our stress-life. Our society is getting increasingly infested with extremism, terrorism and rising criminality, which are additional sources of stress for many.

DETERMINANTS OF SEVERITY

Severity of social stress does not depend on the objective measurements of inflicting influence. It is the perception of the stressor by the stressee, which matters the most, especially its potential to cause damage along with one's ability and confidence to cope with it. Perception refers to the apperceptive process of appraisal or evaluation of the harm-potential of the stressor. Appraisal is a cognitive process, which is subject to many antecedent and concurrent influences. These influences include life experiences intellectual level, temperament, habitual cognitive proclivities including distortions, current social susceptibilities and requirements, perception of coping capacity, and knowledge of likely available social support.

Appraisal: It is a crucial cognitive step, which determines the severity of impact of any stressor on the organism. Therefore, the habitual cognitive style of the concerned person is a very important intermediary step. Various types of cognitive distortions which might enhance the stressogenic potential of environmental variables or be a Suo Moto source of stress itself are overgeneralization, catastrophizing, selective abstraction, magnification, minimization, personalization, blaming, labeling, etc. Basically these are habitual, automatic, faulty pattern of thinking which are irrational and discordant with reality, and therefore are often a source of endless stress. Appraisal process is also influenced by the life experience and circumstances of the individual. Life experiences change the mindset and outlook of the individual through self-validated experiences of life. Since most individuals differ from others as regards "perception" of the same "real" life situation, they will also differ on the dimension of stress-response to a particular stressor.

Coping style: It refers to those individual specific strategies and behaviors which are employed by a person in face of stressful situations with the implied or explicit goal to reduce the impact of the stressor either by favorably optimizing the appraisal process or softening the effect of the stressor through various stress management techniques. Coping ability is acquired through experiences of life in general and of similar situations in past in particular.

Social support: It is integral to the process of everyday living. It is also required in more explicit manner in face of adversity and stress. Social support has been variously defined. National Cancer Institute of USA defines it as a "network of family, friends, neighbours, and community members that is available in times of need to give psychological, physical, and financial help" (NCI Dictionary, 2017). Social support is actually the assistance received from others or even the perception of its availability at the emotional, instrumental, informational, and companionship levels. It has also been clearly observed that just the knowledge of having social support available in case of need proves to provide sufficient psychological strength to buffer the adverse impacts of stressful situations. Social support can be of various kinds and at various levels. At instrumental level, it takes care of required goods and actual services; at informational level, it takes care of providing the right kind of information and guidance at the right time to direct the stress-busting behavior; at emotional and companionship level, it takes care of much needed feelings of warmth, affection, esteem, sense of belonging, and being cared. Different social segments may have somewhat specialized proficiency in providing social support. Wellman and Wortley (1990) have shown that friends are more likely than parents to provide companionship but are less likely to offer financial assistance, and women are more likely than men to provide emotional support. Social support with its reinforcing effects at behavioral and psychological levels also leads to certain physiological and neuroendocrine changes that lead to enhanced internal resistance and resilience.

Gender: It is an evolutionary expression of differentially specialized psychobiological functions, which are most explicitly manifest at the social level as generally dichotomously defined social roles. This is Nature's way of ensuring survival of the individual as well as of the species. The ensuing biopsychosocial disposition makes the female gender relatively more vulnerable to facing greater number of stressors as well as receiving deeper impact of encountered stressors.

Overall, women have higher prevalence of psychological morbidity in general; as regards depression, women are twice as likely to suffer from it during their lifetime as compared to men. Plausible explanations for this gender disparity are many. Firstly, because of their traditional social position in almost all societies, they are likely to be exposed to greater frequency and may also be of greater severity of social stressors. This situation gets further worsened in modern times when women are increasingly stepping out of home to take over additional social roles. Another risk factor for greater impact of stressor is their generally higher temperamental sensitivity as well as their tendency for greater emotional involvement. Women also have a habitual tendency to introject and be nonexpressive about their anger and anguish. Their generally dependent position within family as well as social hierarchy leads to their nonparticipation in decision making and executive processes leading to a sense of nonfulfillment and lower self-esteem, and thereby be in a state of chronic dissatisfaction and thus be stressed. There is another side of the coin also. In the process of stepping outside the gates of their domestic premises, women do experience a sense of social, economic, and emotional empowerment. But this empowerment or the role-enhancing effect of working outside, such as greater personal control, increased earning and wider source of gratification proves insufficient to tilt the balance in their favor from the perspective of susceptibility to stress. The role context that is the environment in which they have to work, either at home or at job is also generally more unfavorable for women, which has a bearing on their total stress level.

Value system: Since the primary source of any social stressor is another individual, any value system relating to interpersonal transactions, which increases emotional and cognitive insensitivity towards another fellow human being, is likely to contribute enormously to stress generation. In this context, the modern trend of placing enormous emphasis on individual-centric values and fostering individualism can easily be pointed as a culprit. Such value-system provides sufficient justification and rationale to people for acting almost exclusively in self-interest to the detriment of others without any feeling of guilt. This leads to reduced social support to everyone because of its nonavailability and lack of readiness by others to come forward to help. This further leads to weakening of every individual and thereby making him/her more vulnerable to stress.

MEASUREMENT OF SEVERITY

Clinical experience and observations have shown that various stressors have a tendency to be cumulative in their effect and also undermine the resilience and buffering capacity of individuals. Therefore, it is important to have an instrument to quantify them. Even though the exact severity of impact of stressors does not depend just on the nature of the event, it is of practical value to count them and develop a system for assessing their severity, at least for the life events. This may not apply to chronic life-strains, since it is much easier to measure and quantify life events than the chronic strains. One highly acclaimed and validated instrument to quantify life events was developed in 1967 by Holme and Rahe, which is known as Social Readjustment Rating Scale or Holmes and Rahe Rating Scale (Holmes & Rahe, 1967). In this scale all major life events have been ascribed a defined number of Life Change Units (LCUs) based on subjective rating of 5,000 medical patients. For example, death of spouse is ranked as the most stressful event with LCU score of 100, followed by divorce, marital separation, imprisonment, and death of a close family member with LCU scores of 73, 65, 63, and 63, respectively. Various other life events like marriage, retirement, pregnancy, child leaving home, change of residence, and others are given different scores depending on their stress generating capacity. A composite LCU score is generated for an an individual, based on the stressful events faced. These observations have been further validated by studies carried out prospectively, and found to have some predictive value for enhanced risk of illness if the total score of LCUs for the preceding year crosses a critical limit.

If the cumulative total of LCUs experienced in previous 1 year adds to 300 or more, it is indicative of definitely increased risk for various kinds of illnesses. If the score falls between 150 and 300, it is indicative of moderately increased risk of illness, 30% less than the previous category. If the score is less than 150, it is indicative of low risk of developing illness. All the same, it has to be kept in mind that such scores cannot be used as mathematical formulas and as such many intervening variables naturally inherent in any biological phenomena would creep in to modify the final outcome.

In our own country a similar Life Event Scale for military personnel was developed in 2001 by Raju et al., on exactly similar pattern at the Armed Forces Medical College (AFMC), Pune, to include the stressors which are typically unique to military life (Raju et al., 2001; Chaudhury et al., 2006). It is known by the name of AFMC Life Events Scale. The AFMC scale has items like spouse having illicit relations, court martial, amputation of body parts, receiving medal for bravery, fighting against enemy during war, sanctioned leave being canceled, and many others. Some other important contributions in the area of measurement of impact of life events on individuals have been by Paykel in 1971, Dubey in 1983 and Presumptive Stressful Life Events scale by Singh et al., (1984) from India.

However, similar strategy of measurement does not seem to work for chronic strain based stressors for various reasons as discussed elsewhere.

HEALTH CONSEQUENCES

Stress can have adverse health consequences, depending on the individual vulnerability and other intervening variables. Stress, accumulated beyond a critical level either on acute or chronic basis, can lead to increased frequency of occurrence of physical and mental disorders as well as increased chances of mortality. At the mental level, anxiety, depression, and irritability are the most common effects; somatic, dissociative, and hypochondriacal symptoms are other important consequences; sleep disturbance, sexual dysfunctions, substance abuse, aggressive, and compulsive behavior are also seen in people who are significantly stressed. Amongst the physical illnesses, hypertension, coronary artery disease, diabetes, asthma, gastrointestinal ulcers, ulcerative colitis, irritable bowel syndrome, various skin disorders, and rheumatoid arthritis are commonly seen as consequences of significant stress, with stress having a causative, precipitating or facilitating role.

Physiological mechanisms, which mediate the appearance of pathological states as a consequence of acute or chronic stress, are generally similar and stereotyped, and also nonspecific, holistic, and organismic. The differences, observed in the nature of consequences of stress in different individuals, may actually be a function of severity and frequency of stressors, as well as on the individual-specific constitutional vulnerabilities and susceptibilities. There are two basic responses: one is activation of sympatho-adreno-medullary (SAM) axis which prepares the organism for fight or flight by hemodynamic changes and changes in the level of response-readiness, and the other is activation of hypothalamic-pituitary-adrenal (HPA) axis which leads to raised cortisol level in the system. Cortisol is a multiedged miracle molecule which may have a permissive, restrictive, or regulatory effect depending on the function concerned. It also has "containment effect" on local inflammatory response, and also influences gene-expression. Other predominant effects of stress are immunosuppression; raised sugar, lipid, and insulin levels; increased platelet coagulability; neurotoxic effects, particularly on hippocampus; inhibition of digestive and sexual functions; increased activation of dopaminergic pathways, and; increased catabolism of tryptophan, thereby to reduced monoaminergic states, which may be responsible for many somatic and other psychiatric symptoms. There is immense amount of activity in motion at the interfaces of neuroendocrine, neuroimmune and immuno-endocrine interfaces to maintain the stability of dynamic milieu interior which is the last-mile determinant of health of cells as well as of the organism. Many of these mechanisms along with altered functioning of different neural circuits underlie the interindividual differences in resilience, adaptation, and susceptibility to stress.

CONCLUSION

Social dimension is inbuilt into the structure of our existence. Social dimension of man is inevitably the source of his origin and is also absolutely essential for his survival. It is also essential for his smooth journey through life and self-actualization. Social dimension is the strongest regulator of human behavior, and is also responsible for some of the most intense pains and pleasures of life. Quite understandably, it is also the source of most powerful stressors. Social stressors are unavoidable and ubiquitous. We cannot wish them away. We have to learn to identify and manage them. All societies need to organize their structure and function in such a way that genesis of social stressors is kept to the minimum.

Awareness of self and the surrounding as well as capacity for personal autonomy seen in human beings, are achievements of highest level for the evolutionary process seen in nature. Both these functions have a social dimension also. It cannot and should not remain limited or confined to the individual alone. Individual awareness and autonomy should be shared with the society in a manner that a mechanism of peaceful and harmonious coexistence prevails in society. The role and importance of family as a primary social unit must be recognized, acknowledged and strengthened. The culturally defined norms and expectations of families must be given more power by other social and legislative means. Families must not be allowed to get fragmented to fulfill whims and fancies of irrational individualistic tendencies, even though the latter situation seems to prevail in the modern times.

As individuals, we owe so much to our obligatory collective way of living, that is conventionally called a society. Therefore, a balance has to be struck between individual and social considerations so that society continues to remain our friend in the most optimal manner. As individuals, we continue to float and swim in the social milieu, meet obstacles sometimes on our way, struggle to overcome them, and sometimes also succumb to them. It is important to realize that these social stressors may not always be overt and obvious; most often they are quite imperceptible and invisible; not always unpredictable and from outside source, often are of our own making at individual or collective levels, and sometimes willfully adopted and predictable. Let us all enlarge our jurisdiction beyond our individual cocoons and own the social dimension collectively. Let us be our masters together to win over all the social stressors.

REFERENCES

Chaudhury S, Srivastava K, Raju MSVK, et al. A life event scale for armed forces personnel. Indian J Psychiatry. 2006;48(3):165-76.

Graboys TB. Stress and the aching heart. N Engl J Med. 1984; 311:594-5.

Holmes TH, Rahe RH. The social readjustment rating scale. J Psychosom Res. 1967; 11(2):213-8.

Ifeld FW Jr. Current social stressors and symptoms of depression. Am J Psychiatry. 1977;134(2):161-6.

Juth V, Dickerson S. Encyclopedia of Behavioural Medicine. New York: Springer; 2013.

NCI Dictionary of cancer terms. [online] Available from https://www.cancer.gov/publications/dictio-naries/cancer-terms?cdrid=440116 [Accessed Dec, 2017].

Paykel ES. Scaling of life events. Arch Gen Psychiatry, 1971;25:340-7.

Raju MS, Srivastava K, Chaudhury S, et al. Quantification of life events in service personnel. Indian J Psychiatry. 2001;43(3):213-8.

Rodin AE, Key JD. William Osler and Aequanimitas: An appraisal of his reactions to adversity. J R Soc Med. 1994; 87(12):758-63.

Singh, G, Kaur D, Kaur H. A new Presumptive Stressful Life Events Scale (PSLES)- a new stressful life events scale for use in India. Indian J Psychiatry 1984;26(2):107-14.

Social Stress[a]. [online] Available from https://en.wikipedia.org/wiki/Social_stress [Accessed Dec, 2017].

Social Stress[b]. [online] Available from http://studylib.net/doc/8707874/social-stress [Accessed Dec, 2017].

Sociology of Health and Medicine. [online] Available from https://quizlet.com/39060725/sociology-of-health-and-medicine-chapter-5-flash-cards/ [Accessed Dec, 2017].

Wadman R, Durkin K, Conti-Ramsden G. Social stress in young people with specific language impairment. J Adolesc. 2011;34(3):421-31.

Wellman B, Wortley S. Different strokes from different folks: Community ties and social support. Am J Sociol. 1990;96(3):558-88.

What is Stress? [online] Available from https://www.stress.org/what-is-stress/ [Accessed Dec, 2017].

WHO: Mental health: A State of Well-being. Geneva: World Health Organization (WHO); 2014.

Wood SK, Bhatnagar S. Resilience to the effects of social stress: Evidence from clinical and preclinical studies on the role of coping strategies. Neurobiol Stress. 2015;1:164-73.

Chapter 14

Spirituality and Mental Health

Anju Dhawan, Monica Mongia

SUMMARY

Spirituality and religion are closely intertwined concepts with some distinctions although research has often addressed them interchangeably. When examined, religious and existential dimensions of spirituality indicate a positive relationship with quality of life, health behaviors such as exercise and healthy diet, and a negative relation with cigarette smoking, risky sexual behaviors, and diseases such as arteriosclerosis. Most evidence on religion/spirituality and health is concerned with mental health. An association of religion/spirituality with better mental health, improved coping, and reduced rates of anxiety, depression, and suicide has been reported. However, there are also reports of an inverse association between spirituality and substance use as well.

Spiritual aspects are often ignored during delivery of mental health care, and increased religiosity may sometimes be a manifestation of psychopathology. As religion/spirituality beliefs may occasionally be associated with distress/conflict, any clinical assessment should look into these facets while addressing religion/spirituality aspects.

A few studies have incorporated and systematically assessed role of or spirituality in mental health treatment and have found it to be beneficial. It is important to note that there are also some interventions such as Mindfulness Based Cognitive Therapy or Twelve-Step Therapy that derive from spiritual/religious traditions. While being sensitive to these issues, it is important to keep ethical considerations and clinical boundaries in mind.

CONCEPT OF SPIRITUALITY

Defining spirituality is complex as it is multifaceted and there may not be agreement regarding the concept. However, an attempt in this regard has been made by different authors. Spirituality has been defined as "the process through which an individual tries to make sense of his/her rootedness to the environment and the transcendent". Spirituality is understood to be basically experiential in nature and individual-oriented, although it may have its roots in social, religious, and cultural dimensions. On the other hand, religion has been regarded as a well-structured system of beliefs and practices, common to a community or institution. This distinction between religion and spirituality is not universally agreed upon, and often the two have been considered closely intertwined. Research on religion and spirituality has also not drawn upon any distinction between the terms.

Some authors have highlighted that the concept of spirituality should include positive psychological constructs such as peacefulness, harmony, meaning, purpose, and satisfaction in life while others think that spirituality should not be equated to these constructs . These may be related but are not synonymous with spirituality (Moreira-Almeida et al., 2014). Spirituality is considered by them to be related to the transcendent and sacrosanct features of the universe or existence. King and Koenig (2009) have attempted to review the concept of spirituality for the purpose of medical research and service provision. One of the definitions reviewed mentions spirituality as a personal need for obtaining answers to vital questions about life, its meaning and about association to the sacred, divine, or transcendent. This could arise from or lead to development of rituals or being connected with a particular community.

Various surveys have shown that spiritual beliefs and experiences occur commonly across various cultures in the world. Stuckelberger in the Geneva Panel Report of the 58th World Health Assembly has mentioned that the link between religion, spirituality, and health has often been neglected or avoided due to irrational reasons, and since these are an integral part of human behavior, these aspects must be integrated into health science. In the paper on Spirituality and Health, Chuengsatiansup (2003) has discussed the understanding of spirituality and health through a discussion on scientific model by Thomas Kuhn. It mentions that scientific thinking has primarily been influenced by a reductionist approach, while spirituality is considered as belonging to a complex living being and can be seen only from a holistic perspective. The author has made a case for the importance of incorporating spiritual assessment into health impact assessment.

SPIRITUALITY AND HEALTH

In 1988, Dr Halfdan Mahler, Director General of WHO consented to a draft resolution which stated: "Health is a state of complete physical, mental, social and spiritual well-being and not merely the absence of disease and infirmity". The draft resolution was presented at the 51st World Health Assembly in 1998 to revise the language of the Constitution in its prologue to include "Spiritual Well-being" but it was decided by the World Health Assembly not to consider the proposed amendment (Panel Report: "Spirituality, Religion, and Social Health", World Health Assembly, 2005). However, the WHO Quality of Life-100 instrument included spirituality, religiousness and personal beliefs (SRPB) as the sixth domain of the instrument (WHOQOL Group, 1998). Another important step in this direction has been the WHOQOL-SRPB field-test scale that included 32 questions, addressing quality of life features related to SRPB. Along with the WHOQOL-100, this instrument produced a quality of life profile and provided in depth information about SRPB related aspects of quality of life. Besides the facets listed in WHOQOL-100, SRPB included eight facets, i.e. spiritual connection, meaning and purpose in life, experiences of awe and wonder, wholeness and integration, spiritual strength, inner peace, hope and optimism and faith.

In addition to the quality of life, religion and spirituality have been linked to health behaviors. Lucchetti and Lucchetti (2014) have reported on the growing evidence of the positive effect of religion and spirituality on health. Their bibliometric analysis found approximately 30,000 articles published in the last 15 years in this area. Religion/spirituality beliefs have been found to be associated with better mental health, physical health, survival, well-being measures and quality of life (Moreira-Almeida et al., 2014), health behaviors such as exercise, diet, and reduced cigarette smoking and risky sexual behaviors with subsequent beneficial effects on diseases such as coronary artery disease, cancer and all-cause mortality, and in persons with special needs such as those with terminal illness (Koenig, 2012).

The literature on the effect of spiritual participation on health behavior is mixed with spirituality serving as a booster as well as an obstruction to health and health behaviors (Isaac et al., 2016). The influence of religion and spirituality is most evident for cigarette smoking. In a review by Koenig (2012) that examined the relationship, among 137 studies 90% reported significant inverse relationship of smoking with religious/spiritual involvement; in 37 studies 68% demonstrated a significant favorable relationship to exercise; of 21 studies that examined relationship with diet, 62% found a positive association with a healthier diet and a relationship with lower cholesterol. However, on the flip side, many of the studies found a positive association with greater weight and religious/spiritual affiliation; in 95 studies 86% found a significant inverse relationship with risky sexual activity.

Koenig (2012) in the review also found that 12/19 studies showed significant inverse relationship with coronary heart disease, 36/63 studies reported significantly lower blood pressure associated with religion/spirituality affiliation and 4/7 studies found lower risk of stroke. Of the 14 studies with highest quality ratings, 8 studies reported positive and 3 reported negative relationship with cognitive functions. There have also been studies that have examined the functioning of the immune system, endocrine system, cancer, physical functioning, self-reported health, pain, somatic symptoms as well as mortality in relation to religious/spiritual involvement. There have been more than 100 studies that have looked into the impact of religious/spiritual association on mortality and more than 75% found an association with greater longevity. It is hypothesized that religious spiritual involvement may influence physical health and longevity through psychological (perhaps due to better coping), social (e.g. through greater social support) and better health behaviors.

Isaac et al. (2016) have made a case for inclusion of spirituality based aspects for the purpose of engagement at the individual and community level for health promotion. They have examined the Health Belief Model to explore how spiritual beliefs could influence help seeking before the appearance of symptoms and in response to symptoms. Best et al. (2015) conducted a systematic review to assess the patients' perspective about discussion related to the spirituality in the course of treatment seeking. Of the 54 studies comprising more than 12,000 patients, more than half the sample thought that such a discussion was appropriate. However, there was a lack of consensus among the patients and doctors as to what constitutes such a discussion. Thus, it becomes important for the doctors to identify which patients would want such a discussion and how to go about it.

RELIGION, SPIRITUALITY VIZ-À-VIZ. MENTAL HEALTH

The Royal College of Psychiatrists of the UK released a position paper in 2011 on "Recommendations for Psychiatrists on Spirituality and Religion". The American Psychiatric Association (APA), additionally, released guidelines regarding the plausible discrepancy between psychiatrists' religious involvement and psychiatric practice in 1990. The section on "Religion, Spirituality and Psychiatry" (SRSP) of the World Psychiatric Association (WPA) has initiated a process in order to facilitate an international agreement on a position paper on religion and spirituality in mental health.

Some important issues in such deliberations are related to acknowledging the importance of addressing religious and spiritual issues as an ingredient of "good clinical practice" while respecting the lack of such inclination among patients. It also involves understanding the boundaries while carrying out such assessment and adequate training of mental health professionals to address these issues during the service delivery (Position Statement, Royal College of Psychiatrists, 2013). Spiritual aspects often get neglected during delivery of mental health care either due to lack of awareness of the existing evidence base and absence of training on strategies to deal with religious or spiritual beliefs in clinical practice (Moreira-Almeida et al., 2014).

More than 80% of the existing literature on religion/spirituality and health is linked with mental health. Weber and Pargament (2014) have discussed several facets of religion, spirituality, and mental health. Research has demonstrated that religious involvement and spirituality may be linked with improved mental health and better quality of life. It has been associated with reduced rates of anxiety, depression, and suicide. Higher level of certainty in belief system has been found to be associated with better psychological status. A negative association among substance use and spirituality has been reported. Positive religious coping may also be linked to improved mental health and has been described to be related to support of community groups, positive reframing of stressors and spiritual connectedness.

More than 100 studies have examined religion/spirituality affiliation with coping in a range of illnesses and different stressful situations, and have found that it is by and large helpful (Koenig, 2012). More than 300 papers reviewed by Koenig (2012) on well-being found a positive relationship. Specifically, 29/40 studies that examined hope, 26/32 studies that assessed optimism, 42/45 studies that looked into meaning and purpose, and 42/69 studies on self-esteem showed a positive association. Contrary to expectation, studies found a relationship with internal locus of control and greater sense of personal control in difficult situations. The relationship of religion/spirituality with social support was examined in 74 studies and 82% studies found a significant positive relationship. Social capital, an indicator of community participation, volunteerism and marital stability also indicated a positive relationship with religion/spirituality. Ten studies that assessed school grades and performance in adolescents/ school students showed better performance (Koenig, 2012).

Bonelli and Koenig (2013) in a review of 43 studies conducted between 1990 and 2010, found that 31 reported an association of the level of religious/spiritual participation with reduced mental disorders, eight demonstrated mixed results and two found more mental disorder. A positive association was found for all available research on dementia, suicide, stress-related ailments, depression, and substance abuse. Studies on schizophrenia and bipolar disorder found no or negative association (Moreira-Almeida et al., 2014). It is also important to remember that increased religiosity may sometimes be a manifestation of psychiatric illness or psychosis. Thus, the belief systems have to be examined carefully in terms of any recent change and the social/cultural milieu needs to adequately addressed.

Some mental health professionals have held the view that religion/spirituality may increase guilt by focussing on sin and thus may lead to depression. However, of the 444 studies reviewed by Koenig (2012), 61% showed an inverse relationship, while only 6% studies showed that religious/spiritual involvement was associated with greater depression. Studies have also found that higher religiosity or spiritual involvement is associated with lower levels of depression, quicker remission of symptoms of depression, improved quality of life, and outcome. Of the 141 studies that examined the association with suicide, 75% reported an inverse relationship, while 4 studies found a positive relationship with religious/spiritual involvement.

The association with anxiety has been studied in 299 studies and although 49% studies showed inverse relationship, 11% reported greater anxiety. Most of these studies were cross-sectional and it is not clear what was the temporal relationship with religious/spiritual involvement.

Religion and spirituality has also been studied in association with personality traits. Overall the studies show lower scores on neuroticism, psychoticism and higher on extraversion, conscientiousness, agreeableness, and openness to experience (Koenig, 2012). Studies on alcohol use, abuse and dependence and drug use/abuse have also by and large depicted a negative association.

There have been efforts made to explain the association between religion/spirituality and mental health. Most important of these are religious coping resources that give meaning to difficult life situations and a sense of purpose. These beliefs may normalize loss and change. Religion and spirituality encourages pro-social behavior and positive values that may themselves help to maintain and enhance social relationships.

However, we must not forget that religion has been also used to justify hatred, aggression, and rigid thinking by some. It may produce conflict and strain related to anxiety and guilt about inability to maintain high religious standards or practices. There is an evidence to suggest that religious challenges can also lead to distress, and have been associated with poor mental health outcome (Weber & Pargamont, 2014). Religious and spiritual beliefs may impact decisions pertaining to treatment and may sometimes interfere with medical advice. Thus, there is a complex interplay between religious beliefs, spirituality, and mental health. In any individual case, it is important to keep this complexity in mind.

CLINICAL APPLICATION OF RELIGION/SPIRITUALITY IN MENTAL HEALTH

The rationale for including spirituality into health care practices includes the finding that many patients have spiritual needs related to their illness and their belief systems may influence their ability to cope with illness, treatment decisions, and the outcome. Moreira-Almeida et al., (2014) searched literature over 15 years and found 985 articles on religion/spirituality and mental health. A significant majority of clinicians approved the need to obtain a comprehensive spiritual history as a part of application of religion/spirituality in health practice. While taking the spiritual aspects of the history, it is important for mental health practitioners to be cognizant that spirituality is a multidimensional concept that is perceived differently by different patients. These include belief systems, practices, values, transcendental/divine experiences, concept of God, etc.

Lucchetti and Lucchetti (2013) have reviewed instruments for taking a spiritual history. They have discussed the strengths and weaknesses of various instruments based on 16 attributes including range of areas related to religion/spirituality and their validation. A majority of the tools were developed for common use while two of them were specifically related to mental health. These included the "Royal College of Psychiatrists" Assessment as well as the Spiritual Assessment Interview'. The Royal College of Psychiatrists Assessment is a comprehensive assessment of psychosocial aspects through an 11 item scale and requires 20–25 minutes. The Faith, Importance, Community, and Address (FICA) has 13 items and requires about five minutes to administer. It is a helpful tool for general as well as psychiatric practice. The questions included in FICA are:

F-Faith and Belief

Do you consider yourself spiritual or religious?
Do you have spiritual beliefs that promote coping with stress?
What gives your life meaning?

I-Importance and Influence

What significance does your faith or belief hold in your life?
Do your beliefs impact the way you care for yourself in this illness?
What role do you think your belief system play in helping you regain your health?

C-Community

Are you associated with a spiritual or religious community?
Is this of support to you and how?
Is there a group of individuals you really like or that are really important to you?

A-Address in Care

How would you want, your healthcare provider to take care of these issues in your care?
The other instruments described by the authors are FAITH (12 items) and HOPE.
The beliefs of patients assessed during the spiritual history or the lack of such beliefs should always be respected. Moreira-Almeida et al. (2014) have suggested certain practice guidelines regarding assessment and integration of religion and spirituality in psychiatry practice. These include maintaining ethical boundaries, person-centered approach, being aware of counter-transference issues, open-minded attitude along with genuine respect of patients' belief system, values, experiences and avoiding self-disclosure of clinicians' perspective related to this aspect.

Strategies to overcome barriers to integrating religious/spiritual issues into interventions include enhancing cultural competence, sharing their understanding about available evidence concerning the impact of religious/spiritual aspects on mental health and training in strategies to address these issues in practice.

Incorporating religion and spirituality in treatment has been systematically assessed in a few studies and has been found to be beneficial (Weber & Pargamont, 2014). Besides generally integrating religious/spiritual aspects in treatment, it is also important to note that there are some interventions that originate from spiritual/religious schools. Mindfulness Based Cognitive Therapy (MBCT) propagated by National Institute for Health and Clinical Excellence (NICE) guidelines for relapse prevention among patients with three or more episodes of depression is one such intervention. Research on twelve step therapy has also shown its effectiveness in alcohol dependence.

There are other interventions such as compassion-focused therapy that are being studied (Position paper Royal College of Psychiatrists, 2013). Christian Cognitive Based Therapy has been demonstrated to be superior to conventional CBT as well as Muslim based psychotherapy for bereavement, anxiety and depression has shown better outcome. Although the number of studies are limited, some of these studies have shown higher patient satisfaction with spiritual/religious based interventions (Weber & Pargamont, 2014).

It is important to mention that a large part of research on religion/spirituality is based on cross-sectional studies and more longitudinal studies need to be carried out. The different faith traditions need to be researched. The negative aspects of religious/spiritual involvement and research on nonbeliefs also needs to be conducted.

FUTURE RESEARCH

Moreira-Almeida et al. (2014) have identified some important areas for further research which include research (a) to explore the possible mechanisms by which religion and spirituality impacts health, (b) feasibility as well as impact of such an assessment in psychiatric care, (c) addressing these aspects across different religious communities and cultures, (d) development and testing of effective spiritual interventions alone or along with standard treatment. They suggest that the outcome should assess positive outcomes besides reduction in psychopathology.

REFERENCES

Best M, Butow P, Olver L. Do patients want doctors to talk about spirituality? A systematic literature review. Patient Educ Couns. 2015;98(11):1320-8.

Bonelli RM, Koenig HG. Mental disorders, religion and spirituality 1990 to 2010: a systematic evidence-based review. J Relig Health. 2013;52(2):657-73.

Chuengsatiansup, K. Spirituality and health: an initial proposal to incorporate spiritual health in health impact assessment. Environ Impact Assess Rev. 2003;23:3-15.

Dhar N, Chaturvedi SK, Nandan D. Spiritual Health Scale 2011: Defining and Measuring 4th Dimension of Health. Indian J Community Med. 2013;36(4):275-82.

Isaac KS, Hay JL, Lubetkin El. Incorporating spirituality in primary care. J Relig Health. 2016;55(3): 1065-77.

King MB, Koenig HG. Conceptualising spirituality for medical research and health service provision. BMC Health Serv Res. 2009;9:116.

Koenig HG. Religion spirituality and health: the research and clinical implications. ISRN Psychiatry. 2012;2012:278730.

Lucchetti G, Bassi RM, Lucchetti ALG. Taking spiritual history in clinical practice: A systematic review of instruments. Explore: J Sci Healing. 2013;9(3):159-70.

Lucchetti G, Lucchetti AL. Spirituality, religion, and health: Over the last 15 years of field research (1999–2013). Int J Psychiatry Med. 2014; 48(3):199–215.

Moreira-Almeida A, Koenig HG, Lucchetti G. Clinical implications of spirituality to mental health: review of evidence and practical guidelines. Revista Brasuleira de Psiquiatria. 2014;36:176-82.

Panel Report. "Spirituality, Religion & Social Health" During the 58th World Health Assembly at the United Nations in Geneva May 2005. http://reseau-crescendo.org/wp-content/uploads/2014/04/SPIRITUALITY.pdf.

Position Statement. Recommendations for psychiatrists on spirituality and religion PS03/2013 November 2013 Royal College of Psychiatrists London Approved by Central Policy Coordination Committee: May 2011. https://www.rcpsych.ac.uk/pdf/PS03_2013.pdf.

Singh NK, Goyal N, Raj J. Role of spirituality in mental health practice. Indian J Psychiatr Soc Work. 2017;8(1):44-9.

The WHOQOL Group. The World Health Organization Quality Of Life Assessment (WHOQOL): development and general psychometric properties. Soc. Sci. Med. 1998;46(12):1569-85.

Weber SR, Pargament KL. The role of religion and spirituality in mental health. Curr Opin Psychiatry. 2014;27(5):358-63.

WHOQOL-SRPB Users Manual. Scoring and Coding for the WHOQOL SRPB Field-Test Instrument, Mental Health: Evidence & Research, Department Of Mental Health & Substance Dependence, World Health Organization Geneva, Switzerland. http://www.who.int/mental_health/evidence/whoqol_srpb_users_manual_rev_2005.pdf.

Chapter 15

Social Aspects of Marriage and Similar Affiliations

Mona Srivastava

SUMMARY

The institution of marriage holds its importance because of various functions related to it like psychological satisfaction, biological function of sexual satiation and procreation. Marriage also fulfils the societal role by enhancing solidarity and preserving the cultural ethos of a community. Multiple definitions for marriage have been put forward but the one which incorporates the legal, social, and biological elements of marriage is the best. Marriage finds its origin along with the civilization and is considered important for social and public recognition of an individual. Over the decades, there has been a major shift in the sociodemographic profile of the institution in that the age of marriage has increased and fewer individuals are keen to tie the knot. The most popular theories of marriage are related to the need for regulation of sexual urges and the procreation. There are personality factors which govern the success of marriage, though education and income also govern the marriage. Marital harmony is a predictor of physical and mental health. Marriage has also an important function of societal integration. Laws are also framed for better integration of marriage. Cohabitation and same sex marriages are emerging as newer social affiliations. These social institutions in some countries are protected by law and given recognition.

MARRIAGE

Introduction

Marriage takes its origin from the French word "marrier" and Latin word "maritare", and both the words carry the same meaning, i.e. to have a spouse (Huston & Melz, 2004). The significance of marriage lies in the purpose it fulfils namely providing a support system of spouse, children, and relatives to an individual; and giving a means to satisfy the physiological need of sex. In the long run, marriage also helps the sustenance of the society and its cultural integrity (Hawkins et al., 2002). Marriage in some places like at certain places in India is not only seen as a relationship between two families but the entire community of villages (Rabbiraj, 2014). Marriage is the institution which gives birth to a family. The family thereafter provides an individual with personal and social security along with caring and procreation (Kamp, 2015). Marriage as an institution has also a great legal significance. Obligations and duties are an integral part of marriage, e.g. matters of inheritance and succession (Coleman, 2000). In the present day urban society, marriage has become individualistic and personal (Gottman, 1998; Gottman & Notarius, 2000).

Definition

Synonymous to marriage is matrimonial alliance or getting into wedlock, and these terms basically signify a union which grants rights and bestows obligations between partners, their offsprings and each set of parents (Bradbury & Karney, 2004).

Different people define marriage in different ways. As per Edward Westermark, "Marriage is a relation of one or more men to one or more women which is recognized by custom or law and involves certain rights and duties both in the case of the parties entering the union and in the case of the children born of it" (Amato et al., 2007). Malinowski defines, "Marriage is a contract for the production and maintenance of children". According to HM Johnson, "Marriage is a stable relationship in which a man and a woman are socially permitted to have children without loss of standing in the community (Amato et al., 2007). There is no one ideal definition and even sociologists do not agree on a single definition. Marriage can be popularly defined as a "legally recognized social contract between two people, traditionally based on a sexual relationship and implying a permanence of the union" (Barlow et al., 2001). To put it simply, marriage is the starting point of society as it gives rise to a family.

Historical Perspective

In olden times, marriage was considered a holy sacrament, a decree of God. The Hindu marriages are elaborate rituals and till date are considered important for performing religious duties. "Till death do us part" is the philosophy of Hindu marriage, and the institution of marriage is a "*sanskar*" (Dinshah & Desai, 2007; Mahajan et al., 2013). The origins of marriage are as obscure as the dawn of civilization. As per Augustine, marriage offers three important social benefits—fidelity, offspring, and a sacred union (Cherlin, 2004). Marriage evolved for the family and gradually took on a religious significance (Coontz, 2005).

The older Hebrew society placed a lot of importance to the wife and she had to be looked after well. The nomadic communities of the Middle East followed the tradition of "beena" wherein the wife owned a tent and had total freedom; this particular ritual is still practised in some parts of Israel (Nazroo, 1997). In ancient Greece, marriage was based on mutual consent of the couple and no civil ceremony was required (Oropesa & Landale, 2004). In the early Christian era (30-325 CE), marriage was considered primarily a private matter and no ceremony was needed for solemnization (Hollinger & Haller, 1990). In the second half of the 16th century, church and parental consent was required for marriage. In England, the passage of Lord Hardwicke's Act in 1753 instituted certain requirements for marriage like presence of a witness and performance of religious ceremony (Rosina & Fraboni, 2004).

Chinese society in 1950 brought in new laws which laid emphasis on monogamy, gender equality, and agreement of both partners for the marriage (Gargan, 2001; Lee & Ono, 2012).

Sociodemographic Characteristics

The dawn of the 20th century has witnessed some shift in the marital institution namely an increase in the age at first marriage, and more couples opting to cohabit than getting married. Studies have shown a fall of 30% in the number of marriages in Europe from 1975 to 2005 (Bardasi & Taylor, 2008). Figures show that about 62% of males and 59% of females are married.

The remarriage rate is 12% in males and 9% in females. Never married rate is 6% and 5% in males and females, respectively. Nine percent of males and 11% of females are divorced and 25% of females are widowed in contrast to 9% of men who are widowers (Bumpass & Sweet, 2001). The rate of marriage is directly proportional to a person's age and educational qualification, like 83% of highly qualified males are married, while the rate is 77% in men educated upto 12th standard (Amato, 2014; Amato, 2015).

Theories of Marriage

There are no specific and accepted theories of marriage. The most popular theories of marriage are related to the need for the regulation of sexual urges and procreation, though a few theories have been put forward to understand other aspects of marital dimensions (Karney & Bradbury, 1997):

1. *Social exchange theory*: The need for an exchange of societal cultures, traditions, and relations lead to the development of the institution of marriage
2. *Attachment theory*: The innate desire in all species to have an attachment was the genesis of marriage and family
3. *Crisis theory*: Tiding over minor and major crisis could be achieved as a collective measure in families, hence marriage and kinship arose
4. *Behavioral theory*: Early attempts at regularizing the society were imbibed as a behavior which passed on and grew stronger with the generations.

   It can be seen that a single theory has not been able to adequately explain the institution of marriage.

Types of Marriage

Popularly marriage takes four main forms depending upon persons involved. There are various ways of categorizing marriage:

1. *Monogamy*: Monogamy is the marriage of one man to one woman. Traditionally and historically, it is the most prevalent form of marriage (Curtice et al., 2001)
2. *Polygamy*: Polygamy is the marriage of one man to two or more wives. It is legally accepted in most of the Asiatic countries, Africa, America, and the Pacific Islands (Ember, 2011)
3. *Polyandry*: In polyandry, one woman has several husbands. The most popular example is of "*Draupadi*" from "Mahabharata" (Mahajan et al., 2013). In Tibet and Southern India, it is practiced. Three subforms of polyandry are identified. In Tibet, the female is married to all the brothers simultaneously. This type of polyandry is called "fraternal" and "Tibetan poly-andry" (Levine, 1998). "Levirate" is the system in monogamous or polygamous marriages wherein the widow of the elder brother marries the next younger brother. "Sororate" is another type, when the husband marries the wife's sister in the event of her death (Hollinger, 1990)
4. *Group marriage*: Group marriage is a kind of marriage when several adults live together and have a collective responsibility regarding money, children, and duties. This particular type of marriage was practised by the people of Polynesia, some parts of Asia and Papua New Guinea (Zeitzen, 2008).

Based on duration, marriages can be:

1. *Permanent*: Marriages which are of long duration
2. *Temporary*: These marriages are short lasting and various cultures practise it under different names, e.g. "hand fasting" in Celtic culture, "NikahMut'ah" in pre-Islamic Arabs (Harknett & McLahanan, 2002) and "walking marriage" in Mouso tribe of China (Stevan, 2001). Since these marriages are easily broken, they are called "brittle" (Fincham, 1987)

Based on the age at marriage, the marriages can be classified as:

1. *Child marriage*: When either of the partners has not reached the age of 18 years, the marriage is called child marriage. In 1900s, this type of marriage was prevalent in USA (Amato et al., 2007). Child marriage is internationally criticized and is banned in India under the Child Marriage Restraint Act of 1929 (Dinshah & Desai, 2007)
2. *Traditional adult marriage*: Both the partners are adults in traditional adult marriage.

Based on the consent, marriages can be divided into two types which are as follows:

1. *Forced marriage*: Marriage in which one or both of the parties are married against their will is called forced marriage. This is practiced in parts of South Asia and Africa (Zeitzen, 2008; Ember, 2011)
2. *Consensual marriage*: In consensual marriage, both parties give their consent.

Another modern type of marriage is called "marriage of convenience" or sham marriage. Examples include "green card marriages" wherein foreign-born individuals marry US citizens to obtain a permanent residency (Green Card). A marriage of convenience is one that is devoid of normal reasons to marry (Kiernan, 2004).

Custom of marrying outside one's family, clan, tribe is called exogamy (Hollinger & Haller, 1990).

Based on the work of Wallerstein and Blackeslee (1996), four types of marriage have been identified:

1. *Romantic marriage*: The couple is attracted to each other even after many years of marriage and are committed to the relationship.
2. *Rescue marriage*: Each spouse had a history of abuse and identifies with the other for solace.
3. *Companionate marriage*: It is characterized by equality in all facets of life. Careers and sharing of responsibilities are central attributes.
4. *Traditional marriage*: In the older form, the husband is a provider and protector and the wife is the nurturer. The newer form has fluid spousal roles.

Religion and Marriage

1. *Hinduism*: The Hindu marriage is considered a holy union and has the consent of family and priests. Hindu marriage is also considered to be essential for performance of *"sanskaras"*
2. *Christianity*: Christianity considers marriage to being faithful to the Lord and fidelity is considered as an important attribute (Mahajan et al., 2013)
3. *Islam*: The holy Quran states that marriage is endogamous, i.e. marriage to a non-Muslim or a nonbeliever is considered void. Polygamy is legal in Islam (Nazroo, 1997)
4. *Jainism*: Jains treat the marriage as a contract which fulfils the need for progeny (Mahajan et al., 2013).
5. *Parsis*: The Parsi community considers the marriage as a righteous act (Mahajan et al., 2013).

6. *Sikhism*: The Sikh scriptures refer to marriage as "Anand Karaj" which literally means "blissful union" (Mahajan et al., 2013).

Factors affecting Success of Marriage

Although there is no absolute guarantee for the success of marriage, Karney and Bradbury's (1997) theory tries to form a model by including factors like personality attributes, family values, life events, and individual resilience. Klagsbrun (1985) has described eight characteristics of successful marriage:

1. Ability and adaptability to develop a positive attitude
2. Adaptability and complete resolution of disagreement
3. Assumption of permanence, commitment, and compromise
4. Trust, security, safety among spouses
5. Balance of dependencies and power
6. Enjoyment, intimacy, and satisfaction among spouses
7. Cherished and shared history between the couple
8. Luck against the unpredictable.

Mackey & O'Brien (1995) identified five factors that appeared to be important to marital longevity. They are as follows:

1. Limiting conflicts
2. Joint decision making
3. Open communication style
4. Mutual trust, respect and understanding
5. Closeness in terms of sexual behavior and day-to-day work.

Stack and Eshelman (1998) studied nonclinical couples from 17 countries who had been married for at least 20 years, so as to identify attributes of lasting marriages. Huston and Melz (2004) also looked at similar attributes. The above two studies found that the personality attributes were important for marital stability and quality. Multiple studies have focused on two primary outcomes: relationship quality and relationship stability for studying the continuation of marriage (Vaillant & Valliant, 1993; Smith & Zick, 1994; Williams & Umberson, 2004; Stanley et al., 2006).

Summarizing from the above studies, predictors of successful marriage include: ethnic background of mother to be from South Asia, maternal religiosity, either of the parents belonging to stable families, either of the parent has not remarried or if done so has no children from previous relationships, both the partners are highly educated, mother's age is at least 20 years, stability of job and house among the partners, time spent with each other and the pregnancy being wanted (Fincham & Bradbury, 1987; Gottman & Korokoff, 1989; Kaufman, 2000; Nazroo, 1997; Gottman & Notarius, 2000; Cutrona, 2002; Popenoe & Whitehead, 2004).

Advantages of Marriage

There is a vigorous debate about the benefits of marriage that has focused on whether formal marriage is a better environment for children? Whether the quality of marriage has an impact upon the children and spouse? (Cohan & Bradbury, 1997; Coleman et al., 2000; Bumpass & Sweet, 2001; Acs, 2007).

The results show that marital harmony is associated with much better sleep, less depression and fewer visits to the doctor (Brown & Booth, 1996; Brown, 2000; Beirman et al., 2006). Williams and Umberson (2004) found that as compared to married men, widowed men have a 44% higher risk of mortality, and divorced men have 60% higher risk of cardiac ailment (Goldman, 1993; Goldman et al., 1995). Health is improved by a good marriage (Mineau et al., 2002). Marriage prevents psychological illness (Soulsby & Bennet, 2015), makes people live much longer (Smith & Zick, 1994), and makes people healthier and happier (Stack & Eshelman, 1998). Men benefit more than women (Zhang & Hayward, 2006), and married people engage in less risky activities (Waite & Gallaghar, 2000).

Functions of Marriage

Marriage gives rise to the family which in turn fulfils the need of physical intimacy which is of utmost importance for societal functioning. The children born out of marriage are given some rights and duties along with the safety of development. The humankind as a race survives through this institution in an ordered way. The growth, social development, sustainability, satisfaction, intimacy, and role attributions are all learned in the family. The continuity of race is also done in an acceptable manner through marriage (Marmot & Wilkinson, 1999; Kim & McKenry, 2002; Hewitt et al., 2010; Musick & Bompass, 2012). Man's need for belonging, love, nesting, and security are fulfilled through marriage (Waite & Gallagher, 2000). The Hindu culture gives an added responsibility of "dharma" to marriage apart from procreation and satisfaction of sexual desires (Mahajan et al., 2013).

Dysfunctions in Marriage

With times, the institution of marriage has changed and is fraught with newer challenges like divorce or spousal separation, remarriage and spousal violence. Conger and Elder (1994) have put forward a "family stress model" (FSM) to understand the decline in marital quality and stability. As per this model, the financial problems and lack of social support lead to a strain in the marriage (Orbuch et al., 2002; Hewitt et al., 2010).

Various dysfunctions which occur in the marriage are as follows:

1. *Divorce and remarriage*: Divorce and remarriage of spouses can lead to tension in the children as well as the partners (Dykstra, 1997; Falke & Larson, 2007). Children may feel fear, loneliness, guilt, and pressure to choose sides (Amato & Rogers, 1999; Faust & McKibben, 1999). It has been frequently reported that couples seeking divorce have some prior psychological disturbances (Gottman, 1994; Orbuch et al., 2002)
2. *Violence and abuse*: Domestic violence is a significant social problem. One in four victims of violent crime are victimized by a spouse or family member (Catalano, 2007). Family sociologists have created the term intimate partner violence (IPV) to explain the phenomenon, it includes physical, sexual, and emotional violence (Centre for Disease Control, 2012; Agarwal et al., 2016).

Preventive Strategy for Saving Marriages

"Prevention and Relationship Enhancement Program" (PREP) developed by Markman et al. (1993) shows that effective communication and conflict resolution can help in marital stability and permanency (McLanahan & Garfinkle, 2002).

Law and Marriage

Multiple laws across the world are related to marriage and its various aspects. Indian legislation related to the subject includes:

1. Hindu Marriage Act is an act of the Parliament of India enacted in 1955 which regulates marriages in Hindus (Dinshah & Desai, 2007)
2. Hindu Succession Act (1956) deals with the inheritance among Hindu citizens (Dinshah & Desai, 2007)
3. Divorce Act deals with annulment of marriage (Dinshah & Desai, 2007)
4. Dowry Prohibition Act, 1961 (Dinshah & Desai, 2007)
5. Special Marriage Act, 1954 (Sharma et al., 2013)
6. Protection of Women from Violence Act, 2005 (Sharma et al., 2013).

There are separate personal laws in India for other religions. For further details, the reader is advised to refer to the specific legislation.

The international laws dealing with the marriage include (Hague, 1978):

1. The Hague Convention that harmonizes different marriage laws and according to it validity of marriage is universal
2. European Union Divorce Law Pact deals with the mutual termination of marriage.

COHABITATION

When unmarried couples live together in an arrangement similar to marriage and share a common bedroom, it is called cohabitation or live-in relationship. The formal marriage does not take place (Eggebeen, 2005). Cohabitation is practiced mostly in the metropolitan cities and is considered a social taboo in many parts of India (Abhang, 2014). Cohabitation may lead to problems like bigamy and multiple partner relationships which may in turn destroy the social fabric (Abhang, 2014). The status of the women in such relationship lacks social approval and sanctity, and therefore chances of their exploitation are higher (Edin, 2000). Studies have shown that child bearing is lesser as cohabiting couples usually prefer not to have children. On the other hand, children in broken relationship are adversely affected due to lack of love and parental care (Ellwood & Jencks, 2002). Litigation on matters pertaining to maintenance, legitimacy of children, and inheritance are the areas of great concern (Kiernan, 2001). Factors like secularization, changing attitudes towards the value of marriage and acceptance of cohabitation have produced changes in the patterns of marriage and cohabitation in the last 40 years (Nazio, 2008). Since this kind of set-up gives an open option of parting ways when desired, it is becoming popular among the present generation. Living apart together (LAT) is also a form of cohabitation (Wu, 2000).

Multiple factors like female independence, availability of contraception, economic independence of women, and feminist ideology have increased the rate of cohabitation in the society (Sweeney, 2002). The acceptability of cohabitation decreases with age as 80% of less than 25 year olds accept cohabitation in contrast to 44% of middle-aged people. The large majority of cohabiting couples marry within 3 years of living together (50%). The couples who cohabit marry late, e.g. 29 years for females and 31 years for males in 2008 in comparison to 23 years for females and 25 years for males in the 1960s–70s (Milan, 2013). It is a known fact that cohabitation decreases the stability of marriage (Jayson, 2010).

Black Caribbean women are less likely to be married at the time of having a baby as compared to White women. Lower educational status, family history of single parents, low income households and personality attributes of impulsivity, and borderline personality traits are some of the factors determining the decision to cohabit (Nazio, 2008). In the Millennium Cohort Study, almost 40% of cohabiting couples had lived together for less than 2 years, as compared with only 8% of married couples. Cohabiting couples have higher maternal depression (Wu, 2000).

Law and Judiciary on the Status of Cohabitation in India

In India, till date there is no specific legislation to deal with the subject matter of cohabitation (Abhang, 2014). The changing scenario of the people moving into cohabitation is an issue of individual right and privacy. Though the number of people supporting such practice may be lesser, there is a genuine concern that in future, people may prefer it over marriage. The Indian laws related to marriage like the Hindu Marriage Act, 1955, the Criminal Procedure Code, 1973, and the Indian Succession Act, 1925, do not lawfully recognize cohabitation (Dinshah & Desai, 2007; Abhang, 2014). However, if the cohabitation is very long, the Supreme Court of India assumes that the couple to be married and deemed to enjoy such rights (Abhang, 2014). Some respite to the cohabiting females is provided by the Protection of Women from Domestic Violence Act, 2005 (Dinshah & Desai, 2007)

Status of Cohabitation Across the World

Across the world, live-in relations are either recognized by law, or some laws are enacted to give the benefit to the children born out of it. In Canada, in the common law, marriage recognition is given to cohabitation; "the family law of Scotland" gives rights to cohabiting couples; UK does not give legal rights to cohabiting couples; Philippines confers property and other rights to cohabiting couples; France allows the cohabiting partners to enter into a pact by signing before the court; Ireland and Australia recognize cohabitation but no clear laws are formulated to address the issue; China allows the partners to sign an agreement for cohabitation and the children out of such a union are given rights equal to the children born out of marriage (Kohm & Groen, 2005).

SAME SEX MARRIAGES

The numbers of same sex marriages have grown significantly in the past decade. In USA, up to 4% marriages are same sex. The phenomenon is growing as a result of more coupling, change in the marriage laws, growing social acceptance of homosexuality, and a subsequent increase in willingness to report it.

As per the statistical report of USA (2012), the same sex marriage percentage ranges from a low of 0.3% to a high of 4%. In Canada, 0.8% of people live in a same sex marriage (US Census Bureau, 2012). Characteristically, the same sex couples are younger in age (25% of couples below 35 years versus 17% below 35 years in opposite sex couples). Male-male couples outnumbered the female-female couples (55% vs. 40%). In terms of parenting, the same sex couples were equal to opposite sex parents. Multiple parenting studies have shown that children in such marriages are well adjusted and have high confidence levels (Biblarz & Stacey, 2010). The Indian law does not recognize same sex marriages (Dinshah & Desai, 2007).

CONCLUSION

The sanctity of the institution of marriage is no longer what it was. Factors like cohabitation, single parenthood, and same sex marriages are posing a challenge on the solidarity of marriage. The change in the family system like emergence of nuclear families and economic independence of women is making the sustainability of the family easy, and hence living apart is also an option which is posing threat on the marital stability. As an impact of globalization, families are breaking up and life partners are bound to stay alone in different cities and countries of the world. The live-in relationship is no longer a novelty to society. It has come to stay, but at the same time institution of marriage is able to hold its own.

REFERENCES

Abhang S. Judicial approach to live- in-relationship in India- Its impact on other related statutes. IOSR J Hum Soc Sci. 2014; 19(12):28-38.

Acs G. Can we promote child well-being by promoting marriage? J Marriage Fam. 2007; 69: 1326-44.

Agarwal A, Sinha SK, Kataria D, Kumar H. Predictors and prevalence of IPV in alcohol use disorder. J Mental Health Hum Behav. 2016;21(1):25-31.

Amato PR. Does social and economic disadvantage moderate the effects of relationship education on unwed couples? An analysis of data from the 15-month Building Strong Families evaluation. Fam Rel. 2014;63(3):343-55.

Amato PR. Marriage, cohabitation and mental health. Fam Matters. 2015;96:5-13.

Amato PR, Booth A, Johnson DR, Rogers SJ. Alone together: How Marriage in America is Changing. Cambridge, MA: Harvard University Press; 2007.

Amato P, Rogers S. Do attitudes toward divorce affect marital quality? J Fam Issues. 1999;20:69-86.

Bardasi E, Taylor M. Marriage and wages: a test of the specialization hypothesis. Economica. 2008;75:569-91.

Barlow A, Duncan S, James G, Park A. Just a piece of paper? Marriage and cohabitation in Britain, in British Social Attitudes. In: Barlow A, Duncan S, James G, Park A, Park J (Eds). New York: Guilford press; 2001. pp. 1097-110.

Biblarz TJ, Stacey J. How does the gender of parents matter? J Marriage Fam. 2010;72:3-22.

Bierman A, Fazio EM, Milkie MA. A multifaceted approach to the mental health advantage of the married. J Fam Issues. 2006;27:554-82.

Bradbury TN, Karney BR. Understanding and altering the longitudinal course of marriage. J Marriage Fam. 2004;66:862-79.

Brown SL, Booth A. Cohabitation versus marriage. A comparison of relationship quality. J Marriage Fam. 1996;58:668-78.

Brown SL. The effect of union type on psychological wellbeing. Depression cohabitants versus marrieds. J Health Soc Behav. 2000;41:241-55.

Bumpass LL, Sweet JA. Marriage, divorce, and intergenerational relationships, In: The Well-Being of Children and Families: Research and Data Needs. Thornton A. Ann Arbor (Ed). University of Michigan Press; 2001. pp. 295-313.

Catalano S. Intimate Partner Violence in the United States. Washington DC: US Department of Justice, Bureau of Justice Statistics; 2007.

Centre for Disease Control. Understanding Intimate Partner Violence. Georgia: CDC; 2012.

Cherlin AJ. The deinstitutionalization of American marriage. J Marriage Fam. 2004;66:848-61.

Cohan CL, Bradbury TN. Negative life events, marital interaction, and the longitudinal course of newly wed marriage. J Pers Soc Psychol. 1997;73(1):114-28.

Coleman M, Fine M, Ganong L. Reinvestigating remarriage: Another decade of progress. J Marriage Fam. 2000;62(4):1288-307.

Coontz S. Marriage, a History. From Obedience to Intimacy, or How Love Conquered Marriage. New York:Viking Press; 2005.

Curtice K, Thomson LJ, Bromley C. British Social Attitudes: Public Policy, Social Ties. The 18th Report. London:Sage Publications; 2001.

Conger RD, Elder H. Families in Troubled Times: Adapting to Change in Rural America. New York, Aldine, 1994.

Cutrona CE, Russell DW, Krebs K. Dimensions of behavior predicting marital outcomes. Invited paper presented at the International Meeting on the Developmental Course of Couples Coping with Stress. Boston College; 2002.

Dinshah FM, Desai SA. Principles of Hindu Law. New Delhi: Lexis Nexis Butterworths; 2007.

Dykstra PA. The effects of divorce on intergenerational exchanges in families. Demogr Res. 1997;11:149-72.

Edin K. What do low-income single mothers say about marriage? Soc Probl. 2000; 47:112-33.

Eggebeen DJ. Cohabitation and exchanges of support. Soc Forces. 2005; 83(3):1097-110.

Ellwood D, Jencks C. The Spread f Singe Parent Families in the United States Since 1960. Cambridge, Massachusetts, Harvard University; 2002.

Ember CR. What we know and what we don't know about variation in social organization: Melvin Ember's approach to the study of kinship. Cross-Cult Res. 2011; 45(1):27-30.

Falke SI, Larson JH. Premarital predictors of remarital quality: Implications for clinicians. Contemporary Fam Ther Journal. 2007;29:9-23.

Faust K, McKibben JN. Divorce, separation, annulment and widowhood. In: Handbook of Marriage and the Family. Sussman MB, Steinmetz S, Peterson GW. New York: Plenum Press, 1999. pp. 475-99.

Fincham FD, Bradbury TN. The impact of attributions in marriage: A longitudinal analysis. J Pers Soc Psychol. 1987;53:510-7.

Gargan EA. China's New Brides Put Freedom First/All perks, No Work in 'Walking Marriages'. Harare, NewsDay, 2001.

Goldman N. Marriage selection and mortality patterns: inferences and fallacies. Demography. 1993;30:189-208.

Goldman N, KorenmanS, Weinstein R. Marital status and health among the elderly. Soc Sci Med. 1995;40:1717-30.

Gottman JM. What Predicts Divorce? The Relationship between Marital Processes and Marital Outcomes. NJ, Lawrence Erlbaum Associates,1994.

Gottman JM. Psychology and the study of marital processes. Annu Rev Clin Psychol. 1998;49:169-97.

Gottman JM, Notarius CI. Decade review: Observing marital interaction. J Marriage Fam. 2000;62:927-47.

Gottman J, Krokoff L. Marital interaction and marital satisfaction: A longitudinal view. J Consult Clin Psychol. 1989;57:47-52.

Hague. Conference on Private International Law: Convention on Celebration and Recognition of the Validity of Marriages. The Hague, Faculty of Law,1978.

Harknett K, McLanahan S. Racial Differences in Marriage Among New, Unmarried Parents: Evidence from the fragile families and child wellbeing study. Princeton, NJ, Center for Research on Child Wellbeing, 2002.

Hawkins A, Wardle L, Coolidge D. Revitalizing the Institution of Marriage for the Twenty-First Century. Westport, Connecticut: Praeger Publishers; 2002.

Hewitt B, Turrell G, Giskes K. Marital loss, mental health and the role of perceived social support: Findings from six waves of an Australian population panel study. J Epidemiol Comm Health. 2010;66:308-14.

Höllinger F, Haller M. Kinship and social networks in modern societies. A cross-cultural comparison among seven nations. Eur Sociol Rev. 1990;6(2):103-24.

Huston TL, Melz H. The case for (promoting) marriage: The devil is in the details. J Marriage Fam. 2004;66:943-58.

Jayson S. Report. Cohabiting has little effect on marriage success. Virginia, USA Today, 2010.

Kamp DC, Amato PR. Relationship happiness, psychological well-being, and the continuum of commitment. J Soc Pers Relatsh. 2005;22:607-28.

Karney BR, Bradbury TN. Neuroticism, marital interaction, and the trajectory of marital satisfaction. J Pers Soc Psychol. 1997;72:1075-92.

Kaufman G. Do gender role attitudes matter? Family formation and dissolution among traditional and egalitarian men and women. J Fam Issues. 2000;21(1):128-44.

Kiernan K. The rise of cohabitation and childbearing outside marriage in western Europe. Int J Law Policy Fam. 2001;15(1):1-21.

Kiernan KE. Redrawing the boundaries of marriage. J Marriage Fam. 2004;66(4):980-7.

Kim HK, McKenry PC. The Relationship between marriage and psychological well- being: A longitudinal analysis. J Fam Issues. 2002;23:885-911.

Klagsbrun F. Married people: staying together in the age of divorce. Toronto, Bantam books,1985.

Kohm LM, Groen KM. Cohabitation and the future of marriage. Virginia, Regent University Law Review. V.17, 2005.

Lee KS, Ono H. Marriage, cohabitation, and happiness: A cross-national analysis of 27 countries. J Marriage Fam. 2012;74:953-72.

Levine N. The Dynamics of Polyandry: Kinship, Domesticity, and Population on the Tibetan Border. Chicago: University of Chicago Press;1998.

Mackey RA, O'Brein BA. Lasting marriages: Men and women growing together. Westport. Connecticut, Praeger,1995.

Mahajan PT, Pimple P, Palsetia D. Indian religious concepts on sexuality and marriage. Indian J Psychiatry. 2013;55(Suppl 2):S256-S262.

Marmot M, Wilkinson R. Social Determinants of Health, New York, Oxford University Press,1999.

McLanahan S, Garfinkel I. Unwed parents in the US: Myths, realities, and policymaking. UK: Cambridge University Press; 2002.

Milan A. Marital status: Overview, 2011. Statistics Canada, 2013.

Mineau GP, Smith KR, Bean LL. 'Historical trends of survival among widows and widowers'. Soc Sci Med. 2002;54:245-54.

Musick K, Bumpass L. Re-examining the case for marriage: Union formation and changes in well-being. J Marriage Fam. 2012;74(1):1-18.

Nazio T. Cohabitation, Family and Society, New York, Routledge, 2008.

Nazroo JY. The Health of Britain's Ethnic Minorities, London: Policy Studies Institute. Neth J Soc Sci. 1997;33:77-93.

Orbuch TL, Veroff J, Hassan H, et al. Who will divorce: A 14-year longitudinal study of black couples and white couples. J Soc Pers Relat. 2002; 19:179-202.

Oropesa RS, Landale NS. The future of marriage and Hispanics. J Marriage Fam. 2004; 66:901-20.

Popenoe D, Whitehead BD. Ten Important Research Findings on Marriage and Choosing a Marriage Partner. Washington DC, University of Virginia, 2004.

Rabbiraj C. Socio-legal dimensions of live-in-relationships in India. IOSR JHSS. 2014; 19(7):25-9.

Rosina A, Fraboni R. Is marriage losing its centrality in Italy? Demographic Res. 2004; 11(6):149-72.

Sharma I, Pandit B, Pathak A, et al. Hinduism, marriage and mental illness. Indian J Psychiatry. 2013;55(S2):243-9.

Smith KR, Zick CD. Linked lives, dependent demise? Survival analysis of husbands and wives. Demography. 1994;31:81-93.

Soulsby KL, Bennett KM. Marriage and psychological wellbeing: The role of social support. Psychology. 2015;6:1349-59.

Stack S, Eshleman JR. Marital status and happiness: A 17 nation study. J Marriage Fam. 1998;60: 527-36.

Stanley SM, Amato PR, Johnson CA, et al. Premarital education, marital quality, and marital stability: Findings from a large, random household Survey. J Fam Psychol. 2006;20:117-26.

Stevan H. Mountain patterns: The survival of Nuosuculture in China. J Am Folklore. 2001;114:451.

US census bureau: Statistical abstracts of United States. US Census Bureau, 2012.

Sweeney MM. Two decades of family change: The shifting economic foundations of marriage. Am Sociol Rev. 2002;67:132-47.

Vaillant CO, Vaillant GE. Is the U-curve of marital satisfaction an illusion? A 40-year study of marriage. J Marriage Fam. 1993;55:230-39.

Waite LJ, Gallagher M. The Case for Marriage: Why Married People Are Happier, Healthier and Better Off Financially. New York, Doubleday, 2000.

Wallerstein JS, Blackeslee S. The Good Marriage: How and Why does Marriage last? US, Grand Central Publishers, 1996.

Williams K, Umberson D. Marital status stability, marital transitions and health: A life course perspective. J Health Soc Behav. 2004;45:81-98.

Wu Z. Cohabitation: An Alternative Form of Family Living. Don Mills, Ontario, Oxford University Press, 2000.

Zeitzen MK. Polygamy: A Cross-Cultural Analysis. New York, Oxford, Berg Publishers, 2008.

Zhang Z, Hayward MD. Gender, the marital life course, and cardiovascular disease in late midlife. J Marriage Fam. 2006; 68:639-57.

Chapter 16

Social Dimensions in Psychiatric Epidemiology

R Padmavati

SUMMARY

Epidemiological methods are necessary to investigate the associations between variation in exposure to external disease-causing agents, resistance of individuals exposed to the disease-causing agents, and in resistance resources in the environments of exposed individuals. While this has been extensively employed in the field of physical illnesses, psychiatric epidemiology has lagged behind due to various difficulties in defining cases, identifying cases, underreporting, and stigma. The interest in social dimensions has gained momentum only since the landmark ecological perspectives of Faris and Dunham (1939). Data from community-based epidemiological studies and refined statistical methods have thrown light on several social factors like gender, age of onset, education, marital status, geography, and poverty, that appear to impact the occurrence of mental disorders. This chapter provides a broad overview of social dimensions across the range of mental disorders throwing some light on possible explanations.

INTRODUCTION

Epidemiological methods help in investigating the association between changes in exposure to external disease-causing agents, resistance of individuals exposed to the disease causing agents, and in resistant resources in the environments of the exposed individuals' environment (Susser, 1973). The focus of epidemiology, whichever branch it may belong to, is to document risk factors and hence help develop preventive interventions (Elwood et al., 1992). However, psychiatric epidemiology still continues to be descriptive as it is often difficult to conceptualize and measure mental disorders to estimate their prevalence. This is the reason that psychiatric epidemiology lags behind other branches (Kessler, 2000). Defining a case, diagnostic interviews to identify cases, underreporting as a result of stigma and cost of surveys are some of the many challenges in psychiatric epidemiology. Additionally, the risk factors, which are often studied in context of psychiatric disorders, are nonspecific, broad, and almost unmodifiable like gender and social class. Studies on modifiable risk factors, which may help plan intervention in other illnesses, are limited in psychiatric epidemiology. Since the period of ending of World War II, there has been a focus on new kind of investigations on mental health, "the socio-medical" enquiry (Faris and Dunham, 1939). Occurrence of mental illness is influenced by various social factors like gender, social class, race and ethnicity, and household patterns; and by social institutions like disability and social security systems, labor markets, and healthcare organizations. Psychiatric epidemiology has seen a gradual progress in methods, incorporating structured tools and statistical techniques and also a move to understand social dimensions of mental health. This chapter provides an overview about the social dimensions of mental illnesses. Subsequent chapters in the book will help us develop better understanding into social dimensions of individual disorders.

GENDER

Gender is an important determinant of mental health and illness. There is a gender difference in the prevalence of common mental illnesses like depression, anxiety, and somatic complaints which are more common in women (World Health Organization, 2017). Higher psychiatric morbidity in women especially for anxiety and depression has been consistently shown in several epidemiological studies over time (Hagnell, 1959; Sethi et al., 1972; Nandi et al., 1980). Data from the National Comorbidity Survey of USA also showed that the rate of occurrence of mood and anxiety disorders is higher in women while the rate of impulse control and substance use was higher in men (Kessler et al., 2005a). In another multinational study from India, Zimbabwe, Chile, and Brazil, which investigated the association of key economic indicators like income, education, and gender with common mental disorders, low education, poverty, and female gender were found to be strongly associated with occurrence of common mental disorders. The prevalence of mental illness, according to the National Mental Health Survey (2015-16) of India is higher among males (13.9%) than among females (7.5%). Prevalence of depression, phobias, agoraphobia, generalized anxiety disorder, and obsessive compulsive disorder was found to be higher in females than males (Gururaj et al., 2016).

Much debate surrounds the gender differences in rates of schizophrenia. Initially it was shown that the prevalence of schizophrenia across genders is the same (Wyatt et al., 1988), but the recent studies have evidenced differences in the incidence of illness across genders. A meta-analysis has shown the median (10 and 90% quantile) rate ratio for incidence of schizophrenia as 1.4 (0.9, 2.4) for male: female estimates (McGrath et al., 2008). Lewine et al., (1984) used six different diagnostic systems to study male to female ratio of schizophrenia among inpatients. The rates of schizophrenia among men and women were estimated to be equal when a diagnostic system which defined schizophrenia broadly was applied. However, when narrow criteria were applied, more numbers of women were excluded from the definition as compared to men. Similarly, when Castle and colleagues (1993) applied different sets of diagnostic criteria to a sample of nonaffective psychosis patients, they found that the gender ratio differed substantially with different criteria. The ratio of female-to-male was found to be 0.41:1 and 0.92:1 on applying restrictive Feighner's criteria and ICD-10 criteria respectively. Aleman and colleagues (2003) carried out a meta-analysis of incidence population studies using standard diagnostic criteria. They confirmed that higher incidence was found in men (ratio 1.42:1) (Aleman et al., 2003). While these gender differences are evident in incidence studies, the prevalence studies done recently showed no differences for schizophrenia as well as for bipolar disorder (Perala et al., 2007; McGrath et al., 2008). Some authors have postulated the reason for this disparity in gender difference in incidence and prevalence lies in higher suicide completion rates and better treatment compliance in men as compared to women (Test et al., 1990).

Brady and Randall (1999) suggest that despite higher prevalence rates of substance abuse and dependence among males as compared to females, the diagnosis of substance abuse is not gender-specific. Yet, until recently, psychoactive substance use has largely been perceived as a male problem. The studies done in western countries on general population as well as in treatment seeking population have shown that the rate of substance use, abuse, and dependence is substantially higher in men than women (Kessler et al., 2005b; Compton et al., 2007). The National Epidemiologic Survey on Alcohol and Related Conditions done in the US evidenced that the rate of substance abuse as well as substance dependence was 2.2 and 1.9 times higher respectively in males as compared to females (Compton et al., 2007). Five percent of women, as compared to 7.7% men, were noted to be using illicit substances according to the data from the National Household Survey on Drug Abuse (NHSDA) in 2000 from the US. However, more recent studies have shown this gap to be narrowing (Grucza et al., 2008).

McHugh and colleagues (2014) emphasized the need for screening of substance use in women universally in primary care settings. Their suggestion was based on the evidence that more than half of the females in reproductive age group reported using alcohol currently, around 20% used tobacco products and around 13% used other drugs. In females, substance use is associated with significant medical, psychiatric, and social consequences. It has been reported in many studies about females using more prescription drugs as compared to men, like narcotic analgesics and tranquilizers (Simoni et al., 2004). In the adolescent age group (12–17 years old), the rates of substance use have been found to be comparable amongst males (9.5%) and females (9.8%). However, the NHSDA report had shown higher rates of tobacco use in adolescent girls as compared to adolescent boys (Epstein, 2002).

In a study from treatment centers of Delhi, Lucknow, and Jodhpur in India, during the period of 1989-1990, only 1–3% of the treatment seekers for drug abuse were women (Lal et al., 2015). According to Drug Abuse Monitoring System (DAMS) report of India, around 2–3% of the new treatment seekers were found to be women (Ray et al., 2012). Another retrospective study done in a de-addiction center in Chandigarh between 1978 and 2008 found that 0.5% of all treatment seekers in the center were women (Basu et al., 2012). Cultural factors including personal and social factors may account for the low rates of substance use as well as treatment seeking in women in India.

AGE OF ONSET

The study of the age of onset, although technically and conceptually difficult, provides significant information to distinguish between lifetime prevalence and projected lifetime risk, and in understanding causes and mechanisms of illness as well as interventions for primary and secondary prevention (Jones, 2013; Kessler, 2005a). This variable has not been addressed adequately in epidemiological studies. A number of recent studies show that most mental illnesses have their onset in adolescence (Kessler, 2007; Jones, 2013).

The data from the National Institute of Mental Health funded Epidemiological Catchment Area program suggested that many psychiatric disorders, including major depression, phobia, and substance dependence, had onset during adolescence or early adulthood. A meta-analysis of anxiety disorders (Lijster et al., 2017) searched seven electronic databases and examined 24 studies, fulfilling inclusion criteria for all anxiety disorders according to DSM-III-R, DSM-IV, or ICD-10 criteria. Anxiety disorder subtypes differed in the mean age of onset, with onsets ranging from early adolescence to young adulthood.

In a review of literature on the World Mental Health Surveys in 28 countries (Kessler, 2007), mood disorder age of onset curves showed low prevalence until the early adolescence, a roughly linear increase through late middle age and a declining increase thereafter. The average age of onset for major depression was 24 years (Kessler, 2007). In India, the mean age of onset of bipolar disorders has been reported to be 27 years (ranging from 12 to 70 years) (Ramdurg et al., 2013).

Differences in the age of onset of schizophrenia have been reported in schizophrenia across gender (Ochoa et al., 2012). Men have been found to develop the illness earlier (18–25 years) than women (25–35 years). The onset distribution curves for men and women have also varied. Women have two peaks, one after menarche and the other peak after the age of 40 years (Castle et al., 1993; Ochoa et al., 2006). A group of researchers have reported that early age of onset shows similar distribution in men and women (Castle et al., 1998). Another group of authors, on the other hand, reported early age of onset in men in first episode psychosis, consistent with the results found in schizophrenia (Larsen et al., 1996; Hafner et al., 1998).

Substance use is found to be universally common in the youth. According to the Treatment Episode Data Set (TEDS) report (2014), the age of onset for substance use disorders is 17 years or younger (SAMHSA, 2014). A study carried out in Nepal showed that a large number of drug users experienced their first drug intake before 20 years of age, with around a third starting it before 15 years (Central Bureau of Statistics, 2013). Onset of regular alcohol use in late childhood and early adolescence as compared to adult onset has been reported to be associated with highest rates of alcohol consumption in the later life (Benegal et al., 1998).

EDUCATION

Lower levels of education are shown to be associated with higher prevalence of common mental diorders (Araya et al., 2003; Patel et al., 2006), schizophrenia (Padmavathi et al., 1988; Yoon & Aziz, 2014), depression and suicide (Lal & Sethi, 1975; Patel et al., 2006). Studies on the impact of mental health on education have been infrequent (Lee et al., 2009). The world mental health survey data suggested that prior substance use disorders in high income (HI) countries were associated with incomplete education attainment at all stages. Similarly, presence of psychiatric illnesses like anxiety disorders, mood disorders, or impulse-control disorders predicted early termination of higher education in high as well as low-income countries (Lee et al., 2009). The same authors also postulated that association between termination of education and presence of psychiatric illness was not as strong in low and middle-income (LAMI) countries as in HI countries. In LAMI countries, probably various other factors like family and community play an important role in attainment or termination of education at various levels, independent of mental health (Buchmann & Hannum, 2001).

MARITAL STATUS

There is little evidence of discussion on marital status in epidemiological studies. Different researchers have reported prevalence rate of psychiatric disorders to be higher in the married group as compared to singles (Mohammadi et al., 2005; Deswal et al., 2012), and in separated and divorced people as compared to others (Sagar et al., 2017). Results from the world mental health survey indicated that marriage acts a protective factor by reducing the risk of most mental disorders in both men and women. The strongest reduction in married females is in substance use disorder, while for married males, it is in depression and panic disorder (Scott et al., 2010). The risk for all disorders was present in both genders, when previously married as against stably married.

POVERTY

Ever since the 1930s, when epidemiological psychiatric studies linked higher rates of schizophrenia to poverty (Faris & Dunham, 1939), research in other psychiatric disorders has also demonstrated similar findings. The role of poverty and socioeconomic status in the epidemiology of mental illness has been debated along several lines like individual experiences, area based deprivation, duration of poverty, and direction of causality (Kuruvilla & Jacob, 2007; Payne et al., 2000).

Associations have been reported between poverty and symptoms of common mental disorders like depression and anxiety. Unemployment and poverty are found to be associated with the duration, rather than with the onset of episodes of common mental disorders (Weich & Lewis, 1998). In the "Personality and Total Health (PATH) through life" survey, financial hardship in the current time was strongly and independently associated with common mental disorders, more than what is found to be associated with other parameters of socioeconomic positions and demographic characteristics (Butterworth et al., 2009). The association between poverty and risk of mental illness was further strengthened by carrying out a study in six LAMI countries. The authors in this study suggested that the experience of hopelessness, insecurity, and rapid social change, as well as the risk of violence and physical ill health were important reasons for making the poor strata of the society more vulnerable to develop common mental disorders (Patel & Kleinman, 2003). The lowest socioeconomic group was twice more at risk for developing major depressive disorder than the highest income group in the analyses of the Epidemiological Catchment Area study (Regire et al., 1993). Ecological analyses indicated that areas of poverty, deprivation, unemployment, and poor education were associated with higher rates of mental illnesses as in the case of higher rates of suicides (Whitley et al., 1999). Contrarily, higher suicide rates have been associated with higher socioeconomic status in Southern states in India (Vijayakumar, 2010).

The association between poverty and schizophrenia has been well reported in several studies globally (Hollingshead & Redleich, 1958; Kessler et al., 2005a; Nandi et al., 1980). Goldberg and Morrison (1963) showed that the actual incidence of schizophrenia did not vary with social class, and lower socioeconomic status was secondary to the psychotic illness. Data from several epidemiological studies, such as the Epidemiological Catchment Area studies (Regire et al., 1993) and the National Comorbidity study (Blazer et al., 1994) have demonstrated the association between low socioeconomic status and the increased risk of major depression in the poor as compared to those who were economically well off. Risk of postpartum depression has been reported to be thrice more common in women belonging to lower socioeconomic status in Pakistan, as compared to those belonging to higher socioeconomic status (Rahman

& Creed, 2006). Review of studies reporting on the relationship between socioeconomic status and bipolar disorders indicate disparities. While older studies noted relatively higher socioeconomic status of those with bipolar disorder as compared to controls or the general population (Lenzi et al., 1993; Verdoux & Bourgeois, 1995), recent epidemiologic studies report a lower social status (Schoeyen et al., 2011; Tsuchiya et al., 2004).

GEOGRAPHY

Research for urban/rural differences in the prevalence of mental disorders has shown mixed results and has been debated widely (Ganguli 2000; Probst et al., 2006; Weaver et al., 2015). Some researchers argue that despite the privilege of better health care access in urban settings, urban dwellers are at a higher risk of developing mental health problems. A report on meta-analysis of 20 population based studies for urban-rural differences in the prevalence of all mental disorders showed a 20–40% increased prevalence in urban areas, a finding that persisted even after adjusting for potential confounders like age, gender, socioeconomic, and marital status (Peen et al., 2010). Weaver and colleagues (2015) reported lower odds for rural African American women to meet criteria for lifetime mood disorder as compared to urban African American women. On the other hand, Probst et al (2006) found a higher rate of depression amongst rural residents as compared to urban residents. In India, reviewing 15 epidemiological studies on prevalence of all psychiatric morbidity, Ganguli (2015) reported a large rural-urban difference for schizophrenia, hysteria, and mental retardation but not for anxiety and depression. He opined that rural-urban difference seems to depend on the disease category and is not unidirectional.

CONCLUSION

Studies of social factors influencing mental health and disease provide a multidimensional understanding of disease occurrence. In the recent years, psychiatric epidemiological studies globally have informed on the different social factors associated with the prevalence and incidence of mental disorders, thus contributing to understanding of not only risk factors studies but also the treatment policies by the mental health services. The immense data on the social factors influencing mental disorders from various epidemiological studies have generated a debate on the possible explanations for the findings. This chapter has provided a bird's eye view on what is to follow in the chapters focusing on individual disorders through the book.

REFERENCES

Aleman A, Kahn RS, Selten JP. Sex differences in the risk of schizophrenia: evidence from meta-analysis. Arch Gen Psychiatry. 2003;60(6):565-71.

Araya R, Lewis G, Rojas G, et al. Education and income: which is more important for mental health? J Epidemiol Comm Health. 2003;57:501-5.

Basu D, Aggarwal M, Das PP, et al. Changing pattern of substance abuse in patients attending a de-addiction centre in north India (1978-2008). Indian J Med Res. 2012;135(6):830-6.

Benegal V, Bhushan K, Seshadri S, et al. Drug abuse among street children in Bangalore: A project in collaboration between NIMHANS, Bangalore and the Bangalore Forum for street and working children, Bangalore, NIMHANS; 1998.

Blazer DG, Kessler KC, McGonagle KA, et al. The prevalence and distribution of major depression in a national community sample: the National Comorbidity Survey. Am J Psychiatry 1994;151:979-86.

Brady KT, Randall CL. Gender differences in substance use disorders. Psychiatr Clin North Am. 1999;22(2):241-52.

Buchmann C, Hannum E. Education and stratification in developing countries: a review of theories. Ann Rev Sociology. 2001;27:77-102.

Butterworth P, Rodgers B, Windsor TD, et al. Financial hardship, socio-economic position and depression: results from the PATH Through Life Survey. Soc Sci Med. 2009;69(2):229-37.

Castle DJ, Wessely S, Murray RM, et al. Sex and schizophrenia: effects of diagnostic stringency, and associations with and premorbid variables. Br J Psychiatry. 1993;162:658-64.

Castle D, Sham P, Murray R, et al. Differences in distribution of ages of onset in males and females with schizophrenia. Schizophr Res. 1998;33(3):179-83.

Central Bureau of Statistics. Survey report on current hard drug users in Nepal-2069. Bijulibazar, Kathmandu: Ministry of Home Affairs; 2013.

Chee KY, Salina AA. A review of schizophrenia research in Malaysia. Med J Malaysia. 2014;69 (Suppl A): 46-54.

Compton WM, Thomas YF, Stinson FS, et al. Prevalence, correlates, disability, and comorbidity of DSM-IV drug abuse and dependence in the United States: results from the national epidemiologic survey on alcohol and related conditions. Arch Gen Psychiat. 2007;64(5):566-76.

Deswal BS, Pawar A. An epidemiological study of mental disorders at Pune, Maharashtra. J Comm Med. 2012;37(2):116-21.

Elwood JM, Little J, Elwood JH. Epidemiology and Control of Neural Tube Defects. New York: Oxford University Press; 1992.

Epstein JF. Substance dependence, abuse and treatment: findings from the 2000 National Household Survey on Drug Abuse. Rockville, MD, Substance Abuse and Mental Health Services Administration, Office of Applied Studies; 2002.

Faris RE, Dunham HW. Mental Disorders in Urban Areas: An Ecological Study of Schizophrenia and Other Psychoses. The University of Chicago, Chicago; 1939.

Ganguli HC. Epidemiological findings on prevalence of mental disorders in India. Indian J Psychiatry. 2000;42(1):14-20.

Grucza RA, Norberg K, Bucholz KK, et al. Correspondence between secular changes in alcohol dependence and age of drinking onset among women in the United States. Alcoholism: Clin Exp Res. 2008;32(8):1493-501.

Goldberg TE, Morrison SL. Schizophrenia and social class. Br J Psychiatry. 1963;109:785-802.

Gururaj G, Varghese M, Benegal V, et al. National Mental Health Survey of India, 2015-16: Summary. Bengaluru, National Institute of Mental Health and Neuro Sciences; 2016.

Hafner H, An Der Heiden W, Behrens S, et al. Causes and consequences of the gender difference in age at onset of schizophrenia. Schizophr Bull. 1998;24(1):99-113.

Hagnell O. Neuroses and other nervous disturbances in a population, living in a rural area of southern Sweden, investigated in 1947 and 1957. Acta Psychiatr Scand Suppl. 1959;34(136):214-20.

Hollingshead AB, Redlich FC. Social Class and Mental Illness: Community Study. New York, NY, US: John Wiley & Sons, Inc; 1958.

Jones PB. Adult mental health disorders and their age at onset. Br J Psychiat. 2013;202 (s54):s5-s10.

Kessler RC. Psychiatric epidemiology: selected recent advances and future directions. Bull World Health Organ. 2000;78(4):464-74.

Kessler RC, Berglund P, Demler O, et al. Lifetime prevalence and age-of-onset distributions of DSM-IV disorders in the National Comorbidity Survey Replication. Arch Gen Psychiatry. 2005;62(6): 593-602.

Kessler RC, Chiu WT, Demler O, et al. Prevalence, severity, and comorbidity of 12-month DSM-IV disorders in the National Comorbidity Survey Replication. Arch Gen Psychiatry. 2005; 62(6):617-27.

Kessler RC, Amminger GP, Aguilar-Gaxiola S, et al. Age of onset of mental disorders: a review of recent literature. Curr Opin Psychiatry. 2007;20(4):359-64.

Kuruvilla A, Jacob KS. Poverty, social stress & mental health. Indian J Med Res. 2007;126(4):273-8.

Lal R, Deb KS, Kedia S, et al. Substance use in women: current status and future directions. Indian J Psychiatry. 2015;57(Suppl 2):S275-85.

Lal N, Sethi BB. Demographic and socio demographic variables in attempted suicide by poisoning. Indian J Psychiatry.1975;17(2):100-7.

Larsen TK, McGlashan TH, Moe LC. et al. First-episode schizophrenia—I. Early course parameters. Schizophr Bull. 1996;22(2):241-56.

Lee S, Tsang A, Breslau J, et al. Mental disorders and termination of education in high-income and low- and middle-income countries: epidemiological study. Br J Psychiatry. 2009;194(5):411-7.

Lenzi A, Lazzerini F, Marazziti D, et al. Social class and mood disorders: clinical features. Soc Psychiatry Psychiatr Epidemiol. 1993;28(2):56-9.

Lewine R, Burbach D, Meltzer HY, et al. Effect of diagnostic criteria on the ratio of male to female schizophrenic patients. Am J Psychiatry. 1984;141(1):84-7.

Lijster JM, Dierckx B, Utens EM, et al. The age of onset of anxiety disorders. Can J Psychiatry. 2017;62(4): 237-46.

McGrath J, Saha S, Chant D, et al. a concise overview of incidence, prevalence, and mortality. Epidemiol Rev. 2008;30:67-76.

McHugh RK, Wigderson S, Greenfield SF. Epidemiology of substance use in reproductive-age women. Obstet Gynecol Clin North Am. 2014;41(2):177-89.

Mohammadi MR, Davidian H, Noorbala AA, et al. An epidemiological survey of psychiatric disorders in Iran. Clin Pract Epidemiol Ment Health. 2005;1:16.

Nandi DN, Mukherjee SP, Boral GC, et al. Socio-economic status and mental morbidity in certain tribes and castes in India—a cross-cultural study. Br J Psychiatry. 1980;136:73-85.

Ochoa S, Usall J, Cobo J, et al. Gender differences in schizophrenia and first-episode psychosis: a comprehensive literature review. Schizophr Res Treatment. 2012;2012:916198.

Ochoa S, Usall J, Villalta GV, et al. Influence of age at onset on social functioning in outpatients with schizophrenia. Eur J Psychiat. 2006;20(3):157-63.

Padmavathi R, Rajkumar S, Kumar N, et al. Prevalence of schizophrenia in an urban community in madras. Indian J Psychiatry. 1988;30(3):233-9.

Patel V, Araya R, de Lima M, et al. Women, poverty and common mental disorders in four restructuring societies. Soc Sci Med. 1999;49(11):1461-71.

Patel V, Kleinman A. Poverty and common mental disorders in developing countries. Bull World Health Organ. 2003;81(8):609-15.

Patel V, Kirkwood BR, Pednekar S, et al. Risk factors for common mental disorders in women: population-based longitudinal study. Br J Psychiatry. 2006;189:547-55.

Payne S. Poverty, social exclusion and mental health: Findings from the 1999 Poverty and Social Exclusion (PSE) survey. Bristol, University of Bristol, 2000.

Peen J, Schoevers RA, Beekman AT, et al. The current status of urban-rural differences in psychiatric disorders. Acta Psychiatr Scand. 2010;121(2):84-93.

Perala J, Suvisaari J, Saarni SI, et al. Lifetime prevalence of psychotic and bipolar I disorders in a general population. Arch Gen Psychiatry. 2007;64(1):19-28.

Probst JC, Laditka SB, Moore CG, et al. Rural-urban differences in depression prevalence: implications for family medicine. Fam Med. 2006;38(9):653-60.

Rahman A, Creed F. Outcome of prenatal depression and risk factors associated with persistence in the first postnatal year: prospective study from Rawalpindi, Pakistan. J Affect Disord. 2007;100 (1-3):115-21.

Ramdurg S, Kumar S. Study of socio-demographic profile, phenomenology, course and outcome of bipolar disorder in Indian population. Int J Health & Allied Sci. 2013;2(4):260.

Ray R, Chopra A. Monitoring of substance abuse in India—Initiatives and experiences. Indian J Med Res. 2012;135(6):806-8.

Regire DA, Farmer ME, Rae DS, et al. One-month prevalence of mental disorders in the United States and sociodemographic characteristics: the Epidemiologic Catchment Area study. Acta Psychiatr Scand. 1993;88(1):35-47.

Sagar R, Pattanayak RD, Chandrasekaran R, et al. Twelve-month prevalence and treatment gap for common mental disorders: Findings from a large-scale epidemiological survey in India. Indian J Psychiatry. 2017;59(1):46-55.

Schoeyen HK, Birkenaes AB, Vaaler AE, et al. Bipolar disorder patients have similar levels of education but lower socio-economic status than the general population. J Affect Disord. 2011;129(1-3):68-74.

Scott KM, Wells JE, Angermeyer M, et al. Gender and the relationship between marital status and first onset of mood, anxiety and substance use disorders. Psychol Med. 2010;40(9):1495-505.

Sethi BB, Gupta SC, Kumar R, et al. A psychiatric survey of 500 rural families. Indian J Psychiat. 1972;14:183.

Simoni WL, Ritter G, Strickler G, et al. Gender and other factors associated with the nonmedical use of abusable prescription drugs. Subst Use Misuse. 2004;39(1):1-23.

Susser M. Causal Thinking in the Health Sciences: Concepts and Strategies of Epidemiology. New York: Oxford University Press; 1973.

SAMHSA. TEDS report—Age of substance use initiation among treatment admissions aged 18 to 30. Rockville MD, Center for Behavioral Health Statistics and Quality, 2014.

Test MA, Senn BS, Wallisch LS, et al. Gender differences of young adults with schizophrenic disorders in community care. Schizophr Bull. 1990;16(2):331-44.

Tsuchiya KJ, Agerbo E, Byrne M, et al. Higher socio-economic status of parents may increase risk for bipolar disorder in the offspring. Psychol Med. 2004;34(5):787-93.

Verdoux H, Bourgeois M. Social class in unipolar and bipolar probands and relatives. J Affect Disord. 1995;33(3):181-7.

Vijayakumar L. Indian research on suicide. Indian J Psychiatry. 2010;52.

Weaver A, Himle JA, Taylor RJ, et al. Urban vs rural residence and the prevalence of depression and mood disorder among African American women and non-Hispanic white women. JAMA Psychiatry. 2015;72(6):576-83.

Weich S, Lewis G. Poverty, unemployment, and common mental disorders: population based cohort study. BMJ. 1998;317(7151):115-9.

Whitley E, Gunnell D, Dorling D, et al. Ecological study of social fragmentation, poverty, and suicide. BMJ. 1999;319(7216):1034-7.

World Health Organization: Gender and Women's Mental Health. Geneva, WHO, 2017.

Wyatt RJ, Alexander RC, Egan MF, et al. Schizophrenia, just the facts—What do we know, how well do we know it? Schizophr Res. 1988;1(1):3-18.

Social Dimensions of Psychiatric Disorders

Chapter 17

Evaluating Well-being and Health

Subho Chakrabarti

SUMMARY

Well-being is complex concept, which refers to optimum psychological functioning and experience. It is multidimensional in its make-up, holistic in its approach, positive in its outlook and predominantly subjective in its nature. The fields of philosophy, economics, sociology, and psychology have all made notable contributions to the construct of well-being. Well-being has an intimate connection with all aspects of health-care including mental health care. Not only has the concept influenced the current positive and holistic conceptualizations of mental health, it also plays a significant role in determining levels of mental health both in the general population as well as in those with psychiatric disorders. It has prompted several efforts to devise interventions and quite a few large-scale initiatives, which enhance the well-being of those with mental health problems. Despite years of research and a voluminous output of evidence, conceptualization, and measurement of well-being is still afflicted by several methodological inadequacies. It is hoped that these will be overcome with future endeavors and the utility of well-being in improving lives as well as health will be truly realized.

INTRODUCTION

Health and well-being are concerns of daily life among people and their families, and for governments and societies. Both health and well-being are intimately connected. Both are multidimensional constructs with similar biological and psychosocial determinants. Yet, health generally focuses on individual conditions while well-being is a broader concept that tries to define what constitutes authentic happiness or a fulfilling life. This chapter deals with the numerous facets of the concept of well-being and its assessment. It also includes the impact of well-being on health, particularly mental health. Research on well-being contains inputs from the fields of philosophy, economics, social sciences, psychology, and health-care. It is not possible to do justice to the vast amount of extant literature regarding well-being from all these perspectives. Moreover, it may not be appropriate to focus on the various controversies and intricacies of the subject in a chapter that intends to serve more as a basic introduction to well-being. Therefore, only a broad overview of the area including different approaches to well-being has been attempted, with mental health being the defining context.

WELL-BEING: EVOLVING PERSPECTIVES AND CONCEPTS

This section deals with the different perspectives of well-being that have evolved over the years, the theories of well-being associated with these perspectives and the concepts of well-being that have arisen from these perspectives. A comprehensive description of these issues is necessary because different conceptualizations of well-being have influenced the process of its evaluation to a large extent. Additionally, these notions of well-being have also determined how the construct has been used to improve the management of health-conditions, especially those relating to mental health.

Philosophical Concepts

The earliest conceptualizations of well-being lie in its philosophical roots, which stretch back to the era of ancient Greece (Ryan & Deci 2001; Brey, 2012; Dodge et al., 2012). What constitutes well-being, or in other words a good life or true happiness, was an important subject of study for Aristotle, Epicurus, and other Greek philosophers. Their ideas influenced the views about well-being and happiness of latter-day philosophers like Bentham and Mill. Many of the philosophical concepts of well-being have been subsequently incorporated in social, economic, and psychological theories of well-being. These have further influenced concepts of well-being and health, including mental health.

Economic Concepts

Economic theories have played a great role in determining the concept of well-being (Juster et al., 1981; Brey, 2012; Salvador-Carulla et al., 2014). Economic theories of well-being originated from neoclassical economics of the 19th century, which advocated the principle of utilitarianism. They were later supplanted by welfare-economic theories of the 1930s, which attempted to conceptualize and improve well-being by adopting a social-welfare approach. This culminated in the birth of "happiness economics" in the 1970s, a new branch devoted to the study of economic conditions for happiness and well-being. Economic theories regarding well-being have also gradually changed their focus once it was realized that income and well-being are not linked, unless the levels of income are very low (Easterlin, 2005). Therefore, objective measures such as the gross domestic product (GDP) were unable to account for well-being or happiness of individuals on a national scale (Conceição & Bandura, 2008). Similarly, once the lack of association between well-being and material resources became apparent, economic theories of well-being devised newer objective methods of measuring well-being by the so called "social indicators" technique, which employed objective indices such as health status or disability-free days to estimate well-being (Juster et al., 1981). However, the link between these objective measures and subjective perceptions of well-being still remained unclear. This led to an increased emphasis on subjective markers, one of which was quality of life (QoL) (Juster et al., 1981; Brey, 2012; Salvador-Carulla et al., 2014). Newer theories such as the capability theory, the preference-satisfaction approach and novel ways to estimate well-being such as the Human Development Index and the indicators such as the Gross National Happiness index have since emerged (Sen, 2002; Easterlin, 2005).

Sociological Concepts

In a sense sociological perspectives of well-being took off from where the initial economic theories ended (Juster et al., 1981; Salvador-Carulla et al., 2014). The beginnings were made by the "social indicators" movement, which emphasized the need to have a measure of the standard of living beyond economic and material indicators. This propelled the research on objective and subjective descriptors of QoL. Sociological conceptualizations of QoL have greatly influenced the research on economic, material, psychological, and health-related aspects of well-being. Social perspectives on well-being have also generated newer theories such as the preference-based ways of life satisfaction or well-being (Easterlin, 2005; Brey, 2012). Thus an individual's choice of a particular state of living (such as health-states) depended on factors such as subjective utility and preference. Sociologists have also contributed to the mental capital approach to mental well-being. Social well-being is now used as a generic term for the family of overlapping concepts including QoL, social satisfaction, social welfare, and the standard of living. An examination of the concept of social well-being found it to consist of five dimensions including social integration, social contribution, social coherence, social actualization and social acceptance (Keyes, 1998). The latent structure of this multidimensional construct of social well-being was confirmed in two studies. The dimensions of social well-being were associated with a number of related social and psychological constructs such as anomie, generativity, social constraints, neighborhood and community living, dysphoric feelings, optimism, physical health, and global well-being.

Psychological Concepts

Psychologists have carried out perhaps the most comprehensive exploration of well-being. Psychological constructs of well-being incorporate a diverse range of constructs including subjective well-being (SWB), psychological well-being (PWB), emotional well-being, mental well-being, and QoL (Diener, 1984; Ryan & Deci, 2001; Miller & Foster, 2007; Dodge et al., 2012). Some of the psychological concepts associated with well-being are described as below:

Subjective focus: Psychological definitions place the greatest stress on examining well-being from the individual's perspective. This stance is diametrically opposite to those social and economic theories that advocate only objective assessments of well-being. Apart from neglecting the experiential aspects of well-being, objective techniques are thought to be overly deterministic and restrictive in their assessments of well-being.

Holistic outlook: All psychological theories follow a holistic outlook toward well-being by integrating rather than separating the three aspects of self, that is mind, body, and spirit.

Positive emphasis: The common basis of psychological theories is their emphasis on the positive aspects of human experience and functioning. Well-being is considered somewhat more than the simple absence of ill-being, psychopathology, or dysfunction. This emphasis on a positive outlook is best exemplified by the positive psychological theories of Seligman and his conceptualizations of well-being.

Dynamic make-up: Psychological theories characterize well-being as a dynamic interplay between its different dimensions like resources and challenges, and over different time-periods. This is in contrast to objective views of well-being, which are deemed to be relatively static.

Multidimensional nature: An important feature of psychological theories is their multidimensionality. The commonest dimensions mentioned across different approaches are physical, psychological (which includes subjective, mental, or emotional elements), social, spiritual, and occupational dimensions. Other common dimensions are economic or material, intellectual, environmental, and cultural. Some authors also make a distinction between personal or individual well-being, family well-being, institutional aspects of well-being, and community well-being (Miller & Foster, 2007; Wollny et al., 2010; Dodge et al., 2012; Salvador-Carulla et al., 2014; Linton et al., 2016).

Stability over time: Most psychological theories are based on the "set-point" assumption. Each person is believed to have a set-point of well-being, which is determined by heredity or personality. Consequently, individuals maintain a reasonably stable level of well-being over time despite deflections below or above the set-point in response to life circumstances (Easterlin, 2005; McMahon et al., 2010).

Theories

There are three major psychological theories of well-being and a number of other theories deriving from these three main approaches. The two most influential standpoints are the theories of SWB and PWB. The former is based on hedonistic conceptualizations and the latter on eudaimonic views of well-being. A third set of theories is based on positive psychology (Ryan & Deci, 2001; Keyes et al., 2002a; Dodge et al., 2012). Not surprisingly, definitions of well-being vary depending on which school of thought they adhere to. Although there is no single definition of the concept, on the whole well-being refers to the happiness or satisfaction derived from "optimal psychological functioning and experience" (Ryan & Deci, 2001). The concept of satisfaction includes emotions such as happiness, contentment, interest, engagement, confidence, and affection. Optimal functioning incorporates fulfilling one's potential, personal growth, environmental mastery, purposeful living, and positive relationships. However, all these are relative rather than absolute requirements, and are based on subjective judgments and aspirations. They do not imply the necessity of either perfect, or sustainable and uniform functioning to define well-being (Huppert, 2009; McDowell, 2010).

Subjective Well-being

The term "subjective well-being" was coined by Diener (1984). The tripartite structure of SWB includes the two affective elements of positive affect (pleasurable feelings) and negative affect (painful feelings), and the cognitive component termed life satisfaction (Ryan & Deci, 2001; Hansen, 2011; Brey, 2012; Dodge et al., 2012; Díaz et al., 2015). The affective component of SWB refers to relatively short-term and ongoing emotional reactions to everyday events. Positive affect includes happiness, contentment or pleasure while negative affective states include depression and loneliness (Hansen, 2011). Positive and negative affective states are considered as relatively independent dimensions rather than being on a continuum (Keyes et al., 2002a; Dodge et al., 2012). Life satisfaction is a cognitive appraisal of the balance between positive and negative effects, and judgments about how life measures up to personal aspirations and social norms. It includes long-term assessments of both overall satisfaction with life and satisfaction in different domains, e.g. health, family, or finances (Hansen, 2011; Brey, 2012). The three-fold structure of SWB has been repeatedly corroborated in many studies (Keyes et al., 2002a). Measurements of SWB commonly take an overall summary approach rather than separating the three components (McDowell, 2010; Lindert et al., 2015). The concept of SWB, particularly its affective dimension is firmly rooted in hedonistic traditions of viewing life as an equilibrium between pleasurable and painful states of existing (Ryan & Deci, 2001; Brey, 2012).

Psychological Well-being

Unlike the hedonistic roots of SWB, theories of PWB are based on another Greek branch of philosophy referred to as the eudaimonic school of thought (Ryan & Deci, 2001; Hansen, 2011; McMahan & Estes, 2011; Brey, 2012; Ryff, 2014). According to Aristotle, the true goal of human life was not about just happiness or satisfaction of pleasures. Instead, it was about striving for virtue and realization of one's true nature (daemon). Recent conceptualizations of PWB have interpreted virtuous living to consist of being engaged in inherently good activities that are congruent with one's deeply held values. Additionally, it has come to include other elements such as personal growth, a sense of purpose, autonomy, self-actualization, and functioning at an optimal level (McDowell, 2010; Hansen, 2011; McMahan & Estes, 2011; Díaz et al., 2015). The eudaimonic tradition was carried forward by proponents of the humanistic school of psychology including Maslow and Erikson. Inspired by these theorists and concepts of positive mental health, Ryff devised a multidimensional construct of PWB. Her model of PWB incorporated six distinct dimensions including self-acceptance (positive evaluations of current and past life), personal growth (development as a person), purpose in life (belief that one's life is purposeful and meaningful), positive relations with others (trusting and lasting relationships), environmental mastery (the capacity to manage life and surroundings), and autonomy (a sense of self-determination) (Ryff & Keyes, 1995; Ryff, 1995; Keyes et al., 2002a; Ryff, 2014). This multifactorial model has been subjected to extensive examination of its reliability and internal consistency. In general the six-factor structure of PWB has been confirmed, though some studies have found a different factorial structure, and modifications to the original list of factors and their constituents have also been suggested (Ryff & Keyes, 1995; Keyes et al., 2002a; van Dierendonck, 2004; van Dierendonck et al., 2008; Ryff, 2014). Age and gender have shown consistent associations with the principal dimensions of this model of PWB. Scales derived from the six-factor model have been used in a variety of cultural, clinical and non-clinical settings to determine the impact of PWB on functioning, to uncover mediating psychosocial processes, or to measure outcome of psychological interventions. The use of the concept of PWB for these purposes has been most frequent in mental health settings. Although Ryff's concept is the most commonly encountered model of PWB, others have suggested simpler versions, which propose that PWB can be defined as fulfillment of three basic needs of autonomy, competence and relatedness (Ryan & Deci, 2001).

Though concepts of SWB and PWB have been conceived of independently, there is ample evidence to show that both are mutually overlapping as well as relatively discrete constructs. Accordingly, the need for greater conceptual integration between SWB and PWB, as well as the hedonistic and eudaimonic traditions has been frequently expressed (Díaz et al., 2015). Nonetheless, over the years there has been a gradual shift in the psychological perspective of well-being from the hedonistic mode of SWB to the eudaimonic approach of PWB (McDowell, 2010).

Positive Psychology

The major proponent of the positive psychological approach toward well-being has been Seligman (Brey, 2012; Dodge et al., 2012). His initial theories were predominantly hedonistic and attempted to explain what constitutes happiness. This has evolved into a theory of well-being with five components including positive emotions, active involvement in life, authentic relationships, a purposeful existence, and a sense of accomplishment. This has been called the PERMA approach (Rusk & Waters, 2015). The positive psychology movement has contributed another concept, which is particularly relevant for mental health. Known as the "flourishing" theory, this conceptualizes mental health in terms of well-being and ill-being by classifying people with or without mental health symptoms into "flourishers" and "languishers" (Keyes, 2002b).

Quality of Life

Quality of life is a complex and somewhat elusive concept, which has been used as an all-embracing term for objective and subjective judgments of functioning in multiple domains such as physical, emotional, social, and material dimensions (Barcaccia et al., 2013). The term originated in the 1960s to capture the different aspects that determine an individual's satisfaction with life. Current conceptualizations of QoL encompass several disciplines including economics, sociology, psychology, and health-care. The "social indicators" movement contributed to the assessment of QoL using both objective and subjective indices (Wollny et al., 2010). QoL has been used interchangeably with well-being, notably SWB (Hansen, 2011; Brey, 2012; Cooke et al., 2016). It seems to share common characteristics with well-being such as its multidimensionality, predominantly subjective focus, and its holistic emphasis (Wollny et al., 2010; Hansen, 2011; Barcaccia et al., 2013; Pinto et al., 2017). QoL assumed importance in the field of health once a holistic model of health was adopted instead of a biomedical one (Karimi & Brazier, 2016). Health-related QoL has been defined by the WHO as "an individual"s perception of their position in life in the context of the culture and value systems in which they live and in relation to their goals, expectations, standards, and concerns. It is a broad ranging concept affected in a complex way by the person's physical health, psychological state, personal beliefs, social relationships, and their relationship to salient features of their environment (WHO, 1997). The development of the WHOQOL scale by the WHO has tremendously boosted the use of QoL as an index of outcome for all health-related interventions, especially those involving psychiatric disorders.

Health and Well-being

In 1948, the WHO accepted a new definition of health, which mooted that it was "a state of complete physical, mental and social well-being and not merely the absence of disease or infirmity" (WHO, 1948). In doing so, the WHO made a radical shift from the disease model of health to a public-health model (Grad, 2002). Moreover, this definition of health highlighted its positive aspects and moved away from defining it negatively as biomedical models of the time did. Though the definition has been subsequently criticized (Saracci, 1997), the WHO was unusually prescient in linking the concept of health to the concept of well-being. Indeed, WHO's holistic view of health was a precursor to similar holistic conceptions of well-being that emerged later (Miller & Foster, 2007). Apart from their holistic outlooks, the concepts of health and well-being share other features such as multidimensionality, subjective focus, positive emphasis, and dynamic nature. Then again, well-being is a much broader concept, which includes several dimensions of living other than health (Salvador-Carulla et al., 2014). Moreover, health-related states do not always correlate with a person's overall sense of well-being (Ryan & Deci, 2001).

Nonetheless, both SWB and PWB have an intimate connection with health. Nowhere is this link more apparent than with mental health. Indeed, the WHO definition of mental health puts far greater weight on the concept of well-being by defining mental health as "a state of well-being in which the individual realizes his or her own abilities, can cope with the normal stresses of life, can work productively and fruitfully, and is able to make a contribution to his or her community" (Herrman et al., 2005). Thus, similar to its definition of health, the WHO highlights the holistic nature, positive outlook and public-health focus of mental health in its definition. Moreover, it provides the much needed emphasis on a move away from treatment-orientated stance to a health-promotional approach to mental health. In keeping with the current developments in research on well-being, the definition is based on an integration of SWB/hedonistic and PWB/eudaimonic concepts of well-being (de Cates et al., 2015). In a review of the influence of SWB on mental health, it was found that while negative emotions could precipitate adverse mental health states such as depression, positive emotions could offer protection from mental health pathology (Ryan & Deci, 2001). A more recent and extensive review of the impact of PWB on mental health has underlined how emotional, psychological, and social well-being, as well as constructs such as self-esteem, mastery, purpose in life, and autonomy are closely associated with mental health (Ryff, 2014). Furthermore, complete recovery from mental illness entails more than amelioration of symptoms or distress and has to incorporate the enhancement of well-being. Several psychological interventions based on this premise of PWB have been successfully used among people suffering from different psychiatric disorders. Resilience is defined as positive adaptation to stressful events and the ability to recover from hardships. A report from the WHO on mental health and resilience found extensive evidence to link positive states of well-being to resilience (Friedli, 2009). Finally, positive psychological concepts such as "flourishing" have been used to define mental health at the population level (Keyes, 2002b; Friedli, 2009; Huppert, 2009). "Flourishing" is a state of positive emotions and positive psychological and social functioning, while "languishing" includes negative states of emotion and experience. Using data from large-scale national-level surveys of Western countries, it was found that states of "flourishing" were prevalent in less than 20% people, while about 10% were in states of "languishing." About half of the people had moderate levels of mental functioning and a fifth was diagnosed with mental disorders.

EVALUATING WELL-BEING

There is an extensive body of literature on the assessment of well-being. Any evaluation of well-being has to be governed by certain principles relating to the characteristics of the concept (Warr, 2013; Linton et al., 2016). Well-being is a multifaceted and multidimensional construct. Therefore, assessments have to be comprehensive and ideally use multidimensional measures. The context, emphasis and scope of measurement, especially the use of measures in different cultural contexts are significant issues in the evaluation of well-being (Hansen, 2011; Warr, 2013). Similarly, the greater emphasis on subjectivity and interactional components of appraisals is of immense consequence. Finally, assessments should have an impact on policies, which could potentially enhance well-being. The evaluation of well-being has both objective and subjective aspects (Conceição & Bandura, 2008; Brey, 2012 ; Lindert et al., 2015). Objective indicators can be economic measures such as GDP, measures of QoL in terms of standards of living or health parameters, and other measures of social well-being such as literacy, job security, or access to public services. Subjective indicators are mainly used to assess social well-being including QoL and psychological constructs such as SWB and PWB (Miller & Foster, 2007; Brey, 2012). Some of the common subjective indices of socio-economic well-being are the Human Development Index, the Gross National Happiness index, the Index of Economic Freedom and the Better Life Index of the Organization for Economic Cooperation and Development. Additionally, there are a number of concept-driven scales to measure social, psychological and health-related aspects of well-being. An assortment of five scales is employed to assess SWB and the six-factor construct of PWB is measured by Ryff's Scales of Psychological Well-Being (Diener et al., 2009; Ryff, 2014). The PERMA-Profiler is a brief multidimensional measure of "flourishing" based on the PERMA approach, while another set of scales are used to measure the five dimensions of social well-being (Keyes, 1998; Butler & Kern, 2016). Finally, there are several scales to measure QoL, including health-related QoL, which is evaluated by using different versions of the WHOQOL scale (Cooke et al., 2016; Karimi & Brazier, 2016). A number of reviews have assessed the instruments used to examine various facets of well-being (Conceição & Bandura, 2008; McDowell, 2010; Hansen, 2011; Warr, 2013; Lindert et al., 2015; Cooke et al., 2016; Linton et al., 2016). These have revealed that there are well over a hundred scales, most of which are used to assess QoL, SWB or PWB. Most of them are multidimensional and evaluate domains such as mental/psychological, social, physical, spiritual, occupational, and personal well-being. These instruments differ a great deal in their structure and length, in their psychometric properties, and in their conception and operational definitions of well-being. Evaluations of SWB and PWB commonly measure affect, life satisfaction and concepts such as autonomy, mastery, and meaning in life. A common refrain across these reviews is the presence of several methodological flaws in the entire process of evaluating well-being. They all note that substantial improvements are required to enhance the utility of currently available tools.

DIFFICULTIES IN CONCEPTUALIZING AND MEASURING WELL-BEING

Despite the long tradition and voluminous output, research on well-being continues to be plagued by several methodological shortcomings, both in the way the construct has been framed and the way it has been evaluated.

Problems with the concept of well-being include lack of clear and agreed upon definitions, the use of different terms to refer to diverse aspects of well-being, interchangeable use of these terms, complex, multidimensional and multilevel operationalizations, lack of consistency, lack of validity particularly cross-cultural validity, lack of empirical examination of constructs used, the predominant emphasis on subjective and personal nature of the concept, and the somewhat excessive preoccupation with well-being of the affluent, mainstream majority in the developed world while neglecting minorities, the marginalized and those from different ethno-cultural backgrounds (Ryan & Deci, 2001; Miller & Foster, 2007; Wollny et al., 2010; Dodge et al., 2012; Ryff, 2014).

Much of the concerns about the concept of well-being spill over into the process of assessment. In fact, many have noted that researchers seem to have put the horse before the cart in first providing operational definitions of the term, and then hoping that a fully-formed concept will emerge. Consequently, evaluation of well-being is not theory-driven and there is a lack of consensus about what is being measured. Added to this is the profusion of scales, many of which lack adequate psychometric qualities. The proliferation of scales each with their own concepts of well-being and attempts to capture different dimensions of the experience add to the confusion, and create difficulties in selecting relevant and useful instruments to assess well-being. The difficulties posed by the differences in objective versus subjective appraisals of well-being also add another dimension of complexity to its evaluation (McDowell, 2010; Hansen, 2011; Barcaccia et al., 2013; Cooke et al., 2016; Linton et al., 2016).

CONCLUSIONS AND IMPLICATIONS

This brief synopsis of the research on well-being demonstrates its long traditions, the considerable amount of research attention devoted to the subject, and the advances that have been made in this field. This review also highlights the methodological lacunae in existing literature that have become apparent over the years. However, regardless of these shortcomings, the concept of well-being has been successful in attracting the attention of policy makers and has played a significant role in guiding social-welfare policies (Miller & Foster, 2007; Cooke et al., 2016). The impact of research on well-being on mental health has been especially notable. Concepts of well-being have aided in gradually shifting the focus from a medical-model approach of reducing psychopathology to a public-health stance that encourages personal growth and promotion of well-being (Ryan & Deci, 2001). The gradually increasing evidence-base, which demonstrates the intimate connections between well-being and mental health, and between well-being and psychological treatment have contributed to this change (Ryff, 2014). The current policies of the WHO have placed well-being at the center of its health-promotional strategies right from the definition of mental health to unraveling the link between absence of well-being and mental illness, and to the development of interventions and initiatives to enhance the well-being of those with mental health problems (Herrman et al., 2005; Friedli, 2009). However, others feel that the research on well-being has not reached a stage where it can dictate public policies to do with mental health (Davies & Mehta, 2013). Therefore, it is evident that while a lot of progress has been made, much remains to be done in this high-priority area of well-being and mental health.

REFERENCES

Barcaccia B, Esposito G, Matarese M, et al. Defining quality of life: a wild-goose chase? Eur J Psychol. 2013;9(1):185-203.

Brey P. Well-being in philosophy, psychology, and economics in the good life in a technological age. In: Brey P, Briggle A, Spence E (Eds). The Good Life in a Technological Age. New York: Routledge, Taylor and Francis Group; 2012. pp. 15-34.

Butler J, Kern ML. The PERMA-Profiler: A brief multidimensional measure of flourishing. Int J Wellbeing. 2016;6(3):1-48.

Cooke PJ, Melchert TP, Connor K. Measuring well-being: a review of instruments. Counsel Psychol. 2016;44(5):730-57.

Conceição P, Bandura R. Measuring subjective wellbeing: a summary review of the literature. UNDP Working Paper. 2008;924:1-24.

Davies SC, Mehta N: Public mental health: evidence based priorities in annual Report of the Chief Medical Officer. In: Mehta N, Murphy O, Lillford-Wildman C (Eds). Public Mental Health Priorities: Investing in the Evidence. 2013. pp. 21-58.

de Cates A, Stranges S, Blake A, et al. Mental well-being: an important outcome for mental health services? Br J Psychiatry. 2015:207(3):195-7.

Díaz D, Stavraki M, Blanco A, et al. The eudaimonic component of satisfaction with life and psychological well-being in Spanish cultures. Psicothema. 2015;27(3):247-53.

Diener E. Subjective well-being. Psychol Bulletin. 1984; 95(3):542-75.

Diener E, Wirtz D, Biswas-Diener R, et al. New measures of well-being; flourishing and positive and negative feelings in assessing Well-Being. In: Diener E (Ed). New York: Springer; 2009. pp. 247-66.

Dodge R, Daly A, Huyton J, et al. The challenge of defining wellbeing. Int J Wellbeing. 2012;2(3):222-35.

Easterlin RA. Building a better theory of well-being, in economics and happiness. In: Bruni L, Porta PL (Eds). Framing the Analysis. Oxford:University Press; 2005. pp. 29-64.

Friedli L. Mental Health, resilience and inequalities. Denmark: World Health Organization; 2009.

Grad FP. The preamble of the constitution of the World Health Organization. Bull World Health Organ. 2002;80(12):981-2.

Hansen T. Subjective well-being in the second half of life: the influence of family and household resources. Phd Thesis. Oslo:University of Oslo; 2011.

Huppert FA. Psychological wellbeing: evidence regarding its causes and consequences. App Psychol Health Wellbeing. 2009;1(2):137-64.

Juster FT, Courant PN, Dow GK. A theoretical framework for the measurement of wellbeing. Rev Income Wealth. 1981;27(1):1-31.

Karimi M, Brazier J. Health, health-related quality of life, and quality of life: what is the difference? Pharmacoeconomics. 2016;34(7):645-9.

Keyes CLM: Social wellbeing. Soc Psychol Q. 1998;61(2):121-40.

Keyes CL, Shmotkin D, Ryff CD. Optimizing well-being: the empirical encounter of two traditions. J Pers Soc Psychol. 2002;82(6):1007-22.

Keyes CLM. The mental health continuum: from languishing to flourishing in life. J Health Soc Behav. 2002;43(2):207-22.

Lindert J, Bain PA, Kubzansky LD, et al. Well-being measurement and the WHO health policy Health 2010: systematic review of measurement scales. Eur J Public Health. 2015;25(4):731-40.

Linton MJ, Dieppe P, Medina-Lara A. Review of 99 self-report measures for assessing wellbeing in adults: exploring dimensions of well-being and developments over time. BMJ Open. 2016;6:e010641.

McDowell I. Measures of self-perceived well-being. J Psychosom Res. 2010; 69(1):69-79.

McMahan EA, Estes D. Hedonic versus eudaimonic conceptions of well-being: evidence of differential associations with self-reported well-being. Soc Indicators Res. 2011;103(1):93-108.

McMahon A, Williams P, Tapsell LC. Reviewing the meanings of wellness and well-being and their implications for food choice. Perspect Public Health. 2010;130(6):282-6.

Miller GD, Foster LT. Defining wellness and its determinants. In: Foster LT, Keller CP. Victoria BC (Eds). The British Columbia Atlas of Wellness, first edition. Western Geographical Press; 2007. pp. 9-20.

Pinto S, Fumincelli L, Mazzo A, et al. Comfort, well-being and quality of life: discussion of the differences and similarities among the concepts. Porto Biomed J. 2017;2:6-12.

Promoting mental health: concepts, emerging evidence, practice: report of the World Health Organization. Department of mental health and substance abuse in collaboration with the victorian health promotion foundation and the University of Melbourne. In: Herrman H, Saxena S, Moodie R (Eds). Geneva: World Health Organization; 2005.

Rusk RD, Waters L. A psycho-social system approach to well-being: empirically deriving the five domains of positive functioning. J Pos Psychol. 2015;10(2):141-52.

Ryan RM, Deci EL. On happiness and human potentials: a review of research on hedonic and eudaimonic well-being. Annu Rev Psychol. 2001; 52:141-66.

Ryff CD. Psychological well-being in adult life. Curr Direc Psychol Sci. 1995;4(4):99-104.

Ryff CD. Psychological well-being revisited: advances in the science and practice of eudaimonia. Psychother Psychosom. 2014;83(1):10-28.

Ryff CD, Keyes CL. The structure of psychological well-being revisited. Journal of Pers Soc Psychol. 1995;69(4):719-27.

Salvador-Carulla L, Lucas R, Ayuso-Mateos JL, et al. Use of the terms "wellbeing" and "quality of life" in health sciences: a conceptual framework. Eur J Psych. 2014;28(1):50-65.

Saracci R. The World Health Organization needs to reconsider its definition of health. BMJ. 1997;314(7091):1409-10.

Sen AK. Health: perception versus observation. BMJ. 2002;324(7342):860-1.

Van Dierendonck D. The construct validity of Ryff's scales of psychological well-being and its extension with spiritual well-being. Pers Ind Diff. 2004;36(3):629-43.

Van Dierendonck D, Diaz D, Rodrıguez-Carvajal R, et al. Ryff's six-factor model of psychological well-being, a Spanish exploration. Soc Ind Res. 2008;87:473-9.

Warr P. How to think about and measure psychological well-being and inequalities, in Research Methods in Occupational Health Psychology. In: Wang M, Tetrick LE, Sinclair RR (Eds). Measurement, Design and Data Analysis. New York, Routledge: Taylor & Francis Group; 2013. pp. 76-90.

Wollny I, Apps J, Henricson C. Can government measure family wellbeing? A literature review. London: Family and Parenting Institute; 2010.

World Health Organization. Constitution of the World Health Organization. Geneva: World Health Organization; 1948.

World Health Organization. WHOQOL: Measuring Quality of Life. Geneva: World Health Organization; 1997.

Chapter 18

Schizophrenia and Other Psychotic Disorders

R Thara, Lakshmi Venkatraman, Subhashini Gopal

SUMMARY

Schizophrenia is a biopsychosocial disorder. This chapter provides an overview of some of the social aspects such as urbanization and immigration, associated with schizophrenia and other psychotic disorders. Social consequences of the illness, such as disability, impaired social functioning, impact on marriage, employment, and stigma have been discussed in some detail. Authors have also explained the role of social cognition, and its relationship to symptomatology and functioning. Possible social interventions like supported employment and social skills training with particular focus on low and middle-income countries have been touched upon. As social media has become popular in the lives of people, the extent of its use by the patients with psychosis is discussed briefly.

INTRODUCTION

The role of social factors in schizophrenia has always been well-recognized and documented. With origins from theories like schizophrenogenic mother, schism and skew, to concepts such as poverty, urbanization, and migration, the current emphasis as shown by research trends seems to be on social cognition and social functioning. It is well-nigh impossible to include all possible social factors in a single chapter. We have therefore confined ourselves to a few important and current issues on causal attributes, outcomes, and interventions.

SOCIAL THEORIES OF SCHIZOPHRENIA

In the mid-20th century, social theories of schizophrenia were very popular. Schizophrenogenic mothers, and marital skew and schism were some of the concepts considered. However, these have not withstood scientific scrutiny and are no longer accepted as causes of schizophrenia.

Incidence of schizophrenia was observed in deprived neighborhoods to be associated with high poverty rates, marital instability, residential mobility, and ethnic heterogeneity as early as in the 1930s by Faris and Dunham (1939). Over the years, arguments have been provided to determine if these were indeed the cause or effect of schizophrenia.

The social causation hypothesis argues that chronic exposure to early adverse neighborhood stressors over a period of time, especially in those with genetic vulnerability, could predispose to schizophrenia.

On the other hand, the social drift hypothesis states that the psychotic features of schizophrenia lead to a downward socioeconomic trajectory. People with schizophrenia have cognitive difficulties and occupational dysfunction, which contribute to the drift into poverty and deprived neighborhood. In England and Wales, a survey by Goldberg and Morrison (1963) noted more patients in the social class V in young men (25–34 years of age) having schizophrenia in their first admission to a mental hospital. The survey found that the fathers' social class distribution was comparable to the general population. The patients during their adolescence had managed various careers and had expectations for professional and technical jobs similar to their home environment. Those with an insidious onset of illness did not attain any professional or technical skills, while those with acute onset dropped in social class shortly before admission.

Sariaslan et al. (2016) argue for a genetic influence on schizophrenia and adulthood neighborhood deprivation association using population, twin, and molecular genetic data. They suggest that genetic liability for schizophrenia also contributes to residing in socioeconomically deprived neighborhood and question the impact of environment in the social drift of patients.

Whilst the above suggest a role for social and economic deprivation in schizophrenia, the contribution of other social factors still seems unclear.

SOCIAL FACTORS CONTRIBUTING TO SCHIZOPHRENIA

Urbanization

Urbanization has been considered an important risk factor in the development of schizophrenia for a long time. Studies have noted a twofold to four-fold increase (most studies show a two-fold increase) in risk of psychosis. A systematic review by Dana March et al. (2008) examines the spatial variation in the distribution of psychotic illnesses. Urbanicity is a broad and ill defined concept. Neighborhood is narrow taking into consideration ethnic density and social capital. Living in an urban neighborhood early in life may be etiologically important than adult urban dwelling. Both risk and protective social factors at the group and individual levels are thought to be etiologically important, according to studies investigating neighborhoods. The spatial variation is consistent with previous studies for nonaffective psychosis. The systematic review however does not address the contextual and social factors that contribute to the variation.

In-utero infection is a proposed mechanism for linking urbanization to schizophrenia. Exposure to infection during gestation, overcrowding and increased person-to-person contact in urban areas could contribute to in-utero infections leading to the offsprings developing psychosis in their adulthood. It is speculated that toxin and pollutant exposure in crowded areas may also play a role.

Migrants and Ethnic Minorities

Ethnic density studies indicate that social processes can also contribute directly to psychosis without relating to physical exposure. "Ethnic density" hypothesis states that ethnic minority groups are more likely to have better mental health when they live in areas with higher proportions of people of the same ethnicity. Social cohesion is the probable protective factor against discrimination and social exclusion.

Kirkbride et al. (2008) found a nonlinear relationship of social cohesion and trust with schizophrenia incidence. A higher incidence of schizophrenia was observed in neighborhoods with low social cohesion and trust and those with high social cohesion and trust compared to the neighborhoods with medial social cohesion and trust. The neighborhood variation in social cohesion and trust were nonlinearly associated with the incidence of schizophrenia. This seems to suggest that social capital is a risk factor. The relationship is complex possibly mediated at the individual level by response to social stress.

A study in London (Boydell et al., 2001) noted that the incidence of schizophrenia in nonwhite ethnic minorities rose significantly as the proportion of the minorities in the local population fell.

The UK studies have observed a significantly increased risk of psychosis in the Afro-Caribbean community specifically in the second-generation immigrants. Two separate studies (Bhugra et al., 1997; Harrison et al., 1997), one in Nottingham and another in London, noted a similar incidence rate (annual incidence 5.9 and 6 per 10,000 respectively). In another study in Holland (Selten et al., 1997), a nearly 4-fold increase was reported in the Dutch Antillean and Surinamese immigrants compared to the general population. As the rates in the Afro-Caribbean immigrant population of the UK is higher compared to the native population from the Caribbean, Jablensky (1999) in his review paper argues against a genetic cause for the increased incidence of psychosis in immigrant population. Selective migration of vulnerable individuals has been considered an unlikely explanation as over half the population moved from Dutch Antilles in Holland. Jablensky postulates that there could be a "strong environmental factor pushing the penetrance of the genetic susceptibility to the disorder upwards".

SOCIAL IMPACT/ OUTCOME FOR SCHIZOPHRENIA

Treatment of schizophrenia can improve social outcome by various mechanisms. Improved symptomatology allows the patient to have better functioning. Improvements in cognition and nonpharmacological interventions such as vocational rehabilitation are other ways in which social outcome can be enhanced. It has also been shown that societal factors play a critical role in determining social outcomes. A society and family which encourage and support people with schizophrenia (robust legal system for people with disability, reduced stigma and discrimination, support and encouragement for competitive employment, ease of availability of jobs) are more likely to see a better outcome (Priebe, 2007).

There are subjective and objective indicators for outcome. Objective indicators are marriage, employment, independent living, and social contacts. Quality of life and social functioning are some of the subjective indicators. There are several factors that influence subjective quality of life. It is less favorable in people with schizophrenia who are younger, male, live alone or are homeless, have a high level of education and are not employed. The factor that appears to be influencing subjective quality of life the most consistently is depressive symptoms. More depressive symptoms relate with poorer subjective quality of life (Priebe et al., 2000).

The western world studies report that those with schizophrenia have lower marriage rates compared to controls and those with other mental illnesses. On the other hand, in a 10-year follow-up study in India that we conducted looking at marital outcome, we observed a high marital rate at about 70%. Good marital outcome was associated with onset of illness after marriage, having children, a shorter illness and auditory hallucinations. Poor marital outcome was associated with flat affect, drop in socioeconomic status, unemployment, and neglecting self (Thara & Srinivasan, 1997).

Employment rates in people with schizophrenia have been variable. A review (Marwaha et al., 2007) found a broad variation ranging from 10 to 20% in European studies. Not surprisingly, people with first episode psychosis are noted to have a higher employment rate. Previous work history is the most consistent predictor of future employment. Being employed correlates better with social functioning, symptom levels, quality of life, and self-esteem, but a clear cause-effect relationship is not possible to establish.

The Madras Longitudinal study showed that male patients with schizophrenia held jobs, more so in the unorganized sector. The authors opined that lack of welfare benefits for the mentally disabled encouraged people to take up jobs (Srinivasan & Thara, 1997).

From China, Yang et al. (2013) reported that people with schizophrenia from a rural background have greater opportunities for employment in rural rather than in urban areas. Agricultural work with its need for survival and individual use, flexibility in terms of seasonality and involvement of the extended kin, all could be the possible factors for this better outcome in rural settings.

SOCIAL COGNITION IN SCHIZOPHRENIA

Capacity to relate to oneself and others, and making use of those representations appropriately in a social situation is referred to as social cognition. Recent research evidences state that social cognition contributes to functional outcome in persons with schizophrenia. When an individual has deficits in this area he/she might face difficulty in relating to their friends, family, and peers, which in turn impact his/her behavior at work, school, etc. The individual fails to recognize other persons' emotions and understand the social cues in social situations, and hence might avoid such interactions. This would have a huge impact on the person's independent living skills. Social cognition comprises of four areas such as facial affect recognition, social perception, theory of mind, and attributional style.

Importance of Social Cognition

Mental health professionals in their regular clinical practice often hear the following statements from family members of persons with schizophrenia:

"He just doesn't understand what my point of view is"

"She looks at him strangely and claims that she is spying on him"

"He doesn't behave properly in front of guests"

"She always blames me for all the problems"

If we carefully examine these statements, we can understand that persons with schizophrenia have impairments in the domains of social cognition which leads to conflicts among family, social, and occupational relationships.

Assessing Social Cognition

There are various tools available to assess social cognitive deficits. Theory of mind deficits were assessed using Sally-Anne, ice cream cookies task, Metaphor Irony, and Faux pas stories (Wimmer & Perner, 1983; Perner & Wimmer, 1985; Drury et al., 1998; Stone et al., 1998). Internal, Personal, and Situational Attribution Questionnaire (IPSAQ) is used to assess attribution styles (Kinderman & Bental, 1996). Social cue recognition test (SCRT) is used to measure social perception and emotional recognition (Corrigan & Green, 1993). These tools were developed to suit the western culture and have clear limitations for use with Indian patients. The team from National Institute of Mental Health and Neuro Sciences, Bangalore adapted these independent tests without modifying the original constructs and validated the tool named Social Cognition Rating Tool in Indian setting (SOCRATIS) whose psychometric properties are found to be satisfactory (Mehta et al., 2011). The topic has been discussed in chapter 6.

Intervention for Deficits in Social Cognition

Social cognitive deficits are intervened using various psychosocial approaches such as cognitive remediation, social skill training, social cognitive skill building, etc. Research has shown promising evidence but all these methods have their own limitations.

David Penn and his team has developed a 24-week intervention module called social cognition and interaction training (SCIT) for persons with schizophrenia. The preliminary study using SCIT has shown promising results. In a study on 31 outpatients with schizophrenia, who underwent SCIT, significant improvement was observed in facial affect recognition (FAR) but not in the other domains. The efficacy of SCIT has to be studied with larger sample size and across different settings (Penn et al., 2005).

Kurtz and Richardson (2008) conducted a meta-analysis on social cognition training in schizophrenia. They identified around 19 controlled studies. The results were consistent with the hypotheses that these interventions produced moderate to large effect on FAR and smaller but significant effect on theory of mind. The meta-analysis did not find any improvement with regard to positive and negative symptoms.

Social cognition being a significant predictor of functional outcome, its relationship with symptom dimensions and functioning needs to be studied intensively with larger sample size in Low and Middle Income (LAMI) countries. Based on the results, appropriate culturally relevant interventions can be developed.

SOCIAL STIGMA

Stigma is a social phenomenon, which has historically been associated with a number of disorders such as tuberculosis, leprosy, sexually transmitted illnesses, and mental disorders. It results in a person experiencing a sense of shame and disgrace, which often results in social isolation. Although Rabkin (1974) and Bhugra (1989) have stated that more information on the illness improves stigma, research has not revealed any efficacy of patient centered interventions on stigma.

In many developing countries, the severely mentally ill continue to live with their families. The family members who are the primary carers, experience as much if not greater stigma than the patients. A study at the Schizophrenia Research Foundation at Chennai (Thara & Srinivasan, 2000) looked at the nature and degree of stigma experienced by 159 urban dwellers with schizophrenia. The Family Interview Schedule of the International Study of Schizophrenia was used to measure stigma and divide the group into high and low stigma groups. The most stigmatized areas of concern were marriage, acquiring jobs, and fear that neighbors would treat them differently. The family members often had to make special efforts to hide the fact of mental illness from others.

With most of the marriages being arranged by the families, the disclosure of mental illness by one of the partners is often fraught with the danger of the breakup of the marriage. It can also jeopardize the chances of marriage of other members in the family. It was also found in our study that stigma was higher in female patients and carers, which was irrespective of what causes they attributed to have led to the disorder.

Another study by the group (Thara et al., 2003) focused on the status of women with schizophrenia whose marriages had been broken. This was viewed by the families as a "dual tragedy" and they felt very stigmatized. Most of these women did not receive any support from their husbands, either emotional or financial. The break in marriage was considered more stigmatizing than the mental disorder since they felt socially ostracized. Inability of some of the mentally ill women to bear a child also adds up to the stigma.

Jadhav et al. (2007) demonstrated that stigma is not confined to urban areas. Using a vignette based scale to measure stigma, they found that rural Indians showed significantly higher stigma scores than their urban counterparts. This was more in those who were manual workers, while the urban sample displayed a less punitive and more liberal view of severe mental illness. Urban Indians however showed reluctance to have the mentally ill as their work colleagues, which was not the case in rural areas. Yet another study of Loganathan and Murthy (2008) on stigma in rural areas found that persons with mental disorders and their families experienced ridicule, shame, and discrimination.

Do explanatory models held by families influence attitudes and stigma? The study of Srinivasan and Thara (2001) involved interview of key relatives living with 254 chronic schizophrenia patients and asking them of their explanatory models. Only 12% of the families named a supernatural cause. The commonest reason cited was psychosocial stress followed by personality defect and heredity illness. In another study from Vellore in South India, multiple and contradictory beliefs about causation of illness and its treatment were held by patients and relatives. Majority had used more than one system of healing including allopathy and traditional, magico-religious, and religious modes. Karma, evil spirits as causes of mental illnesses and belief in disease models influenced stigma scores of patients. Thus, the belief systems can play a part in coping with the illness (Charles et al., 2007).

People who plan mental health services should keep in mind the factors that influence help seeking behavior of patients and families.

IMPROVING SOCIAL FUNCTIONING: SOCIAL SKILLS TRAINING, VOCATIONAL REHABILITATION, AND SOCIAL MEDIA

Mental health professionals have recommended psychosocial interventions in the comprehensive management of schizophrenia. The Schizophrenia Patient Outcomes Research Team (PORT, 2009) psychosocial treatment recommendations provide a comprehensive summary of current evidence-based psychosocial treatment interventions for persons with schizophrenia. The latest summary of recommendations (Dixon et al., 2010) makes eight treatment recommendations including Assertive Community Treatment (ACT), supported employment, skills training, cognitive behavioral therapy, token economy interventions, family-based services, psychosocial interventions for comorbid alcohol and substance use disorders, and psychosocial interventions for weight management.

Supported Employment

Increasing emphasis is placed on finding competitive employment for patients with schizophrenia, moving away from the earlier models of sheltered workshops and day care. Whilst the latter still have a role to play for some patients, finding real work in the real world goes a long way in improving self-esteem and quality of life for patients with schizophrenia. Those, who want to work, will require support to find and maintain employment. They need to find jobs, that suit and interest them to enable motivation to work. PORT evidence summary reports the effectiveness of supported employment in helping persons with schizophrenia to achieve competitive employment, work more hours, and earn more wages than persons who did not receive supported employment. Evidence favors a quick search for jobs rather than elaborate prevocational preparation. Patients who find competitive employment will need continued support to maintain their employment and the role of mental health services in this regard is important to monitor mental health and provide help to sustain in the job. Evidence does not indicate that supported employment leads to exacerbation of symptoms, increased stress or other negative clinical outcomes. Hence all patients, who aim to work, should be offered supported employment. LAMI countries are more likely to find people with schizophrenia being employed than those in the Western countries. In our study, we observed two-thirds to one-fourth annual employment rate in the first 10 years of follow-up in a cohort of 90 people with first-episode schizophrenia (Srinivasan & Thara, 1997).

Social Skills Training

Patients with schizophrenia who have deficits require training in areas like social interactions and independent living. Social skills training programs should have a major emphasis on behavioral approach with role plays, modeling, rehearsal, corrective feedback, and positive reinforcement. Patients should be encouraged to practice the skills in real life situations when they receive clinic-based training. Involving families and training family members to participate in skills training efforts is an emerging strategy.

Social skills training produces significant effects on skills as observed in role-play tests, and also in community functioning. Evidence does not support indirect effects on relapse or general psychopathology. Evidence indicates that learnt skills are retained up to a year. There is not enough data looking at long-term follow-up in this area, and so sustainability of benefits is not known (Kurtz & Mueser, 2008).

Social Media

All around the world, social media has gathered pace as an inevitable part of people's lives. Patients with schizophrenia have difficulty in interacting with others and hence find it easier using the developing technology for their social contacts. Miller et al. (2015) conducted a survey of 80 inpatients and outpatients with schizophrenia. They found that more than half of the subjects (56%) use text messaging and just under half (48%) have an email account. Facebook was the most popular social media site. In their review and meta-analysis, Firth et al. (2016) observed an overall mobile phone ownership rate of 66.4% (95% CI = 54.1–77.6%). They noted that mobile phone ownership amongst patients has been increasing since 2007 and is not far behind the general population. As access to technology is no longer proving a barrier, many patients are likely to be using social media and it is imperative that technology and social media are used to help people with schizophrenia. Current evidence base does not support worsening of psychosis due to the use of social media though this is a potential side effect. Work is already happening to harness this resource in providing help with symptom management, adherence to treatment, online peer support, and social interactions.

CONCLUSION

Whilst the biological underpinnings of schizophrenia are becoming clearer, one has to accept the significant role of social factors in the development of the disorder. Understanding the social factors in operation and the impact of the disorder on the social outcome allows us to carefully plan a biopsychosocial intervention plan for people with this disorder. More studies evaluating psychosocial interventions in the LAMI countries are essential to improve the quality of life of those with this disorder.

REFERENCES

Bhugra D, Leff J, Mallett R, et al. Incidence and outcome of schizophrenia in Whites, African-Caribbeans and Asians in London. Psychol Med. 1997;27:791-8.

Bhugra D. Attitudes towards mental illness—A review of the literature. Acta Psychiatr Scand. 1989;80(1): 1-12.

Boydell J, van Os J, McKenzie K, et al. Incidence of schizophrenia in ethnic minorities in London: ecological study into interactions with environment. BMJ. 2001;323:1-4.

Charles H, Manoranjitham SD, Jacob KS. Stigma and explanatory models among people with schizophrenia and their relatives in Vellore, south India. Int J Soc Psychiatry. 2007;53(4):325-32

Corrigan PW, Green MF. Schizophrenic patients' sensitivity to social cues: the role of abstraction. Am J Psychiatry. 1993;150:589-4.

Dixon LB, Dickerson F, Bellack AS, et al. The 2009 schizophrenia PORT psychosocial treatment recommendations and summary statements. Schizophr Bull. 2010;36:48-70.

Drury VM, Robinson EJ, Birchwood M. Theory of mind skills during an acute episode of psychosis and following recovery. Psychol Med. 1998;28:1101-12.

Faris REL, Dunham WW. Mental disorders in urban areas. Chicago, University of Chicago Press, 1939.

Firth J, Cotter J, Torous J, et al. Mobile phone ownership and endorsement of "mhealth" among people with psychosis: a meta-analysis of cross-sectional studies. Schizophr Bull. 2016;42(2): 448-55.

Goldberg EM, Morrison SL. Schizophrenia and social class. Br J Psychiatry. 1963;109(463):785-802.

Harrison G, Glazebrook C, Brewin J, et al. Increased incidence of psychotic disorders in migrants from the Caribbean to the United Kingdom. Psychol Med. 1997;27:799-806.

Jablensky A. Schizophrenia: epidemiology. Curr Opin Psychiatry. 1999;12:19-26.

Jadhav S, Littlewood R, Ryder AG, et al. Stigmatization of severe mental illness in India: Against the simple industrialization hypothesis. Indian J Psychiatry. 2007;49(3):189-94.

Kinderman P, Bentall RP. A new measure of causal locus: the internal, personal and situational attributions questionnaire. Pers Ind Differ. 1996;261-4.

Kirkbride JB, Boydell J, Ploubidis GB, et al. Testing the association between the incidence of schizophrenia and social capital in an urban area. Psychol Med. 2008;38:1083-94.

Kurtz MM, Mueser K. A meta-analysis of controlled research on social skills training for schizophrenia. J Consult Clin Psychol. 2008;76(3):491-504.

Kurtz MM, Richardson CL. Social cognitive training for schizophrenia: A meta-analytic investigation of controlled research. Schizophr Bull. 2012;38(5):1092-104.

Loganathan S, Murthy RS. Prevalence and pattern of mental disability using Indian disability evaluation assessment scale in a rural community of Karnataka. Indian J Psychiatry. 2008;50(1): 21-3.

March D, Hatch SL, Morgan C, et al. Psychosis and Place. Epidemiol Rev. 2008;30(1):84-100.

Marwaha S, Johnson S, Bebbington P, et al. Rates and correlates of employment in people with schizophrenia in the UK, France and Germany. Br J Psychiatry. 2007;191:30-7.

Mehta UM, Thirthalli J, Kumar CN, et al. Validation of Social Cognition Rating Tools in Indian Setting (SOCRATIS): A new test-battery to assess social cognition. Asian J Psychiatry. 2011;4: 203-09.

Miller BJ, Stewart A, Schrimsher J, et al. How connected are people with schizophrenia? Cell phone, computer, email, and social media use. Psychiatry Res. 2015;225(3):458-63.

Penn DL, Roberts DL, Munt E, et al. A pilot study of Social Cognition and Interaction Training (SCIT) for schizophrenia. Schizophr Res. 2005;80(2-3):357-9.

Perner J, Wimmer H. "John thinks that Mary thinks that..." attribution of second order beliefs by 5-10-year-old children. J Exp Child Psychol. 1985;437-71.

Priebe S, Roder-Wanner UU, Kaiser W. Quality of life in first admitted schizophrenia patients: follow-up study. Psychol Med. 2000;30:225-30.

Priebe S. Social outcomes in schizophrenia. Br J Psychiatry. 2007;191(suppl 50):s15-s20.

Rabkin J. Public attitudes toward mental illness: a review of the literature. Schizophr Bull. 1974;10:9-33.

Sariaslan A, Fazel S, D'Onofrio BM, et al. Schizophrenia and subsequent neighbourhood deprivation: revisiting the social drift hypothesis using population, twin and molecular genetic data. Trans Psychiatry. 2016;6(5):e796

Selten JP, Slaets JPJ, Kahn RS. Schizophrenia in Surinamese and Dutch Antillean immigrants to The Netherlands: evidence of an increased incidence. Psychol Med. 1997;27:807-10.

Srinivasan TN, Thara R. Beliefs about causation of schizophrenia: do Indian families believe in supernatural causes? Soc Psychiatry Psychiatr Epidemiol. 2001;36(3):134-40.

Srinivasan TN, Thara R. How do men with schizophrenia fare at work? A follow up study from India. Schizophr Res. 1997;25:149-54.

Stone VE, Baron-Cohen S, Knight RT. Frontal lobe contributions to theory of mind. J Cog Neurosci. 1998;10:640-56.

Thara R, Kamath S, Kumar S. Women with schizophrenia and broken marriages-doubly disadvantaged? Part II: Family perspective. Int J Soc Psychiatry. 2003;49(3):233-40.

Thara R, Srinivasan TN. How stigmatizing is schizophrenia in India?. International Journal of Social Psychiatry. 2000;46(2):135-41.

Thara R, Srinivasan TN. Outcome of marriage in schizophrenia. Soc Psychiatry Psychiatr Epidemiol. 1997;32:416-20.

Wimmer H, Perner J. Beliefs about beliefs: representation and constraining function of wrong beliefs in young children's understanding of deception. Cognition. 1983;13:103-28.

Yang LH, Phillips MR, Li X, et al. Employment outcome for people with schizophrenia in rural v. urban China: population-based study. Br J Psychiatry. 2013;203:272-9.

Chapter 19

Social Dimensions of Depressive and Bipolar Disorders

Uday Chaudhuri, Ranjan Bhattacharyya, Ishan Chaudhuri, Rituparna Biswas

SUMMARY

The current trends in psychiatry show that psychiatrists focus their clinical practice on psychopharmacological treatments as the lynchpin of care. Psychotherapy and psychosocial interventions take the back seat. Effectiveness studies like Systematic Treatment Enhancement Program for Bipolar Disorder (STEP-BD) in bipolar disorders and Sequenced Treatment Alternatives to Relieve Depression (STAR*D) in depression highlight the limitations of a bio-bio model and the need for a biopsychosocial model. The importance of a resilience-based mindset beyond a pathology deficit mindset will aid in bringing back functional recovery in patients suffering from mood disorders. The focus, modus, and goal of treatment should not just be symptomatic recovery, but also the promotion of functional recovery. It is a journey from patienthood to personhood, and toward human excellence.

INTRODUCTION

Every fifth female and every tenth male are affected by depressive disorder at sometime in their lives. It is estimated that by 2020, depression will be the second most common cause of worldwide morbidity across the globe, only after ischemic heart disease, and will contribute to 5.7% of the total disease burden (Lopez et al., 2006) which is why the theme of World Health Day, on 7th April 2017 was kept as "Depression: Let's talk" by the World Health Organization (WHO). Grover and colleagues (2010) estimate one year prevalence of unipolar depressive disorder at 5.8% and 9.5% in males and females respectively.

In a review bipolar disorder, though less common than unipolar depression, is likely to have much higher prevalence at 3–5% than the earlier estimates of 1%, which excluded the bipolar II and other subtypes (Rao, 2010). Disability associated with mood disorders is huge, despite effective treatment being available. Suicide rate is as high as 15% in patients of depression. Bipolar depression accounts for one of the highest suicide rates in any illness especially in young and elderly males. Middle-aged women are another risk group with increasing rates of suicide in whom mood disorders are often associated with psychosocial stressors. Apart from hormonal and physiological differences, a woman's morbidity and mortality depend on traumatic events related to development and lifecycle.

There is a need to address socio-economic factors in the research done on mood disorders. Certain authors have postulated that the incidence of mood disorders may be rising in youth,

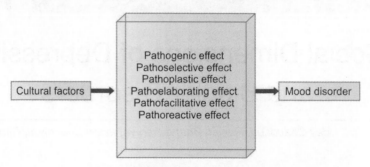

Figure 1: The influences of cultural factors in mood disorder.

due to various psychosocial factors like alcohol and other substances. Cultural factors have also been suggested to play an important role in epidemiology, clinical presentation as well as management of mood disorders. The role of cultural factors in mood disorders is multidirectional, as depicted in **Figure 1**.

EPIDEMIOLOGICAL STUDIES OF MOOD DISORDERS IN INDIAN CONTEXT

In Indian studies, the researchers have focused on various issues including prevalence, impact of life events, comorbidities, demographic and cultural factors, outcome, management, nosology, prevention, diagnosis and therapeutic issues related to mood disorders. Depression is more common in women, single, divorced and widowed, and those who hail from lower socio-economic background with poor nutritional status residing in urban region and in nuclear families, in young adults, and amongst Muslims (Mohandas et al., 2009). Geriatric depression is more common in elderly females in community samples and among elderly males in clinic-based samples, and in those having lower socio-economic status, lower educational attainment, single, widowed, unemployed, or living in nuclear family (Sharma et al., 1985). The depressed individuals suffer from significantly more number of life events (e.g. bereavement, death in the family, personal life events, interpersonal relationship issues) than the patients suffering from schizophrenia in 6–12 months prior to their illness (Prakash et al., 1980). Patients with moderate-to-severe depression use avoidance and maladaptive coping strategies more commonly during stressful situation (Satija et al., 1998). Parental disharmony, marital dispute, foster parents, and single parenthood make the eldest sibling vulnerable for depression in early life in Indian context (Bagadia et al., 1973). The risk factors of childhood and adolescent depression include death in the family, frequent change in school and residence, inability to adjust with new peer group, failure in examination, mental and chronic physical illness in the family (Krishnakumar et al., 2006). Women of child bearing age experience more depression due to use of tobacco, poverty, having leucorrhea, partner violence, relationship problems, having a girl child, and during antenatal and postnatal period (Patel et al., 2006). The patients suffering from depression have specific attribution style, and make more stable and global attributions in comparison to schizophrenia or other mental disorders. The cognitive errors as attributed by Beck have been challenged by the study findings that significant proportions of patients during remission do not show any cognitive distortions but patients, who show significant cognitive distortions are more vulnerable to early relapse (Venkoba Rao et al., 1989). People suffering from neurotic disorders including depression suffer from more unpleasant type of reaction rather than pleasant type of reactions (Srivastava et al., 2006). The higher "hardiness" score in personality trait is inversely correlated with depression (Sinha & Singh, 2009). Some of the salient findings of Indian research are given in the **Table 1**.

A follow-up study by Venkoba Rao and Nammalvar (1977) of 122 cases of depression at an interval of 3–13 years found that 28 subjects had no recurrence. Half of the cases of unipolar depression turned into bipolar (21 out of 42). They also found manic episodes to be more in number as compared to depressive episodes with the number of episodes of depression occurring before mania ranging from 1 to 3. The risk of recurrence was higher if the age of onset of depression was before 40 years, while if the onset of depression was after 40 years, the risk of chronicity was higher.

Table 1: Epidemiological studies of mood disorders in Indian context

Study	Prevalence rate	Methodology
Reddy and Chandrasekhar, 1998	7.9–8.9 per 1000	Meta-analysis of 13 studies with 33, 572 subjects found prevalence in urban areas two times higher than in rural areas
Nandi et al., 2000	1.7–74 per 1000	The study focuses on depression in community samples
Poongothai et al., 2009	15.1% after adjusting for age using the 2001 census data	Screening of 24,000 subjects in Chennai using Patient Health Questionnaire (PHQ)-12. (CURES 70)
Nandi et al., 1997	Depression was the most common illness of old age, the rate being 522/1000. Women had a higher rate of depression-704/1000	The study was carried out in rural Bengal with highest comorbidities in widowhood
Dey et al., 2001	Depression was the most common psychiatric diagnosis among the 1,586 elderly subjects (age ≥60 years)	Patients attending Geriatric Clinic of the AIIMS, New Delhi
Srinath et al., 2005	Prevalence 0.1% in the 4–16 years age group and no child in the age group 0–3 was diagnosed to have depression	Childhood and adolescent clinic in South India.
Chandran et al., 2002	Incidence of postnatal depression is 11%.	Community-based epidemiological data collected from last trimester pregnancy and 6–12 weeks after delivery
Guha and Valdiya, 2000	Major depression (13.4%) the most common diagnosis	Old age home

On comparing dermatoglyphics in groups of unipolar and bipolar depression with normal subjects, significant findings were obtained in bipolar subjects with positive family history (Balgir et al., 1978). Bipolar disorders is a heterogeneous condition and does not follow simple Mendelian inheritance as social factors modify the course and outcome of the illness (Kumar et al., 2001).

Neuropsychological and neurocognitive impairments have been studied in patients with bipolar disorder in remission and maintenance phases by Taj and Padmavathi (2005) and impairments found in attention, memory and executive functions. The social and occupational impairments can be minimized by psychoeducation and cognitive rehabilitation.

Recent literature suggests association of behavioral addictions with mood disorders in children and adolescents. In contrast to Emil Kraepelin's postulated idea that no more than 5% cases of mood disorders in Germany had a chronic course, recent data suggests mood disorders to be more chronic, recurrent, and refractory to treatment. The present scenario has changed nowadays, chronicity is reported to be around 1 in 3 mood disorder patients. Cognitive decline in cases of poorly controlled depression and bipolar disorders pose a diagnostic and therapeutic challenge. The early and effective treatment of mood disorders has been advocated by researchers across the globe in the primary prevention of dementia.

Hundreds of studies have suggested that behavioral, cognitive, cognitive behavioral, psychodynamic, interpersonal, and social rhythm therapies, and psychosocial treatments are effective for mood disorders. A combination of medication and psychosocial intervention is often better than either alone. The brain changes associated with various evidence-based psychotherapies allow therapy responders to be differentiated from non-responders based on brain imaging (Lazar, 2010). Inspite of evidence of effectiveness, current trends in psychiatry show that psychiatrists focus their practice on psychopharmacological treatment as the lynchpin of care. Psychotherapy and psychosocial interventions take the back seat (Perry et al., 2012).

The concept of vulnerability genes and plasticity genes by Belsky and colleagues (2009) offers potentially "paradigm shifting observations". So far we have studied and researched on vulnerability genes for depression and bipolar disorder. We have ignored the plasticity model, a genuine blind spot in psychiatry. A plasticity model with its links to concepts such as resilience, makes room for importance of remote and recent beneficial environments and relationships highlighting the potential values of psychosocial intervention in mood disorders. Having both pathology-deficit and resilience-based mindset will promote functional recovery. The heuristic value of attending to plasticity versus vulnerability in the thinking about mental disorders provides a link to concepts such as resilience.

Environmental factors interact with genes to shape individuals by turning genes on and off (Holmes, 2013). It is more gene and environment (G x E) or epigenetics rather than genes alone. As per Holmes, epigenetics is another way to say "biopsychosocial". Phenotype does not come only from genes, but rather $Phe = GE^2$. Here Holmes mirrors Einstein's transformative equation $E = mc^2$ and thought that energy and mass are different manifestations of the same and even a small amount of mass can produce a huge amount of energy. In his transformative $Phe = GE^2$ equation, Holmes suggests that phenotype is a function not only of genes but also the environment squared (i.e. a function of both early and recent environments).

BEYOND PILLS—PRESCRIPTIONS FOR THE MIND

In case of bipolar disorder, prescription of mood stabilizers and/or second generation antipsychotics (SGAs) is not associated with functional recovery. It just gives rise to symptom removal, that too to some extent. Psychosocial approaches need to be integrated for recovery of function. In the STEP – BD, only 58% of index cases recovered within 6 months and half had recurrences within 2 years (Perlis et al., 2006). Thus there is something more to bipolar disorder than only the need for medication. Similarly, in major depressive disorder, the STAR*D study shows that many patients fail to respond to initial treatment of depression or to switch or augmentation strategies including cognitive and behavioral therapies (CBT) (Thase et al., 2007). Once again the data highlights the limitation of the "bio-bio-model". The need is a holistic combination of biopsychosocial model with integration of psychosocial intervention.

Another issue is importance of personality disorders as a comorbidity in mood disorders. In the Collaborative Longitudinal Personality Disorders Study (CPLS) (Skodol et al., 2005), personality disorders co-occurring with mood disorders carried a bad prognosis for both. It leads to persistent functional impairment, higher rates of suicide, and more treatment utilization. Cluster B personality disorders like borderline personality disorder specifically have been predictive of persistent major depressive disorder. The authors, hence, suggested assessment of personality disorders to be essential in patients having major depressive disorder. The primary treatment in personality disorders remains psychotherapy. Psychopharmacologic treatment integrated with psychotherapy, and additional resilience-based psychosocial assessment and intervention can take the patient from a state of patienthood to personhood and toward human excellence.

Are Pills the Best Treatment?

Contemporary psychiatric medications are undoubtedly effective and powerful treatment agents, but are not a cure. Even when effective, antidepressants may leave patients symptomatic and understandably seeking more treatment. Some authors note that the effect size of psychotherapy is greater than the effect size of medications. There is some evidence that the patients with chronic and comorbid depression, perhaps those with a history of early adversity, respond well to CBT and long-term psychodynamic psychotherapy. Nemeroff and colleagues (2003) concluded that psychotherapy is an essential treatment in patients having persistent major depressive disorder along with childhood history of trauma.

PSYCHOSOCIAL FACTORS IN MOOD DISORDERS

- **Developmental issues:** Parents suffering from mood disorders are often found to be having interpersonal conflicts resulting in separation, divorce, or suicide of either. A child who is born in such an environment, according to epigenetic researchers, is biologically predisposed to develop mood disorder (Jacob, 2015). Object loss during developmental phase may modify the illness expression by causing earlier onset, higher severity, increased likelihood of personality disorders, and suicide attempts. Polymorphism of serotonin transporter has been implicated in mediating early trauma and depression (short allele of serotonin transporter), suicidal attempts, and comorbid anxiety features.

- **Stressful life events:** First episode of mood disorder, rather than subsequent episodes is often preceded by stressful life events. It is hypothesized that stress which accompanies the first episode results in long-standing biological changes in the brain. These changes alter the interneuronal signaling and neurotransmitter system of the brain. It may even lead to neuronal loss or synaptic contact reduction. This leads to occurrence of subsequent mood disorders even in absence of external stressors. Stressful life events may play a primary role in depressive disorder, one of the most important being loss of parent before the age of 11 years. Other important life events having a similar impact include loss of a spouse, and unemployment. It has been seen that unemployed individuals are at three times higher risk for developing depression than employed individuals. Guilt also plays an important role. Recent stressful events are more predictive of an episode. From a psychodynamic perspective, the psychiatrist needs to understand the subjective meaning of the stressor for the patient, as a stressor may hold special idiosyncratic meaning for the bearer which may appear trivial or insignificant to a third person. It has been seen that stressors which reflect negatively on an individual's self-esteem are the most predictive. Patients with certain personality disorders like anankastic, histrionic, and borderline types are more predisposed to develop depression. Patients with dysthymia and cyclothymia are predisposed to develop depressive disorder and bipolar disorder respectively.

PSYCHODYNAMIC FACTORS

Sigmund Freud's theory which was later expanded by Karl Abraham is known as the classic view of depression. It states that depression is a result of disturbance in the infant-mother relationship during the oral phase of psychosexual development. It also links depression to introjection of a lost object (real or imaginary) to deal with the distress. This brings a feeling of love and hatred toward object (which was introjected) leading to inwards turning of anger.

John Bowlby in his elaboration of attachment theory stated that early attachments and traumatic separation during childhood predispose an individual to develop depression. Subsequently, adult losses revive the childhood losses leading to depressive episodes. Melanie Klein's theory states that an expression of aggression toward loved ones turned inwards leads to depression.

Aaron T Beck gave the cognitive theory of depression where he stated that the depression results from certain cognitive distortions labeled as "depressogenic schemata" which predispose vulnerable individuals. These distortions are the way an individual perceives his external as well as internal environment as illustrated in Beck's cognitive triad of depression (negative perception of self, environment, and future). Cognitive behaviour therapy works by correcting these distortions.

Learned helplessness theory of depression—Based on learning theories of classic and operant conditioning, the learned helplessness theory of depression connects depressive phenomenon to the experience of uncontrollable events, e.g. domestic and social traumatic life events leading to depression in women, children, and adolescents (by the stress diathesis model). In context of depression in humans, learned helplessness internally leads to lowered self-esteem after adverse external events. Clinical improvement in depression is evidenced when a person achieves self-control and masters his control over the environment.

Psychodynamic theory for mania—Mania is viewed as defense against underlying depression by many authors. According to Karl Abraham, inability to tolerate developmental tragedy like early loss of a parent predisposes an individual to develop manic episode. According to Melanie Klein, manic defences like omnipotence (evidenced in delusion of grandeur) act as defense against depression.

Psychiatry has become increasingly biologically focused. Today psychiatrists focus their practice mostly on psychopharmacological treatment. The great thinker Leon Eisenberg (1986) has rightly pointed out, "neither brainlessness nor mindlessness, brain – mindfulness" should be the paradigm in psychiatry in the 21st century. To make the point clear, prior to the 1950s, we did not know much about the brain and active psychopharmacologic agents. The entire approach focused on psychoanalysis and psychosocial theory and practices. 1990s was the decade of the brain—the pendulum swung toward psychopharmacological agents. Today psychiatrists focus their practice on psychopharmacological agents and costly brain imaging. Psychiatry now suffers from "mindlessness". The paradigm of psychiatry in the 21st century should echo Leon Eisenberg's concept – "neither brainlessness nor mindlessness, brain – mindfulness". This is a harmonious integration of biological and psychosocial approaches for patient care.

Despite evidence of the effectiveness of psychotherapy and psychosocial treatments, the place of psychosocial intervention in psychiatry is endangered (Laska et al., 2014; Plakun et al., 2009; Weerasekera, 2013). The future of psychotherapy and psychosocial treatments in psychiatry depends on the matters of social policy, law and on whether psychiatry broadens its bio-medical focus to a biopsychosocial model. Should we focus on a reductionistic "bio-bio model" or integrative biopsychosocial model? Mental health care too needs that broader perspective of integration of biological and psychosocial interventions.

In the understanding and management of mood disorders, prescribing psychopharmacological agents (backed by the considerable influence and financial power of the pharmacological industry) should be harmonized and integrated with the psychosocial interventions. This is the lynchpin of patient care in the journey beyond symptomatic recovery and toward functional recovery. The journey from patienthood to personhood and toward human excellence is only possible through the formulation of a care pathway, network therapy, psychoeducation and psychotherapy in mood disorders. This will definitely put a smile on the faces of patients and their families. The whole is more than the sum of its parts.

The WHO definition of health states that health is not merely an absence of disease or infirmity but a harmonious state of physical, mental, and social well-being. Some thinkers also add the dimension of spiritual well-being into the concept of health. We have also been trying to divide psychiatry into biological psychiatry and social psychiatry. Worth mentioning here also is the concept of epigenetics – gene and environment interaction that ultimately leads to a whole (the phenotype). As in the transformative equation of Einstein, $E = mc^2$, energy and mass are different manifestations of the same thing. Similarly, social cognition resides in the brain areas namely temporal lobes, posterior superior temporal sulcus, and medial prefrontal cortex. The paradigm of psychiatric care in the 21st century will be based on the integration of biological and social dimensions into a holistic model. Leon Eisenberg (2000) has rightly pointed out that the paradigm of psychiatric care in the 21st century should be an integration of biological and psychosocial dimensions of care. The concept of "whole" has been beautifully expressed in the opening invocation to the famous *Isa Upanishads*, written in Sanskrit "*purnamadah, purnamidam, purnatpurnamudacyate purnasya, purnamadaya purnamevavasisyate*". This means "that is whole, this is whole, from the whole emerges the whole. The whole is taken from the whole but the whole remains".

Worldwide literature suggests that depression and mood disorders often go undetected (similar to adult onset diabetes mellitus) and are often undertreated. As a result, patient advocacy groups along with national psychiatric organizations and government mental health sector are making efforts to increase public awareness about mood disorders.

Another challenging task would be to provide all physicians in primary care adequate experience in detecting mood disorders. Availability of easy-to-apply and user-friendly tools in general medical sector for detection of suicide may further enhance efforts in preventing it. There is a need to change the structure of health care at primary as well as district level by improving the participation of nursing staff, social workers, and clinical psychologists. This will act as a liaison in primary mental health and may help in continuing the care for depressed and suicidal patients.

Suicide prevention: Suicide is a major complication of mood disorders which underlie 50–70% of all suicides. Hence, treatment of mood disorders will eventually help in reducing the suicide rates. It is necessary that antidepressants, mood stabilizers, and depression-specific psychotherapy are made available adequately. Physician's exposure to mood disorder clinically is suboptimal not only in primary care (general medical training) but in psychiatric care (specialized training) as well. Hence, mood disorders being highly prevalent and a a leading cause of death by suicide by suicide, warrant greater teaching hours in curriculum of both psychiatrists as well as general medical practitioners. Young doctors must be trained at mood disorder clinics as these are chronic relapsing conditions and one is highly likely to witness these in the clinical practice. This should include learning about aspects such as lithium prophylaxis for suicide prevention, use of user—friendly antidepressants and depression and specific psychotherapy. Crisis intervention for suicide as well as training in the management of patients with acute mania should form an integral part of the medical training.

CONCLUSION

Mood disorders including depression and bipolar disorder have a multifactorial etiology and are a major contributor to the global burden of disease. Psychosocial interventions are often ignored in management of mood disorders. The mental health professionals need to follow the biopsychosocial model of etiology in the management of mood disorders and should not ignore psychosocial interventions while treating patients with mood disorders.

REFERENCES

Balgir RS, Ghosh A, Murthy RS, et al. Dermatoglyphics in manic-depressive psychosis. Indian J Psychiatry. 1978;21:384-9.

Bagadia VN, Jeste DV, Dave KP, et al. Depression: Family and psychodynamic study of 233 cases. Indian J Psychiatry. 1973;15:217-23.

Belsky J, Jonassaint C, Pluess M, et al. Vulnerability genes or plasticity genes? Mol Psychiatry. 2009;14(8):746-54.

Chandran M, Tharyan P, Muliyil J, et al. Post-partum depression in a cohort of women from a rural area of Tamil Nadu, India Incidence and risk factors. Br J Psychiatry. 2002;181:499-504.

Dey AB, Soneja S, Nagarkar KM, et al. Evaluation of the health and functional status of older Indians as a prelude to the development of a health programme. Natl Med J India. 2001;14(3):135-8.

Eisenberg L. Mindlessness and brainfullness in psychiatry. Br J Psychiatry. 1986;148:497-508.

Eisenberg L. Is psychiatry more mindful and brains than it was a decade ago? Br J Psychiatry. 2000;176(1):1-5.

Grover S, Dutt A, Avasthi A. An overview of Indian research in depression. Indian J Psychiatry. 2010;52(S1):S178-88.

Guha S, Valdiya PS. Psychiatric morbidity amongst the inmates of old age home. Indian J Psychiatry. 2000;42:S44.

Holmes J. An attachment model of depression: integrating findings from the mood disorder laboratory. Psychiatry. 2013;76(1):68-86.

Jacobs RH, Orr JL, Gowins JR, et al. Biomarkers for Intergenerational risk for depression: a review of mechanisms in longitudinal high-risk studies. J Affect Disord. 2015;175:494-506.

Kraepelin E. 100 years of psychiatry. Vertex. 2010;21(91):317-20.

Krishnakumar P, Geeta MG. Clinical profile of depressive disorder in children. Indian Pediatr. 2006;43(6):521-6.

Kumar R, Sinha BN, Chakrabarti N, et al. Phenomenology of mania – A factor analysis approach. Indian J Psychiatry. 2001;43(1):46-51.

Laska KM, Gurman AS, Wampold BE. Expanding the lens of evidence-based practice in psychotherapy: a common factors perspective. Psychother. 2014;51(4):467-81.

Lazar SG. Psychotherapy is Worth It: A Comprehensive Review of its Cost-effectiveness. Washington DC: American Psychiatric Publishing, 2010.

Lopez AD, Mathers CD, Ezzati M, et al. Global Burden of Disease and Risk Factors. Washington: The World Bank; 2006.

Mohandas E. Roadmap to Indian psychiatry. Indian J Psychiatry. 2009;51:173-9.

Nandi DN, Banerjee G, Mukherjee SP, et al. Psychiatric morbidity of a rural Indian community changes over a 20 year interval. Br J Psychiatry. 2000;176:351-6.

Nandi PS, Banerjee G, Mukherjee SP, et al. A study of psychiatric morbidity of the elderly population of a rural community in West Bengal. Indian J Psychiatry. 1997;39(2):122-9.

Nemeroff CB, Heim CM, Thase ME, et al. Differential response to psychotherapy versus pharmacotherapy in patients with chronic forms of major depression and childhood trauma. Proc Natl Acad Sci USA. 2003;100(24):14293-6.

Patel V, Kirkwood BR, Pednekar S, et al. Risk factors for common mental disorders in women Population-based longitudinal study. Br J Psychiatry. 2006;189:547-55.

Perlis RH, Ostacher MJ, Patel JK, et al. Predictors of recurrence in bipolar disorder: primary outcomes from the Systematic Treatment Enhancement Program for Bipolar Disorder (STEP-BD). Am J Psychiatry. 2006;163(2):217-24.

Perry JC, West J, Plakun EM. Why psychiatrists don't do therapy even though it works. Workshop presentation at APA Institute on Psychiatric Services. New York, October 7, 2012.

Plakun EM, Sudak DM, Goldberg D. The Y model: an integrated, evidence-based approach to teaching psychotherapy competencies. J Psychiatr Pract. 2009;15(1):5-11.

Poongothai S, Pradeepa R, Ganesan A, et al. Prevalence of depression in a large urban South Indian population - The Chennai Urban Rural Epidemiology Study (CURES-70). PLoS One. 2009;4(9):E7185.

Prakash R, Trivedi JK, Sethi BB. Life events in depression. Indian J Psychiatry. 1980;22(1):56-60.

Rao GP. An overview of Indian research in bipolar mood disorder. Indian J Psychiatry. 2010;52(suppl 1): S173-7.

Reddy MV, Chandrashekhar CR. Prevalence of mental and behavioural disorders in India: A metaanalysis. Indian J Psychiatry. 1998;40(2):149-57.

Satija YK, Advani GB, Nathawat SS. Influence of stressful life events and coping strategies in depression. Indian J Psychiatry. 1998;40(2):165-71.

Sharma DK, Satija DC, Nathawat SS. Psychological determinants of depression in old age. Indian J Psychiatry. 1985;27(1):83-90.

Sinha V, Singh RN. Immunological Role of Hardiness on Depression. Indian J Psychol Med. 2009;31(1): 39-44.

Skodol AE, Gunderson JG, Shea MT, et al. The Collaborative Longitudinal Personality Disorders Study (CLPS): overview and implications. Acta Psychiatr Scand. 2005;112(3):208-14.

Srinath S, Girimaji SC, Gururaj G, et al. Epidemiological study of child and adolescent psychiatric disorders in urban and rural areas of Bangalore, India. Indian J Med Res. 2005;122(1):67-9.

Srivastava S. Deficiencies in social relationships of individuals with neurosis. Indian J Psychiatry. 2006; 48(3):154-8.

Taj M, Padmavati R. Neuropsychological impairment in bipolar affective disorder. Indian J Psychiatry. 2005;47:48-50.

Thase ME, Friedman ES, Biggs MM, et al. Cognitive therapy versus medication in augmentation and switch strategies as second-step treatments: a STAR*D report. Am J Psychiatry. 2007;164(5):739-52.

Venkoba Rao A, Nammalvar N. The course and outcome in depressive illness. A follow-up study of 122 cases in Madurai, India. Br J Psychiatry. 1977;130:392-6.

Venkoba Rao A, Reddy TK, Prabakar ER, et al. Cognitive disorder and Depression (An Analysis of the Causal Relationship and Susceptibility to Relapses). Indian J Psychiatry. 1989;31(3):201-7.

Weerasekera P. Psychotherapy Training e-Resources (PTeR): on-line psychotherapy education. Acad Psychiatry. 2013;37(1):51-4.

Chapter 20

Anxiety Disorders

Ramandeep Pattanayak, Saurabh Kumar

SUMMARY

Anxiety is an anticipatory and adaptive response of an individual in response to a challenging or stressful situation in the external environment. Pathological anxiety is excessive, disproportionate to the situation and is associated with distress and disability. Anxiety disorders have a complex multifactorial etiology with evidence for biological underpinnings which often interact with psychological and social risk factors during the genesis and progression. Anxiety disorders assume a social and public health significance in view of their chronic course and tendency to cause substantial socioeconomic burden. Even though effective treatment strategies exist, only a fraction of individuals receive any form of help resulting in a huge treatment gap especially in the developing countries. Anxiety disorders also need to be understood from a cross-cultural perspective. Anxiety symptoms are often expressed and experienced within socio-cultural contexts. Understanding that context can help in managing the cultural diversity in clinical presentation and symptom expression.

INTRODUCTION

Anxiety is an anticipatory and adaptive response of an individual in response to a challenging or stressful situation in the external environment. It is considered to be a normal human emotion and a necessary cue for adaptation and coping. Anxiety qualifies to be a disorder when it arises in the absence of any stressful situation or is out of proportion to the situation, thereby causing significant distress and impairment (Trivedi & Gupta, 2010). Anxiety is manifested in physical, affective, cognitive, and behavioral domains. Pathologic anxiety symptoms may be inaccurately attributed to other physical causes leading to unnecessary investigations, or may be prematurely dismissed as insignificant or normal response.

Anxiety disorders are important from a social and public health perspective due to their high prevalence, chronic course, and tendency to cause substantial disability, poor quality of life (QoL) and tremendous costs to the society (Mendlowicz & Stein, 2000). Even though effective treatment strategies exist, only a fraction of individuals with anxiety disorders are able to receive any form of help resulting in a huge "treatment gap", which is even more marked in the developing countries (Kohn et al., 2004).

This chapter attempts to provide an evidence based review of epidemiological, social, cultural, and public health dimensions of anxiety disorders specifically focusing on the developing countries. The chapter does not venture into core clinical or treatment aspects in keeping with the scope of this section.

CONCEPT AND BACKGROUND

Historical Context

Older medical texts (including Burton's The Anatomy of Melancholy) carry references to anxiety like states, though the term anxiety was not used till much later (Berrios & Link, 1995). Initial attention was directed only to the manifest or "objective" symptoms of anxiety which were considered as separate disease conditions (e.g. difficulty breathing as related to pulmonary abnormality, dizziness as vertigo, etc). Possible connection between manifestations of body and mind began to be described only later on. Anxiety was initially subsumed as a part of melancholia descriptions. Over the 19th century, there was a wider recognition of anxiety, and various forms of anxiety disorders began to be unified. This position was further consolidated in the 20th century with anxiety seen as the "common thread" for a group of conditions, such as panic disorder, agoraphobia, and social anxiety (Stone, 2009; Berrios & Link, 1995).

Fear versus Anxiety

From an evolutionary viewpoint, the emotion of fear appears to be hard-wired into organisms and is designed to avoid danger. Typically, fear is directed at a concrete, external, overtly dangerous stimulus and is an acute immediate reaction to such a threat. Unlike fear, anxiety persists over a period of time even when the threat is spatially or temporally remote (Merikangas et al., 2017). The term anxiety tends to be reserved for reactions to a perceived threat or impending danger that are excessive or exaggerated reactions.

Explanatory Models and Causal Attributions

Anxiety disorders often have a complex multifactorial etiology with evidence for biological underpinnings which interact with psychological and social factors during the genesis and/ or progression. Principal explanatory models for anxiety have ranged from predominantly biological (with emphasis on constitutional vulnerability) to cognitive-behavioral (with emphasis on self-perpetuating patterns of cognitions and behaviors) and psychodynamic (with emphasis on meanings and internal representations). From a pragmatic standpoint, a clinician may follow more than one model to suit the patient needs and some models may not be mutually exclusive. For example, in some individuals, the dysregulated (anxiety-prone) networks may remain homeostatic until major life events or stressors disturb them. An integrated model has been proposed, wherein the risk prediction for manifest anxiety disorders can be construed as a consequence of biological vulnerability, developmental risk/ protective factors, and internal psychological and extraneous factors (Stein & Williams, 2009).

Among the causal attributions, considerable cross-cultural variation is seen among patients. In the Asian and African cultures, the mental health problems may be related to the supernatural forces, angry spirits of forefathers or black magic. Attempts to argue with patients holding these culturally-derived beliefs is often a futile exercise and may lead to more harm than benefit to the therapeutic relationship especially when it is still being built. Patients often hold multiple, simultaneous causative explanations and may continue to seek treatment from mental health care settings in addition to various faith healers.

Current Nosology

The classification and boundaries of anxiety disorders has been the subject of several controversies. There are several debates pertaining to the boundaries of anxiety disorders with mood disorders (Merikangas et al., 2017). Other issues are an unusually high prevalence of symptomatic yet clinically subthreshold anxiety states and culturally linked somatic presentations of anxiety disorders in low and middle income countries.

The DSM-5 categorizes various anxiety disorders as panic disorder (with or without agoraphobia), agoraphobia (without a history of panic disorder), specific phobia, social phobia, and generalized anxiety disorder (GAD). It has excluded obsessive-compulsive disorder and posttraumatic disorder from the category of anxiety disorders, and also delinked agoraphobia from panic disorder. These changes now concur better with the ICD-10 classification of anxiety disorders. Other modifications in DSM-5 were a lifespan perspective by inclusion of separation anxiety disorder and selective mutism, and assigning a specifier of panic attacks for a wide range of diagnoses (Kupfer, 2015).

The ICD-10 classified anxiety disorders along with other stress and neurotic disorders, however, the ICD-11 draft attempts to bring all disorders with anxiety or fear as a central theme in a new grouping of anxiety and fear-related disorders. A key differentiating feature is disorder-specific focus of apprehension, i.e. triggering stimuli. GAD has been elaborated further so that it is no longer a diagnosis of exclusion. In addition, more flexibility has been provided for cultural variation and clinical judgment for diagnosis of anxiety disorders (Kogan et al., 2016).

PREVALENCE AND RISK FACTORS OF ANXIETY DISORDERS: GLOBAL AND INDIAN PERSPECTIVE

Anxiety disorders are recognized as highly prevalent disorders across countries (Üstün & Sartorius, 1995). The World Health Organization (WHO) in its global estimates reported that 3.6% of the world population suffers from anxiety disorders over a year which translates to an estimated 264 million people living with these disorders during the year 2015 alone (World Health Organization, 2017).

A systematic review of the international studies (1980–2004, 41 prevalence studies and 5 incidence studies) estimated pooled lifetime and current year prevalence at 16.6% and 10.6% respectively for any anxiety disorder (Somers, 2006). More recently, a systematic review of 48 reviews (Remes et al., 2016) reported a high prevalence (3.8–25%), particularly among women, youth and individuals from Euro/Anglo cultures compared to Eastern cultures (Remes et al., 2016).

The World Mental Health Surveys (WMHS), the largest cross-national community epidemiological surveys conducted in more than 25 countries with over 130,000 sample, reported that any anxiety disorder affects 2.4–18.2% in past 1 year across nations. Lifetime prevalence varied widely from 4.8% in China to 31% in USA (Kessler et al., 2005; Kessler et al., 2009).

Some key observations from cross-national WMHS findings (Kessler et al., 2005; Kessler et al., 2007; Kessler et al., 2009) were:

- Lifetime and 12 months prevalence in the Asian (e.g. China, India) and African (e.g. Nigeria) regions was on lower side (probably figures are reflective of survey not being able to capture the culturally linked differences rather than truly vast differences in prevalence)
- Certain anxiety disorders are more prevalent (e.g. specific phobia and social anxiety) than others (e.g. agoraphobia) globally. Lifetime prevalence in order of frequency is as follows: specific phobia: 7.7–12.5%; social phobia: 2.5–12.1%; GAD: 2.8–5.7%; panic disorder: 2.1–4.7% and agoraphobia: 1–1.4%, as per WMHS data from western countries (Michael et al., 2007)
- Anxiety disorders have a relatively early age of onset with phobia and separation anxiety having median age of onset between 7–14 years, while it is later for GAD and panic disorder (24–50 years) with a relatively wide variation across countries
- Anxiety disorders do co-occur with one another as well as with other psychiatric disorders
- Treatment seeking usually does not occur until at least a decade after onset, even in well-resourced countries
- WMHS data convincingly demonstrated that separation anxiety is found in adults in addition to children, and is prevalent around the globe. Around one-third of childhood-onset cases persist into adulthood, whereas the majority of adult respondents report adult onset of symptoms. These data provided evidence base to include separation anxiety disorder as a new entity in the DSM-5.

Several local and regional epidemiological studies are available from India which were reviewed by Reddy and Chandrashekhar (1998), and Ganguli (2000). However, there were several methodological heterogeneities in individual studies and relatively smaller sample sizes. No large scale study was available in India till WMH Indian epidemiological survey was conducted in year 2005. In the recently published findings from that survey (with nearly 25,000 adult household sample assessed using WHO-CIDI instrument), the past year prevalence of anxiety disorders was 3.4% (Sagar et al., 2017). A variety of factors like under reporting, cultural variations in presentation, threshold of detection, etc probably contributed to the lower prevalence rates in India and other developing countries (Baxter et al., 2013). While it is possible that the prevalence rates may be different across cultures, many experts agree that a limited validity and sensitivity of survey instruments and cultural differences in symptom expressions result in a lack of measurement equivalence. These findings allude to the fact that one should be cautious while comparing prevalence data across countries.

The female preponderance for anxiety disorders (1.5-2:1) is a well-established finding in epidemiological studies across all the countries (Comer & Olfson, 2010; WHO, 2017). Several factors including biological and psychosocial factors, e.g. low education, recent intimate partner violence, spousal substance use, etc. have been associated with poorer outcome among women (McLean et al., 2011). In addition to gender, additional risk factors include being widowed, separated or divorced, being unemployed, having a low education, living in an urban area, poverty, and presence of lifetime/recent negative life events (Comer & Olfson, 2010; Stone, 2009; Trivedi & Gupta, 2010). These findings indicate that the different societal and cultural factors play an important role in the manifestation of anxiety disorders.

Several long-term prospective community studies are now available that have followed community samples for more than a decade (Zurich Cohort Study for 19–20 years old, Early

Development Stages of Psychopathology Study for 14–24 years old and the Great Smoky Mountain Study for 9–26 years old). These three longitudinal cohort studies (Copeland et al., 2014; Angst et al., 2015; Beesdo-Baum et al., 2015) add information on an overall prevalence of 30% for anxiety disorders which confirms the same rates from cross sectional studies. All these studies showed that there is a substantial fluctuation across subtypes of anxiety disorders, and across diagnostic thresholds overtime. In general, phobic disorders are far more stable than panic disorder and GAD, that tend to resemble mood disorders in their waxing and waning across the lifespan.

ECONOMIC AND HUMAN BURDEN

Anxiety disorders pose a significant burden on individuals, families, and communities. The impaired role functioning and QoL as a result of disorder contributes to the disability and disease burden.

Measurement of disability and disease burden associated with anxiety disorders is of extreme importance for public health policies (Whiteford et al., 2010). Anxiety disorders accounted for 10.4% proportion of the disability (as measured by DALYs) associated with mental, substance use and neurological disorders in the Global Burden of Disease (GBD) study of 2010. Anxiety disorders figure in the top ten contributors to non-fatal health loss and disability (as measured by YLD-Years of life lived with disability). The highest burden was seen in the age group 15–34 years which is the most productive time in an individuals' lifespan (Baxtor et al., 2014, Whiteford et al., 2010).

Economic burden of any disorder is usually calculated measuring both the direct and indirect cost (includes lost productivity, excessive absenteeism, or reduced work capacity) (Tolin et al., 2009). In a study by Greenberg et al., (1999), anxiety disorders accounted for nearly one-third of economic burden due to mental illnesses. These and several other recent study estimates suggest that anxiety disorders impose a huge financial burden on the society (Stuhldreher et al., 2014).

A review by Hoffman et al. (2008) pointed to high economic costs because of both low work productivity and high use of medical resources. Studies typically show that human burden in GAD is comparable to depressive disorders (Hoffman et al., 2008; Bereza et al., 2009).

Individuals with anxiety disorders have been shown to have impaired QoL across almost all domains (Tolin et al., 2009). Several studies have also shown that familial burden posed by anxiety disorders viz. agoraphobbia and panic disorder is similar to that seen with severe mental illnesses (Borgo et al., 2017). However, it should be noted that most of the earlier family burden research was restricted to obsessive-compulsive disorder (which is no longer considered under anxiety disorders), and comparatively less research is available for anxiety disorders such as panic disorder or GAD. The chronic distressing and disabling anxiety symptoms tends to have negative effect on familial relationships and lead to increased caregiver burden.

CROSS CULTURAL PERSPECTIVES ON ANXIETY DISORDERS

Emerging evidence shows that the anxiety disorders have certain universal biological mechanisms, though these disorders are often expressed and experienced within sociocultural contexts. Understanding that context can help in managing the cultural diversity in clinical presentation and symptom expression (Stein et al., 2009). The "idioms of distress" may also differ across cultures (Nichter, 1981; Hoffman & Hinton, 2014).

Attempts to understand the intersection between anxiety disorders and culture should take the ethnopsychology/ethnophysiology as well as contextual factors and cultural variations in symptoms into account (Hoffman & Hinton, 2014).

Ethnopsychological Interpretations

These factors are the meanings or beliefs that any cultural group attributes to bodily systems or psychiatric symptoms and signs (Hoffman & Hinton, 2014). For example, traditional Chinese medicine believes that anxiety states results from a "weak" kidney (*shen xu*) or heart (*xin xu*). Cultural beliefs in Cambodia attribute panic attacks (which occur upon rising from lying to standing) to a condition called "wind overload" (*khyal ko*). The underlying belief is that standing results in an increase in the wind and blood flow upwards in the body of predisposed individuals resulting in a panic attack. In Africa, anxiety was associated with fear of bewitchment and poisoning or as a result of breaking any rituals. The somatic symptoms of anxiety are also interpreted differently in different cultures. In Nigeria, the somatic symptoms of anxiety are believed to be due to an insect crawling through the head or other body parts.

The level of tolerance to the symptoms in a given culture can also result in delay in treatment seeking. Illness causation beliefs also mediate the treatment seeking efforts and may impact prognosis of these disorders.

Contextual Factors

Contextual factors refer to the prevailing social norms or context in which the behavior is expressed. Individualism and collectivism is a widely used paradigm to understand cultural differences across different societies. In a collectivist society, preference is given to interdependence and group goals. Behavior of an individual is guided by group norms rather than personal attitudes, and is focused on maintaining relationships with others and avoiding conflicts. Caldwell-Harris and Ayçiçegi (2006) tried to analyze the relationship between psychopathology across individualism-collectivism societies, and found that having a personality which conflicts with societal norms is associated with mental disorders including anxiety disorders.

Various sociocultural factors can modulate the different facets of anxiety disorder. Therefore, it is pertinent for clinicians to be aware of these factors while treating patients with anxiety disorders.

Phenomenology: Variations in Symptom Expression

Individuals suffering from anxiety disorders from the Asian countries have a somatic preponderance of symptoms. In Indian studies too, a similar pattern is observed. Srinivasan and Neerakal (2002) found that Indian patients with panic disorder reported fewer cognitive symptoms such as fear of loss of control and depersonalization, than patients in the western countries. A WHO collaborative study of primary healthcare settings across 14 countries found that musculoskeletal pain and fatigue were the most common somatic presentations for both anxiety and depression (Simon et al., 1996).

Some variations have been reported in the phenomenology of anxiety disorders between Eastern and Western settings (Stein & Williams, 2009; Hoffman & Hinton, 2014; Khambaty & Parikh, 2017). In Asian cultures, shame and anxiety have been closely linked. Studies have found that shame has a more important effect on social anxiety in the Asian individuals. Taijin kyofusho which is commonly seen in Japan, is characterized by fear of offending or embarrassing others rather than fear of embarrassing themselves. This may reflect important cultural differences.

Culture also influences the severity and content of phobias. In general, girls experience more fear than boys. In Western cultures, fears about burglars and getting lost are reported, whereas in Asian cultures, themes of fear relate to animals, ghosts, deep waters, dark, imaginary things, and supernatural things (Marques et al., 2011).

Cultural concepts of distress may cover anxiety symptoms, for example, dhat syndrome is culture-specific to the Indian subcontinent and is seen to be associated with hypochondriacal anxiety. Though it is not a classic anxiety disorder, substantial number of patients do present with anxiety symptoms or comorbid anxiety disorder. The local and regional culture specific factors across various parts of India do exercise influence on the manner of clinical presentation and treatment of anxiety disorders.

PUBLIC HEALTH ASPECTS: CLOSING THE TREATMENT GAP

Majority of patients with anxiety disorder fail to receive any treatment. The treatment gap for anxiety disorders is much higher in the low and middle income countries estimated at nearly 95% in India, where only about 5% patients sought any treatment in past 12 months. The treatment seeking varied from 1.66% for specific phobia to 11.55% for panic disorder (Sagar et al., 2017)

The delay in treatment seeking appears to be a norm for anxiety disorders ranging from 3 years to 3 decades (Wang et al., 2007). Lack of awareness and accessibility to services are major barriers in the treatment seeking. Patients with anxiety disorders usually visit other health care professionals before coming in contact with mental health professionals. Studies have found that there is a low detection rate of anxiety disorders amongst the general physicians (Collins et al., 2004) which could be improved through physician training.

Although the research on stigma has majorly focused on severe mental illnesses, a recent review found that stigma (specifically internalized stigma) lowers the self-esteem and self-efficacy of the patients with anxiety disorders and results in hopelessness toward recovery (Ociskova et al., 2013). Management of patients with anxiety disorders should include interventions to reduce stigma and educational interventions, promoting awareness about the disorder and its treatment aspects. Improving public awareness through various education campaigns through participation of various stakeholders can help in early identification of the problem and may lead to increase in help-seeking behavior. For example, there has been a recent focus on depression with several key themes and campaigns devoted to depression awareness throughout the year 2017. Similarly, one of the proposed strategies involves organizing national screening days for anxiety disorders (Collins et al., 2004).

No healthcare system can deliver without suitably trained human resources. In India, the number of psychiatrists, psychologists, nurses, and social workers are abysmally low compared to the West (World Health Organization, 2011). Multisectoral collaborations are required to deal with the social factors which may modify the course of anxiety disorders. Giving more work and responsibilities to the lay trained workers based in the community after their optimum orientation and training is one of the strategies to enhance the workforce (Beaglehole et al., 2008).

For depression and anxiety disorders, the net value of investments and expected returns was calculated for the period from 2016-2030 (Chisholm et al., 2016). The resulting benefit to cost ratio was 2–3 more when economic benefits only were considered and increased further to 3–7 times when health benefits were also included. The returns are likely to be higher than the investments making a case for investment in mental health.

PREVENTION OF ANXIETY DISORDERS

The conceptual models of prevention for anxiety disorders can be based on similar broad principles of prevention that are used in non-communicable disorders. There is a need to conceptualize the prevention of anxiety disorders by linking it with positive mental health promotion as well as the overall health promotion with a developmental and lifespan perspective. The thrust of prevention activities for common mental disorders may be placed on information and awareness campaigns, workplace prevention, and multisectoral collaborations with cultural relevance, and use of smart technological tools for cost-effective solutions for a wider reach (Pattanayak, 2017). The effect sizes are, however, rather small (Ahlen et al., 2015) and further research is needed.

CONCLUSION

Anxiety disorders are prevalent across different countries, though the prevalence rates have shown wide variations in cross-national epidemiological research. Anxiety disorders have a chronic course, low treatment seeking and are responsible for a substantial disability, and socioeconomic burden. Recent revisions in classificatory systems have shown some flexibility for cultural variations in anxiety disorders. Anxiety symptoms are often expressed and experienced within socio-cultural contexts. Understanding those contexts can help in managing the cultural diversity in clinical presentations. For a comprehensive viewpoint, there is a need to conceptualize and understand the clinical, social, economic, public health, and cultural dimensions of anxiety disorders which can help us to effectively deal with the problem.

REFERENCES

Ahlen J, Lenhard F, Ghaderi A. Universal prevention for anxiety and depressive symptoms in children: a meta-analysis of randomized and cluster-randomized trials. J Prim Prev. 2015;36(6):387-403.

Angst J, Paksarian D, Cui L, et al. The epidemiology of common mental disorders from age 20 to 50: results from the prospective Zurich cohort study. Epidemiol Psychiatr Sci. 2015;24:1-9.

Baxter AJ, Scott KM, Vos T, et al. Global prevalence of anxiety disorders: a systematic review and meta-regression. Psychol Med. 2013;43(5):897-910.

Baxter AJ, Vos T, Scott KM, et al. The global burden of anxiety disorders in 2010. Psychol Med. 2014;44(11):2363-74.

Beaglehole R, Epping-Jordan J, Patel V, et al. Improving the prevention and management of chronic disease in low-income and middle-income countries: a priority for primary health care. Lancet. 2008;372(9642):940-9.

Beesdo-Baum K, Knappe S, Asselmann E, et al. The early developmental stages of psychopathology (EDSP) study: a 20-year review of methods and findings. Soc Psychiatry Psychiatr Epidemiol. 2015;50(6):851-66.

Bereza BG, Machado M, Einarson TR. Systematic review and quality assessment of economic evaluations and quality-of-life studies related to generalized anxiety disorder. Clin Ther. 2009;31(6):1279-308.

Berrios G, Link C. Anxiety disorders in A History of Clinical Psychiatry. Edited by Berrios G, Porter R. New York, New York University Press; 1995. Pp. 545-62.

Borgo EL, Ramos-Cerqueira AT, Torres AR. Burden and distress in caregivers of patients with panic disorder and agoraphobia. J Nerv Ment Dis. 2017;205(1):23-30.

Caldwell-Harris CL, Ayçiçegi A. When personality and culture clash: The psychological distress of allocentrics in an individualist culture and idiocentrics in a collectivist culture. Transcult Psychiatry. 2006;43(3):331-61.

Chisholm D, Sweeny K, Sheehan P, et al. Scaling-up treatment of depression and anxiety: a global return on investment analysis. Lancet Psychiatry. 2016; 3(5):415-24.

Collins KA, Westra HA, Dozois DJ, et al. Gaps in accessing treatment for anxiety and depression: challenges for the delivery of care. Clin psychol Rev. 2004;24(5):583-616.

Comer JS, Olfson M. The epidemiology of anxiety disorders. In: Simpson HB, Neria Y, Lewis-Fernández R, Schneier F (Eds). Anxiety disorders: Theory, research and clinical perspectives. London: Cambridge University Press; 2010. pp. 6-19.

Copeland WE, Angold A, Shanahan L, et al. Longitudinal patterns of anxiety from childhood to adulthood: the Great Smoky Mountains Study. J Am Acad Child Adolesc Psychiatry. 2014;53(1):21-33.

Ganguli HC. Epidemiological findings on prevalence of mental disorders in India. Indian J Psychiatry. 2000;42(1):14.

Greenberg PE, Sisitsky T, Kessler RC, et al. The economic burden of anxiety disorders in the 1990s. J Clin Psychiatry. 1999;60(7):427-35.

Hoffman DL, Dukes EM, Wittchen HU. Human and economic burden of generalized anxiety disorder. Depress Anxiety. 2008;25(1):72-90.

Hofmann SG, Hinton DE. Cross-cultural aspects of anxiety disorders. Curr Psychiatry Rep. 2014;16(6):450.

Kessler RC, Aguilar-Gaxiola S, Alonso J, et al. The global burden of mental disorders: An update from the WHO World Mental Health (WMH) Surveys. Epidemiol Psichiatr Soc. 2009;18(1):23-33.

Kessler RC, Angermeyer M, Anthony JC, et al. Lifetime prevalence and age-of-onset distributions of mental disorders in the World Health Organization's World Mental Health Survey Initiative. World Psychiatry. 2007;6(3):168-76.

Kessler RC, Chiu WT, Demler O, et al. Prevalence, severity, and comorbidity of 12-month DSM-IV disorders in the National Comorbidity Survey Replication. Arch Gen Psychiatry. 2005;62(6):617-27.

Khambaty M, Parikh RM. Cultural aspects of anxiety disorders in India. Dialogues Clin Neurosci. 2017;19(2):117-26.

Kogan CS, Stein DJ, Maj M, et al. The classification of anxiety and fear-related disorders in the ICD-11. Depress Anxiety. 2016;33(12):1141-54.

Kohn R, Saxena S, Levav I, et al. The treatment gap in mental health care. Bull World health Organ. 2004;82(11):858-66.

Kupfer DJ. Anxiety and DSM-5. Dialogues Clin Neurosci. 2015;17(3):245-6.

Marques L, Robinaugh DJ, LeBlanc NJ, et al. Cross-cultural variations in the prevalence and presentation of anxiety disorders. Expert Rev Neurother. 2011;11(2):313-22.

McLean CP, Asnaani A, Litz BT, et al. Gender differences in anxiety disorders: prevalence, course of illness, comorbidity and burden of illness. J Psychiatr Res. 2011;45(8):1027-35.

Mendlowicz MV, Stein MB. Quality of life in individuals with anxiety disorders. Am J Psychiatry. 2000;157(5):669-82.

Merikangas KR. Anxiety disorders: Introduction and overview. In: Sadock BJ, Sadock VA, Ruiz P (Eds). Kaplan and Sadock's Comprehensive Textbook of Psychiatry, 10th edition. Philadelphia: Wolters Kluwers publishers; 2017. Pp. 4407-14.

Michael T, Zetsche U, Margraf J. Epidemiology of anxiety disorders. Psychiatry. 2007; 6: 136-42.

Nichter M. Idioms of distress: Alternatives in the expression of psychosocial distress: A case study from South India. Cult Med Psychiatry. 1981;5(4):379-408.

Ociskova M, Prasko J, Sedlackova Z. Stigma and self-stigma in patients with anxiety disorders. Activitas Nervosa Superior Rediviva. 2013;55(1-2):12-8.

Pattanayak RD. Prevention for common mental disorders in low resource settings. Indian J Soc Psychiatry. 2017;33(2):91-4.

Reddy VM, Chandrashekar CR. Prevalence of mental and behavioural disorders in India: A meta-analysis. Indian J Psychiatry. 1998;40(2):149-57.

Remes O, Brayne C, van der Linde R, et al. A systematic review of reviews on the prevalence of anxiety disorders in adult populations. Brain Behav. 2016;6(7):e00497.

Sagar R, Pattanayak RD, Chandrasekaran R, et al. Twelve-month prevalence and treatment gap for common mental disorders: Findings from a large-scale epidemiological survey in India. Indian J Psychiatry. 2017;59(1):46-55.

Simon G, Gater R, Kisely S, et al. Somatic symptoms of distress: an international primary care study. Psychosom Med. 1996;58(5):481-8.

Somers JM, Goldner EM, Waraich P, et al. Prevalence and incidence studies of anxiety disorders: a systematic review of the literature. Can J Psychiatry. 2006;51(2):100-13.

Srinivasan K, Neerakal I. A study of panic patients with and without depression. Indian J Psychiatry. 2002;44(3):246-2.

Stein DJ, Williams D. Cultural and Social Aspects of Anxiety Disorders. In: Stein DJ, Hollander E, Rothbaum BO (Eds). Textbook of Anxiety Disorders. Washington DC: American Psychiatric Publishers; 2009. Pp. 742-55.

Stone MH. History of Anxiety Disorders. In: Stein DJ, Hollander E, Rothbaum BO (Eds). Textbook of Anxiety Disorders. Washington DC: American Psychiatric Publishers; 2009. Pp. 3-15.

Stuhldreher N, Leibing E, Leichsenring F, et al. The costs of social anxiety disorder: the role of symptom severity and comorbidities. J Affect Disord. 2014;165:87-94.

Tolin FD, Gilliam CM, Dufrense D. The Economic and Social Burden of Anxiety Disorders. In: Stein DJ, Hollander E, Rothbaum BO (Eds). Textbook of Anxiety Disorders. Washington DC: American Psychiatric Publishers; 2009. pp. 756-71.

Trivedi JK, Gupta PK. An overview of Indian research in anxiety disorders. Indian J Psychiatry. 2010;52(S1):S210-8.

Üstün TB, Sartorius N. Mental illness in general health care: an international study. New Jersey, John Wiley and Sons, 1995.

Wang PS, Angermeyer M, Borges G, et al. Delay and failure in treatment seeking after first onset of mental disorders in the World Health Organization's World Mental Health Survey Initiative. World Psychiatry. 2007;6(3):177-85.

Whiteford HA, Ferrari AJ, Degenhardt L, et al. The global burden of mental, neurological and substance use disorders: an analysis from the Global Burden of Disease Study 2010. PLoS One. 2015;10(2):e0116820.

World Health Organization. World Mental Health Atlas 2011: Geneva: WHO; 2011

World Health Organization. Depression and Other Common Mental Disorders: Global Estimates. Geneva: WHO; 2017.

Chapter 21

Somatoform and Dissociative Disorders

Rajiv Gupta, Krishan Kumar

SUMMARY

Somatoform disorders comprise of a group of disorders characterized by the presence of somatic symptoms suggestive of physical illness in the absence of any diagnosable physical ailment. Dissociative disorders, on the other hand, comprise of a disjunction of consciousness, identity, memory, and motor functions. "Somatoform disorder" is an umbrella term which comprises of several disorders. Several theories have been proposed for the etiopathogenesis of this group of disorders, and several psychosocial risk factors have been identified, but the concept is still evolving and remains a fertile ground for controversy. The same applies to dissociative disorders. Both these groups of disorders have been found to be prevalent in the general population, and pose a large burden in terms of distress and disability. These disorders tend to be chronic with changing symptomatology and high morbidity. Management involves a combination of psychological, behavioral, and pharmacological approaches.

INTRODUCTION

Somatoform and dissociative disorders are two independent groups of mental disorders, which historically came in the broad rubric of hysteria, and hence have been put together in this book. The disorders are termed somatoform disorders, if the symptoms occur in physical domain, suggesting a physical illness in the absence of any evidence, and dissociative disorders, if there is a disturbance in one or more of the personality functions of consciousness, personal identity or motor behavior. The symptom formation shares the mental mechanism of dissociation in the pathogenesis.

CONCEPTUAL FRAMEWORK

Somatoform Disorders

Somatoform disorders are a group of disorders with persistent physical symptoms, such as discomfort, immobility, and pain as the predominant presenting features. The overlying feature is preoccupation with physical symptoms with no evidence of a physical illness on history, examination or investigations. The umbrella term of "somatoform disorders" includes several disorders which include pain disorder, somatization disorder, hypochondriasis, undifferentiated somatoform disorder, somatoform autonomic dysfunction, and somatoform disorder not otherwise specified. The definition and classification of these disorders remains difficult and controversial. This has led to frequent revisions of nomenclatures that constantly move the target used to designate "cases" and complicate the clinical recognition and management of these syndromes (American Psychiatric Association, 2000, 2013; World Health Organization, 1992). Clinicians and researchers have proposed a wide range of theories for their etiology, diagnosis and treatment. However, reaching to a consensus has been almost an impossible proposition. Ever evolving ideas and concepts have been just as varied as the unexplained symptoms themselves. So, the controversy regarding their diagnosis has been a rule rather than exception (Kroenke et al., 1998). Diagnosis of somatoform disorders has undergone a metamorphosis over the years but this has been shrouded with controversies at every stage. Current controversy regarding somatoform disorders in DSM-5 and the upcoming ICD-11 is between a radicalist and a "go-slow" approach. Recommendations have varied from total abolishment of the category as in DSM-5 to expansion and relaxation of the criteria to encompass the less severe versions in the community with minor regroupings of subcategories. It is worth considering the changing nomenclature, organization, and criteria of the section dealing with somatoform disorders in the DSM-5 and ICD-10. The improvement in healthcare of the people suffering from somatic symptoms in clinics requires modification not only in the systems of healthcare delivery, but also in changing of attitudes of healthcare providers.

Dissociative Disorders

Dissociative disorders comprise of a person's state of interruption or dissociation from his/her basic tenets of consciousness. The concept of dissociative disorders has taken new significance nowadays in current clinical practice. According to Steinberg (1994), dissociative experiences entail the functional isolation of certain aspects of consciousness (viz. emotions, memories, perception, thoughts, motor activity, and identity) from one another, when they would normally be expected to occur together, so much so that in some scenarios, they become inaccessible to the conscious mind. The category includes dissociative convulsions, stupor, mutism, amnesia, fugue, multiple personality, and others.

CATEGORIZATION OF SOMATOFORM AND DISSOCIATIVE DISORDERS

Somatoform disorders can be categorized under four broad categories:
a. *Somatization disorder:* Historically, somatization disorder has been known as a form of hysteria and Briquet's syndrome. This syndrome is characterized by a person experiencing multiple physical symptoms, which are not caused by any underlying physical pathology. The underlying phenomenon of somatization has been conceptualized by Lipowski as the patient misattributing the physical symptoms to some physical illness, and seeking medical help for the same (Lipowski, 1988). A fact worthy of note is that these symptoms are not merely "reported", but in fact "experienced" as those of a physical illness, i.e. patients with somatization do not merely feign symptoms; this differentiates somatization disorder from malingering and factitious disorders
b. *Hypochondriasis:* This disorder is characterized by the patient being unrealistically fearful of (or believing himself to be) suffering from some serious medical ailment based on a

heightened awareness of bodily function. The person tends to misinterpret normal bodily sensations as pathological. The patient continues to hold this preoccupation despite being reassured repeatedly, and being shown that the results of investigations are normal

c. *Pain disorder:* Although pain rooted in the psyche is listed separately from somatization in the DSM-IV, chronic pain is observed to be the most common manifestation of somatization (Katon et al., 1984). Diagnosing this disorder becomes challenging especially in the presence of physical ailment/injury, for example, in case of partially understood illnesses (e.g. complex regional pain syndrome)

d. *Somatoform autonomic dysfunction:* The disorder is characterized by the presence of symptoms of autonomic arousal, which may involve cardiovascular, gastrointestinal, respiratory or genitourinary systems. Symptoms may occur in the form of palpitations, excessive sweating, pain in the chest, hyperventilation, hiccups, nervous diarrhea, vomiting, frequency of micturition or dysuria, etc. in the absence of a primary physical illness.

Dissociative disorders can be classified under five types:

a. *Conversion disorder:* Historically it has been known as hysterical neurosis, conversion type. A normal function of the body is lost/altered as a part of this disorder which is inexplicable by physical findings. This loss/alteration is usually rooted in psychological conflicts and issues. DSM-IV included it under the group of somatoform disorders, while ICD-10 categorized it in dissociative disorders. In DSM-5, the category is included in somatic symptom and related disorders.

b. *Dissociative amnesia:* It is a classical functional illness in which episodic memory is lost. Dissociative amnesia may be localized, selective, continuous, generalized or systematized, and has no involvement of the storage of memory, or certain types of memory such as procedural memory. It may develop in an acute or gradual manner following trauma.

     Often there is a dramatic and florid clinical disturbance, characterized by complete loss of life memories and identity (the classic presentation). Such amnesia usually includes the memories of stressful events, or those of trauma (e.g. rape or combat) (Loweinstein & Putnam, 2005).

c. *Dissociative fugue:* Fugue typically presents with episodes of sudden, unexpected travel, which appear purposeful in contrast to the confused wandering that may be seen in psychogenic amnesia. The patients are usually unable to recall sections of current and past life, and have either a lost identity, or assume a new one, which is simple and incompletely developed. In rare cases, the new identity is so perfect that the presence of mental disorder is not suspected. Some aspects of a person's personal memory fail to integrate, and the person presents with a lost/altered identity, accompanied with motor automatisms.

d. *Dissociative identity disorder (DID):* The DID is a relatively uncommon disorder, though the most prolifically discussed among all dissociative disorders. It is characterized by the "presence of two or more distinct identities or personality states" (American Psychiatric Association, 2000). In simple words, a person with DID shows attributes of many personalities. A single person exhibits numerous personalities that are distinct from one another. As is the case with healthy people, these multiple personalities too interact with their environment in a unique manner. When a person watches a movie, he/she is able to relate to different characters, and is able to experience to some extent what the characters are experiencing, while at the same time maintaining one's own objectivity and personal identity. A similar phenomenon happens with patients of DID with the difference that they are unable to maintain their primary identity. By completely assuming the identity of a different personality, these patients experience a relief from suppressed emotions/feelings/conflicts. This disorder requires the presence of at least two distinct personalities (though there may be more); of all the distinct personalities, two must repeatedly take control of that patient's behavior. These patients are typically reticent about revealing their dissociative symptoms especially hallucinations, amnesia, and identity. The most common presentation is relatively inhibited and obsessional behavior with affective and somatic complaints. Also, these patients are unable to recall significant information about their personal self, and this inability is not explicable by routine forgetfulness (American Psychiatric Association, 2013)

e. *Depersonalization disorder*: In depersonalization disorder, different aspects of perception fail to integrate. The disorder is characterized by a continued sense of detachment, unreality and estrangement from one's person or body, and is often accompanied by the feeling that the patient himself is observing his own mental process from outside (American Psychiatric Association, 2013). In depersonalization, there is a disturbance in person's perception of oneself; whereas in derealization, it is external environment which is perceived in a distorted way. The presentation may include a sense of change in body, being cut off from others or being cut off form one's emotion (Loweinstein, 2005). All these distorted perceptions are experienced as unpleasant and may be accompanied by anxiety, depression, or fear of becoming insane.

CHANGES IN DSM-5

In DSM-5, the section on somatic symptom and related disorders includes the subcategories of somatoform disorders. In order to avoid overlapping, DSM-5 has merged the subcategories such as pain disorder, hypochondriasis, somatization disorder, and undifferentiated somatoform disorder. Conditions, which were earlier diagnosed as somatization disorder, undifferentiated somatoform disorder or pain disorder usually meet the criteria for "somatic symptom disorder" of the DSM-5, provided the patient has maladaptive thoughts, feelings, and behaviors along with somatic symptoms. DSM-5 also merges undifferentiated somatoform disorder with the rubric of somatization disorder, as previously the distinction between the two was based on arbitrary criteria. Conversely, patients with few somatic symptoms, but a higher degree of anxiety related to health who would previously be diagnosed as having hypochondriasis are diagnosed as "illness anxiety disorder" according to DSM-5 (with the caveat that this anxiety should not be better explained by a primary anxiety disorder, such as generalized anxiety disorder).

EPIDEMIOLOGY AND PUBLIC HEALTH ISSUES OF SOMATOFORM AND DISSOCIATIVE DISORDER

Somatoform disorders are the most prevalent mental illness encountered by the medical practitioners in attending general practice. In an investigation of more than 1000 people attending general physicians, 16% were found to be suffering from severe form of somatoform disorder, a rate which was 22% if those with the milder form of the illness were included. Frequently, anxiety and depression too were found to be comorbid in such people. For example, in an investigation of patients from a hospital setting, a comorbid psychiatric illness such as anxiety or depression was found in around 36% of the people who were found to be suffering from any somatoform disorder. Depression, anxiety or concurrent substance misuse, and other medically unexplained (somatic) symptoms are common in primary care. Chronic somatic symptoms are usually less common, but result in a significant workload. In a general practice sample from Southampton, 19% of the patients attending their practice were considered by their general practitioners to be suffering from medically unexplained symptoms for at least 3 months duration (Preveler et al., 1997).

Ross et al. (1990) in a study on 1055 adults from Canada found 2.8% of the subjects to have depersonalization disorder, 6% to have dissociative amnesia, 1.3% to suffer from dissociative identity disorder, and 0.2% to have unspecified dissociative disorder. The prevalence of the above-mentioned disorders was found to be 1.8%, 1.5%, 0.8%, and 4.4%, respectively in 658 adults sampled from the community (Johnson et al., 2006). In another study on patients sampled from an outpatient clinic 10% were found to have dissociative amnesia, 6% had dissociative identity disorder, 5% had depersonalization disorder, and 9% had unspecified dissociative disorder (Foote et al., 2006). Interestingly, not one case of dissociative fugue was observed in any of the above-mentioned studies. Thus, dissociative symptoms are not so uncommon even in the Western settings.

RISK FACTORS: PSYCHOLOGICAL/SOCIAL THEORIES EXPLAINING SOMATOFORM AND DISSOCIATIVE DISORDERS

Psychological Factors

Psychological factors play a significant role in a number of somatoform syndromes. Traits like suggestibility, dramatic demeanor, flair, and flamboyance are related to the classic notion of hysteria. Some of these traits survived in more recent nomenclatures and were included in the personality disorders category ("hysterical personality" and more recently "histrionic personality"). The concept of "alexithymia," is used to describe an inability to express and normally process emotions, that has also been associated with a tendency to emphasize somatic rather than psychological symptom presentations.

Psychodynamic Theories

Janet and Freud were the two major contributors who conceptualized the theories that explain the underlying phenomena of dissociation processes. For both, the appearance of amnesia was considered to be the result of the removal of a cluster of mental associations from consciousness accompanied by an inability of the person to recall them voluntarily from their conscious mind. For Janet, the process of dissociation was based on the ultimate physiological concept of a constitutional lowering of nervous energies of such a magnitude that the forces normally binding brain and mental functions into an integrated whole could no longer keep them together. As a consequence, some of those functions escaped central control. When memory was affected by this disintegration, a dissociation of memory clusters followed, and the dissociation placed them beyond the purview of consciousness resulting in amnesia and other related symptoms.

Freud, on the other hand, proposed the concept of repression, a psychic force that actively removed contents from conscious awareness. The mental contents are unacceptable to the person and are pushed away from consciousness by the specific psychic force of repression and are actively kept in an unconscious mind. For Freud, amnesia and the related symptoms were the result of active mental processes as opposed to Janet's passive mental processes.

Some patients when faced with a situation that had aroused overwhelming grief, despair, or anxiety, may respond by a total repression of the memories of the disturbing events, accompanied by a disappearance of the painful affect. That is frequently the reason for the amnesia that develops in soldiers who have been exposed to intolerable battle stress, and it certainly accounts for some of the cases found in the general civilian population (Nemiah, 1985).

In patients with multiple personality disorder and psychogenic fugue, a drive that is usually repressed or patterns of behavior that are normally under control may emerge into open expression in a dissociative state. The psychological conflicts in the adult patients that lead to dissociative symptoms are viewed as being ultimately the result of early disturbance during the course of growth and development. Both oedipal and preoedipal elements contribute to the pathogenesis of dissociative disorders, but those elements are in no way different from what are found in conversion disorder.

Role of Social Factors

The risk of mental illnesses is increased by stressful life events, which also lead to a reduction in the quality of life of people. Stressors, which are psychosocial in nature, have been shown to have a strong association with somatic symptoms. Psychosocial stressors commonly encountered in adults' life include relationships issues, death of a near and dear one, financial problems, and discrimination on the basis of factors such as race (Hotoph et al., 1998). Sexual abuse has been found to be a major and frequent life stressor in many female patients with somatization disorder (Morrison, 1989). Women, who had a history of severe sexual abuse in childhood, are at a higher risk of having a life-time diagnosis of disorders such as phobias, panic disorder, depression, and dissociative disorder (Walker et al., 1992).

COURSE AND OUTCOME

The course of most somatoform disorders tends to be chronic, which is to be expected in the case of syndromes so closely associated with personality and cognitive styles. It has often been observed that there is a qualitative and quantitative change in the somatic symptoms during follow-up, suggesting a certain inconsistency in symptom presentation. However, according to international studies, although idiopathic symptoms change, the number of symptoms present appears to remain high. The presence of high levels of idiopathic physical symptoms appears to be very disabling, leading to higher levels of disability than those reported for most medical and psychiatric disorders. Research in primary care has shown that mental illnesses, for example, anxiety or depression become more severe and disabling if they are associated with severe somatic symptoms.

Childhood abuse, trauma, or other forms of negative experiences are often found to be associated with dissociative disorder. Clinically significant dissociative disorder may become apparent at any age including a very young or advanced age. Juvenile dissociative disorder may present with complaints related to concentration, memory or attachment, but identity changes are rarely seen. Older individuals may present with mood disorders or symptoms which mimic mood disorders, psychotic mood, or paranoia.

MANAGEMENT

Establishing an Alliance

Building a trusting alliance in this context must begin with respect for the patient's symptoms and an acknowledgement of their validity. Active and receptive listening, tolerance for repetition, and a "neutral" approach (avoiding being dismissive, confrontational, or overly reassuring) are essential skills. It takes time and persistence to develop a trusting, therapeutic partnership.

Taking the History

Somatizing patients usually bring with them "thick" charts. These include descriptions of many clinical encounters and multiple tests and procedures that are often redundant and ordered without clear rationale. The prospect of reviewing these medical records is challenging and often leads to a negative attitude from the physician. The physician should keep an open mind, despite forewarnings in the medical records, and perform an independent assessment of the patient. An emphasis on psychological questioning and interpretations should be avoided at this stage. Premature reassurance, although seemingly appropriate from the physician's perspective, may be perceived by the patient as disinterest or dismissiveness.

Reassurance

Reassurance simply means letting patients know that their symptoms do not appear to be caused by physical disease. It may not work well in many patients presenting with "idiopathic" physical symptoms. The timing and degree of reassurance must be based on an adequacy of data and trust and security of the relationship.

Physical versus Psychological Focus

Somatizing patients appear to feel most comfortable providing details of symptoms in physical or somatic terms. However, they may also bring a repertoire of significant events (e.g. losses, trauma, disappointments, and deprivations) that may be related to the onset or persistence of symptoms and need to be explored at some point. However, many patients do not readily acknowledge or recognize emotional issues and will feel more comfortable dealing with questions related to their physical symptoms than questions related to psychological issues. Taking a history of multiple physical complaints can be carried over into subsequent appointments. A thorough physical examination should follow history taking at the initial visit, and briefer physical assessments should be performed in subsequent visits. An inclusive drug history including prescription and nonprescription remedies should also be completed. As the history taking moves along, attitudes, beliefs, and attributions should become clearer and patterns of interaction and illness behavior discernible. Distorted beliefs, contradictory ideas, and fears can be addressed at several points during the process of gathering historical data.

PSYCHOSOCIAL AND BEHAVIORAL INTERVENTIONS FOR SOMATOFORM DISORDERS

Treating somatoform disorders needs a multidisciplinary team approach (comprising of psychiatrist, psychologist, and a physician). It is important to avoid interventions and procedures (both therapeutic or diagnostic), which are not necessary. If a specific cognitive distortion can be identified, e.g. in body dysmorphic disorder or hypochondriasis, cognitive therapy focused on correcting these distortions can be undertaken in addition to behavioral therapy for changing maladaptive behavior, e.g. repeated reassurance seeking. Managing expectancy, suggestion and reassurance can be helpful in treating conversion disorder. These general techniques may be complemented by physical and behavioral techniques. Pharmacotherapy seems to be the best option for pain disorder, along with cognitive behavioral therapy (CBT).

Though various disorders, which are classified under the rubric of somatoform disorders, have been the center of attention for psychotherapists from the psychodynamic school, in common experience such therapy is not used frequently. What has shown results in such disorders are techniques such as relaxation training, problem solving, assertiveness training, and emotional expression, all of which can be delivered under group cognitive therapy (Kashner et al., 1995). Individual CBT has also shown similar success in undifferentiated somatoform disorder. CBT combines behavior therapy with cognitive therapy. Examining how thoughts of a person regarding self, others, or environment interact with their mental illness is the purview of cognitive therapy. To complement this, examination of a person's behavior and how it affects the illness , is required. By the combination of these therapies, CBT helps patients to modify the thoughts and behaviors, which help to improve their quality of life and ameliorate their distress (Looper & Kirmayer, 2002).

INTERVENTIONS FOR DISSOCIATIVE DISORDERS

Psychotherapy

A supportive contact with the patient going into the details of the genesis of symptoms, exploring into the history and stressors may help in identifying the conflict associated with the symptoms. A collaborative approach may be followed with the patient for conflict resolution. One may also go for brief dynamic therapy. Generally, it is possible to identify the stressors being faced by the patient over a course of therapy sessions, and attempts should be targeted at resolving them.

Hypnosis

Patients suffering from dissociative disorder are found to have a high degree of suggestibility, and hypnotic techniques often work well in such cases.

Abreaction

If the dissociative disorder is associated with trauma, abreaction may help the patient to express the unconscious emotions by eliciting repressed memories. Though not harmful, such techniques may not be very efficacious. Psychotherapeutic help is needed by such patients to integrate such memories and the associated affect into their consciousness.

CONCLUSION

Although the concept of somatoform and dissociative disorders has evolved with better understanding, many questions still remain unanswered. Two key features for establishing diagnosis of somatoform disorders are that there must not be any physical findings or known physiological mechanism that might account for the symptoms, and there must be direct or strong presumptive evidence of their psychological origin. The dissociative disorders on the other hand are group of psychiatric syndromes characterized by sudden, temporary disruption of some aspect of consciousness, identity, or motor behavior. The causes of somatoform and dissociative disorders are not clearly or specifically defined but psychological theory of causation is widely accepted. Traditionally, these disorders have been attributed to trauma and other psychological stress. The relationship between the dissociative disorders and trauma is currently well accepted. The treatment of these disorders is poorly understood and not always effective.

REFERENCES

American Psychiatric Association. Diagnostic and Statistical Manual of Mental Disorders, 4th edition (DSM-IV). Washington, DC: American Psychiatric Association; 1994.

American Psychiatric Association. Diagnostic and Statistical Manual of Mental Disorders, 4th edition, text revision (DSM-IV-TR). Washington, DC: American Psychiatric Association; 2000.

American Psychiatric Association. Diagnostic and Statistical Manual of Mental Disorders, 5th edition (DSM-5). Washington, DC: American Psychiatric Association; 2013.

Foote B, Smolin Y, Kaplan M. Prevalence of dissociative disorders in psychiatric outpatients. Am J Psychiatry. 2006;163:623-9.

Hotoph M, Carr S, Mayou R. The somatoform disorders and stress. BMJ.1998;316:1196-200.

Johnson JG, Cohen P, Kasen S, et al. Dissociative disorders among adults in the community, impaired functioning, and axis I and II comorbidity. J Psychiatr Res. 2006;40:131-40.

Kashner TM, Rost K, Cohen B, et al. Enhancing the health of somatization disorder patients: effectiveness of short-term group therapy. Psychosomatics. 1995;36:462-70.

Katon W, Ries R, Kleinman A. The prevalence of somatization in primary care. Compr Psychiatry. 1984;25:208-15.

Kroenke K, Spitler RL, De Gruif V, et al. Multi-somatoform disorder: an alternative to undifferentiated somatoform disorders for the somatizing patient in primary care. Arch Gen Psychiatry. 1998;55:352-8.

Lipowski Z. Somatization: the concept and its clinical applications. Am J Psychiatry. 1988;145:1358-68.

Loweinstein RJ. Psychopharmacologic treatment for dissociative identity disorder. Psychiatr Ann. 2005;35(8):666-73.

Loweinstein RJ, Putnam FW: Dissociative disorders. In: In: Sadock BJ, Sadock va (Eds). Comprehensive Textbook of Psychiatry, 8th edition. New York, Lipincott Williams & Wilkins, 2005; pp. 1844-901.

Looper KJ, Kirmayer LJ. Behavioral medicine approaches to somatoform disorders. J Consult Clin Psychol. 2002;70:810-27.

Morrison J. Managing somatization disorders. Disease-a-month. 1989;36(100):537-91.

Nemiah JC. Dissociative disorders. In: Kaplan H, Sadock B (Eds). Comprehensive Textbook of Psychiatry, 4th edition. Baltimore: Williams & Wilkins; 1985. pp. 942-57.

Preveler R, Kilkenney L, Kinmouth A. Medically unexplained physical symptoms in primary care. J Psychosom Res. 1997;42:245-52.

Ross, CA, Joshi S, Currie R. Dissociative experiences in the general population. Am J Psychiatry. 1990;147:1547-52.

Steinberg M. Structured Clinical Interview for DSM-IV Dissociative Disorder-Revised (SCID-D-R). Washington DC: American Psychiatric Press; 1994.

Walker EA, Hanson, J, Holm L, et al. Medical and psychiatric symptoms in women with childhood sexual abuse. Psychosom Med. 1992;54(6):658-64.

Chapter 22

Social Dimensions of Substance Use Disorders

Anju Dhawan, Shalini Singh

SUMMARY

Substance use disorders (SUDs) are a significant problem in society. There are several social and cultural determinants of SUDs. Social factors such as peer pressure and changing risk perceptions in the society regarding substance use influence drug use in the adolescent age group. A lack of religious and cultural beliefs, discrimination, and family dysfunction too are important risk factors. Women face severe social consequences due to drug use and are also more vulnerable due to higher risk of violence, interpersonal conflict, and social isolation as compared to men. India being a developing economy typically had a large male to female ratio for SUDs, and lower prevalence of drug use in the younger age group. However, due to rapid economic advances, the drug use patterns are changing. Culturally distinct patterns of drug use are gradually disappearing due to globalization and new social problems such as forced migration have led to increased prevalence of substance use.

Social theories attempt to explain the individual and population-based drug use behavior, and have helped to create psychosocial and policy-based interventions to manage the SUDs. Families of substance users have to deal with strained relationships, violence, and social marginalization. Stigma due to drug use is experienced both by the patient and their family members, and leads to lack of rehabilitative opportunities and greater distancing from the society. Social cost of SUDs has been calculated in many parts of the world including India and confirm the massive burden of SUDs on the society and individual.

Social therapies for SUDs are useful in long-term management. Self-help groups, network therapy, community reinforcement approach, therapeutic community, and family based interventions have been found to be effective interventions. In India, some of these interventions have been adapted to various treatment settings. Further research is needed to understand their effectiveness in the Indian population and to develop newer evidence-based psychosocial interventions that target social risk factors specific to this region.

INTRODUCTION

According to the World Drug Report (2017), there are around 2 billion alcohol users, and nearly 255 million people used illicit drugs in 2015 (United Nations Office on Drugs and Crime, 2017). According to the National Household Survey on drug use in India by Ray et al. (2004), the prevalence of current alcohol use, opioid use and cannabis use in the 12–60 age group is 21%, 0.7%, and 3% respectively.

The SUDs can be better understood by examining the social factors that impact drug use, social interventions that are effective in its management, and their social complications. This chapter explores the various social dimensions of SUDs.

DRUG USE TRENDS FROM A SOCIAL PERSPECTIVE

This section examines the extent of drug use and trends in the context of age, gender, economic status, and cultural influences.

Adolescents and Young Adults

Trends in drug use patterns in the younger age group correlate with certain social factors: increased perceived risk from using drugs, disapproval of drug use by peers, high exposure to advertising campaigns against use, and reduced availability of some drugs (Bachman et al., 2014). Concurrently, environmental factors such as increased variety of tobacco products (Abad-Vivero et al., 2016), reduced risk perception of smokeless tobacco use (Callery et al., 2011), and increased restrictions on public smoking have led to a rebound increase in the use of smokeless tobacco. Vaping has quickly become one of the most common forms of adolescent substance use because e-cigarettes have some of the lowest levels of perceived risk (Patrick et al., 2016). Similarly for marijuana, lowering perceived risk and changing legal status are consistent with the rising prevalence of its use in the adolescent population (Shi et al., 2015). Other known risk factors include peer influences (Byrd et al., 2016), trouble with the law (Leslie et al., 2013), academic and disciplinary issues (Gauffin et al., 2013), lack of religious beliefs (Luk et al., 2013), family dysfunction (Vanassche et al., 2014), immigrant status (Pavarin et al., 2016), racial discrimination (Hurd et al., 2014), and poor parenting practices (Trapl et al., 2015). Adolescent girls are more prone to these social risk factors than boys (Schinke et al., 2008).

An authoritarian parenting style (Calafat et al., 2014), strong cultural and religious beliefs, and strong family values are protective social factors that prevent substance use in adolescents (Kim-Spoon et al., 2015). Strong neighborhood support confers a protective resiliency to adolescents exposed to other risk factors (Jones et al., 2016). A review of longitudinal studies (n = 17) by Kwan et al. (2014) shows a protective role of involvement in socially integrating activities such as sports. High parental socio-economic status and early transition of the adolescent into desired life course protects them from SUDs (Pampel et al., 2014).

Gender

The social consequences of drug use are more severe for women than men. The World Drug Report (WDR) 2016 indicates a higher rate of increase in disease burden from SUDs among women (+25%) than in men (+19%) in 2015 as compared to 2005 (United Nations Office on Drugs and Crime, 2016). Globally, changing gender roles and greater economic parity between men and women have resulted in an increase in substance use by women, but still the prevalence of substance use in females is comparatively lower with some exceptions (Wagner & Anthony, 2007).

Besides alcohol (used by about 2% of Indian women—with large regional variation), use of other substances has also been reported among women in India. A countrywide survey by

Murthy et al. (2008) of 1865 women substance users showed that 61% used opioids, and 25% had used injecting drugs once in their lifetime. Treatment seeking is low among women as compared to men, probably due to a lower prevalence as well as more prominent barriers to treatment seeking. However, there has been some increase in treatment seeking among women substance users in India recently (Nebhinani et al., 2013).

A review of the social risk and protective factors partly explains the distinctive prevalence and impact of SUDs in men and women (Cotto et al., 2010). Men are more prone to risk factors such as greater cultural acceptability of substance use, greater social sanction for substance use by men in some cultures, and a greater positive expectancy from drug and alcohol use, for example drinking to relieve stress (Castro et al., 2014). Conversely, societies that disapprove of drug use in women, play a protective role (Erol et al., 2015). According to the Global Alcohol Report 2014, women abstain from alcohol use in many parts of the world due to prevalent social norms (World Health Organization, 2014). Women across the world are held to a higher standard than men in regard to substance use, and these social expectations from women also act as treatment-seeking barrier (Sielski, 2011).

The greater severity of SUDs among female drug users can be understood by examining the social risk factors. A history of violence predisposes both women and men to an increased risk of developing SUDs, but women are more vulnerable (Evans et al., 2017). Women who abuse drugs are more likely to suffer intimate partner violence (IPV), therefore exposing them to a lifetime of cyclical trauma and abuse. A cross sectional evaluation by Malik et al. (2015) of psychosocial profiles of Indian women seeking treatment for drug abuse showed that 20% of them were abused as children, and 70% had experienced marital discord and interpersonal conflict at home or work. Marriage has greater impact on women substance use patterns than on men (Rodriguez et al., 2014). Women mimic the substance use pattern of their spouse and relapse due to partner's substance use (Finkelstein et al., 2011).

Economic Status

A region's socio-economic status has a complex relationship with the prevalence of substance abuse (Singer et al., 2008). Developing economies are rapidly urbanizing, leading to overcrowding, poverty, unemployment, high levels of violence and increasing alienation within a community. Coupled with aggressive marketing of licit drugs, these changes have increased the rate of SUDs (Bryden et al., 2011). Cannabis is now a widely used illicit drug among adolescents in developing countries with similar social predictors of early use as in developed nations, which include peer pressure, poor academic performance, and antisocial behavior (Degenhart & Hall, 2007). A comparison between substance use patterns of developing economies such as India and China and high-income countries highlights distinctive socio-demographic patterns. High-income countries have a smaller male-to-female ratio for SUDs, and higher prevalence in young adults and in those with lower socioeconomic status. Cheng et al. (2016) reviewed literature on SUD epidemiology in India and China published between 1990 and 2015, and showed that the two countries by contrast have a large male-to-female ratio for SUDs, increasing prevalence with age, low prevalence in college students, and little association with income.

Recent rapid economic transition in China has altered the substance use pattern, quite similar to what is seen in the developed countries. There is now a negative association between income and alcohol/tobacco use and increased substance use in women (Yang et al., 2017). The National Family Health Survey (2010) of India too shows a negative correlation between alcohol use and socio-economic status. Reduced drug use among affluent class could be due to rising health awareness, investment in education rather than in pleasure, and other socio-cultural transformations that accompany economic growth (Kimbro et al., 2009). The increased substance use among women is due to a more liberalized and modern identity of women (Gilbert, 2007). Alternatively, substance use might also be a self-medicating tool of the expanding women workforce to cope with the stress of striking the right work-life balance (Glaser et al., 2015).

Culture

Cultural variations and social customs modulate drug use rates and pattern. Traditional use of psychoactive plants such as opium, cannabis and coca in indigenous communities is restricted to special occasions and rarely leads to SUDs (Durrant & Thakker, 2003). Disappearance of traditional societies and rapid industrialization has led to rising rate of SUDs. For example, the dry and wet culture dichotomy of alcohol use in the world might soon cease to exist due to dissolution of cultural differences across regions like greater lifestyle homogeneity, urbanization, female liberalization, globalized marketing of alcoholic beverages, and greater uniformity in legislations pertaining to licit drugs (Jernigan et al., 2009). Similarly, greater level of cultural and spiritual engagement plays a protective role against development of SUDs and also improves the treatment outcome (Allen et al., 2010). Anomie has also been identified as a risk factor for developing SUDs (Tam et al., 2012). Forced migration has also led to a significant increase in lifetime prevalence of SUDs in the migrant population (Horyniak et al., 2016).

SOCIOLOGICAL THEORIES OF SUBSTANCE USE DISORDERS

The sociological theories incorporate the society and the external environment into the causative model of the SUDs. The stress and coping theories demonstrates how substance use is a result of alienation from the society and poor coping with stressful situations. Imitation theories such as the social learning theory and modeling explain the impact of the peer group and immediate social environment on one's substance use behaviors (Heyes, 2011). The pathway model by Blaszczynski et al. (2002) outlines the process by which social and environmental factors interact with personal characteristics to increase the possibility of engaging in a particular behavior. Population-based theories such as the social network and social control theory describe the protective effects of a well-knit social network where the interpersonal interactions are healthy and improve self-image (Christakis et al., 2013). The systems theory shows how SUDs are a product of mutual interactions between various stakeholders (government policy, drug supply chain, and community). Some of these theories have been used for development of interventions for the management of SUDs.

SOCIAL IMPLICATIONS OF SUBSTANCE USE DISORDERS

Impact on the Family

Family members, who have been impacted by addiction, are the silent sufferers of the consequences of SUDs. SUD in a family is associated with dysfunctional relationships, draining of family resources on drugs and health care, and violence. Based on the ethnographic research on different social-cultural groups, Orford et al. (2013) describe a stress-strain-coping-support model to describe the impact of drug use on family members. The affected family experiences disempowerment and social marginalization. The impact of substance use on the children in the family is a major concern. Family dynamics get distorted due to loss of healthy family interactions, feelings of anger, hatred, bitterness and being let down, and open conflict, that seeps into all family ties. Indian women with drug dependent spouses demonstrate high rates (81.6%) of codependency, defined as a type of dysfunctional helping relationship, where one person supports or enables another person's drug addiction (Anderson et al., 1994). The degree of codependence correlates with the addiction severity scores of their husbands (Bhowmick et al., 2001). Similar to the findings by Orford et al. coping behavior of wives of the alcohol dependent males in India includes avoidance, indulgence, and fearful withdrawal (Rao et al., 1992).

Stigma and Substance Use

Substance users face three different kinds of stigma: enacted, perceived, and self-stigma (Link et al., 2004). Enacted stigma is the directly experienced social discrimination such as not being able to get a job, and rejection by non-drug using peers. Perceived stigma is the set of beliefs held by a stigmatized group about how they are perceived by the society. Self-stigma refers to the self-directed negative feeling (remorse, shame, and anger) that results in certain behaviors such as not seeking treatment and alienating self from the existing social networks. A multisite cross-sectional study by Luoma et al. (2007) on 197 patients of SUDs who were in the recovery phase reported that the participants experienced high levels of all the three kinds of stigma, and that greater number of treatment attempts and high-risk behaviors such as injecting drug use was associated with higher levels of stigma. Mattoo et al. (2015) in a cross-sectional study among treatment seekers at a de-addiction center in North India found that those with alcohol dependence reported a significantly higher degree of stigma than opioid dependent individuals. Longer duration of dependence was associated with greater degree of perceived stigma, and being employed and having a higher per capita income was associated with lesser degree of perceived stigma.

SOCIAL COST OF SUBSTANCE USE DISORDERS

The negative consequences of substance use on the society can be quantified by determining the social costs of substance abuse. The method of arriving at the cost of SUDs is complex and involves measuring the loss of resources due to SUDs, e.g. gross national product reduced by the morbidity, early death of substance abusers and the cost of medical care for substance use related illness. It takes into account the additional costs such as expenses incurred by the criminal justice system, insurance costs due to property damage, etc. While these approaches have rightly been criticized for being unable to quantify the entire social impact of substance use, they are a useful objective measure to measure the extent of social burden due to substance use. According to a review by Mohapatra and colleagues (2010), the social cost due to alcohol use in 14 high-income countries is 1% or more of their Gross Domestic Product (GDP), indicative of an enormous burden on public health. One of the earliest reports of social costs due to drug use comes from Japan by Nakamura et al. (1993), which estimated the social cost due to alcohol use at 1.9% of GDP in 1987. In India, the per capita social cost of alcohol use in India has been estimated at 29,886 rupees per annum by Benegal et al. (2000).

SOCIAL TREATMENTS FOR SUBSTANCE USE DISORDERS

Psychosocial therapies and socially grounded treatment strategies have been used as management strategies for SUDs. The nature of psychosocial intervention is decided after evaluating the psychological status of the client and social issues associated with substance use. The social issues in an individual's life that can be modified are taken up and treated through various social interventions.

Successful psychosocial interventions encourage large, diverse social networks, and promote social networks that have a greater number of abstainers in it (Panebianco et al., 2016). Social interventions need to be culturally adapted to the needs of diverse populations, while maintaining fidelity to the treatment program's active ingredients. Some of these factors are race, gender, ethnicity, sexual orientation, and the client's degree of acculturation and alienation in society (Castro et al., 2007). Some of the social interventions used for SUDs are discussed as below:

1. **Self-help groups (SHGs):** Alcoholic Anonymous (AA) and Narcotics Anonymous (NA) are mutual support programs and examples of SHGs, that rely upon the protective social networks and spiritual inclinations of the 12-step approach to ensure abstinence among drug dependent individuals (Borman, 1998). Data on the 12-step effectiveness comes from membership surveys, observational studies and analysis of longitudinal studies (Kelly et al., 2017). These reports indicate that the median length of abstinence is over 5 years with approximately 30% subjects having between 1 and 5 years of abstinence. Studies have shown better outcomes in other psychosocial dimensions as well. The acceptance of SHGs in India and their effectiveness is not known at this point. In Japan, the SHG model has been indigenously adapted into the Danshukai model for alcohol dependent patients as described by Chenhall and Oka (2006)

2. **Network therapy (NT):** There are three elements in NT: cognitive behavioral approach for relapse prevention, social network support to promote treatment engagement, and a central orchestrating figure, the therapist, who ensures proper utilization of the available psycho-social resources. In a multisite, randomized, controlled trial (UK alcohol treatment trial- UKATT, 2005) on 742 clients, NT was compared to Motivational Enhancement Therapy (MET). Both groups had a similar reduction in drug use, but the NT method was found to be more cost-effective. While there are no examples of NT in the Indian scenario, it could be a useful social intervention

3. **Community reinforcement approach (CRA) and family training (CRAFT):** The CRA is a psychosocial intervention that utilizes the client's community, i.e. family, friends, and colleagues as a source of reinforcement to compete with substance use. Behavioral therapy is used in conjunction to mitigate reinforcing behaviors associated with drug use. In the CRAFT therapy, the therapist instructs family members on how to motivate treatment-refusing clients to come for treatment and abstain from drug use. The preliminary step is to make family members emotionally capable of handling client's drug use. Empirical evidence supports use of CRA and CRAFT for treatment of most SUDs and in diverse populations (Smith et al., 2001). Web-based delivery has also found acceptability (Campbell et al., 2015). A randomized controlled trial by Brigham et al. (2014) on opioid dependent patients found that CRAFT led to greater treatment retention. Assadbeigi et al. (2016) showed that CRAFT approach significantly improves the family's quality of life (QoL). CRA is useful in management of SUDs in adolescents and in improving their school performance (McGarvey et al., 2014)

4. **Therapeutic community (TC):** It is a recovery oriented program where recovery is broadly defined as a change in one's lifestyle and identity through community-oriented techniques. The concept of "community as a method", as given by De Leon (2010), can be used to summarize the TC approach. The approach uses community as a method or mechanism to teach individuals how to improve their lives by using community. There is evidence of effectiveness of TC in reviews by De Leon (2010) and Vanderplasschen et al. (2013) that show effectiveness to be proportional to the duration of treatment retention. However, a review of data on relapse rates as an outcome variable concluded that the effect of TCs is short-term (Malivert et al., 2012). TCs are an effective and cost-effective social therapy especially for the subjects with more severe psychosocial dysfunction. Worldwide, the TC approach has been adapted to match the socio-cultural needs of clients. In cultures, where sexes cannot mingle, there are segregated TCs. At places, religious practices have been integrated into TCs like in the East. In Malaysia and Indonesia, TCs have strong family involvement with some of the TCs being run by parents of subjects who had originally been sent there (De Leon et al., 2015). In India, TCs have mushroomed in the urban areas but there is no evidence available about their fidelity and success rate. A 3-month yoga-based retreat for drug-dependent individuals in Punjab has shown improved psychological wellbeing of the residents at the end of their stay, as shown in a cross sectional survey by Khalsa et al. (2008)

5. **Family-based interventions:** People who abuse substances, get increasingly isolated from their families, and similarly families with a substance-using individual suffer consequences due to substance use. The goal of family based interventions is to:
   a. Help the family make changes that promote sobriety in the substance user
   b. Provide a neutral forum in which family meets to understand and solve problems
   c. Use the family's strengths and resources to help find or develop ways to live without substances of abuse
   d. Ameliorate the impact of SUDs on the client and family.

Family intervention therapy has been tried in patients with alcohol dependence in India with satisfactory results. Kumar et al. (2007) evaluated 50 patients of alcohol dependence after

1 year of initiating customized family therapy. The therapy led to reduced alcohol use and lesser number of stressful life events in the family.

There are many kinds of family based interventions. One of these is multisystemic therapy (MST). MST is an intensive family and community based treatment program that has been found to be especially useful for families dealing with adolescent substance use and anti-social behavior. The problematic behavior of adolescents (substance use, conduct problems, and criminal activity) is driven by the social risk factors, found in their family, community, peer group, and school. During the MST process, the client's social risk factors that are embedded in the multiple systems (home, school, peer group, and the community), are addressed while concomitantly building social protective factors. The family, especially the parents along with the school authorities and officials of the juvenile justice department act as a unit to determine the treatment goals. The therapist works towards bringing about these changes using intervention strategies, such as strategic family therapy, structural family therapy, behavioral parent training, and cognitive behavior therapy (Henngeler et al., 2002). The therapist carries out the therapy where the client lives (home, school, and community), and is available to the client and the family round the clock. The therapeutic alliance needs to be strong to maintain and cultivate the family's engagement with the process. The therapy lasts for an average of 4 months and consists of individual and family sessions as required. The cultural context of recovery for the adolescents and their families are kept in mind while designing the interventions. In a review by Huey and Polo (2008), MST has been successfully implemented in families from different cultural backgrounds in many countries, and is supported by a strong empirical evidence base (Henngeler, 2009). A meta-analysis of 11 studies by Curtis et al. (2005) involving 708 participants showed that MST is able to successfully impact the youth's natural environments, and results in most improvement in family relations when compared to other interventions.

CONCLUSION

Substance use disorders pose a significant public health problem in the world and in India. The development of SUDs is a complex interplay of individual and social risk factors. Interventions that address only the individual risk factors would have a limited impact if the social risk factors remain unchanged and continue to wield influence. Thus identifying and targeting the social determinants of SUDs is essential to have effective strategies for dealing with the SUDs.

REFERENCES

Abad-Vivero EN, Thrasher JF, Arillo-Santillán E, et al. Recall, appeal and willingness to try cigarettes with flavour capsules: assessing the impact of a tobacco product innovation among early adolescents. Tob Control. 2016;25(e2):e113–9.

Allen TM, Lo CC. Religiosity, spirituality, and substance abuse. J Drug Issues. 2010;40(2):433-59.

Anderson SC. A critical analysis of the concept of codependency. Soc Work. 1994;39(6):677-85.

Assadbeigi H, Pourshahbaz A, Mohamadkhani P, Farhoudian A. Effectiveness of Community Reinforcement and Family Training (CRAFT) on quality of life and depression in families with drug abuse. Global J Health Sci. 2016;9(3):167-75.

Bachman JG, O'Malley PM, Schulenberg JE, Johnston LD, Bryant AL, Merline AC. The Decline of Substance Use in Young Adulthood: Changes in Social Activities, Roles, and Beliefs. Psychology Press; 2014. pp. 313.

Benegal V, Velayudhan A, Jain S. The social cost of alcoholism (Karnataka). NIMHANS J. 2000;18(1/2): 67-76.

Bhowmick P, Tripathi BM, Jhingan HP, Pandey RM. Social support, coping resources and codependence in spouses of individuals with alcohol and drug dependence. Indian J Psychiatry. 2001;43(3): 219-24.

Blaszczynski A, Nower L. A pathways model of problem and pathological gambling. Addiction. 2002;97(5):487-99.

Borman PD, Dixon DN. Spirituality and the 12 steps of substance abuse recovery. Journal of Psychology and Theology. 1998.

Brigham GS, Slesnick N, Winhusen TM, Lewis DF, Guo X, Somoza E. A randomized pilot clinical trial to evaluate the efficacy of Community Reinforcement and Family Training for Treatment Retention (CRAFT-T) for improving outcomes for patients completing opioid detoxification. Drug Alcohol Depend. 2014;138:240-3.

Bryden A, Roberts B, McKee M, Petticrew M. A systematic review of the influence on alcohol use of community level availability and marketing of alcohol. Health Place. 2012;18(2):349-57.

Byrd KM. Binge drinking in and out of college: An examination of social control and differential association on binge drinking behaviors between college students and their non-college peers. Sociol Spectrum. 2016;36(4):191-207.

Calafat A, García F, Juan M, Becoña E, Fernández-Hermida JR. Which parenting style is more protective against adolescent substance use? Evidence within the European context. Drug Alcohol Depend. 2014;138:185-92.

Callery WE, Hammond D, O'Connor RJ, Fong GT. The appeal of smokeless tobacco products among young Canadian smokers: The impact of pictorial health warnings and relative risk messages. Nicotine Tob Res. 2011;13(5):373-83.

Campbell AN, Turrigiano E, Moore M, et al. Acceptability of a web-based community reinforcement approach for substance use disorders with treatment-seeking American Indians/Alaska natives. Com Mental Health J. 2015;51(4):393-403.

Castro FG, Nichols E, Kater K. Relapse Prevention with Hispanic and Other Racial/Ethnic Populations. Can Cultural Resilience Promote Relapse Prevention?. In Therapist's Guide to Evidence-Based Relapse Prevention 2007. Elsevier Inc.

Cheng HG, Shidhaye R, Charlson F, et al. Social correlates of mental, neurological, and substance use disorders in China and India: a review. Lancet Psychiatry. 2016;3(9):882-99.

Chenhall RD, Oka T. An initial view of self-help groups for Japanese alcoholics: Danshukai in its historical, social, and cultural contexts. Int J Self-Help Self-Care. 2006;5(2):111-52.

Christakis NA, Fowler JH. Social contagion theory: examining dynamic social networks and human behavior. Stats Med. 2013;32(4):556-77.

Cotto JH, Davis E, Dowling GJ, Elcano JC, Staton AB, Weiss SR. Gender effects on drug use, abuse, and dependence: a special analysis of results from the National Survey on Drug Use and Health. Gender Med. 2010;7(5):402-13.

Curtis NM, Ronan KR, Borduin CM. Multisystemic treatment: A meta-analysis of outcome studies. J Fam Psychol. 2004;18(3):411-9.

De Leon G, Perfas FB, Joseph A, Bunt G. Therapeutic Communities for Addictions: Essential Elements, Cultural, and Current Issues. In: el-Guebaly N., Carrà G., Galanter M. (eds) Textbook of Addiction Treatment: International Perspectives. Springer, Milano, 2015. pp. 1033-47.

De Leon G. Is the therapeutic community an evidence-based treatment? What the evidence says. Ther Com. 2010;31(2):104-28.

Durrant R, Thakker J. Substance Use and Abuse: Cultural and Historical Perspectives. SAGE; 2003. p. 325.

Erol A, Karpyak VM. Sex and gender-related differences in alcohol use and its consequences: contemporary knowledge and future research considerations. Drug Alcohol Depend. 2015;156:1-3.

Evans EA, Grella CE, Upchurch DM. Gender differences in the effects of childhood adversity on alcohol, drug, and polysubstance-related disorders. Soc Psychiatry Psychiatr Epidemiol. 2017; 3:1-2.

Finkelstein NB. Substance abuse treatment: addressing the specific needs of women. Diane Publishing; 2011.

Gauffin K, Vinnerljung B, Fridell M, Hesse M, Hjern A. Childhood socio-economic status, school failure and drug abuse: a Swedish national cohort study. Addiction. 2013;108(8):1441-9.

Gilbert E. Performing femininity: Young women's gendered practice of cigarette smoking. J Gender Studies. 2007;16(2):121-37.

Glaser G. Her best-kept secret: Why Women Drink- and How They can Regain Control. Simon and Schuster; 2014.

Hall W, Degenhardt L. Prevalence and correlates of cannabis use in developed and developing countries. Curr Opin Psychiatry. 2007;20(4):393-7.

Henggeler SW, Clingempeel WG, Brondino MJ, Pickrel SG. Four-year follow-up of multisystemic therapy with substance-abusing and substance-dependent juvenile offenders. J Am Acad Child Adolesc Psychiatry. 2002;41(7):868-74.

Henggeler SW, Schoenwald SK, Borduin CM, Rowland MD, Cunningham PB. Multisystemic Therapy for Antisocial Behavior in Children and Adolescents. Guilford Press; New York. 2009.

Heyes C. Automatic imitation. Psychol Bulletin. 2011;137(3):463–83.

Horyniak D, Melo JS, Farrell RM, Ojeda VD, Strathdee SA. Epidemiology of substance use among forced migrants: a global systematic review. PLoS ONE. 2016;11(7):e0159134.

Huey Jr SJ, Polo AJ. Evidence-based psychosocial treatments for ethnic minority youth. J Clin Child Adolescent Psychol. 2008;37(1):262-301.

Hurd NM, Varner FA, Caldwell CH, Zimmerman MA. Does perceived racial discrimination predict changes in psychological distress and substance use over time? An examination among Black emerging adults. Dev Psychol. 2014;50(7):1910-8.

Jernigan D. The global alcohol industry: an overview. Addiction 2009;104(Suppl. 1):6e12.

Jones TM, Hill KG, Epstein M, Lee JO, Hawkins JD, Catalano RF. Understanding the interplay of individual and social–developmental factors in the progression of substance use and mental health from childhood to adulthood. Dev Psychopath. 2016;28(3):721-41.

Kelly JF. Is Alcoholics Anonymous religious, spiritual, neither? Findings from 25 years of mechanisms of behavior change research. Addiction. 2017;112(6):929-36.

Khalsa SB, Khalsa GS, Khalsa HK, Khalsa MK. Evaluation of a residential Kundalini yoga lifestyle pilot program for addiction in India. J Ethn Subs Abuse. 2008;7(1):67-79.

Kim-Spoon J, McCullough ME, Bickel WK, Farley JP, Longo GS. Longitudinal associations among religiousness, delay discounting, and substance use initiation in early adolescence. J Res Adolesc. 2015;25(1):36-43.

Kimbro RT. Acculturation in context: Gender, age at migration, neighborhood ethnicity, and health behaviors. Soc Sci Q. 2009;90(5):1145-66.

Kwan M, Bobko S, Faulkner G, Donnelly P, Cairney J. Sport participation and alcohol and illicit drug use in adolescents and young adults: A systematic review of longitudinal studies. Addict Behav. 2014 Mar 31;39(3):497-506.

Leslie EM, Cherney A, Smirnov A, Wells H, Kemp R, Najman JM. Willingness to cooperate with police: A population-based study of Australian young adult illicit stimulant users. Criminol Crim Justice. 2017;17(3):301-18.

Link BG, Yang LH, Phelan JC, Collins PY. Measuring mental illness stigma. Schizophr Bull. 2004;30(3):511-41.

Luk JW, Emery RL, Karyadi KA, Patock-Peckham JA, King KM. Religiosity and substance use among Asian American college students: Moderated effects of race and acculturation. Drug Alcohol Depend. 2013;130(1):142-9.

Luoma JB, Twohig MP, Waltz T, et al. An investigation of stigma in individuals receiving treatment for substance abuse. Addict Behav. 2007;32(7):1331-46.

Malik K, Benegal V, Murthy P, Chand P, Arun K, Suman LN. Clinical audit of women with substance use disorders: findings and implications. Indian J Psychol Med. 2015;37(2):195-200.

Malivert M, Fatséas M, Denis C, Langlois E, Auriacombe M. Effectiveness of therapeutic communities: a systematic review. Eur Addic Res. 2012;18(1):1-11.

Mattoo SK, Sarkar S, Gupta S, Nebhinani N, Parakh P, Basu D. Stigma towards substance use: comparing treatment seeking alcohol and opioid dependent men. Int J Mental Health Addic. 2015;13(1):73-81.

Mattoo SK, Sarkar S, Nebhinani N, Gupta S, Parakh P, Basu D. How do Indian substance users perceive stigma towards substance use vis-à-vis their family members? J Ethn Subst Abuse. 2015;14(3): 223-31.

McGarvey EL, Leon-Verdin M, Bloomfield K, et al. Effectiveness of A-CRA/ACC in treating adolescents with cannabis-use disorders. Community Ment Health J. 2014;50(2):150-7.

Mohapatra S, Patra J, Popova S, et al. Social cost of heavy drinking and alcohol dependence in high-income countries. Int J public Health. 2010;55(3):149-57.

Murthy P. (2008). Women and Drug Use in India: Substance, Women and High-Risk Assessment Study. United Nations Office on Drugs and Crime, Ministry of Social Justice and Empowerment, United Nations Development Fund for Women. [Online] Available from http://www.unodc.org/documents/southasia/reports/UNODC_Book_Women_and _Drug_Use_in_India_2008pdf [Accessed January 2018].

Nakamura K, Tanaka A, Takano T. The social cost of alcohol abuse in Japan. J Stud Alcohol. 1993;54(5): 618-25.

National family health survey (NFHS-4) 2012–14. Mumbai: International Institute for Population Sciences (IIPS) and Macro International; 2010. [Accessed January 2018].

Nebhinani N, Sarkar S, Gupta S, et al. Demographic and clinical profile of substance abusing women seeking treatment at a de-addiction center in north India. Ind J Psychiatry. 2013;22(1):12-6.

Orford J, Velleman R, Natera G, et al. Addiction in the family is a major but neglected contributor to the global burden of adult ill-health. Soc Sci Med. 2013;78:70-7.

Pampel FC, Mollborn S, Lawrence EM. Life course transitions in early adulthood and SES disparities in tobacco use. Soc Sci Res. 2014;43:45-59.

Panebianco D, Gallupe O, Carrington PJ, et al. Personal support networks, social capital, and risk of relapse among individuals treated for substance use issues. Int J Drug Policy. 2016;27:146-53.

Patrick ME, Miech RA, Carlier C, et al. Self-reported reasons for vaping among 8th, 10th, and 12th graders in the US: nationally-representative results. Drug Alcohol Depend. 2016;165:275-8.

Pavarin RM, Pavarin RM, Emiliani F, et al. Risky consumption, reasons for use, migratory status and normalization: the results of an Italian study on minors aged between 13 and 16. Int J Migration Health Soc Care. 2016;12(4):264-77.

Rao TS, Kuruvilla K. A study on the coping behaviors of wives of alcoholics. Indian J Psychiatry. 1992;34(4):359-65.

Ray R. The Extent, Pattern and Trends of Drug Abuse in India, National Survey, Ministry of Social Justice and Empowerment, Government of India and United Nations Office on Drugs and Crime, Regional Office For South Asia, 2004.

Rodriguez LM, Neighbors C, Knee CR. Problematic alcohol use and marital distress: An interdependence theory perspective. Addiction Res Theory. 2014;22(4):294-312.

Schinke SP, Fang L, Cole KCA. Substance Use among Early Adolescent Girls: Risk and Protective Factors. J Adolesc Health. 2008;43(2):191-4.

Shi Y, Lenzi M, An R. Cannabis liberalization and adolescent cannabis use: a cross-national study in 38 countries. PloS One. 2015;10(11):e0143562.

Sielski CL. Women, Girls, and Addiction. Celebrating the Feminine in Counseling Treatment and Recovery, by Cynthia A. Briggs and Jennifer L. Pepperell. J Soc Work Pract Addictions. 2011;11(3):287-9.

Singer M. Drugs and development. The global impact of drug use and trafficking on social and economic development. Int J Drug Policy. 2008;19(6):467-78.

Smith JE, Meyers RJ, Miller WR. The community reinforcement approach to the treatment of substance use disorders. Am J Addict. 2001;10(suppl):51-9.

Smith, JE, Meyers RJ. The community reinforcement approach, 1995.

Suresh Kumar PN, Thomas B. Family intervention therapy in alcohol dependence syndrome: One-year follow-up study. Indian J Psychiatry. 2007;49(3):200-4.

Tam FW, Zhou H, Harel-Fisch Y. Hidden school disengagement and its relationship to youth risk behaviors: A cross-sectional study in China. Int J Educ. 2012;4(2):87.

Trapl ES, Yoder LD, Frank JL, et al. Individual, parental, and environmental correlates of cigar, cigarillo, and little cigar use among middle school adolescents. Nicotine Tob Res. 2015;18(5):834-41.

UKATT Research Team. Effectiveness of treatment for alcohol problems: findings of the randomized UK alcohol treatment trial (UKATT). BMJ. 2005;331(7516):541.

United Nations Office on Drugs and Crime. World Drug Report 2016 (Vol. 1). United Nations Publications, 2016.

United Nations Office on Drugs and Crime. World Drug Report 2017 (Vol. 1). United Nations Publications, 2017.

Vanassche S, Sodermans AK, Matthijs K, et al. The effects of family type, family relationships and parental role models on delinquency and alcohol use among Flemish adolescents. J Child Family Stud. 2014;23(1):128-43.

Vanderplasschen W, Colpaert K, Autrique M, et al. Therapeutic communities for addictions: a review of their effectiveness from a recovery-oriented perspective. Scientific World Journal. 2013;(15):427817.

Wagner FA, Anthony JC. Male–female differences in the risk of progression from first use to dependence upon cannabis, cocaine, and alcohol. Drug Alcohol Depend. 2007;86(2):191-8.

World Health Organization. Management of Substance Abuse Unit. Global status report on alcohol and health. World Health Organization; 2014.

Yang XY. How community-level social and economic developments have changed the patterns of substance use in a transition economy? Health Place. 2017;46:91-100.

Chapter 23

Psychosexual Disorders: Social Perspective

*Abhinav Tandon, TS Sathyanarayan Rao, Shivanand Manohar,
Manju George, Suhas Chandran, Shreemit Maheshwari*

SUMMARY

Sexual health is an important component of health and well being. Sexual health has been an area of neglect for long by health professionals and patients alike, either due to incomplete assessment by the clinicians or due to hesitation shown by the patients. Social psychiatry deals with interpersonal and cultural context of mental health and its associated problems, and thus can play a crucial role in improving sexual health and ameliorating psychosexual disorders. This chapter takes a look at the various aspects of psychosexual disorders from a social psychiatry perspective.

INTRODUCTION

The World Psychiatric Association has defined sexual health as "a dynamic and harmonious state involving erotic and reproductive experiences and fulfilment, within a broader physical, emotional, interpersonal, social, and spiritual sense of well-being, in a culturally informed, freely and responsibly chosen and ethical framework, and not merely the absence of sexual disorders" (Mezzich & Hernandez-Serrano, 2006). Sexual health has been an area of neglect for long by health professionals and patients alike, either due to incomplete assessment by the clinicians or due to hesitation shown by the patients. Social psychiatry deals with interpersonal and cultural context of mental health and its associated problems; by adopting an educative approach, it can help in promotion of mental health and prevention of mental illness. Sexual dysfunctions are strongly influenced by relationships and get flavored by cultural aspects of the society. Strong cultural beliefs may lead to anxiety and influence sexual performance of an individual. Social expectations from the female population may also contribute to sexual dysfunction.

However, there has been a lot of debate on what constitutes "normal" or healthy sexual behavior. Considering a patient centered approach, a sexual problem is said to exist if an individual presents with behavioral, cognitive, or emotional problems associated with sexual functioning. In 1966, Masters and Johnson described the EPOR (Excitement, Plateau, Orgasmic and Resolution phases) Model of sexual response cycle. Kaplan elaborated the DEOR [Desire, Excitement (Arousal), Orgasm and Resolution phases] Model (Avasthi et al., 2006). "Sexual dysfunction was referred to a problem during any phase of the sexual response cycle that prevents the individual or couple from experiencing satisfaction from the sexual activity" (Avasthi et al., 2006). The term "psychosexual", as described by Merriam-Webster dictionary, describes the mental, behavioral, and emotional aspects of sexual development. It suggests that the individual's personality development is influenced by his/her sexuality. It is not defined in the same way as libido was by Freud. Four factors are included in sexuality, viz., sexual orientation, sexual behavior, sexual identity, and gender identity (Sadock, 2009).

Sexual dysfunctions as defined by DSM-5 are "a heterogeneous group of disorders that are typically characterized by a clinically significant disturbance in a person's ability to respond sexually or to sexual pleasure". The dysfunctions are divided into subtypes based on the time of acquiring the dysfunction (lifelong vs. acquired) and the situations of expression (generalized vs. situational) (Bhugra & DeSilva, 1993; American Psychiatric Association, 2013).

EPIDEMIOLOGY AND ETIOLOGY

The frequency of reporting and seeking help for sexual problems is strongly influenced by social and cultural factors; hence, many epidemiological studies may have unknowingly under reported sexual dysfunctions. In 1970, Masters and Johnson concluded that sexual problems exist in 50% of all Americans during some point in their lifetime (Hatzichristou et al., 2004; Avasthi et al., 2006; Sadock, 2009). A Southeast Asian study done in Chandigarh, India in 1977, found sexual problems to be present in 10% males attending OPD (psychiatry and medical) (Nakra et al., 1977). A 2-year retrospective study of psychiatric OPDs of a general hospital and private clinic revealed that 50% of the patients had *Dhat* syndrome while the follow-up attendance was poor in majority of the cases. A study done in Beijing, China on 6000 women concluded that female sexual problems are highly prevalent in Beijing. This was associated with dissatisfaction of the individuals with the spouse's sexual ability and poor marital relationship. Not satisfied with one's marriage, rural life, chronic pelvic pain, and postmenopausal status are other factors associated with female sexual dysfunction (Lou et al., 2017). A few of the epidemiological studies have been briefed in **Table 1**.

In the study done by Rao and colleagues in South India (Suttur village) among males, erectile dysfunction was the most common disorder, whereas arousal disorder was the most common female dysfunction noted, implicating that biology plays an important role in men,

Table 1: Epidemiological studies of sexual dysfunction	
Rao and colleagues in South India: Suttur village (above 60 years and sexually active) (Rao et al., 2015)	• Prevalence: female hypoactive sexual desire disorder – 16% • Female sexual arousal dysfunction – 28%, female anorgasmia – 20% • Dyspareunia -8% • 43.5% of the male subjects had erectile dysfunction • 10.9% premature ejaculation • 0.77% male hypoactive sexual desire disorder • 0.38% male anorgasmia
Singh and colleagues (cross-sectional survey; 149 married women; medical outpatient clinic of a tertiary care hospital) (Singh et al., 2009)	• Female sexual dysfunction – 73.2% • Difficulties with desire – 77.2% • Arousal problems – 91.3% • Lubrication problem – 96.6% • Orgasmic problems – 86.6% • Dissatisfaction – 81.2% • Pain – 64.4%

whereas psychology plays an important role in women with respect to sexual functioning (Rao et al., 2015).

Important postulations reported by various authors for being associated with sexual dysfunction include ignorance, superstitions, and guilt feelings (Bagadia et al., 1959). The most common sexual worries amongst the unmarried group included nocturnal emission (65%), and passing semen in urine (47%). On the other hand, impotence (48%), premature ejaculation (43%), and passing semen in urine (47%) were the common complaints amongst married males (Bagadia et al., 1972). The common psychiatric diagnosis included anxiety (57%), schizophrenia (16%) and reactive depression (16%) (Bagadia et al., 1972). Nakra and colleagues studied male population in a hospital in Chandigarh, and reported that 10% males had sexual complaints (Nakra et al., 1977). A retrospective analysis of 1242 patient records from 1979 to 2005 reported that premature ejaculation was the most common complaint by the patients and the most common diagnosis made by the clinicians in marriage and sex clinic, which was followed by erectile problems and *Dhat* syndrome (Kendurkar et al., 2008).

Avasthi et al. (2008), interviewed 100 women attending pediatrics outpatient department for the care of their children and concluded that 17% of the subjects encountered difficulties during sexual activity including painful intercourse (7%), difficulty in reaching orgasm (9%), lack of vaginal lubrication (5%), vaginal tightness (5%), bleeding after intercourse (3%), and vaginal infection (2%).

ETIOLOGY OF SEXUAL DISORDERS

Human sexual response is a complex phenomenon and therefore sexual dysfunctions are of multifactorial origin and involve biological and psychosocial factors. Masters and Johnson in 1970 described a two-tier model for etiology of sexual dysfunction **(Table 2)**. **Table 3** gives an overview of the etiology of sexual dysfunctions (Avasthi et al., 2006; Fazio & Brock, 2004; Levine, 2000; Butcher., 1999a; Swerdloff & Kandeel, 1992). Significant associations were found between problems of sexual desire, arousal, and pain with decreased physical, emotional and overall life satisfaction, and arousal dysfunction in females was particularly predicted by poor relationship as well as overall life satisfaction (Laumann et al., 1999).

Sexual learning and psychological factors: Childhood is the time when sexual learning begins through child-parent interaction reinforcing or discouraging gender-associated activities. Genital self-stimulation is considered to be a normal activity of babies between 15 and 19 months of age. Abusive incidents may negatively affect sexual learning dwuring

Table 2: Masters and Johnson (1970) two-tier model for etiology of sexual dysfunction

1. Immediate causes
   - Performance fear
   - Adoption of spectator role
   - Observer vs. participant

2. Distal (historical) causes
   - Sociocultural
   - Biological
   - Sexual trauma
   - Homosexual orientation

Table 3: Etiology of sexual disorders

Psychological factors	Depression/anxiety Performance pressure/monotonous routine Poor self-esteem/rigid attitude/negative thoughts Lack of privacy Relationship issues
Physical factors	Cardiovascular morbidity, diabetes, vascular insufficiency, penile disease Neurological problems, urogenital disorders, endocrinal disorders Alcohol/smoking Drugs
Sociocultural factors	Conflict with religious, personal or family values Societal taboos

childhood. Sex play during early adolescence may include experiments among the same sex for a short period. Establishing a sexual identity in adolescence is a conflicting process and controlling sexual impulses produces a physiological sexual tension, which is released by masturbation as a part of normal sexual development. In adolescence, the body image is more firmly established and sexual desire begins to develop. Peer acceptance forms an important part and experimenting with a partner or partners is part of the normal learning process. Association between traumatic sexual experiences in early childhood and sexual and relationship preferences in later adulthood has been found. In adults, a mature sexual relationship includes strong bonding, intimacy, and love for one's partner (Sadock, 2009). Sexual desire constitutes three interactive components, which include sexual drive (biological component), sexual motivation (psychological component), and sexual wish (social component). Psychological factors such as body image disturbances, intimacy, knowledge about sexual needs of partner and self-esteem have an impact on sexual functioning (Levine, 2003). Drugs leading to sexual dysfunction in males and females are mentioned in **Table 4**.

OTHER SEXUAL DISORDERS/DYSFUNCTIONS IN INDIAN CONTEXT

The nosological systems don't include all sexual disorders which are influenced by culture and commonly seen in the Indian subcontinent. Indian researchers have consistently found

Table 4: Drugs leading to sexual dysfunction

Males	*Females*
Antihypertensive medications: Diuretics, beta blockers **Antiandrogenic:** Digoxin, H2 blockers **Others:** Alcohol, ketoconazole, phenytoin/other antiepileptics **Psychotropics:** Antipsychotics, antidepressants, benzodiazepines	**Antihypertensive medications:** Diuretics, beta blockers, calcium channel blockers **Psychotropics:** Antipsychotics, antidepressants, benzodiazepines, buspirone, lithium **Other Drugs:** Digoxin, histamine H2-receptor blockers, alcohol, ketoconazole, phenobarbital/other antiepileptics, GnRH agonists, OCPs

GnRH, gonadotropin-releasing hormone; OCPs, oral contraceptive pills.

certain sexual clinical conditions such as, *Dhat syndrome* and *apprehension about potency*. *Dhat syndrome* finds mention in ICD-10 under other neurotic disorders (F48.8) category whereas the diagnosis of apprehension about potency does not find mention.

Dhat syndrome (first described in 1960) refers to a clinical condition which is culture bound and characterized by guilt about loss of semen particularly in young men. This is associated with excessive concern with loss of semen causing a debilitating effect on physical and psychological health. There is subjective reporting of loss of semen during micturition or while straining to pass stools, with no evidence regarding the same. Patient presents with vague and multiple somatic complaints, pain, generalized fatiguability, poor memory, anxiety, or depressive symptoms (Wig, 1960).

DIAGNOSTIC EVALUATION AND TREATMENT ISSUES

A patient-centered approach should be followed for evaluation and treatment. Privacy should be maintained during assessment with focus on medical, sexual, and psychosocial history. A strong rapport, non-judgemental attitude, and comfort of the patient should be the focus while taking history which in majority of cases is a very sensitive issue for the patient.

Sexual History

A comprehensive sexual history along with an evaluation of the patient's current sexual functioning should be recorded. Issues related to maintaining confidentiality should be addressed. Some of the key information to be obtained while taking the history includes stressors if any, duration of the problem, whether problem is specific to any time, place or partner, decrease or loss in sexual drive, decreased interest in sexual contact, problems in relationship, physical complaints like pain, weakness, and psychiatric symptoms like anxiety or depression (Tomlinson, 1998). Some important questions for males/females are mentioned in **Table 5** (Butcher, 1999a; Gregoire, 1999; Kandeel et al., 2001; Basson et al., 2004; Lue et al., 2004; Avasthi et al., 2006).

It is important to take into account the fact that women play different roles at different times in their lives like professional, daughter, wife, and mother. While playing different roles, a woman has to devote time to her family, her work, as well as extended family (parents and relations). Apart from that, social time, personal time, and relationship time spent with the partner during different phases of life is helpful in evaluating sexual problems (Butcher, 1999a; Butcher, 1999b).

Table 5: Important questions to be asked in males/females	
Males	*Females*
• Interest in sexual activity, fantasy, sex drive • Performance problems; initiation and maintenance of erection; partner specific erection problems; loss of erection before penetration • Ejaculation, orgasm, satisfaction	• Interest in sexual activity, fantasy, sex drive • Arousal, performance problems • Orgasm, satisfaction, stimulation (with partner/masturbation) • Pain (during penetration or thrusting, duration; during riding bicycle, touching)

Treatment

The psychological treatment steps are common for most of the disorders. Further specific behavioural measures for the specific disorders are usually based on the type of disorder.

Assessment and treatment gets channelized depending on one's specialty and the type of the problem encountered by the client. Intensive therapy involves primarily sensitization and desensitization techniques (Hawton, 1989; Hengeveld, 1991). The general principles of treatment are applicable to most of the inadequacies which needs to be tailored further depending upon the type of problem. During sex therapy, therapeutic involvement of the partner is an important determinant of the outcome of treatment. Therapy should de-emphasize blaming of oneself or one's partner. Sex is something a man and woman do together and cannot proceed if one of the partners is not dedicated during the act. It can be a form of intimate interpersonal communication which also benefits the relationship in general (Avasthi & Banerjee, 2002). Annon (1974) proposed a graded intervention popularly called as PLISSIT Model **(Figure 1)** (Meuleman et al., 1995). Sensate focus exercises include structured exercises of 3–5 sessions, assigned between the visits. These help the couple to recognize the fact that sexual activity is not limited to sexual intercourse; the couple can enjoy through "Pleasuring" and "Receiving Pleasure" without it being regarded as foreplay or a preliminary to sexual intercourse. Slow progress is made from nondemanding pleasure (i.e. pleasing to explore one's own feelings about the experience) from non-genital areas to breasts and then to penile pleasure (American Urological Association, 1996). Systematic sensitization and desensitization is a technique particularly helpful for premature ejaculation. "Start-Stop Sensitization" technique can be used by the partner to provide manual stimulation to the male; the partner stops at a signal from him when orgasm becomes imminent. This exercise is repeated. After some degree of control is achieved, partners should try intravaginal containment, usually in

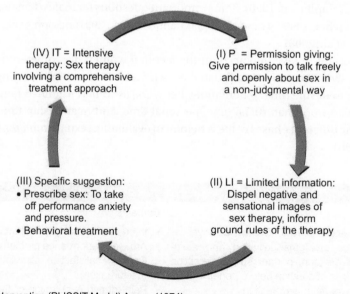

(IV) IT = Intensive therapy: Sex therapy involving a comprehensive treatment approach

(I) P = Permission giving: Give permission to talk freely and openly about sex in a non-judgmental way

(III) Specific suggestion:
• Prescribe sex: To take off performance anxiety and pressure.
• Behavioral treatment

(II) LI = Limited information: Dispel negative and sensational images of sex therapy, inform ground rules of the therapy

Figure 1: Graded intervention (PLISSIT Model) Annon (1974)

female superior position. Partner is advised to increase the rhythmic movements until the man gives the signal to stop. The activity is stopped and then restarted again; with time the couple learns how to prolong the pleasure of intercourse while containing the urge to ejaculate (Guiliano et al., 1997). Similar techniques of desensitization and sensitization can be utilized in treating psychogenic erectile and orgasmic dysfunctions in men and arousal and orgasmic dysfunctions in women. With progressive stimulation of clitoris and other genital areas by partner, arousal is experienced without demand or pressure of intercourse.

SOME OTHER SEXUAL ISSUES

A brief account about homosexuality, gender dysphoria, and paraphilia is included here.

Homosexuality has gradually come to be considered as a variation of sexual activity rather than deviation. It is a component of identity that includes a person's sexual and emotional attraction to another person and the behavior and/or social affiliation that may result from this attraction. Sexual orientation categories are broadly divided into: (i) gay men or lesbian women (i.e. attraction to members of one's own sex), (ii) heterosexuals (i.e. attraction to members of the other sex), and (iii) bisexuals (i.e. attraction to members of both sexes). A number of people identify their sexual orientation as queer or pansexual (i.e. sexual orientation lying outside of the gender bifurcation of "male" and "female" only). It has been postulated in the recent research that sexual orientation is not categorical in its definition, but occurs on a continuum. Sexual orientation has been suggested to be fluid for some people especially women.

For some individuals, the lived role in society cannot be attributed to the biological characteristics of the individual. Hence the term "gender" was introduced. Gender is defined as the role lived by the individual in the society as a boy or a man and a girl or a woman. If a person feels discontent with his/her "assigned" gender both at the emotional as well as the cognitive level, it is termed as **gender dysphoria**. The affected person experiences incongruence between one's expressed (which is experienced by the person) and one's assigned (which is perceived by the society) gender. Another reason for this distress is unavailability of options for therapies at physical level to match assigned gender to expressed gender, e.g. hormonal or surgical interventions. The change brought in DSM-5 from DSM-IV was changing the term from "gender identity disorder" to "gender dysphoria". as the latter is a more descriptive term emphasizing on the dysphoria rather than identity problem. Gender dysphoria in children has to be differentiated from that in adults. Any of the following six symptoms should be present for 6 months for making a diagnosis in children (including criterion i): (i) desire to be of the other gender, (ii) cross-dressing, (iii/iv) cross gender fantasy or play, (v) cross gender playmates, (vi) rejection of toys, games or activities of his/her assigned gender, (vii) dislike of anatomy, (viii) desire to have other sex characteristics. For diagnosing gender dysphoria in adults/adolescents, any of the following two symptoms should be present for 6 months: (i) incongruence between gender identity and primary/ secondary sex characteristics, (ii/iii) wish or desire to have sex characteristics of the other gender, or to change one's own to the other (iv/v) desire to be of the other gender and desire to be treated as other gender, and (vi) convinced about having the feelings of the other gender.

As per DSM-5 "The term *paraphilia* denotes any intense and persistent sexual interest other than sexual interest in genital stimulation or preparatory fondling with phenotypically normal, physically mature, consenting human partners." Often, in persons who are elderly, or medically ill, the criteria of "intense and persistent" may be difficult to apply. Hence in such cases, any kind of sexual interest which is greater than or equal to normophilic sexual interests, the term "paraphilia" may be applied. When paraphilia causes distress to the individual whether or not associated with harm to self or others, it is termed as "**paraphilic disorder**". While paraphilia in itself is not sufficient to diagnose paraphilic disorder and per se does not require any clinical intervention, it is a necessary condition for diagnosing paraphilic disorder.

CONCLUSION

From a patient centered approach, a sexual problem occurs when an individual presents with behavioral, cognitive, or emotional problems associated with sexual functioning. A substantial number of individuals suffer from psychosexual problems during their lifetimes, though many a times it is not reported and treatment is not sought. The types and relative frequencies of psychoseuxal problems differ between the two genders. Cultural aspects play a role in expression and genesis of psychosexual problems as well, as exemplified by the occurrence of Dhat syndrome in the Indian subcontinent. Sexual problems can have diverse etiology and the treatment is often directed at the underlying cause. Variations do occur in sexual expression and affiliation, though it falls under the purview of psychiatry only when it causes significant distress.

REFERENCES

American Psychiatric Association (APA). Diagnostic and Statistical Manual of Mental Disorders, 5th edition: DSM-5. Washington DC: American Psychiatric Publishing; 2013.

American Urological Association. Erectile Dysfunction. Clinical Guidelines Panel. Treatment of Organic Clinical Practice Guidelines, 1996.

Anastasiadis AG, Salomon L, Ghafar MA, et al. Female sexual dysfunction: State of the art. Curr Urol Rep. 2002;3:484-91.

Avasthi A, Banerjee ST. Guidebook on sex education. Marital and Psychosexual Clinic; Chandigarh: 2002.

Avasthi A, Kaur R, Prakash O, et al. Sexual behavior of married young women: A preliminary study from north India. Indian J Community Med. 2008;33(3):163-7.

Avasthi A, Rao TSS, Grover S, et al. Clinical practice guidelines for management of sexual dysfunctions. In: Gautham S, Avasthi A. Clinical practice guidelines for management of substance abuse disorders, sexual dysfunctions and sleep disorders. India: Indian Psychiatric Society; 2006. pp 144-32.

Bagadia VN, Dave KP, Pradhan PV, et al. Study of 258 male patients with sexual problems. Indian J Psychiatry. 1972;14:143-51.

Bagadia VN, Vardhachari KS, Mehta BC, et al. Educational group psychotherapy for certain minor sex disorders of males. Indian J Psychiatry. 1959;1:237-40.

Basson R, Althof S, Davis S, et al. Summary of the recommendations on sexual dysfunctions in women. J Sex Med. 2004;1(1):24-34.

Bhugra D, DeSilva P: Sexual dysfunction across cultures. Int Rev Psychiatry. 1993;5(2-3):243-52.

Butcher J. ABC of sexual health Female sexual problems I: Loss of desire—what about the fun? BMJ. 1999a;318:41-3.

Butcher J. ABC of sexual health Female sexual problems II: Sexual pain and sexual fears. BMJ. 1999b;318:110-2.

Cho MC, Paick JS. Udenafil for the treatment of erectile dysfunction. Ther Clin Risk Manag. 2014;10:341-54.

Fazio L, Brock G. Erectile dysfunction: management update. CMAJ. 2004;170:1429-37.

Gregoire A. ABC of sexual health: Assessing and managing male sexual problems. BMJ. 1999;318:315-7.

Guiliano F, Jardin A, Gingell CJ, et al. Sildenafil (VIAGRA), an oral treatment for erectile dysfunction: a 1-year, open label extension study. Br J Urol. 1997; 80:93.

Hatzichristou D, Rosen RC, Broderick G, et al. Clinical evaluation and management strategy for sexual dysfunction in men and women. J Sex Med. 2004;1:49-57.

Hawton K. Sexual dysfunctions. In: Cognitive Behaviour Therapy for Psychiatric Problems: A Practical Guide. New York: Oxford University Press; 1989.

Hengeveld MW. Erectile dysfunction. In: Jonas U, Thon WF, Stief CG (Eds). Erectile disorders. A psychosexological review. Berlin: Springer-Verlag; 1991. pp 14-22.

Kandeel FR, Koussa VKT, Swerdloff RS. Male sexual function and its disorders: physiology, pathophysiology, clinical investigation, and treatment. Endocr Rev. 2001;22(3):342-88.

Kendurkar A, Kaur B, Agarwal AK, et al. Profile of adult patients attending a marriage and sex clinic in India. Int J Soc Psychiatry. 2008;54(6):486-93.

Laumann EO, Paik A, Rosen RC. Sexual dysfunction in the United States; prevalence and predictors. JAMA. 1999;281(6):537-44.

Levine LA: Diagnosis and Treatment of erectile dysfunction. Am J Med. 2000;109:S3-12.

Levine SB: Sexual Disorders, in Psychiatry. Edited by Tasman A, Kay J, Liberman JA. New Jersey: John Wiley & sons; 2003. p 1475.

Lou WJ, Chen B, Zhu L, et al. Prevalence and factors associated with female sexual dysfunction in Beijing, China. Chin Med J. 2017; 130(12):1389-94.

Lue TF, Giuliano F, Montorsi F, et al: Summary of the recommendations on sexual dysfunctions in men. J Sex Med. 2004; 1:1-23.

Mezzich JE, Serrano RH. Comprehensive definition of sexual health. In: Mezzich JE. Psychiatry and Sexual Health—An Integrated Approach. Lanham, Jason Aronson Inc, 2006, pp 3-13.

Nakra BR, Wig NN, Varma VK. A study of male potency disorders. Indian J Psychiatry. 1977;19:13-8.

Rao TSS, Darshan MS, Tandon A. Sexual disorders among elderly: An epidemiological study in South Indian rural population. Indian J Psychiatry. 2015;57(3):236-41.

Sadock VA. Normal human sexuality and sexual and gender identity disorders. In: Sadock BJ, Sadock VA, Ruiz P. Kaplan and Sadock's Comprehensive Textbook of Psychiatry. New York, Lippincott Williams & Wilkins, 2009, pp 2027-41.

Singh JC, Tharyan P, Kekre NS, et al. Prevalence and risk factors for female sexual dysfunction in women attending a medical clinic in south India. J Postgrad Med. 2009; 55:113-20.

Swerdloff RS, Kandeel FR. Textbook of Internal Medicine. New York: Lippincott Co; 1992.

Tomlinson J. ABC of sexual health: taking a sexual history. BMJ. 1998;317(7172):1573-6.

Van Ahlen H, Piechota HJ, Kias HJ, et al. Opiate antagonistsin erectile dysfunction: a possible new treatment option? Results of a pilot study with naltrexone. Eur Urol. 1995;28:246-50.

Wig N. Problems of mental health in India. J Clin Soc Psychol. 1960;17:48-53.

World Health Organization (WHO). ICD 10 Classification of Mental and Behavioral Disorders: Diagnostic Criteria for Research. Geneva, World Health Organization, 1993.

Yuan J, Zhang R, Yang Z, et al. Comparative effectiveness and safety of oral phosphodiesterase type 5 inhibitors for erectile dysfunction: a systematic review and network meta-analysis. Euro Urol. 2013;63(5):902-12.

Chapter 24

Sociocultural Dimensions of Personality Disorders

Pratap Sharan, Saurabh Kumar

SUMMARY

Personality disorders have complex multifactorial etiology with social and cultural factors playing a significant role in their genesis. The prevalence and manifestations of personality disorders varies across different countries emphasizing the need for cross-cultural studies to understand these differences. The chapter describes various sociocultural factors that impact the development of personality disorders. The chapter also underscores the need to take a multipronged approach to protect children from various forms of maltreatment, as a prevention strategy against the development of personality disorders. Important social dimensions like violence in the context of personality disorders and stigma faced by individuals with personality disorders has also been discussed. Sociocultural issues in relation to assessment and treatment of personality disorders are also mentioned.

INTRODUCTION

Personality disorders are of significant public health importance as they are relatively common, but often unrecognized in different clinical settings. It leads to adverse social outcomes comparable to other mental disorders. Patients suffering from personality disorders are known to have higher rates of separation and divorce, difficulty in keeping their jobs and poorer quality of life (Sharan, 2010).

Personality disorders have complex multifactorial etiology with social and cultural factors playing a significant role in their genesis (Paris, 1998). The different personality characteristics and behavioral patterns can only be assessed in proper societal context, and existence of relatively culture independent personality traits is questionable (Church, 2000). In this chapter, we will discuss various cross-cultural issues related with personality disorders. The chapter will also focus on maltreatment experienced by children, as it is considered to be an important risk factor for development of personality disorders. Important social dimensions like violence in context of personality disorders and stigma faced by individuals with personality disorders will also be addressed.

CROSS-CULTURAL EPIDEMIOLOGY

The understanding of personality largely depends upon how a certain society or culture views any behavior. Different researchers have tried to study universality of the personality construct.

Cross-national studies suggest that the Three Factor Model of Eysenck (Eysenck, 1982) and Five Factor Model (Costa & Widiger, 1994) were invariant across cultures. However, these studies have mostly utilized western concepts in different cultural settings. As a result, they do not establish the cross-cultural validity or usefulness of the Western diagnostic categories or personality dimensions (Lewis-Fernández & Kleinman, 1994). It should be remembered that personality and personality disorders are relatively recent Western concepts [the present understanding crystallized in the 1920s according to Berrios (1993)]. They are still foreign to other cultures (Tang & Huang, 1995). Cultural studies help researchers in understanding the effect of various individual and ecological factors on personality and in mitigating the various cultural stereotypes. Appreciating the cultural backdrop of a particular behavior will provide better understanding of consistency and coherence in individual differences and patterns of personality. It will enable the various stake holders in better understanding and managing the cultural diversity that characterizes our society (Benet-Martinez, 2007).

Epidemiology

There is limited number of studies available comparing the cross national prevalence and correlates of personality disorders. Most of the studies are from Western countries where prevalence estimates for any personality disorder range from 3.9 to 15.7% (Huang et al., 2009). The studies are limited by having small sample sizes and nonrepresentative study population. This hampers cross-cultural comparison of various facets of personality disorders.

Though not an epidemiological study, the International Pilot Study of Personality Disorders assessed personality disorders in multiple countries around the world utilizing the International Personality Disorder Examination (IPDE) (Loranger et al., 1994). The authors found that majority of personality disorder subtypes were diagnosed in most countries. The exceptions were India where no diagnosis of avoidant personality disorder were made and Kenya where borderline personality disorder were not diagnosed. In a recent study using IPDE screen across 13 different countries, cluster A personality disorders were found to be most prevalent whereas cluster B personality disorders were least prevalent (Huang et al., 2009). The prevalence estimates for any personality disorder were lowest in Western Europe (2.4%) and Nigeria (2.7%) and were highest in Colombia (7.9%) and the USA (7.6%). The authors proposed several reasons for this between country differences: lack of validity of IPDE screening questions across different countries, variation in concordance of screening questions with clinical diagnosis in different countries and failure of three cluster models to characterize personality disorders equally in all countries.

Prevalence of individual personality disorders have been shown to vary greatly between different countries. The lifetime prevalence of borderline personality disorder in the USA was found to be 5.9% (Grant et al., 2008), whereas point prevalence rates in European national community samples were around 0.7% (Torgersen et al., 2001). Similarly the most common personality disorder found in the United States and Australia was obsessive-compulsive personality disorder, whereas schizotypal personality disorder was the most common in Iceland (Sansone & Sansone, 2011). These variations indicate that different societal and cultural factors play an important role in manifestation of personality disorders. Rapid social changes and social disintegration resulting in transition from traditional to modern social structures can also explain differences in prevalence of personality disorders in different societies (Paris, 1997). The authors feel that rapid technological development, increased residential mobility, disruption of family systems, and weakening interpersonal ties can result in rising prevalence of personality disorders. This is an interesting idea which needs further evaluation in different settings like India which is witnessing large-scale changes in its societal structure. However, there is limited existing literature on personality disorders in India (Sharan, 2010).

Clinical Features

Western authors have postulated that the lower rates of personality disorders seen in Asian countries could be due to lack of understanding of characteristics of personality disorders in Asian cultural context (Ryder et al., 2014). However, though limited in number, studies conducted in Asia suggest cross-cultural variations in clinical features of personality disorders as a probable reason for difference in identification of personality disorders in different countries. Patients suffering from borderline personality disorder in Japan were more likely to show symptoms of derealization or depersonalization and were less likely to indulge in substance abuse compared to their American counterparts (Moriya et al., 1993). Similarly repeated self-injurious behaviors seen in persons with borderline personality disorder is more frequent in Western societies (Paris, 2002) where the healthcare systems is highly developed and the behavior can be understood as an effective attempt at "cry for help" (Ziegenbein et al., 2008). In a study in China, it was found that presence of cluster B personality disorders did not confer increased risk of suicide attempts relative to the other clusters (Tong et al., 2016).

SOCIOCULTURAL DETERMINANTS

It is important to take both etic and emic approaches like open-ended clinical interview and ethnographic methods to understand the various social contexts and to test locally generated hypothesis to understand cultural variations in personality (Ryder et al., 2015). But such efforts are few.

Individualism and Collectivism

Individualism and collectivism is a widely used paradigm to understand cultural differences across different societies. Within an individualist society, emphasis is on independence of person from the society, as a result of which priority is given to personal goals, and the behavior of an individual is based on personal attitudes rather than group norms. Conversely, in a collectivist society, preference is given to interdependence and group goals. The behavior of an individual is guided by group norms rather than personal attitudes, and is focused on maintaining relationships with others and avoiding conflicts (Triandis, 2001). The impact of individualism-collectivism on personality could be understood from the different effects, it has on the various determinants of personality. A meta-analysis found that individualism-collectivism has moderate effects on self-concept and relationality, and large effects on attribution and cognitive style (Oyserman et al., 2002). Although the concept of individualism-collectivism appears to have profound influence on expression of personality psychopathology across cultures, there have been a limited number of studies to examine this relationship (Mulder, 2012).

Childhood Maltreatment

Child abuse or neglect is a significant global problem with almost forty million children between age group 0–14 years suffering from it. The various societal risk factors for childhood maltreatment are: lack of adequate housing or services to support families and institutions; high levels of unemployment or poverty; easy availability of alcohol and drugs, and child prostitution and labor (World Health Organization, 2017). It is well documented that exposure to childhood adversities poses a significant risk factor for development of personality disorders. Empirical research has identified a great degree of social dysfunction in the families of the individuals who are diagnosed with personality disorders (Paris, 1998). In a longitudinal study, almost three-quarters of the individuals with personality disorder reported both neglect and abuse (Battle et al., 2004). The study also found that amongst all personality disorders, borderline personality disorder was most commonly associated with childhood maltreatment. Another longitudinal study showed that childhood emotional, physical, and supervision neglect were associated with elevated rates of personality disorders in early adulthood. Emotional neglect was associated with increased risk of avoidant personality disorder whereas physical neglect was associated with schizotypal personality disorder. Childhood supervision neglect was associated with increased risk for passive-aggressive and cluster B personality disorders (Johnson et al., 2000). Both physical as well as sexual abuse and emotional neglect are significantly associated with wide array of personality disorders (Tyrka et al., 2009). Studies have shown that children who are at risk of maltreatment develop fewer secure and more disorganized patterns of attachment than children living in low-risk families (Cyr et al., 2010).

Given the intricate relationship between child abuse and personality disorders, a multipronged approach needs to be taken to address this risk factor. In a systematic review, it was found that several interventions like home visiting, parent education, and multi-component programs have the highest evidence in preventing child maltreatment (Mikton & Butchart, 2009). Studies have also shown that programs that target maltreating families rather than at-risk families and those with at least moderate number of sessions (16–30) were more effective (Euser et al., 2015). A problem with literature on interventions is that there is very little evidence from low- and middle-income countries; making up only 0.6% of the total evidence base (Mikton & Butchart, 2009).

SOCIOCULTURAL CONSEQUENCES

Violence

Personality disorders have been shown to have close association with violence. There is higher prevalence of personality disorders in offenders and individuals convicted especially for violent offences (Logan & Johnstone, 2010). A recent meta-analysis found that there was three-fold increased risk of violence in individuals with personality disorders when compared with general population (Yu et al., 2012). The study also highlighted the increased probability of repeat offences by offenders with personality disorders. It is difficult to establish the temporal precedence of personality disorder to the risk of violence and to rule out any alternative explanation or the role of other/third variables like substance use in causing violence (Duggan & Howard, 2009). Evidence suggests that certain intrapersonal factors like emotional impulsiveness, psychopathy, and delusional ideation provide a link between personality disorders and violence (Howard, 2015).

Some form of violence like domestic violence poses special risk as it is mostly hidden and occurs in relationships which are expected to provide protection and care (Fountoulakis et al., 2008). There is wide variation in lifetime prevalence rates of domestic violence in different regions, e.g. the rates varied from 1.9% in Washington to 70% in Hispanic Latinas in Southeast United States (Alhabib et al., 2010). The geographical bias in prevalence studies for domestic violence is obvious with more than 60% of the studies coming from North America and Europe. The National Family Health Survey done in India shows more than one-third of women experiencing domestic violence (International Institute for Population Sciences (IIPS) and Macro International, 2017).

In a study examining the prevalence of personality disorders amongst men convicted for severe partner violence, more than 85% of the study population had at least one personality disorder. The study also showed that almost 15% of the sample also met the criteria for psychopathy (Fernández & Echeburúa, 2008). Another study found that antisocial batterers when compared with other antisocial offenders had deficient affective experience (Swogger et al., 2007). In a large community sample of United Kingdom, borderline personality disorder was significantly associated with intimate partner violence. Anger and impulsivity features of borderline personality disorder were independently associated with most violent outcomes (González et al., 2016). Individual personality disorders have been shown to be differentially associated with the type of violence; where proactive violence was associated with antisocial personality disorder; and reactive violence was more associated with borderline personality disorders (Ross & Babcock, 2009).

Domestic violence is a public health priority and needs to be addressed. More research is needed in the area to explain how personality characteristics and violence are correlated. One such effort is the use of General Aggression Model to understand the individual variations in propensity of aggression (Gilbert & Daffern, 2011). Such efforts can successfully help in better understanding of the problem, and eventually will help in focusing violence reduction efforts on relevant psychological constructs.

Stigma and Discrimination

Stigma can be described as a sociocultural process in which specific social groups are devalued, rejected, and excluded on the basis of a socially discredited health condition (Weiss et al., 2006). Personality disorders have been found to be highly stigmatizing condition in existing literature (Nehls, 1998; Catthoor et al., 2015). Several studies have reported that the stigma associated with personality disorders is even higher than other mental illnesses (Rüsch et al., 2006; Sheehan et al., 2016). Individuals with borderline personality disorder experience stigma due to various reasons like difficulties in interpersonal relations and presence of visible devaluating signs such as self-mutilation scars (Rüsch et al., 2006). It is felt that the individuals with personality disorders are manipulative and do not want help as they are believed to be purposefully indulging in the problematic behaviors (Aviram et al., 2006). A potential reason for discrimination against individuals with personality disorders could be poor understanding of the disorder by the general public. In a case vignette based study, only 2.3% of respondents were able to correctly identify borderline personality disorder in comparison to 72.5% respondents correctly identifying depressive disorders (Furnham et al., 2015).

The very diagnosis of personality disorder can decrease the empathy of healthcare professionals toward individuals with personality disorders (Gallop et al., 1989). They experience discrimination when they contact health service system for admission during crisis periods. A study also found that the patients with personality disorders have to wait for longer duration when they present to emergency departments with self-harm attempts (Lawn & McMahon, 2015). Another study conducted in Israel showed that psychiatrists and nurses have lesser empathy and more negative attitude towards individuals with borderline personality disorder compared to psychologists and social workers (Bodner et al., 2015).

Young proposed "five faces" of oppression seen in any society (Young, 2009). These include cultural imperialism (in the sense of being pathologized, normalized, and stereotyped), marginalization, powerlessness, exploitation, and violence (psychological and physical). Findings of a qualitative study highlighted that individuals with borderline personality disorder experience four of these (except exploitation) (Bonnington & Rose, 2014). The study also found that patients with personality disorders also experience stigma in healthcare settings. This is a worrisome fact as it can reduce the amount and quality of service and can also dissuade people from seeking and continuing treatment (Sheehan et al., 2016).

Providing education and meaningful interpersonal contact with individuals suffering from mental illness can be effective in reducing the stigma associated with these disorders (Corrigan et al., 2012). There are limited number of studies which have tried to investigate effective anti-stigma interventions specifically for this population. Lack of fund allocation and poor advocacy could be hampering research in this area (Zimmerman, 2015).

SOCIOCULTURAL ISSUES IN ASSESSMENT

Patients with personality disorders do not usually present with complaints directly related to their core disorder but rather with the consequences of their maladaptive relationship patterns with anxiety, depression, marital problems, or drug or alcohol dependence. It is only subsequently that the repetitive self-defeating behavior pattern becomes clear to both the patient, and mental health professional.

Data from World Mental Health Survey has shown that failures and delayed treatment was generally higher in developing countries which could be due to financial and structural barriers in accessing healthcare in these countries (Wang et al., 2007). It is important to consider the role of sociocultural factors in evaluating and managing individuals suffering from personality disorders. In a study, when cultural factors were evaluated in conjugation with the standard diagnostic procedure, more than half of original diagnoses had to be revised (Bäärnhielm et al., 2015).

Assessment Instruments

Most of the assessment instruments in personality evaluation have been developed in Western countries and translated for local use without taking into account possible effects of different cultural contexts. Several studies have shown the limitation of using such approach in personality assessment. In a study conducted in China with an objective to replicate the five-factor model, the five factors that emerged on the use of a lexicon of Chinese trait descriptors, were different from the factors extracted from the Chinese translation of English words from an established five-factor questionnaire (Yang & Bond, 1990). The ICD-10 IPDE was translated into Hindi following a standard translation protocol, and joint rater reliability and applicability of the Hindi version was established in non-psychotic adult outpatients in North Indian Hindi speaking population (Sharan et al., 2002). The authors highlighted several cultural issues faced by them while translating the instrument. The patients found the questions related to self-image, internal preferences, emptiness, and emotional shallowness as most difficult to understand. Further, there were several items which were difficult for the interviewers to rate because of cultural variation in what can be considered a norm. Ethnocentric work of this kind is required before it is assumed that assessment instruments developed in western countries function alike in all cultures.

The pattern of rating any item in an instrument can vary across the cultures. In a Chinese study, it was seen that the participants rated items more at the midpoint. The authors postulated that it could be due to strong norm of moderation and high degree of public self-consciousness (Hamid et al., 2001). When Chinese Minnesota Multiphasic Personality Inventory (MMPI) was applied to normal Chinese participants, it was found that mean scores on several MMPI-2 clinical and content scales were higher than their American counterparts (Cheung et al., 1996; Kwan, 1999). Careful examination of the contents of the MMPI-2 scale suggested differences in the endorsement rate between the two study populations for some of the items in the scale. The social desirability rating of the items indicated that there was difference in how psychopathology was reflected in both cultures. For example, one of the items which was endorsed by most of the Chinese participants was "Most anytime I would rather sit and daydream than do anything else", was also rated as socially desirable indicating that it is not considered as a psychopathology in Chinese culture. These studies suggest that a systematic approach is needed for cross cultural validation of scales (Cheung et al., 2011).

SOCIOCULTURAL FACTORS IN MANAGEMENT OF PERSONALITY DISORDERS

Management of individuals suffering from personality disorders is considered quite challenging as pharmacotherapy has been shown to be of limited value in this subset of patients (Silk, 2015). Specialized forms of psychotherapy like dialectical behavior therapy and mentalization-based treatment have been shown to be effective in large number of patients with personality disorder (Paris, 2015). Sociocultural factors are important determinants of effectiveness of psychotherapy. For example, many researchers have used different concept of self as an organizing construct of personality disorders especially borderline personality disorder (Kerr et al., 2015). The concept of self has been shown to be different in individualistic and collectivist societies. The diversity of beliefs within different cultures and regions makes it mandatory for the therapist to understand the individual patient's perspective. Similarly, cultural factors can also determine the acceptance of any therapeutic modality. Studies have shown that ethnic-minority groups in the UK and US are less likely to accept psychotherapy as treatment modality and drop out of treatment than the majority white population (McGilloway et al., 2010). This could be due to difference in understanding and belief about efficacy of various treatment strategies amongst patients with different cultural background. Therapists should enquire about such beliefs before offering any treatment plan.

The concept of illness and symptom expression is largely affected by cultural beliefs. Hence it is important to assess the prevalent explanatory model in the society and elicit the patient's causal and treatment beliefs. It is essential for the success of the therapy to integrate the apparent contradictions between the patient's explanatory model and the guiding principles of various forms of psychotherapy (Jacob & Kuruvilla, 2012).

CONCLUSION

Empirical studies have shown the variations in different facets of personality across cultures. Sociocultural factors play a role in shaping the psychopathology of the personality disorders as also in management of these disorders. There is a need to develop culturally validated assessment instruments to gauge the differences in presentation of personality disorders across cultures. The personality disorders have been shown to have close association with violence especially intimate partner violence. This association between the two does not necessarily imply causality of personality disorders in violence but emphasizes the need to incorporate personality disorder assessments for both the perpetrators and victims of violence. Personality disorders have been found to be highly stigmatizing condition and studies have shown that even healthcare providers have discriminatory attitudes towards individuals with personality disorders. This is a worrisome fact which needs to be addressed through anti-stigma programs.

REFERENCES

Alhabib S, Nur U, Jones R. Domestic violence against women: systematic review of prevalence studies. J Fam Violence. 2010;25(4):369-82.

Aviram RB, Brodsky BS, Stanley B. Borderline personality disorder, stigma, and treatment implications. Harv Rev Psychiatry. 2006;14(5):249-56.

Bäärnhielm S, ÅbergWistedt A, Rosso MS. Revising psychiatric diagnostic categorisation of immigrant patients after using the Cultural Formulation in DSM-IV. Transcult Psychiatry. 2015;52(3):287-310.

Battle CL, Shea MT, Johnson DM, et al. Childhood maltreatment associated with adult personality disorders: findings from the Collaborative Longitudinal Personality Disorders Study. J Pers Disord. 2004;18(2):193-211.

Benet-Martinez V. Cross-cultural personality research: conceptual and methodological issues. In: Robins RW, Fraley CR, Krueger RF (Eds). Handbook of Research Methods in Personality Psychology. New York: Guilford; 2007. pp. 170-89.

Berrios GE. European views on personality disorders: a conceptual history. Comprehensive Psychiatry. 1993;34(1):14-30.

Bodner E, Cohen-Fridel S, Mashiah M, et al. The attitudes of psychiatric hospital staff toward hospitalization and treatment of patients with borderline personality disorder. BMC Psychiatry. 2015;15(1):2.

Bonnington O, Rose D. Exploring stigmatisation among people diagnosed with either bipolar disorder or borderline personality disorder: a critical realist analysis. Soc Sci Med. 2014;123:7-17.

Catthoor K, Feenstra DJ, Hutsebaut J, et al. Adolescents with personality disorders suffer from severe psychiatric stigma: evidence from a sample of 131 patients. Adolesc Health Med Ther. 2015;6:81-9.

Cheung FM, Leung K, Fan RM, et al. Development of the Chinese personality assessment inventory. J Cross-Cult Psychol. 1996;27(2):181-99.

Cheung FM, van de Vijver FJ, Leong FT. Toward a new approach to the study of personality in culture. Am Psychol. 2011;66(7):593-603.

Church AT. Culture and personality: toward an integrated cultural trait psychology. J Pers. 2000;68(4): 651-703.

Corrigan PW, Morris SB, Michaels PJ, et al. Challenging the public stigma of mental illness: a meta-analysis of outcome studies. Psychiatr Serv. 2012;63(10):963-73.

Costa PT, Widiger TA. Personality Disorders and the Five-factor Model of Personality. Washington DC: American Psychological Association; 1994.

Cyr C, Euser EM, Bakermans-Kranenburg MJ, et al. Attachment security and disorganization in maltreating and high-risk families: a series of meta-analyses. Dev Psychopathol. 2010;22(1):87-108.

Duggan C, Howard R. The 'functional link' between personality disorder and violence: A critical appraisal. In: McMurran M, Howard R. Wiley-Blackwell (Eds). Personality, Personality Disorder and Violence: An Evidence Based Approach; 2009. pp. 19-37.

Euser S, Alink LR, Stoltenborgh M, et al. A gloomy picture: a meta-analysis of randomized controlled trials reveals disappointing effectiveness of programs aiming at preventing child maltreatment. BMC Public Health. 2015;15(1):1068.

Eysenck H. Culture and personality abnormality. In: Al-Issa (Eds). Culture and Psychopathology. Baltimore: University Park Press; 1982. pp. 277-308.

Fernández-Montalvo J, Echeburúa E. Trastornos de personalidad y psicopatíaen hombres condenado-sporviolencia grave contra la pareja. Psicothema. 2008;20(2):193-8.

Fountoulakis KN, Leucht S, Kaprinis GS. Personality disorders and violence. Curr Opin Psychiatry. 2008;21(1):84-92.

Furnham A, Lee V, Kolzeev V. Mental health literacy and borderline personality disorder (BPD): what do the public "make" of those with BPD? Soc Psychiatry Psychiatr Epidemiol. 2015;50(2):317-24.

Gallop R, Lancee WJ, Garfinkel P. How nursing staff respond to the label "borderline personality disorder." Psychiatr Serv. 1989;40(8):815-9.

Gilbert F, Daffern M. Illuminating the relationship between personality disorder and violence: Contributions of the General Aggression Model. Psychol Violence. 2011;1(3):230-44.

González RA, Igoumenou A, Kallis C, et al. Borderline personality disorder and violence in the UK population: categorical and dimensional trait assessment. BMC Psychiatry. 2016;16(1):180.

Grant BF, Chou SP, Goldstein RB, et al. Prevalence, correlates, disability, and comorbidity of DSM-IV borderline personality disorder: results from the Wave 2 National Epidemiologic Survey on Alcohol and Related Conditions. J Clin Psychiatry. 2008;69(4):533-45.

Hamid PN, Lai JC, Cheng ST. Response bias and public and private self-consciousness in Chinese. Soc Behav Pers. 2001;29(8):733-42.

Howard R. Personality disorders and violence: what is the link? Borderline Personal Disord Emot Dysregu. 2015;2(1):12.

Huang Y, Kotov R, De Girolamo G, et al. DSM-IV personality disorders in the WHO World Mental Health Surveys. Br J Psychiatry. 2009;195(1):46-53.

Jacob KS, Kuruvilla A. Psychotherapy across cultures: the form–content dichotomy. Clin Psychol Psychothen. 2012;19(1):91-5.

Johnson JG, Smailes EM, Cohen P, et al. Associations between four types of childhood neglect and personality disorder symptoms during adolescence and early adulthood: findings of a community-based longitudinal study. J Pers Disord. 2000;14(2):171-87.

Kerr IB, Finlayson-Short L, McCutcheon LK, et al. The 'Self' and borderline personality disorder: conceptual and clinical considerations. Psychopathology. 2015;48(5):339-48.

Kwan KL. MMPI and MMPI-2 performance of the Chinese: cross-cultural applicability. Professional Psychology - Research and Practice. 1999;30(3):260-8.

Lawn S, McMahon J. Experiences of care by Australians with a diagnosis of borderline personality disorder. J Psychiatr Ment Health Nurs. 2015;22(7):510-21.

Lewis-Fernández R, Kleinman A. Culture, personality, and psychopathology. J Abnorm Psychol. 1994;103(1):67-71.

Logan C, Johnstone L. Personality disorder and violence: making the link through risk formulation. J Pers Disord. 2010;24(5):610-33.

Loranger AW, Sartorius N, Andreoli A, et al. The international personality disorder examination: The World Health Organization/Alcohol, Drug Abuse, and Mental Health Administration international pilot study of personality disorders. Arch Gen Psychiatry. 1994;51(3):215-24.

McGilloway A, Hall RE, Lee T, et al. A systematic review of personality disorder, race and ethnicity: prevalence, aetiology and treatment. BMC Psychiatry. 2010;10(1):33.

Mikton C, Butchart A. Child maltreatment prevention: a systematic review of reviews. Bull World Health Organ. 2009;87(5):353-61.

Moriya N, Miyake Y, Minakawa K, et al. Diagnosis and clinical features of borderline personality disorder in the East and West: a preliminary report. Compr Psychiatry. 1993;34(6):418-23.

Mulder RT. Cultural aspects of personality disorder. In: Widinger TA (Ed). The Oxford Handbook of Personality Disorders. Widinger TA: Oxford University Press; 2012. pp. 260-72.

Nehls N. Borderline personality disorder: gender stereotypes, stigma, and limited system of care. Issues Ment Health Nurs. 1998;19(2):97-112.

International Institute for Population Sciences (IIPS) and Macro International, 2007. National Family Health Survey (NFHS-3), 2005–06: India. Volume I. Mumbai: IIPS.

Oyserman D, Coon HM, Kemmelmeier M. Rethinking individualism and collectivism: evaluation of theoretical assumptions and meta-analyses. Psychol Bull. 2002;128(1):3-72.

Paris J. Chronic suicidality among patients with borderline personality disorder. Psychiatr Serv. 2002;53(6):738-42.

Paris J. Personality disorders in sociocultural perspective. J Pers Disord. 1998;12(4):289-301.

Paris J. Social factors in the personality disorders. Transcult Psychiatry. 1997;34(4):421-52.

Paris J. Why patients with severe personality disorders are overmedicated. J Clin Psychiatry. 2015;76(4):e521.

Ross JM, Babcock JC. Proactive and reactive violence among intimate partner violent men diagnosed with antisocial and borderline personality disorder. J Fam Violence. 2009;24(8):607-17.

Rüsch N, Lieb K, Bohus M, et al. Brief reports: self-stigma, empowerment, and perceived legitimacy of discrimination among women with mental illness. Psychiatr Serv. 2006;57(3):399-402.

Ryder AG, Sun J, Dere J, et al. Personality disorders in Asians: summary, and a call for cultural research. Asian J Psychiatry. 2014;7:86-8.

Ryder AG, Sunohara M, Kirmayer LJ. Culture and personality disorder: from a fragmented literature to a contextually grounded alternative. Curr Opin Psychiatry. 2015;28(1):40-5.

Sansone RA, Sansone LA. Personality disorders: a nation-based perspective on prevalence. Innov Clin Neurosci. 2011;8(4):13-18.

Sharan P, Kulhara P, Verma SK, et al. Reliability of the ICD-10 international personality disorder examination (IPDE - hindi version): a preliminary study. Indian J Psychiatry. 2002;44(4):362-4.

Sharan P. An overview of Indian research in personality disorders. Indian J Psychiatry. 2010;52(Suppl1):s250.

Sheehan L, Nieweglowski K, Corrigan P. The stigma of personality disorders. Curr Psychiatry Rep. 2016;18(1):11.

Silk KR. Management and effectiveness of psychopharmacology in emotionally unstable and borderline personality disorder. J Clin Psychiatry. 2015;76(4):e524-5.

Swogger MT, Walsh Z, Kosson DS. Domestic violence and psychopathic traits: distinguishing the antisocial batterer from other antisocial offenders. Aggressive Behav. 2007;33(3):253-60.

Tang SW, Huang Y. Diagnosing personality disorders in China. Int Med J. 1995;2:291-7.

Tong Y, Phillips MR, Conner KR. DSM-IV Axis II personality disorders and suicide and attempted suicide in China. Br J Psychiatry. 2016;209(4):319-26.

Torgersen S, Kringlen E, Cramer V. The prevalence of personality disorders in a community sample. Arch Gen Psychiatry. 2001;58(6):590-6.

Triandis HC. Individualism, collectivism and personality. J Pers. 2001;69(6):907-24.

Tyrka AR, Wyche MC, Kelly MM, et al. Childhood maltreatment and adult personality disorder symptoms: influence of maltreatment type. Psychiatry Res. 2009;165(3):281-7.

Wang PS, Angermeyer M, Borges G, et al. Delay and failure in treatment seeking after first onset of mental disorders in the World Health Organization's World Mental Health Survey Initiative. World Psychiatry. 2007;6(3):177-85.

Weiss MG, Ramakrishna J, Somma D. Health-related stigma: Rethinking concepts and interventions. Psychol Health Med. 2006;11(3):277-87.

World Health Organization. Child maltreatment [Internet]: Retrieved from www.who.int/mediacentre/factsheets/fs150/en/. Accessed on 10th June, 2017.

Yang KS, Bond MH. Exploring implicit personality theories with indigenous or imported constructs: the Chinese case. J Pers Soc Psychol. 1990;58(6):1087-95.

Young IM. Five faces of oppression: Geographic thought. A praxis perspective. 2009;55-71.

Yu R, Geddes JR, Fazel S. Personality disorders, violence, and antisocial behavior: a systematic review and meta-regression analysis. J Pers Disord. 2012;26(5):775-92.

Ziegenbein M, Calliess IT, Sieberer M, et al. Personality disorders in a cross-cultural perspective: Impact of culture and migration on diagnosis and etiological aspects. Curr Psychiatry Rev. 2008;4(1):39-47.

Zimmerman M. Borderline personality disorder: a disorder in search of advocacy. J Nerv Ment Dis. 2015;203(1):8-12.

Chapter 25

Suicide and Similar Behaviors

Sandeep Grover, Swapnajeet Sahoo

SUMMARY

Suicide is a major public health problem, with no part of the world remaining untouched by it. Various terms are used interchangeably to describe different types of suicidal behaviors. Existing literature suggests an overlap between suicide and different forms of suicidal behaviors (nonsuicidal self-injury, parasuicide, suicidal attempt, etc.) and suggests that these lie in a continuum. Significant evidence exists that suggest indulgence in any form of nonsuicidal self-injury increases the risk of suicide attempt which further increases the risk of completed suicide in future. There is a substantial overlap in the risk factors (social, psychological, genetic, and biological factors) for suicide, suicide attempt and nonsuicidal self-injurious behaviors. Effective liaison psychiatry services are required for management of patients presenting with self-harm. Proper assessment and evaluation of an individual presenting with self-harm is very essential as it can be therapeutic. Depending on the need and assessment, various pharmacological and nonpharmacological agents can be used. There is an urgent need for developing special treatment approaches based upon the psychosocial, biological, socioeconomical and sociocultural characteristics of individuals presenting with self-harm.

INTRODUCTION

No part of the globe has remained untouched by suicide. As per recent suicide statistics, 78% of suicide across the world occurs in low and middle income (LAMI) countries. Suicide was the 17th leading cause of mortality worldwide in 2015 (WHO, 2015) and remains one of the preventable causes of mortality. Suicide and suicidal behaviors have been considered to be in a continuum and multifactorial in origin.

Different definitions have been given to define suicide and associated suicidal behaviors. Simply speaking, suicide is defined as the act of deliberately causing one's own death. However, the most well-accepted definition of suicide is *"a conscious act of self-induced annihilation best understood as a multidimensional malaise in a needful individual who defines an issue for which the suicide is perceived as the best solution"* (Shneidman, 1985). Suicide is the final act of self-harm and is usually associated with behaviors which often precede the completed suicide, and are understood as suicidal behaviors which occur in continuum with the completed suicide.

Classification of Suicidal Behaviors

The main problem in the existing literature on suicide and similar behaviors is interchangeable use of the terms to describe the same behavior and there is variation in the use of terms across different countries, both of which leads to confusion among the researchers to reach to a definite conclusion on the usage of a commonly accepted terminology for the same behavior. Of all these terminologies, the term "deliberate self-harm (DSH)" is considered to be the most accepted. DSH has been defined by World Health Organisation (Platt et al., 1992) as *"an act with nonfatal outcome, in which an individual deliberately initiates a nonhabitual behavior that, without intervention from others, will cause self-harm, or deliberately ingests a substance in excess of the prescribed or generally recognized therapeutic dosage, and which is aimed at realising changes which the subject desired via the actual or expected physical consequences"*.

However, there is a great degree of confusion over the terminology and it has been described by several authors in different manner. **Table 1** lists out the definitions of some of the commonly used terms which are used interchangeably to describe the self-harming behaviors. Some of the authors have acknowledged the problem in classifying nonfatal self-harm because of several methodological issues (Stanley et al., 1992). The basic problem centers around ascertainment of deliberation, intent to die and lethality of the act. Broadly the suicidal and self-injurious behaviors are classified as suicidal behavior and nonsuicidal self-injury (NSSI) (**Flowchart 1**). NSSI is considered to be often repetitive without any intent to die and the act is of low lethality. Suicidal behaviors are understood as thoughts or acts which have associated intent to die and if the act occurs, then these are of moderate to high lethality and are usually

Table 1: Commonly used terms associated with self-harm

Term	Definition	Reference
Attempted suicide	Any nonfatal act of self-damage inflicted with intention of death	(Stengel, 1952)
Parasuicide	Behavioral equivalent of suicide without considering psychological orientation towards death	(Kreitman et al., 1969)
Deliberate self-harm	A careful nonfatal act, whether drug overdose, poisoning, physical, done with the awareness that it was potentially damaging and in the case of drug overdose, the amount taken was extreme	(Morgan et al., 1976)
Nonsuicidal self-injury	Self-directed deliberate damage or alteration of bodily tissues in the absence of suicidal intent; includes behaviors such as self-cutting, burning, self-hitting, and scratching to the point of bleeding and interfering with wound healing	(Heath et al., 2008; Nock et al., 2008)
Self-mutilation	Serious bodily mutilation or any repetitive superficial bodily harm without suicidal intent	(Favazza, 1998)
Self-poisoning/self-injury	Self-harm by these methods irrespective of suicidal intent	(Kessel, 1965)

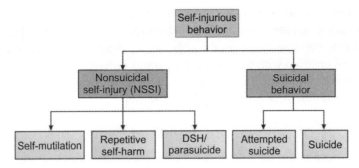

Flowchart 1: Classification of self-injurious behaviors.

Table 2: Differentiating features between parasuicide and suicidal attempt (Hjelmeland et al., 2002; Kurz et al., 1987)		
Features	*Parasuicide*	*Suicidal attempt*
Effort	Less definite and conscious	Very definite and conscious
Determination	Less determined	Strongly determined but failed in execution
Seriousness of attempt	Less serious	Very serious and but failed
Survival	Often easy	By chance or by intervention
Relation to suicide	Does not overlap with suicide but may overlap with attempted suicide	Overlaps with suicide but is a distinct act
Homogeneousity	Nonhomogeneous as it is based on seriousness and manipulative nature	More homogeneous group based on seriousness
Wish to die	Usually absent	Genuine
Intent	Change in life/cry for help	Die
Planning	Less planned	Usually well planned
Secretive	Freely expresses suicidal ideations	Can be secretive
Nature of the act	Less violent act	Can be violent
Termination	Need not necessarily progress to consummated suicide	Can go into consummated suicide requiring medical attention

less repetitive in nature. Behaviors such as self-mutilation, repetitive self-harm and deliberate self-harm (DSH)/parasuicide are often categorized under NSSI whereas attempted suicide and completed suicide are included under suicidal behavior. Often there is confusion while understanding the terms parasuicide, suicidal attempt and suicide. Some of the differences between these behaviors are listed in the **Table 2.**

Flowchart 1 depicts the classification of self-injurious behaviors.

Over the last few decades, there is reasonable evidence to suggest that those who indulge in NSSI and suicide attempts have higher risk of completed suicide (Huang et al., 2017). Accordingly the researchers have suggested that these behaviors lie in a continuum and have common risk factors. Suicide is actually a range of interrelated overlying attitudes and activities, including suicide attempts, suicidal gestures and ideations (Hawton & Harriss, 2007). The suicide continuum ranges through passive death wish, suicidal ideation without method, suicidal ideation with method, self-injurious behavior with unclear intent, suicidal attempt and then finally completed suicide. Both theoretically and clinically, various clinical parameters suggest that there exists a significant overlap.

Epidemiology of Suicide and Suicidal Behaviors

About 800,000 people die by suicide per year worldwide, which amounts to an annual age-standardized suicide rate of 10.7/100,000 population. Based on the available statistics, it is projected that global annual suicide rates could rise to 1.5 million by 2020 (WHO, 2014). As per the current statistics, suicide is among the three most common causes of death in the age group of 15–44 years. In terms of age, data from low and middle income countries suggest that suicide is more common in young adults and elderly women, whereas data from high income countries suggests that suicide is more prevalent in middle-aged men (WHO, 2014). However, all over the world, only a small proportion of individuals who attempt self-harm, present to the healthcare set ups, and a major proportion of such behaviors largely remain hidden from clinical services which has been described as the iceberg phenomenon.

Epidemiological data on exact prevalence of suicide in India is very limited. Statistics on suicide rates in India is recorded by the National Crime Records Bureau (NCRB). It has been reported that the NCRB data on suicide rates is quite less as compared to the suicide rates estimated by WHO (Patel et al., 2012). A study from Vellore estimated average suicide rate for young women to be 148/100,000 and for young men to be 58/100,000 of population in a rural area in South India (Aaron et al., 2004). Similarly, another study from South India had estimated that age group of 15–24 years, the female suicide rate was 109/100,000 which exceeded the male suicide rate of 78/100,000 (Gajalakshmi & Peto, 2007). There is also a report of average annual suicide rate of 189/100,000 population in elderly individuals in an area in South India, which is too high as compared to general population (Abraham et al., 2005). Additionally, studies have reported three times higher suicide rate in Southern part of India than the national average of 11.2/100,000 (Joshi et al., 2015). However, some of the studies from North India have also reported suicide rate of 24.4/100,000 of population, which is higher than the national figures (Salve et al., 2013). These findings contradict the lower suicide rates data as recorded by the NCRB.

The Million Death Study (MDS) is one of the limited nationally illustrative studies of the causes of death in India (Jha et al., 2006), which evaluated the underlying cause of death and key risk factors (behavioral, environmental, physical, and genetic) by using verbal autopsy method. Another national level representative survey found out that about 3% of the surveyed deaths in population greater than equals to 15 years are due to suicide. It estimated cumulative risk of 1.3% in 15-year old to die before the age of 80 by suicide, with higher risk for men (1.7%) than women (1.0%); with higher figures from south India (3.5% in men and 1.8% in women) (Patel et al., 2012). Poisoning (mainly ingestions of pesticides) is the most common method used for suicide in India. However, more public attention in India is towards farmer suicides (Münster, 2012). Still there exists significant lacunae in estimating the exact incidence and prevalence of suicide in India and more research is required in this aspect.

There exists a lacuna on the exact prevalence of DSH/suicide attempts in India. However, few studies have tried to estimate the rate of DSH/attempted suicide across different parts of India (Radhakrishnan & Andrade, 2012). Rate of attempted suicide in males has been reported to be 3.2–3.8/1000 population and in females to be 3.3–3.7/1000 population (Saddichha et al., 2010). A substantial proportion of individuals who attempt suicide had a psychiatric disorder (Kar, 2010; Sharma, 1998). Social adversities like joblessness, lack of formal schooling, presence of stressful life events and comorbid pain/physical illness have been reported to be reason for attempting suicide (Srivastava et al., 2004). However, some studies from India which have evaluated patients with self-harm attempts/DSH in an emergency setting have found that nearly half of such patients do not satisfy criteria for any Axis I or Axis II disorder at the time of assessment for psychiatric disorder (Das et al., 2008; Grover et al., 2015; Grover et al., 2016).

Nosological Aspects of Suicide and Similar Behaviors

In the Diagnostic and Statistical Manual of Mental Disorders-IV (DSM-IV) and the International Statistical Classification of Diseases and Related Health Problems 10th Edition (ICD-10), DSH is mentioned as one of the diagnostic criterion for borderline personality disorder (BPD). However, subjects who indulge in self-harm behavior are diagnostically diverse and can suffer from a range of psychiatric disorders ranging from alcohol and substance abuse, dissociative disorders, eating disorders, anxiety disorders, body dysmorphic disorder (BDD), depressive disorder, schizophrenia, post-traumatic stress disorder, bipolar disorder, and several personality disorders. While in DSM-IV, self-harm behavior is included under impulse disorder not otherwise specified, ICD-10 has an additional Z code for a personal history of self-harm. Masked self-harm with an aim of playing a sick role is a distinguished symptom found in the diagnostic description of factitious disorder (Fliege et al., 2002). In DSM-5, suicidal behavior disorder and NSSI are included under the heading of conditions for further study category.

Theories of Suicide Suggesting Overlap between Various Suicidal Behaviors

There are many ancient theories about suicide such as the famous Durkheim's theory, Menninger's theory, and Shneidman's theory. The famous Durkheim's theory focused on the influence of society and culture on suicide and classified suicide as egoistic, altruistic, and anomic (Durkheim, 1966). Karl Menninger postulated his theory of suicide based on Freud's ideas as inverted homicide because of a patient's anger toward another person and described suicide as a self-directed death instinct along with presence of wish to kill, the wish to be killed, and the wish to die (Menninger, 1985). Shneidman considered suicide as an outcome of "psychache," which was understood as a strong psychic pain, tension and suffering, which made the life intolerable. However, in recent years with better understanding of the overlap of NSSI with suicide, researchers have proposed the gateway theory, the third variable theory and Joiner's theory, which clearly explain the overlap between various suicidal behaviors (Hamza et al., 2012).

According to the Gateway theory, NSSI heralds the development of suicidal behaviors, because suicidal behaviors stem from mounting NSSI behaviors and thereby NSSI may be a gateway to more dangerous forms of self-injury, similar to the way cannabis is regarded as a gateway drug to more extreme hard drug usage. This theory also suggests that the age of onset keeps on increasing from NSSI to suicide and the frequency of NSSI predicts the frequency and lethality of suicidal attempts. In other words, NSSI precedes suicide attempt and suicidal attempt precedes suicide (Nock et al., 2008). The main limitation of this theory is that the hypothesis of gateway theory can only be tested on a longitudinal design.

As per the third variable theory, the association between NSSI and suicidal behavior is spurious and a third variable can possibly account for the co-occurrence of NSSI and suicidal behaviors. NSSI may not escalate the risk for suicidal behavior, but rather, possibly a joint third variable, such as having a psychiatric disorder such as BPD, perceived psychological distress and biological factors which increases risk for both NSSI and suicidal behavior (Jacobson et al., 2008), may be liable for the co-occurrence of these behaviors.

Joiner's theory of acquired capability suggests that suicide is a terrifying and life-threatening action and most people are initially unable to engage in suicide attempts. However, with repeated NSSI, individuals tend to familiarize to the distress and physical pain associated with self-injury, and thus acquire the capability to complete lethal self-injury. When acquired capability is united with perceived social isolation and burdensomeness, suicidal attempts may result. Based on this theory, it has been reported that more frequent NSSI and a longer duration of indulgence in NSSI are predictive of more lethal suicidal attempts. However, this theory is criticized as the supportive findings are based on cross-sectional studies, and longitudinal studies evaluating this hypothesis are lacking. Secondly, NSSI and suicidal behavior often involve dissimilar means (i.e. cutting vs. drug overdose), and familiarizing to self-harming behavior may not essentially accustom an individual to another form of self-harm behavior (Joiner, 2003).

Risk Factors for Suicide and Suicidal Behaviors

Suicide and similar behaviors have a complex multifactorial etiology. Almost all the suicide related behaviors have similar type of risk factors. Over the years, researchers have shown that none of this risk factor can be considered as a sole causative factor. Further, the authors have tried to categorize these risk factors as proximal versus distal depending on the level at which these act (Turecki & Brent, 2016). The distal risk factors commonly reported/evaluated include genetic loading, personality characteristics, early traumatic life events, neurobiological disturbances like hypothalamic-pituitary axis hyperactivity and serotonergic dysfunction. The common proximal risk factors for suicide and suicidal behaviors include presence of a psychiatric disorder and/or physical disorder, psychosocial crisis and availability of means.

The commonly reported (demographic, social, and psychological) risk factors associated with suicide and suicidal behaviors are depicted in **Table 3**.

Psychiatric disorders: Studies from across the world have found that most individuals who end their life by suicide, attempt self-harm or show some degree of suicidal behavior, and have an underlying psychiatric disorder (Hawton et al., 2013). Almost all psychiatric diagnoses have been linked with suicide and suicidal behaviors (Haw et al., 2001). The prevalence and characteristics of various psychiatric disorders linked with suicidal behaviors are depicted in **Table 4**. In patients with schizophrenia and bipolar disorder, DSH has been found to be a strong predictor for suicide. In individuals with schizophrenia, presence of past or recent

Table 3: Risk factors for suicide and suicidal behaviors

Risk factors	NSSI	DSH/Suicidal attempt	Suicide
Age	Peak age of NSSI has been reported from age 13 years onwards (Hawton & Harriss, 2008)	DSH in children and young adolescents (below 15 years of age) is associated with a relatively low long-term risk of suicide and is generally of low suicidal intent (Hawton & Harriss, 2008)	Reported in the adulthood and mostly in the age group of 25–34 years (Hamza et al., 2012) but elderly are about 60 times more likely to commit suicide later after an initial DSH/suicidal attempt (Murphy et al., 2012).
Gender	Female ≥ male (Hawton et al., 2012)	Female > male (Hawton et al., 2012)	Male > female (Hamza et al., 2012; Wasserman et al., 2005)
Sexual orientation	Lesbian, gay or those with bisexual orientation more probable to self-harm than are heterosexuals (Hamza et al., 2012).	Gays > lesbians (Skegg, 2005)	4-fold lifetime risk in gays and bisexual men for suicide (Tabaac et al., 2016)
Marital status	More in single/unmarried individuals (Hamza et al., 2012)	Separated/divorced > married and single individuals (Hamza et al., 2012; Hawton et al., 2012)	Divorced > married (Nock et al., 2008)
Occupation	–	High-risk of DSH/attempted suicide in persons with precarious employment or those who are unemployed (Milner et al., 2013).	Greater risk of suicide is found in those with low skilled occupation (Milner et al., 2013)
Socioeconomic status	–	Socioeconomic disadvantage/poverty (Iemmi et al., 2016)	Low socioeconomic class (Iemmi et al., 2016)
Religion	–	Less religious (Dervic et al., 2004)	Lower rates in religious communities (Hamza et al., 2012) (Hamza et al, 2012)
Stressful life events	No such association noted between NSSI and stressful life events	Traumatic life events predict the transition from suicidal ideation to suicide attempts in adolescents (Hawton et al., 2012)	Negative life events (Liu & Miller, 2014)
Childhood sexual abuse	Significant risk factor (Maniglio, 2011)	Significant risk factor (Maniglio, 2011)	Significant risk factor (Maniglio, 2011)

Contd...

Contd...

Risk factors	NSSI	DSH/Suicidal attempt	Suicide
Familial factors	Dysfunctional families (Kokkevi et al., 2011)	Familial and marital discord, maladaptive parenting, domestic violence, parent with psychiatric disorder (Kokkevi et al., 2011)	Familial conflicts, marital problems (Hawton et al., 2012; Wasserman et al., 2005)
Psychological factors	Impulsivity, novelty seeking, impaired problem solving (Anestis et al., 2014)	Impulsivity, impaired problem solving (Anestis et al., 2014), higher neuroticism, higher extroversion, higher openness, low conscientiousness and low agreeableness (Brown, 2009)	Impulsivity (Lockwood et al., 2017) and perfectionism (Flamenbaum & Holden, 2007)

DSH, deliberate self-harm; NSSI, nonsurgical self-injury.

suicidal ideations, past history of depression, previous history of DSH, comorbid substance abuse or dependence and high mean number of hospital admissions have been found to be strongly associated with an amplified risk of DSH or completed suicide (Haw et al., 2005). In individuals with bipolar disorder, there exists a very high lethality of suicidal acts as proposed by a considerable lower ratio of attempts: suicide (3:1) than in the general population (30:1) (Baldessarini et al., 2006a). Higher number of lifetime mood (mixed and depressive) episodes, comorbid substance use disorder, early onset of illness, personality disorder and poor social support in patients with bipolar disorder are some of the risk factors for suicide (Tidemalm et al., 2014).

Antidepressants and Suicidal Behavior

The association between antidepressants usage and emergence of suicidal behavior has always been a controversial issue ever since the Food and Drug Administration (FDA) had issued a black-box warning on antidepressants suggesting that the use of antidepressants was associated with an amplified risk of suicidal thinking, feeling, and behavior in young persons (Friedman, 2014). The black-box warning led to confusion among the mental health professionals, discouraging them from prescribing antidepressants when they were clinically indicated. Even after 12 years of the FDA warning, there exists no strong evidence to promote this association. Some researchers have highlighted the fact that most of the evidence for and against antidepressants use and suicidality is circumstantial as most of the suicidal and severely depressed patients were excluded from the studies which have led to the inference of the black box warning of antidepressant use and suicide (McCain, 2009). Meta-analysis of double blind randomized controlled trials have found out that the suicide rate associated with the use of antidepressants is strongly dependent on age of the individual and higher rates are reported among children and adolescents (Stone et al., 2009). However, the use of antidepressants have

Table 4: Association of psychiatric disorders with suicidal behaviors				
Item	NSSI	DSH/Attempted suicide	Suicide	Remarks/References
Prevalence of at least one psychiatric diagnosis	80–90%	80–90%	80–85%	No difference in the prevalence in terms of diagnosis made clinically or based on structured instruments (Chesney et al., 2014; Gómez-Durán et al., 2016)
Most common diagnosis	Mood disorder	Depression followed by substance abuse and anxiety disorders	Depression followed by substance abuse and anxiety disorders	Mood disorder commonest type of psychiatric disorder (Hawton et al., 2013)
Severity of psychopathology	Higher level of psychopathology—higher risk	Higher level of psychopathology—higher risk	Higher level of psychopathology—higher risk	Same in all types of suicidal behaviors (Hamza et al., 2012) including NSSI
Comorbidity of affective disorders and alcohol abuse/personality disorder	Increased risk	Increased risk	Increased risk	Comorbidity poses an increased risk for any type of suicidal behavior (Hawton & James, 2005)
Most common Personality disorder	Borderline personality disorder	Borderline and antisocial personality disorder	Borderline, anankastic and narcissistic personality disorder	Borderline personality disorder poses a higher risk for any type of suicidal behavior (Hawton et al., 2013; Hawton et al., 2012)
Repetition of self-harm	More in cases of borderline personality disorder	More in cases of depression, alcohol dependence, and personality disorders	Higher risk in females	More in females with personality disorders (Hawton & Harriss, 2007)

DSH, deliberate self-harm; NSSI, nonsurgical self-injury.

been found to be possibly protective for suicidal ideation in adults aged 25–64 years and to decrease the risk of both suicidality and suicidal behavior in those greater than equals to 65 years/elderly (Stone et al., 2009).

However, what one needs to know is that most of the studies have shown that in only an insignificant subset of young subjects with depression, antidepressants can lead to emergence of suicidal thinking and behavior, and there is a need to establish the possible biological mechanisms for development of such an adverse effect (Perlis et al., 2007). Among elderly, antidepressant use can possibly lead to an increased risk of suicidality because of antidepressant induced akathisia (Crumpacker, 2008). Hence, though controversial, yet all possible measures should be taken during evaluation of individuals on antidepressants for suicidality.

Risk Factors and the Journey from NSSI–DSH to Suicide

It has been postulated by various researchers that suicide and suicidal behaviors lie in a continuum. Genetic and biological factors of an individual may interplay with the personality factors (aggression/impulsivity) and psychological construct (perfectionism /low optimism), which when faced with any negative life events or psychiatric disorder or any type of psychological distress/hopelessness, may lead to development of suicidal ideation. Suicidal ideations further prompt an individual to carry out any self-harm attempt. Depending on the cognitive rigidity and psychosocial parameters along with the availability of method (lethal/nonlethal), the outcome of the self-harm attempt can be either DSH/nonfatal or suicide/fatal (Hawton et al., 2012). Hence, there is a significant overlap in the risk factors for suicide, suicide attempt and NSSI but it is clearly evident from the existing literature that indulgence in any form of NSSI increases the risk of suicide attempt, which further increases the risk of completed suicide.

Management

Management of patients presenting with self-harm includes assessment of DSH, psychiatric treatment and prevention of further similar suicidal attempt by specific interventions.

Assessment of Patient Presenting with Self-harm

Assessment of suicidal behavior is always an ongoing process and cannot be just done cross-sectionally. Ideally, it should be done in a calm environment but nevertheless it can be done even in a busy emergency setup. Assessment for suicidal behavior needs to be done when someone is brought with intentional harm to self or a suicidal attempt, when family member/others express concern of suicidality, whenever there is a change in psychiatric condition, while making a shift in treatment plan, making a change in level of care, and when discharging the patient. General principles of assessment in case of a suicidal attempt should be applied, whatever may be the seriousness/lethality of the attempt. Every person must be taken seriously, enquiry should be done from all possible available informants and sources, and all assessments done should be properly documented.

Assessment for future risk of self-harm should include assessment of potential risk factors, protective factors and specific suicide inquiry. The risk factors assessment should include various domains like demographic data, psychosocial history, psychiatric history, presence of any physical illness, psychological dimensions (impulsivity, aggression, hopelessness, etc.), cognitive dimensions (polarized thinking, thought constriction), childhood trauma, and any positive family history of suicide (*see* **Table 3**). Possible protective factors should also be enquired like positive coping skills, any deterrent religious beliefs, satisfaction with life, positive social support, self-efficacy, supportive living arrangements, hope for future, and fear of the act of suicide (Meadows et al., 2005). Specific suicide enquiry should be done with regard to current suicidal ideation, suicidal plans, lethality of the act, intent to die, feelings of ambivalence, efforts taken to conceal the attempt, preparation for the attempt and any past attempts. It is also mandatory to enquire regarding patient's expectations about the lethality and accessibility of the method used. Specific psychiatric signs and symptoms suggesting any psychopathology should also be documented. Assessment is incomplete if the patient is not asked for his/her reasons for living and any specific plans for his/her future. There is always a controversy regarding whether asking about suicidal ideation further implants the same issue in patient's mind or it can provide an opportunity to feel understood. Recent studies have demonstrated that asking about current suicidal ideations and planning does not increase suicidiality (Crawford et al., 2011). It has been suggested that not all attempts are with the intent to die. Therefore, it should be enquired routinely.

Assessment of proximal risk factors like agitation (panic attacks, aggression, poor concentration), specific ideation, depressive thinking, drug/alcohol abuse, loss of any family member or availability of any lethal agents should be documented/recorded. Similarly, distal risk factors like personal and family history of suicide, impulsive aggression, hopelessness, BPD, history of abuse and trauma and comorbid substance abuse should also be included in assessment. Psychiatric disorder should be careful diagnosed keeping in view previous treatment history and previous suicide attempt. Any comorbid medical illness and family history of suicide and suicidal attempt should also be documented. It is always advisable to detect immediate and continuing psychosocial stressors and patient's cultural and religious beliefs about death and suicide. Individual assets and susceptibilities can also be assessed after stabilization, and assessment of coping skills, personality traits and past response to stress can be done so as to plan future specific strategies to prevent repetition of DSH.

The question regarding who should be doing the assessment has been raised by many researchers and it has been finally inferred that other than mental health professionals, if given proper training, even psychiatric nursing staff can reasonably do assessment of self-harm and predict future risk too (Murphy et al., 2011). Similarly, another big question is the timing of assessment. It has been seen that nearly 75% of patients with self-harm seek help in the evening when only emergency services are available. In this regard, suicide prevention guidelines suggest that patient should be kept admitted overnight with a view to complete the psychosocial assessment on the very next day so as to ensure after care and prevent drop out from services. Some have even suggested that nearly half of the patients usually consume alcohol or drugs hindering the assessment during evening hours and hence assessment in morning hours is more helpful (National Collaborating Centre for Mental Health (UK), 2004). Proper psychosocial assessment following an index episode of DSH has been found to reduce the rate of repetition by more than 50% (Carroll et al., 2016). People around the patient, i.e. family members and hospital staff should not be critical, should not blame the person or his/her parents or any significant others for the act, and should not discuss about the social or legal consequences in front of the person who attempted suicide. It is rather expected that the staff and family members should try to talk about the things which had led to the act of self-harm as it may be the first opportunity of the person to discuss his/her problems.

Various assessment scales **(Table 5)** have been developed to ease out the assessment procedure as well as to estimate the severity of the attempt, and to predict future risk of repetition. These assessment scales can give a rough idea of future risk for suicide but for

Table 5: Scales for assessment of suicide behaviors

Scale	No. of items	Reference
Hopelessness scale	21	(Beck et al., 1974)
Suicide intent score	21	(Beck et al., 1979)
Risk of repetition scale	6	(Buglass & Horton, 1974)
Edinburgh risk of repetition scale	11	(Kreitman & Foster, 1991)
Suicide assessment-SAD PERSONS	10	(Patterson et al., 1983)
Modified intent score	12	(Pierce, 1977)
The Columbia Suicide severity rating scale	6 broad	(Posner et al., 2011)
Suicide assessment checklist	21	(Rogers et al., 1994)

prediction of suicide, these tools have extremely weak predictive power because of their low specificity and low prevalence of the expected outcome (Borschmann et al., 2012).

Psychiatric Management

Establishment of therapeutic alliance is the key and initial step in the management of a patient presenting with DSH/attempted suicide. Therapeutic alliance with appropriate empathy helps the patient to feel emotionally supported in a holding environment. Patient's safety should be given priority. There should be observation of patient on one to one basis with removal of potentially hazardous items from his/her vicinity. There should not be any guess work approach and DSH should be treated as a medical and psychiatric emergency with appropriate promptness and urgency.

The treatment setting should be decided promptly, based on the severity of the attempt and severity of the specific psychiatric disorder, level of functioning, available support system, estimation of suicide risk and potentiality of the dangerousness to significant others. The choice of treatment settings, i.e. inpatient /outpatient/emergency usually rely on the balance between the above mentioned elements. Hospitalization is not a treatment although it may prevent further attempt in the near future by facilitating evaluation and observation in the present situation. Next step in management is to develop a plan of treatment by selecting the modality of treatment, i.e. somatic/pharmacological/nonpharmacological therapy depending on the nature of the psychiatric disorder and its severity. The treatment strategy should be modified as per the individual's responses and preferences. There is a need of more intensive management during the early stages with involvement of family members and significant others. Coordinating with other clinicians and providing proper psycho-education to the patient and family are other aspects of a holistic treatment strategy.

In the acute phase, high-risk management should be instituted **(Box 1)**. All potential risk factors along with all possible resources, which can reduce risk should be identified. If the risk of self-harm outweighs available resources then hospitalization should be considered as mandatory. Studies have found some important factors, which indicate hospitalization, are male gender, age above 12 years, presence of depression, hopelessness, social withdrawal, substance intoxication, persisting suicidal ideation, potentially lethal attempt, previous suicide attempt and absence of caring or responsible social support.

> **Box 1:** High-risk management
>
> - Two to three attendents to accompany the patient
> - Scissors, razors, and other potentially lethal objects should be removed and plastic utensil to be used
> - No medicines to be kept with the patient
> - Patient should not to be left alone, to be assisted even to toilet
> - Constant supervision by staff
> - Bed should be located close to the nursing station within easy view
> - Shatter proof window of the room
> - Doors of the room without latches/bolts from inside
> - Patients to be protected from jumping from upper story windows and from falling down open stair
> - Repeated search of the patient
> - Consultation with family members to be done to deal with their reaction and feeling about the attempt
> - Physician should pay particular attention to the nurse's notes which often report the patient's talk of wanting to die or symptom of depression

Supervision and monitoring of the patient at various levels such as 24 hour supervision versus intermittent supervision, arm length supervision versus at-distance supervision as well as video monitoring should be done depending on the severity of the attempt. The supervision level may change with time depending on the clinical status of the patient. All potential dangerous items in vicinity like medications, sharp objects, ropes etc. should be kept away. It is a general principle that admitted patients with DSH be preferably given a bed as close to the nursing station or need to be placed in such a way that he/she is visible to the nursing staff. Patient should be assisted to toilets in which bolts should not be used.

No suicide contract has often been used as a tool to prevent self-harm attempts (Drye et al., 1973). It comprises of a contract between patient and the therapist. The patient has to sign the contract which states that he/she would not try to harm self and will let others know if having suicidal ideations. Though it is not legally binding, it helps in establishing a good therapeutic relationship. It is anticipated that such a contract will increase the individual's and family's obligation to treatment, but it should never be considered as a substitute for other types of strategies.

Specific Interventions

Pharmacological interventions: There is no specific medication for DSH/self-harm per se. The pharmacological treatment is usually directed towards treating the underlying Axis I and Axis II disorder. Some psychotropics like lithium (Baldessarini et al., 2006b) and clozapine (Reid et al., 1998) have been well documented to help in prevention of further self-harm attempts in patients with mood disorder, psychosis, and personality disorder. But still the evidence is not strong enough to recommend these agents in all cases of DSH. Electroconvulsive therapy has also been recommended to treat acute suicidal behavior due to any underlying psychiatric disorder like depression or psychosis. Few studies have found the favorable role of omega-3 fatty acids supplementation in patients with repeated self-harm with significant improvement in depressive symptoms, suicidiality and daily stresses (Hallahan et al., 2007). However, further research is required in this aspect to reach to a definite conclusion.

Psychological interventions: Usually self-harm attempts are precipitated by personal and interpersonal problems and the aim of the psychological interventions in patients with self-harm is to improve the social functioning and to reduce the self-harm behavior in future (Calear et al., 2016). Commonly followed psychological interventions which have been shown to be efficacious in patients with self-harm include problem-solving, dialectical behavior therapy, cognitive behavior therapy and mentalization based treatment (MBT).

Psychosocial interventions: Many types of psychosocial interventions have been developed with a focus to improve contact and engagement with the services after the index episode of self-harm so as to prevent drop out from ongoing therapy and to prevent further similar attempt in near future. Some of the well-established psychosocial interventions are intensive intervention, emergency card/green card intervention, postcard intervention, telephone supportive contact, brief intervention and contact (BIC) and no self-harm contract.

Suicide Prevention

Suicide prevention can be done at various levels, i.e. primary (at the level of society), secondary (early diagnosis and treatment), and tertiary levels.

Primary prevention includes changes to be done at the level of the society to modify or rectify the risks associated with suicide. Some of the modifiable risk factors like poverty, low education, unemployment, acculturation stress, marital conflicts, and substance abuse can be taken care by appropriate strategies by various Government and Nongovernmental Organizations (NGOs). Stigma reduction programs are necessary to promote awareness among the public regarding mental disorders as well as for better identification and management of potential suicidal persons by the primary care physicians and family members. Another important aspect of primary prevention is strengthening of legal enforcement by banning over the counter sale of potentially dangerous drugs like sedatives/hypnotics, tranquilizers, etc, as well as banning the easy availability of organophosphorous compounds. Strict dispensing of large quantities should also be restricted and public should be made aware about the dangers associated with these compounds/chemicals. Community-based suicide prevention services have also been established such as crisis hot lines, suicide method restrictions (firearms security laws, raising minimum drinking age limit) and indirect case finding through educational programs. Role of media in suicide prevention is also very essential as media has a very responsible role to play in this regard. Not only media can help in increasing public awareness but can also reduce the impact of suicide on public by desensationalizing such acts or not glorifying such individuals, as sensationalization often results in many "copycat" suicides. Earlier, suicide attempt was considered legally punishable in India, thereby preventing people from seeking treatment due to fear of medico-legal proceedings. However, as now the new Mental Health Care Act (2017) has been approved in the Lok Sabha and suicide has been decriminalized, it is expected to improve reporting of suicide attempts (The Gazette of India, 2017).

Secondary prevention involves identifying the individuals at high-risk of suicide and instituting treatment or psychosocial interventions as early as possible. Individuals and family members should be educated about the symptoms of mental illness and should be properly counseled regarding timely interventions so as to reduce any self-harm attempt. Emergency and crisis helplines as well as counseling services should be made available 24 × 7 to patients and their family members.

Tertiary prevention is aimed at avoiding suicide in survivors of attempted suicide. It has been often seen that suicide survivors and their family face guilt and shame, and experience long-term social and legal problems. They should be well-equipped with coping skills and nonpharmacological interventions should be carried out so as to improve their quality of life and strengthen their rehabilitation.

Indian Scenario

Studies conducted from different parts of the country have revealed that the rates of DSH are 8–10 times higher than the suicide rates in India (Chowdhary et al., 2007). Suicide rate in South India has been found to be more than North India (Vijayakumar, 2010). Better literacy, better and more accurate reporting system, higher socioeconomic status, lower external hostility and higher opportunities are the possible explanations for the higher suicide rates in the southern states of India (Aggarwal, 2015). Poisoning is the most commonly reported method followed by hanging and self-immolation to commit suicide in India (Vijayakumar, 2010). With regard to gender and method of self-harm, males usually tend to use hanging and pesticide ingestion, and females tend to use self-immolation and hanging to commit suicide (Saddichha et al., 2010).

Cross-cultural variation as compared to West: Data from the Western part of the World suggests that self-harm is more prevalent in women who were living alone, separated or deserted by their partner. In contrast, most of the suicide attempters in India continued to live in an extended family setup. There is almost no alcohol consumption by female suicide attempters. The commonest agents used in India are organophosphorous compounds and other household poisons as compared to firearms in the West. Domestic violence, dowry demands, and intimate partner violence by husband are the most common reasons revealed for suicidal attempts (Chowdhury et al., 2009). Additionally, poverty, unemployment and illiteracy are much more common along with almost nonexistent of social security system in India as compared to the West. Indians also rely heavily on religious beliefs, holy rites, fasting, and confidence in the almighty to provide solace and maintain optimism.

Suicide prevention services in India: The healthcare infrastructure in India is heterogenous and the provision and quality of services provided vary enormously. The psychiatric services available in the country are currently inadequate and patchy to provide suicide prevention services (Kumar et al., 2012). Additionally, it has been seen that there are attitudinal problems among the hospital staff dealing with patients with suicide attempt when they present to emergency services and very less staff have any training in assessment of self-harm survivors (Kumar et al., 2016). Several NGOs have taken initiative to provide support to suicidal individuals, and in providing education and raising awareness in the public and media. Many websites and blogs have been developed to raise awareness about suicide too.

Conclusions and Future Directions

Deliberate self-harm is common, causes considerable distress to the person, family and friends. Various self-harming behaviors lie in continuum with NSSI at the one end and suicide at the other end, with NSSI shown to increase the risk of suicide attempt, which further increases the risk of suicide. Existing literature suggest that there is significant overlap in the risk factors between those indulging in self-harm and suicide. Provision of services necessary for management of DSH is costly but essential.

Proper assessment of a patient presenting with self-harm can be therapeutic. However, adequate numbers of trained persons are not available to carry out thorough evaluation of all the patients presenting with self-harm. Training in assessing suicide risk should be made widely available to nonmental health professionals. Effective liaison psychiatry services are required for management of patients presenting with self-harm. There is a need for the development of further interventions based upon the psychosocial, cultural, and biological characteristics of patients and also to take into account individual socioeconomic and sociocultural aspects too. Lastly, there is a need for large sample, multicentric longitudinal studies spread across different countries with adequate control of potential confounders while reporting the association of various risk factors with different self-harming behaviors.

REFERENCES

Aaron R, Joseph A, Abraham S, et al. Suicides in young people in rural southern India. Lancet. 2004;363(9415):1117-8.

Abraham VJ, Abraham S, Jacob KS. Suicide in the elderly in Kaniyambadi block, Tamil Nadu, South India. Int J Geriatr Psychiatry. 2005;20(10):953-5.

Aggarwal S. Suicide in India. Br Med Bull. 2015;114:127-34.

Anestis MD, Soberay KA, Gutierrez PM, et al. Reconsidering the link between impulsivity and suicidal behavior. Personal Soc Psychol Rev. 2014;18(4):366-86.

Baldessarini RJ, Pompili M, Tondo L. Suicide in bipolar disorder: Risks and management. CNS Spectr. 2006;11(6):465-71.

Baldessarini RJ, Tondo L, Davis P, et al. Decreased risk of suicides and attempts during long-term lithium treatment: a meta-analytic review. Bipolar Disord. 2006;8(5 Pt 2):625-39.

Beck AT, Kovacs M, Weissman A. Assessment of suicidal intention: the Scale for Suicide Ideation. J. Consult. Clin. Psychol. 1979;47(2):343-52.

Beck AT, Weissman A, Lester D, et al. The measurement of pessimism: the hopelessness scale. J Consult Clin Psychol. 1974;42(6):861-5.

Brown SA. Personality and non-suicidal deliberate self-harm: Trait differences among a non-clinical population. Psychiatry Res. 2009;169(1):28-32.

Buglass D, Horton J. A scale for predicting subsequent suicidal behavior. Br J Psychiatry. 1974;124(0),573-8.

Calear AL, Christensen H, Freeman A, et al. A systematic review of psychosocial suicide prevention interventions for youth. Eur Child Adolesc Psychiatry. 2016;25(5):467-82.

Carroll R, Metcalfe C, Steeg S, et al. Psychosocial assessment of self-harm patients and risk of repeat presentation: An instrumental variable analysis using time of hospital presentation. PLOS ONE. 2016;11(2):e0149713.

Chesney E, Goodwin GM, Fazel S. Risks of all-cause and suicide mortality in mental disorders: a meta-review. World Psychiatry. 2014;13:153-60.

Chowdhary AN, Banerjee S, Brahma A, et al. Pesticide poisoning in nonfatal, deliberate self-harm: A public health issue. Indian J Psychiatry. 2007;49(2):117-20.

Chowdhury AN, Brahma A, Banerjee S, et al. Pattern of domestic violence amongst non-fatal deliberate self-harm attempters: A study from primary care of West Bengal. Indian J Psychiatry. 2009;51(2):96-100.

Crawford MJ, Thana L, Methuen C, et al. Impact of screening for risk of suicide: Randomized controlled trial. Br J Psychiatry. 2011;198(5):379-84.

Crumpacker DW. Suicidality and antidepressants in the elderly. Proc Bayl Univ Med Cent. 2008;21:373-7.

Das PP, Grover S, Avasthi A, et al. Intentional self-harm seen in psychiatric referrals in a tertiary care hospital. Indian J Psychiatry 2008;50(3):187-91.

Dervic K, Oquendo MA, Grunebaum M.F, et al. Religious affiliation and suicide attempt. Am J Psychiatry. 2004;161:2303-8.

Drye RC, Goulding RL, Goulding ME. No-suicide decisions: Patient monitoring of suicidal risk. Am J Psychiatry. 1973;130(2):171-4.

Durkheim É. Suicide; a Study in Sociology. Free Press; 1966.

Favazza AR. The coming of age of self-mutilation. J Nerv Ment Dis. 1998;186 (5):259-68.

Flamenbaum R, Holden RR. Psychache as a mediator in the relationship between perfectionism and suicidality. J Couns Psychol. 2007;54:51-61.

Fliege H, Scholler G, Rose M, et al. Factitious disorders and pathological self-harm in a hospital population: An interdisciplinary challenge. Gen Hosp Psychiatry. 2002;24(3):164-71.

Friedman RA. Antidepressants' black-box warning – 10 years later. N Engl J Med. 2014;371(18):1666-8.

Gajalakshmi V, Peto R. Suicide rates in rural Tamil Nadu, South India: verbal autopsy of 39 000 deaths in 1997-98. Int J Epidemiol. 2007;36(1):203-7.

Gómez-Durán EL, Forti-Buratti MA, Gutiérrez-López B, et al. Psychiatric disorders in cases of completed suicide in a hospital area in Spain between 2007 and 2010. Rev Psiquiatr Salud Ment. 2016;9(1):31-8.

Grover S, Sarkar S, Bhalla A, et al. Demographic, clinical and psychological characteristics of patients with self-harm behaviors attending an emergency department of a tertiary care hospital. Asian J Psychiatry 2016;20:3-10.

Grover S, Sarkar S, Chakrabarti S, et al. Intentional self-harm in children and adolescents: A study from psychiatry consultation liaison services of a tertiary care hospital. Indian J. Psychol Med. 2015;37(1):12.

Hallahan B, Hibbeln JR, Davis JM, et al. Omega-3 fatty acid supplementation in patients with recurrent self-harm. Single-centre double-blind randomised controlled trial. Br J Psychiatry. 2007;190: 118-22.

Hamza CA, Stewart SL, Willoughby T. Examining the link between nonsuicidal self-injury and suicidal behavior: a review of the literature and an integrated model. Clin Psychol Rev. 2012;32(6):482-95.

Haw C, Hawton K, Houston K, et al. Psychiatric and personality disorders in deliberate self-harm patients. Br J Psychiatry. 2001;178(1):48-54.

Haw C, Hawton K, Sutton L, et al. Schizophrenia and deliberate self-harm: A systematic review of risk factors. Suicide Life Threat Behav. 2005;35:50-62.

Hawton K, Harriss L. Deliberate self-harm by under-15-year-olds: characteristics, trends and outcome. J Child Psychol Psychiatry. 2008;49(4):441-8.

Hawton K, Harriss L. Deliberate self-harm in young people: characteristics and subsequent mortality in a 20-year cohort of patients presenting to hospital. J Clin Psychiatry. 2007;68(10):1574-83.

Hawton K, James A. Suicide and deliberate self harm in young people. BMJ. 2005;330(7496):891-4.

Hawton K, Saunders K, Topiwala A, et al. Psychiatric disorders in patients presenting to hospital following self-harm: A systematic review. J Affect Disord. 2013;151(3):821-30.

Hawton K, Saunders KE, O'Connor RC. Self-harm and suicide in adolescents. Lancet. 2012;379 (9834):2373-82.

Heath N, Toste J, Nedecheva T, et al. An examination of nonsuicidal self-injury among college students. J Ment Health Couns. 2008;30(2):137-56.

Hjelmeland H, Hawton K, Nordvik H, et al. Why people engage in parasuicide: a cross-cultural study of intentions. Suicide Life Threat Behav. 2002;32(4):380-93.

Huang Y-H, Liu H-C, Sun F-J, et al. Relationship between predictors of incident deliberate self-harm and suicide attempts among adolescents. J Adolesc Health. 2017;60(5):612-8.

Iemmi V, Bantjes J, Coast E, et al. Suicide and poverty in low-income and middle-income countries: a systematic review. Lancet Psychiatry. 2016;3(8):774-83.

Jacobson CM, Muehlenkamp JJ, Miller AL, et al. Psychiatric impairment among adolescents engaging in different types of deliberate self-harm. J Clin Child Adolesc Psychol. 2008;53:37(2), 363-75.

Jha P, Gajalakshmi V, Gupta PC, et al. Prospective study of one million deaths in India: Rationale, design, and validation results. PLoS Med. 2006;3(2).

Joiner TE. Contagion of suicidal symptoms as a function of assortative relating and shared relationship stress in college roommates. J Adolesc. 2003;26(4):495-504.

Joshi R, Guggilla R, Praveen D, et al. Suicide deaths in rural Andhra Pradesh—a cause for global health action. Trop Med Int Health. 2015;20(2):188-93.

Kar N. Profile of risk factors associated with suicide attempts: A study from Orissa, India. Indian J Psychiatry. 2010;52(1):48-56.

Kessel N. Self-poisoning. II. Br Med J. 1956;2(5474):1336-40.

Kokkevi A, Rotsika V, Arapaki A, et al. Changes in associations between psychosocial factors and suicide attempts by adolescents in Greece from 1984 to 2007. Eur J Public Health. 2011;21(6):694-8.

Kreitman N, Foster J. The construction and selection of predictive scales, with special reference to para-suicide. Br J Psychiatry. 1991;159:185-92.

Kreitman N, Philip AE, Greer S, et al. Parasuicide. Br J Psychiatry. 1996;115:746-7.

Kumar CTS, Tharayil HM, Kumar TVA, et al. A survey of psychiatric services for people who attempt suicide in south India. Indian J Psychiatry. 2012;54:352-5.

Kumar N, Rajendra R, Majgi SM, et al. Attitudes of general hospital staff toward patients who self-harm in South India: A cross-sectional study. Indian J Psychol Med. 2016;38(6):547.

Kurz A, Möller HJ, Baindl G, et al. Classification of parasuicide by cluster analysis. Types of suicidal behavior, therapeutic and prognostic implications. Br J Psychiatry. 1987;150:520-5.

Liu RT, Miller I. Life events and suicidal ideation and behavior: a systematic review. Clin Psychol Rev. 2014;34(3):181-92.

Lockwood J, Daley D, Townsend E, et al. Impulsivity and self-harm in adolescence: a systematic review. Eur Child Adolesc Psychiatry. 2017;26(4):387-402.

Maniglio R. The role of child sexual abuse in the etiology of suicide and non-suicidal self-injury. Acta Psychiatr Scand. 2011;124(1):30-41.

McCain JA. Antidepressants and suicide in adolescents and adults. Pharm Ther. 2009;34(7):355-78.

Meadows LA, Kaslow NJ, Thompson MP, et al. Protective factors against suicide attempt risk among African American women experiencing intimate partner violence. Am J Community Psychol. 2005;36(1-2):109-21.

Menninger KA. Man Against Himself. Harcourt Brace Jovanovich;1985.

Milner A, Page A, LaMontagne AD. Long-term unemployment and suicide: A systematic review and meta-analysis. PLOS ONE. 2013;8(1),:e51333.

Morgan HG, Barton J, Pottle S, et al. Deliberate self-harm: a follow-up study of 279 patients. Br J Psychiatry. 1976;128:361-8.

Münster D. Farmers' suicides and the state in India: Conceptual and ethnographic notes from Wayanad, Kerala. Contrib Indian Sociol. 2012;46:181-208.

Murphy E, Kapur N, Webb R, et al. Risk assessment following self-harm: comparison of mental health nurses and psychiatrists. J Adv Nurs. 2011;67(1):127-39.

Murphy E, Kapur N, Webb R, et al. Risk factors for repetition and suicide following self-harm in older adults: multicentre cohort study. Br J Psychiatry. 2012;200(5):399-404.

National Collaborating Centre for Mental Health (UK). Self-Harm: The short-term physical and psychological management and secondary prevention of self-harm in primary and secondary care. National institute for Health and Clinical Excellence: Guidance. British Psychological Society, Leicester (UK); 2004.

Nock MK, Borges G, Bromet EJ, et al. Suicide and Suicidal Behaviour. Epidemiol. Rev. 2008;30(1):133-54.

Patel V, Ramasundarahettige C, Vijayakumar L, et al. Suicide mortality in India: A nationally representative survey. Lancet. 2012;379(9834):2343-51.

Patterson WM, Dohn HH, Bird J, et al. Evaluation of suicidal patients: the SAD PERSONS scale. Psychosomatics. 1983;24(4):343-5, 348-9.

Perlis RH, Beasley CM, Wines JD, et al. Treatment-associated suicidal ideation and adverse effects in an open, multicenter trial of fluoxetine for major depressive episodes. Psychother Psychosom. 2007;76(1):40-6.

Pierce DW. Suicidal intent in self-injury. Br J Psychiatry. 1977;130:377-85.

Platt S, Bille-Brahe U, Kerkhof A, et al. Parasuicide in Europe: the WHO/EURO multicentre study on parasuicide. I. Introduction and preliminary analysis for 1989. Acta Psychiatr Scand. 1992;85(2):97-104.

Posner K, Brown GK, Stanley B, et al. The Columbia-Suicide Severity Rating Scale: Initial validity and internal consistency findings from three multisite studies with adolescents and adults. Am J Psychiatry. 2011;168(12):1266-77.

Radhakrishnan R, Andrade C. Suicide: An Indian perspective. Indian J Psychiatry. 2012;54(4):304-19.

Reid WH, Mason M, Hogan T. Suicide prevention effects associated with clozapine therapy in schizophrenia and schizoaffective disorder. Psychiatr Serv. 1998;49(8):1029-33.

Rogers JR, Alexander R, Subich L. Development and psychometric analysis of the suicide assessment checklist. J Ment Health Couns.1994;16:352-68.

Saddichha S, Vibha P, Saxena MK, et al. Behavioural emergencies in India: a population based epidemiological study. Soc Psychiatry Psychiatr Epidemiol. 2010;45(5):589-93.

Salve H, Kumar R, Sinha S, et al. Suicide an emerging public health problem: evidence from rural Haryana, India. Indian J Public Health. 2013;57(1):40-2.

Sharma RC. Attempted suicide in Himachal Pradesh. Indian J Psychiatry. 1998;40(1):50-4.

Shneidman ES. Definition of Suicide. New York: John Wiley; 1985.

Skegg K. Self-harm. Lancet. 2005;366(9495):1471-83.

Srivastava MK, Sahoo RN, Ghotekar LH, et al. Risk factors associated with attempted suicide: a case control study. Indian J Psychiatry. 2004;46(1):33-8.

Stanley B, Winchel R, Molcho A, et al. Suicide and the self-harm continuum: phenomenological and biochemical evidence. Int Rev Psychiatry. 1992;4:149-55.

Stengel E. Enquiries into attempted suicide. Proc R Soc Med. 1952;45(9):613-20.

Stone M, Laughren T, Jones ML, et al. Risk of suicidality in clinical trials of antidepressants in adults: analysis of proprietary data submitted to US Food and Drug Administration. BMJ. 2009;339:b2880.

Tabaac AR, Perrin PB, Rabinovitch AE. The relationship between social support and suicide risk in a National sample of ethnically diverse sexual minority women. J Gay Lesbian Ment Health. 2016;20(2):116-26.

The Gazette of India, 2017. Mental Health Care Act; 2017.

Tidemalm D, Haglund A, Karanti A, et al. Attempted suicide in bipolar disorder: Risk factors in a cohort of 6086 patients. PLOS ONE. 2014;9(4):e94097.

Turecki G, Brent DA. Suicide and suicidal behaviour. Lencet. 2016;387(10024):1227-39.

Vijayakumar L. Indian research on suicide. Indian J Psychiatry 2010;52(Suppl1):S291-6.

Wasserman D, Cheng Q, Jiang G-X. Global suicide rates among young people aged 15-19. World Psychiatry. 2005;4(2):114-20.

WHO. Preventing suicide: A global imperative. World Health Organization, Luxembourg, 2014.

Chapter 26

Social Dimensions of Childhood and Adolescent Psychiatric Disorders

Vivek Agarwal, Chhitij Srivastava

SUMMARY

Childhood development is dependent on a complex interaction between genes and environment. Environmental influences have the potential to modify the effects of genes and even change gene expression. Nourishing childhood environment is therefore very important for healthy development. On the other hand, psychosocial stressors can negatively affect childhood development and increase the risk of a number of emotional and behavioral problems. The most important environmental factors include the family, parenting, peer group, and school. Acute events including natural disasters, war, and terrorism can have a major impact both acutely and in the long-term due to the secondary changes in circumstances of life. In the Indian context, a lot of stressors arise in background of poverty and homelessness. India, together with the developing world, is witnessing a shift from rural to urban living, which is translating into nuclear families and decreasing social support. Together with urban unemployment, poverty, beggary, poor living conditions and exposure to crime, this shift potentially poses a serious risk to the mental well-being of children and adolescents. In this chapter, we shall introduce the childhood characteristics that contribute to one's resilience, and study the various psychosocial factors that interact with these characteristics to shape a child's development and affect his/her mental health. We shall also endeavor to understand and interpret the psychosocial factors within the Indian sociocultural context.

INTRODUCTION

Childhood is the most crucial period of human development. A child's development is shaped by the interaction of biological characteristics and environmental factors in multiple ways. Adaptation to environment depends upon the individual's resilience and vulnerability as well as the severity of environmental adversity. Adaptation to an apparently similar environment may be uniquely different for each individual. Siblings or even twins who have faced the same adverse event may have a completely different reaction to that particular event. Also, environmental influences not only add to one's genetic makeup but also modulate gene expression through a phenomenon called epigenetics. Therefore, biological, psychological, and social aspects are interdependent on each other.

Psychosocial factors have to be understood in context of the changing sociocultural milieu that India, along with the developing world, is witnessing. There is a shift from rural to urban living, which is translating into nuclear families and decreasing social support. Together with urban unemployment, poverty, beggary, poor living conditions and exposure to crime, this shift potentially poses a serious risk to the mental well-being of children and adolescents. This assumes even more importance in developing countries like India where 40% of the population is aged 0–19 years (Census of India, 2011). Although extremely relevant and important, these factors have not been systematically studied using robust scientific research methodology in India. In this chapter, we shall introduce the childhood characteristics that contribute to one's resilience, and discuss various psychosocial factors that interact with these characteristics to shape a child's development and affect his/her mental health. We shall also endeavor to understand and interpret psychosocial factors within the Indian sociocultural context.

RESILIENCE VERSUS VULNERABILITY

There is a growing body of evidence on various factors that increase one's resilience as compared to those that make one vulnerable to mental health disorders. Psychological resilience is conceptualized as a multidimensional construct that includes characteristics of tenacity, self-efficacy, emotional and cognitive control under pressure, adaptability, tolerance of negative affect, and goal orientation (Connor & Davidson, 2003). A person resilient in one situation may not be resilient in another. Resilience is a modifiable construct (Montpetit et al., 2010), mediated by adaptive changes in several neural circuits that regulate reward, fear, emotional reactivity, and social behavior. These changes are mediated through complex interactions between environmental and genetic influences (Feder et al., 2009). These interactions start in the prenatal period to shape the child's temperament at birth. Our understanding of childhood temperament comes to a large extent from the work done in the 1970s (Thomas & Chess, 1977) which found that 65% of children can be classified into easy (40%), difficult (10%), and slow-to-warm-up (15%). Thomas and Chess suggested that easy babies are energetic, readily adapt to new experiences and generally display positive emotions. Difficult babies tend to be very emotional, irritable, and fussy. Slow-to-warm-up babies have a low activity level, tend to withdraw but adapt after repeated exposure. During early development, a number of environmental factors interact with the child's temperament to promote resilience or make the child more vulnerable (Feder et al., 2009). Those that promote resilience include a stimulating environment and close relationship with a caring adult while early and prolonged maternal separation, and physical and sexual abuse is associated with increased vulnerability to psychiatric disorders. It is also likely that exposure to manageable stressors during development is associated with resilience.

Childhood disorders and disabilities also increase vulnerability to psychiatric problems. Not only children with intellectual disabilities have limited skills to cope with stressors, they are also more likely to face stressors like bullying, and critical and harsh parenting. They have a much higher risk of developing psychiatric disorders in adulthood with rates ranging from 13.9 to 75.2% (Buckles et al., 2013). A child with specific learning disabilities may also experience the above issues but to a lesser extent. Similarly, a child with a physical disability is also disadvantaged and is more vulnerable to psychosocial stressors. Certain disorders like attention deficit hyperactivity disorder (ADHD) may make one either resilient or vulnerable, depending on the extent of symptoms. ADHD traits have made the humans explore different things, take calculated risks (that benefit the society as a whole) and be creative. However, when these traits become excessive and take the shape of a disorder, risk taking becomes excessive and makes the individual vulnerable.

ROLE OF FAMILY AND PARENTING

Family environment and parenting are perhaps the most important modifiable influences on a child's development and behavior. Parenting styles are influenced by cultural norms, and, parents' own childhood experiences, beliefs and understanding about parenting. Different parenting dimensions have been associated with child's mental health. Warm and responsive parenting leads to a good overall development of the child. Such parents provide a rich and cognitively stimulating environment to the child. They respond to the child's needs promptly, are available in distress and also, encourage the child's independence and promote autonomy. Parental warmth also moderates the effect of adversities on children. This parenting style is effective in adolescence too as it improves communication between the parent and the child. On the other hand, harsh and punitive parenting with over criticism, lack of praise for good behavior, verbal aggression and physical punishment leads to problems like aggression, conduct symptoms, low self-esteem, irritability and emotional problems in children (Jenkins et al., 2015).

There are certain cultural differences in Indian parenting as compared to the West. It is generally quite authoritarian. Indian parents wish to control and plan their child's life without considering the child's opinion. This sometimes continues even into adulthood. Males are pampered while females are subjected to lots of restrictions. A traditional Indian family is a joint family in which uncles, aunts, grandparents also have a role in parenting. Consistency is therefore often missing and children can get very conflicting messages related to their behavior. It is common in such families that the mother gets overruled by the grandmother. This can lead to externalizing symptoms in the child. Children in joint families are often compared with others and criticized for not being able to fulfil expectations. This can lead to internalizing problems in the child and sibling rivalry, which can persist for a long time. Also, problems in one or two members of a joint family can affect the overall environment of the family. A joint family also has some advantages. It means more children to play with. With multiple parents, children benefit from a more stimulating environment and different parenting approaches. So, while the mother might consistently give a negative response to a hyperactive, impulsive or irritable child, the grandfather might be able to deal with him in a much better manner. Also, social support from close relationships with siblings and relatives is protective for children at times of adversities.

Due to rapid urbanization, Indian families are becoming smaller. Often both parents in an urban family are working with much less time to spend with children (Deb et al., 2010). Consequently, children now spend more time in front of electronic devices. They also have more demands placed on them. The effects of these cultural changes on Indian children need to be studied in carefully designed studies (Bornstein, 2013).

FACTORS AFFECTING PARENTING AND FAMILY ENVIRONMENT

Marital Conflict and Separation

Marital conflicts can seriously affect the child's upbringing and give rise to a number of mood and behavioral problems. The association with behavioral problems is particularly robust and these children can become quite aggressive themselves. Open hostility and aggression is most harmful but inconsistent parenting and poor emotional support for the child also has significant negative effects. Directly witnessing domestic violence or being a victim can seriously traumatize the child. The adverse effects also depend on the reason of marital conflicts which may include parental personality problems, psychiatric disorders, deprived living conditions, psychosocial stressors, or child-related factors. Conflicts that are about the child are perhaps more distressing (Grych & Fincham, 1993). Chronic conflicts have chronic effects and can make a child fearful, anxious, and depressed. In the long-term, these children grow up into adults who have poor self-esteem, poor emotional control, and resultant relationship difficulties (Waldfogel et al., 2010; Roberts et al., 2013). Marital conflicts may lead to parental separation and divorce. In some cases, this may be a welcome change for the child if it signifies the end of the conflictual relationship. However, children react more negatively if there has been apparently little marital conflict before separation. The initial shock-like reactions includes anger, denial, and guilt. However, the initial reaction does not reflect the long-term outcome which to an extent depends on factors like absence of one parent, quality of parenting by single parent, social support, and associated financial constraints.

Parental Psychiatric Illness

Parental psychiatric disorder confers both an increased genetic and environmental risk. Environmental effects include chaotic parenting style, problems with attachment and maladaptive social learning through observation of parental behavior. A depressed mother may be emotionally and even physically absent. This could result in the child taking on the role of a carer for the mother and a parent for the younger siblings. Anxious parents may be overprotective and therefore limit the opportunities that their child gets. Such parents also express lots of fears and apprehensions, which these children learn. They start to perceive danger in seemingly normal day-to-day situations and become anxious themselves. Parental psychotic or a manic episode can be extremely frightful for the child. A parent who has a personality disorder can be very unpredictable, inconsistent and chaotic. Generally, the effects of parental mood swings, impulsivity, anger outbursts, over protectiveness or unavailability due to any psychiatric illness can seriously affect the emotional, social, and cognitive development of children. Such effects are seen more with low socioeconomic status, single parents and girl child. Parental substance use can desensitize children and make them more vulnerable to early substance use. It also leads to inconsistent parenting and abnormal behavior especially during intoxicated state, which can give rise to behavioral problems (Stein & Harold, 2015). These effects are not limited to maternal illness; paternal mental health problems equally affect children (Stephen et al., 2014).

Parental Death

Early parental death appears to increase one's vulnerability and has been known to be associated with an increased overall risk of depressive and anxiety disorders in adulthood (Tyrka et al., 2008). The risk of depression is higher immediately after death, in those with a previous history of depression and following maternal as compared to paternal death (Brent &

Maalouf, 2015). The effects are greater if bereavement leads to financial constraints, change of school, home, friends, and extracurricular activities (Jenkins et al., 2015). Suicidal ideation can be reportedly present in 35% of bereaved children (Jenkins et al., 2015). High socioeconomic status and better coping with the surviving parent is associated with better outcome (Jenkins et al., 2015).

Children Living in Deprivation

Low socioeconomic status of family and deprived neighborhood significantly affect the child's well-being. India has a large population of children living in extremely deprived conditions with very little adult support. The reasons include extreme poverty, death of parents, accidental separation, abandonment by caregivers and absconding from home to avoid abuse. Children who have lost both their parents may live with extended families that provide adequate care; however, some continue living in their parental home with little or no adult supervision. Some of these children end up in orphanages and lucky ones get adopted. Generally, adopted children may grow up normally as other children. However, there are several factors that make them more vulnerable to psychological problems including higher genetic risk, inadequate care during perinatal and postnatal periods, and exposure to abuse and neglect before adoption. Good adjustment depends both on the child's temperament and on the adopting family.

Children living in deprived and overcrowded neighborhoods face multiple challenges in terms of availability of food, shelter, clothes, sanitation, school and health care. They also suffer from inconsistent and harsh parenting with low cognitive stimulation and are exposed to aggression and crime. Children that end up on the streets have the worst outcome. A study undertaken by the Ministry of Women and Child Development (2007) found that 18.7% of the child respondents lived on the streets; 65.9% of these street children lived with their families but still had to earn their own living. This results in a lack of education, forced child labor, beggary, criminal activities, prostitution, and physical and sexual abuse. There are 4.5 million child laborers in India between 5 and 14 years of age (Census of India, 2011). Majority of them are unpaid as they work along with their parents. These children are exposed to harsh working conditions with the risk of exposure to poisonous substances, injury (Shendell et al., 2016) and all sorts of abuse. They also faced harassment from people who are expected to help them including law enforcement agencies, other children on street, relatives, etc. Because of the chronic neglect and abuse, these children are exposed to medical problems, infections, poor nutrition, injuries, etc. All these factors contribute to the development of a range of internalizing and externalizing problems along with low achievement (Jenkins et al., 2015). Substance abuse is rampant in up to 90% of these children and includes tobacco, alcohol, cannabis, inhalant, and opioids (Pacione et al., 2014; Abdullah et al., 2014; Islam et al., 2014).

PEER GROUP AND SIBLINGS

Peer group and siblings can influence each other's behavior in both positive and negative ways. Bullying in peer group is a major risk to the well-being of children and is quite prevalent in Indian schools (Malhi et al., 2014). Recurrent bullying leads to behavioral and emotional problems, school refusal and increases the chances of self-harm and suicide. School can also be a source of negative peer influences like drug abuse, truancy, and antisocial behavior. Aggression in the peer group leads to more aggression and delinquency in children over time. Parental monitoring of daily functioning of child and peer group activities helps in reducing the risk of externalizing behaviors and substance use (Jenkins et al., 2015).

SCHOOLING

There are over 8.15 million children aged 6–14 years in India who do not go to school (Census of India, 2011). This is despite the legal provision through the "Right to Education Act". Absence of schooling often goes hand in hand with child labor, abuse and neglect, exposure to antisocial activities and drug/alcohol use, as discussed in other sections.

The quality of education is also unsatisfactory in a significant proportion of government and private schools in India. Huge population density, limited resources and the resultant competition make it difficult to look beyond exams and career. However, this defeats the basic purpose of education and ends up producing rote learners who try to fit into the society without questioning its basic tenets. A lot of teachers in Indian schools use harsh discipline and even physical punishment, which can instill a sense of fear in the child. School-related factors such as academic difficulties, school absenteeism, pressure to achieve, control by teacher, and poor peer acceptance are important risk factors for emotional and behavioral disorders in adolescents in India (Aggarwal et al., 2015). A significant number of children also present to physicians with medically unexplained symptoms that are stress-related.

Most schools in India are not well equipped to cope with the needs of children who require special help for their educational, social, emotional, and behavioral difficulties. Poor teacher-student ratio, lack of awareness, and poor resources make this an almost impossible task for most schools. This often means that a child with mental health problems like depression, anxiety, and stress-related disorders does not get any validation for his/her difficulties and also gets bullied by peers. School refusal and subsequent drop out are sometimes the outcome for these children, which further accentuate their difficulties. Children with autism and intellectual disabilities often are not able to access any meaningful education, as there are very few schools to meet their needs. Children with ADHD are seen as bad and disobedient children who end up as backbenchers. These children also have a higher rate of specific learning difficulties, which often do not get the necessary attention required. As a result, they end up being more vulnerable to all sorts of bad peer influences and secondary mental health problems.

MEDIA AND INTERNET

The increased exposure to the media and internet in the last two decades appears to be having a significantly negative effect on the overall development and functioning of children and adolescents. It appears to have led to an increase in the prevalence of aggression, substance use, early sexual activity, obesity, eating disorders, and sleep problems (Strasburger et al., 2012).

Children watching violent cartoons or playing violent video games become more aggressive and risk taking over time. Portrayal of aggression with humor and bravery desensitises children to aggression (Hopf et al., 2008; Fischer et al., 2009). Display of explicit sexual content in the media has increased significantly and pornographic content is easily accessible. Vulnerable young people can naively share too much personal information on social networking sites, including inappropriate pictures of themselves, making them a potential prey to stalkers and pedophiles. Such exposure in the absence of sex education leads to early initiation of sexual activity with associated complications like teen pregnancy, sexually transmitted diseases, etc.

Spending more time online promotes a sedentary lifestyle with unhealthy eating habits. Also, advertisement of unhealthy food promotes its consumption by youth leading to obesity (Hingle & Kunkel, 2012). Studies have demonstrated a deleterious effect of excessive use of media on academic performance. However, if used under supervision for time and content, media can be a great learning tool also (Strasburger et al., 2012).

DISASTER AND WAR

Rates of mental health problems are significantly higher in populations that are exposed to disasters. These include natural (e.g. tsunami, earthquake, flooding) and man-made disasters (war, terrorism). In terrorism-affected areas, children never feel secure as terrorist activities are unpredictable. There is always a real threat to them, their family members or their friends being killed. These exposures affect the whole family or even the whole community. The effects of these traumas are both acute and chronic. Acute events like witnessing a disaster, injury, loss, or threat to safety can lead to acute stress reactions whose outcomes depend on the support from family, community and resilience of the child.

Chronic effects occur due to secondary factors like loss of school and friends, lack of adequate adult support in the family, poor social support and a chronic sense of insecurity following a major adverse event. Sometimes a family or an individual tries to escape and immigrate to a different state or country. There also have been occasions when an entire community has been forced to leave their homeland and immigrate. The issues around migration can be divided into three distinct phases (Kirmayer et al., 2011): **Firstly**, families emigrating from troubled regions often have mental health issues due to the trauma they have faced. **Secondly**, a lot of families especially when they are escaping from areas of chronic conflict have to face unimaginable difficulties which pose a serious threat to their lives and drain them financially. **Thirdly**, even after migration, there are ongoing problems including uncertainties about citizenship status, exposure to violence, poor quality of life, communication difficulties, cultural differences, and rejection by the receiving community. Children may remain out of school, feel isolated, struggle to get a sense of their identity and get bullied by their peers.

Such stresses may lead to post-traumatic stress disorder, depression, anxiety, externalizing symptoms, or substance use (Kar et al., 2007; Chrisman & Dougherty, 2014; Mushtaq et al., 2016).

CHILD ABUSE

Child abuse refers to the intended, unintended and perceived maltreatment, whether habitual or not, including emotional, physical and sexual maltreatment towards a person below the age of 18 years. Child neglect is an act of omission or commission leading to the denial of child's basic needs. A study undertaken to understand the extent and magnitude of child abuse in India found that children in the 5–12 years age group are most at-risk for different kinds of abuse and exploitation (Ministry of Women and Child Development, 2007). Key findings from this study are summarized under different headings:

Physical Abuse

An overwhelming majority, 68.99% reported physical abuse, out of which more than half (54.68%) were boys. This figure was higher (72.20%) in the 5–12 years age group. Children were more likely to be abused by their own family members (48.7%) as compared to others (34.0%). Amongst family members, parents were the most likely offenders in 89% of cases.

Sexual Abuse

About 53.22% of the children reported having faced one or more forms of sexual abuse. The overall percentage of boys (52.94%) was much higher than that of girls. The study found that abuse starts at an early age of 5 years, gains momentum at around 10 years and peaks at 12–15 years after which it starts to decline. Out of the total child respondents, 20.90% were subjected to severe forms of sexual abuse that included making the child exhibit or fondle private body parts, being photographed in the nude and penetrative sexual assault. Reports of sexual assault were high (5.69%). Working children living on the streets, and those in institutional care reported the highest incidence. Contrary to the public perception, 50% of the abusers were known to the child or in a position of trust and responsibility including cousins, uncles, friends, and class fellows. Seventy two percent of children in this study said that they had not reported the matter to anyone.

Effects of Abuse and Neglect

Child abuse and neglect are often accompanied by multiple other problems that operate together like poverty, marital conflict, living on the streets, and parental mental illness which have their own adverse effects on the child's upbringing. Sexual abuse especially starting at an early age can be extremely traumatic. These children often end up blaming themselves and are left with a sense of shame and guilt. Legal proceedings like repeated court appearances, doubts on the child's account due to lack of evidence and poor parental support add to the trauma. Consequences of abuse are more if it is recurrent, severe and associated with breach of trust (Glaser, 2015). These children subsequently may display inappropriate sexualized behavior. They are at a significantly increased risk of developing post-traumatic stress disorder, depression, anxiety disorders, oppositional defiant disorder, and conduct disorder. The resultant shame and guilt together with an inability to make trusting relationships often translates into personality problems in adulthood. They report a higher incidence of self harm and suicidal ideation, and have an elevated risk of committing suicide in their lifetime (Danese & McCrory, 2015; Glaser, 2015).

CONCLUSION

Exposure to a range of psychosocial adversities affects the development of children and increases the risk of mental health problems. The severity and the number of events occurring together negatively affect the individual more. However, generally the negative effects are at least partly moderated by the individual's temperament and other factors like family and social support. A lot of psychosocial adversity in India and other developing countries is linked with poverty, poor access to education, homelessness and related factors. This makes it preventable to an extent and hopefully concerted government efforts will make a difference. Targeted interventions can help build on the resilience factors and reduce the negative effects of adverse environmental conditions. India is going through a period of cultural change, which potentially appears to be having an effect on the quality of child upbringing both in negative and positive ways. Also, training in psychiatry and allied sciences in India focuses largely on biological aspects of illness, while it is evident that psychosocial factors play an equally important role in the illness. There is a need to change the focus of training and sensitization of trainees about the effects of psychosocial factors in illness and its management. Future research in this area should aim to study these factors in carefully designed naturalistic studies.

REFERENCES

Abdullah MA, Basharat Z, Lodhi O, et al. A qualitative exploration of Pakistan's street children, as a consequence of the poverty-disease cycle. Infect Dis Poverty. 2014;3:11.

Aggarwal S, Berk M. Evolution of adolescent mental health in a rapidly changing socioeconomic environment: a review of mental health studies in adolescents in India over last 10 years. Asian J Psychiatry. 2015;13:3-12.

Bornstein MH. Parenting and child mental health: a cross-cultural perspective. World Psychiatry. 2013;12:258-65.

Brent D, Maalouf F. Depressive disorders in childhood and adolescence. In: Thapar A, Pine DS, Leckman JF, Scott S, Snowling MJ, Taylor E (Eds). Rutter's Child and Adolescent Psychiatry. West Sussex, John Wiley & Sons; 2015. pp. 874-92.

Buckles J, Luckasson R, Keefe E. A systematic review of the prevalence of psychiatric disorders in adults with intellectual disability, 2003–2010. J Mental Health Res Intellec Disabil. 2013;6:181-207.

Chrisman AK, Dougherty JG. Mass trauma: disasters, terrorism, and war. Child Adolesc Psychiatr Clin N Am. 2014;23:257-79.

Connor KM, Davidson JR. Development of a new resilience scale: the Connor-Davidson resilience scale (CD-RISC). Depress Anxiety. 2003;18(2):76-82.

Danese A, McCrory E. Child maltreatment. In: Thapar A, Pine DS, Leckman JF, Scott S, Snowling MJ, Taylor E (Eds). Rutter's Child and Adolescent Psychiatry. West Sussex, John Wiley & Sons; 2015. pp. 364-75.

Deb S, Chatterjee P, Walsh K. Anxiety among high school students in India: comparisons across gender, school type, social strata and perceptions of quality time with parents. Australian J Educ Dev Psychol. 2010;10:18-31.

Feder A, Nestler EJ, Charney DS. Psychobiology and molecular genetics of resilience. Nature Rev Neurosci. 2009;10(6):446-57.

Fischer P, Greitemeyer T, Morton T, et al. The racing-game effect: why do video racing games increase risk-taking inclinations? Pers Soc Psychol Bull. 2009;35(10):1395-409.

Glaser D. Child sexual abuse. In: Thapar A, Pine DS, Leckman JF, Scott S, Snowling MJ, Taylor E (Eds). Rutter's Child and Adolescent Psychiatry. West Sussex, John Wiley & Sons; 2015. pp. 376-88.

Grych JH, Fincham FD. Children's appraisals of marital conflict: initial investigations of the cognitive-contextual framework. Child Dev. 1993;64:215-30.

Hingle M, Kunkel D. Childhood obesity and the media. Pediatr Clin N Am. 2012;59:677-92.

Hopf WH, Huber GL, Weiss RH. Media violence and youth violence. J Media Psychol. 2008;20:79-96.

Islam F, Kar S, Debroy A, et al. Substance abuse amongst the street-children in Guwahati City, Assam. Ann Med Health Sciences Res. 2014;4(Suppl 3):S233-8.

Jenkins J, Madigan S, Arseneault L. Psychosocial adversity. In: Thapar A, Pine DS, Leckman JF, Scott S, Snowling MJ, Taylor E (Eds). Rutter's Child and Adolescent Psychiatry. West Sussex, John Wiley & Sons; 2015. pp. 330-40.

Kar N, Mohapatra PK, Nayak KC, et al. Post-traumatic stress disorder in children and adolescents one year after a super-cyclone in Odisha, India: exploring cross cultural validity and vulnerability factors. BMC Psychiatry. 2007;14:7-8.

Kirmayer LJ, Narasiah L, Munoz M, et al. Common mental health problems in immigrants and refugees: general approach in primary care. CMAJ. 2011;183(12):E959-67.

Malhi P, Bharti B, Sidhu M. Aggression in schools: psychosocial outcomes of bullying among Indian adolescents. Indian J Pediatr. 2014;81(11):1171-6.

Ministry of Home Affairs (Office of Registrar General India). Census of India 2011. Gazette of India.

Ministry of Women and Child Development Government of India: Study on Child Abuse: India 2007. Kriti, New Delhi, 2007.

Montpetit MA, Bergeman CS, Deboeck PR, et al. Resilience-as-process: negative affect, stress, and coupled dynamical systems. Psychol Aging. 2010;25(3):631-40.

Mushtaq R, Shah T, Mushtaq S. Post-traumatic stress disorder (PTSD) in children of conflict region of Kashmir (India): a review. J Clin Diag Res. 2016;10(1):VE01-3.

Pacione L, Measham T, Kronick R, et al. The mental health of children facing collective adversity, poverty, homelessness, war and displacement. In: Rey JM (Ed). IACAPAP e-textbook of Child and Adolescent Mental Health. Geneva, International Association for Child and Adolescent Psychiatry and Allied Professions; 2014. J4, pp. 1-35.

Roberts YH, Campbell CA, Ferguson M, et al. The role of parenting stress in young children's mental health functioning after exposure to family violence. J Traumat Stress. 2013;26(5):605-12.

Shendell DG, Noomnual S, Chishti S, et al. Exposures resulting in safety and health concerns for child laborers in less developed countries. J Environ Public Health. 2016; http://dx.doi.org/10.1155/2016/3985498

Stein A, Harold G. Impact of parental psychiatric disorder and physical illness. In Thapar A, Pine DS, Leckman JF, Scott S, Snowling MJ, Taylor E (Eds). Rutter's Child and Adolescent Psychiatry. West Sussex, John Wiley & Sons; 2015. pp. 352-63.

Stephen M, Amrock SM, Weitzman M. Parental psychological distress and children's mental health: results of a national survey. Acad Pediatr. 2014;14:375-81.

Strasburger VC, Jordan AB, Donnerstein E. Children, adolescents, and the media: health effects. Pediatr Clin N Am. 2012;59:533-87.

Thomas A, Chess S. The Temperament Trap: Recognizing and Accommodating Children's Personalities. New York, Brunner/Mazel, 1977.

Tyrka AR, Wier L, Price LH, et al. Childhood parental loss and adult psychopathology: effects of loss characteristics and contextual factors. Int J Psychiatry Med. 2008;38(3):329-44.

Waldfogel J, Craigie T, Brooks-Gunn J. Fragile families and child wellbeing. Future Child. 2010;20(2): 87-112.

Chapter 27

Psychiatric Disorders in Elderly: An Indian Overview

G Prasad Rao, SC Tiwari, Damodar Chari, Parmod Kumar, Sriramya Vemulokonda

SUMMARY

The geriatric population has shown a steady increase all over the world including India. Mental health problems are more common in old age as compared to the younger population. The elderly population because of poor physical health and aging is often dependent on the society. Because of the breakup of the joint family system in our country, the formal support system has gradually come down. There are very limited formal health care and welfare set up for the geriatric population. There is also need of research into the mental health issues of the elderly and to create formal support institutions.

INTRODUCTION

India has seen a gradual transition in its demographic and social profile since its independence in 1947. Improvement in health care setup has led to increasing life expectancy, better health outcomes and enhanced quality of life. There is a wide disparity in the difference between the falling birth rate and falling mortality rates over last six decades. This has contributed to the rise of overall population of India, specifically a tremendous increase in the proportion of elderly people (Government of India, 2011).

A closer look at statistics gives us a better idea of the changes in Indian population. In 1950, infant mortality rate (IMR) was 193.14 per 1000 live births, and crude birth rate (CBR) was 43.97 per 1000 population. While in 2011, IMR fell to 43.82 per 1000 live births and CBR reduced to 21.12 per 1000 population. As is evident from these figures, the rate of fall in mortality is much higher than fall of birth rates. This has led to rise in population from 361,088,000 in 1950 to 1,210,726,932 in 2011 (Chandramouli, 2011).

There is a steady incline in the proportion of elderly individuals as well. As of 2013, there are 103.9 million persons above the age of 60 years, which stands for 9% of the total population of India (Government of India, 2016). The projected trends predict that during the period 2000–2050, while the total population will rise by 55%, the number of people above 60 years of age will rise by 326%, and those above 80 years of age by 700% (United Nations, 2002). In terms of absolute numbers, the population of those aged 60 years or above rise from 20 million (1951) to 77 million (2001) and 83.58 million (2006), and is predicted to further increase to 173 million by the year 2026. Thus, it is expected that the population of the elderly in 2026 will be double of what it was in 2006 (National Institute of Social Defense, 2008).

According to the national population census of the year 2011, there are a total of 104 million people aged 60 years or above, including 51 million men and 53 million women. In

India, the old-age dependency ratio increased from 10.9% in 1961 to 14.2% in 2011. This ratio was 13.6% and 14.9% for men and women respectively in the year 2011. As per a 2016 estimate, the rates of employment are 66% and 28% for elderly rural men and women respectively, and 46% and 11% for their urban counterparts (Government of India, 2016). The literacy rates in this population also increased from 27% in 1991 to 44% in 2011 (Government of India, 2011). The literacy rates for the elderly men are more than double (59%) of the elderly women (28%). Almost 65% of the elderly were dependent on someone else for their day to day care. Though most of the elderly men were economically independent, less than a fifth of the elderly women enjoyed this privilege.

HEALTH-RELATED ISSUES IN ELDERLY

Aging is considered a natural and universal process. It is regarded as an inevitable biological phenomenon. Elderly people suffer from various physical, mental, social, and economic problems. A greater burden of disease is faced by the elderly compared to other age groups, irrespective of gender or place of residence (Agrawal, 2016).

In the geriatric population, the most prevalent illnesses are cancers, cardiovascular illnesses, osteoarthritis, sensory deficits, cognitive deterioration, respiratory problems, prostate hypertrophy, and so on. In India, the geriatric population commonly suffers from noncommunicable illnesses in the form of metabolic, degenerative, and cardiovascular disorders, in addition to communicable diseases (Reddy, 1996). Of these, cardiovascular causes top the list of causes of mortality in this age group.

The elderly are highly prone to different infectious diseases. Prevalence of tuberculosis has been reported to be higher in elderly compared to the younger population. They are also likely to suffer due to chronic use of substances such as tobacco and alcohol (Arora & Bedi, 1989). Elderly population suffers further misery due to sensory impairment. Hearing disability, followed by visual impairment, are the two most prevalent sensory impairments observed (Government of India, 2006). The elderly population is also liable to be abused in the household and institutional settings. The abuse may be physical, psychological, emotional, or sexual in nature (Shankardass, 2009).

MENTAL HEALTH OF ELDERLY

Elderly are significantly prone to suffer due to the increasing burden of different mental health issues. They are particularly vulnerable owing to many factors, such as presence of medical complications, progressive brain pathology, substance abuse, and social factors like increasing dependency needs, social isolation, family breakdowns, being subjected to abuse, economic insecurity, etc. (Guha, 1994). For the greater part of past century, hardly any studies were conducted focusing on the mental health status of elderly. Though the scenario is changing now, still the literature on the health status of the geriatric population remains scarce. Whatever literature is available, is derived from studies conducted in the general population, and not community-based studies targeted to investigate this particular population (Shaji et al., 2010).

Reports obtained from different epidemiological studies indicate a variable degree of mental health morbidity in older adults. Various studies suggest the prevalence of mental disorders to be in the range of 2.3–44% (Ramchandran et al., 1979; Premarajan et al., 1993). A study conducted in Pondicherry revealed the prevalence of psychiatric disorders to be around 17.4% in older adults (Premarajan et al., 1993). Another study in Northern India found 43.3% of elderly to be suffering from psychiatric disorders compared to 4.7% of the adults (Tiwari, 2000). Mood disorders and dementia are frequently encountered mental illnesses. Delirium, substance abuse, neurotic illnesses, personality disorders, and psychosis are some of the other conditions observed (Seby et al., 2011). Female gender, loss of spouse, poor education, poor socioeconomic status, medical illnesses, and chronic disability are common risk factors which have an association with the development of psychiatric illnesses in the elderly (Harris et al., 2003).

Depression has been noted to be the most prevalent mental illness, based on studies from old age homes, community settings, and hospital settings (Seby et al., 2011). Depression was ranked the third top contributor to the burden of illness in WHO's Global Burden of Disease Report, 2004 (Mathers, 2008). Prevalence of depression in the elderly can range from 17–55% (Tiple et al., 2006; Seby et al., 2011). A study done in North Indian state of Punjab reported the prevalence of depression to be 17% in elderly individuals (Goyal & Kajal, 2014). Several factors which increase the risk of depression in the geriatric population include lack of adequate social support, adverse life events (divorce, poverty, bereavement, social isolation, and separation), dependent/anxious/avoidant personality traits, limitations in the activities of daily living, chronic pain and disability, and genetic predisposition (Mathers, 2008). Among the constellation of depressive symptoms which may amount to either minor or major depression, the elderly are also more likely to experience somatic and atypical symptoms (Fiske et al., 2009).

It has been found in numerous studies that the suicide rate in persons aged above 65 years is as high as that in the general population, if not higher (Shah, 2007). A study originating from South India observed a suicide rate of 189/100,000 in people aged 55 years and above (Hall et al., 1999). Approximately, a fifth of all successful suicides were committed by the elderly. A few predictors of suicide which have been identified in the elderly are mental illnesses (notably depression), physical morbidity, functional impairment, and stressful life events. Also, the suicides attempted by the elderly are more likely to be well-planned ones, with a high intent and lethality (Conwell & Thompson, 2008).

With the prevalence of dementia in India being reported in the range of 0.84–4.1%, it is emerging as the next silent epidemic (Das et al., 2012). Alzheimer's dementia is the most prevalent type of dementia, as in the rest of the world. In a study originating from west India, poor literacy, advancing age, positive family history, and low socioeconomic status have been identified as risk factors for dementia, while marriage has been found to have a protective role (Saldanha et al., 2010).

Schizophrenia like symptoms can present in different forms in the elderly. Firstly, early onset schizophrenia can progress into late adulthood. Other than that, new onset psychotic symptoms that resemble schizophrenia can occur after the age of 60 years, which is called very late-onset psychosis (Nebhinani et al., 2014). Studies on the prevalence of psychosis are scarce in the Indian context. In one of the review studies, it was observed that elderly patients having psychosis were found to be more commonly females, having neurocognitive impairment and brain structural abnormalities and had higher risk of developing tardive dyskinesia (Nebhinani et al., 2014).

Studies focusing on substance use in elderly are comparatively infrequent. An epidemiological study found alcohol misuse of 11.3% in the 55–64 years age group and 16.8% in the 65–74 years age group (Sethi & Trivedi, 1979). The prevalence of alcohol use disorders is generally higher in the urban population as compared to the rural elderly population in India (Nadkarni et al., 2013). Tobacco and alcohol use can further increase the incidence of cardiovascular, pulmonary or malignant diseases, and cause impairment of quality of life at late age (Murthy et al., 2010).

Although anxiety disorders are less common in the elderly than the younger population, these nonetheless affect a significant proportion of the elderly population. Research into this topic in India has been limited. Prevalence of anxiety disorders can range from 4–21%. Generalized anxiety disorder is the commonest entity found in this population (Prakash & Rajkumar, 2009).

GERIATRIC MENTAL HEALTH CARE SYSTEM IN INDIA

Geriatric mental health issues are faced and dealt with at various levels, state and central government hospitals under psychiatry department, private psychiatry setups, old age and rehabilitation setups, and at the level of family members, providing the social and emotional support to the patients (Ingle & Nath, 2008).

Currently, professional and trained psychiatrists are catering to over 21 million geriatric patients (Thirunavukarasu & Thirunavukarasu, 2010). Although some tertiary hospitals have separate geriatric outpatient department (OPD) dedicated the specific group, mostly the patients are treated in general psychiatric OPDs. Government run hospitals have multiple drawbacks like lack of infrastructure, lack of funds, and limited availability of drugs and equipment, and an overburdened staff, thus contributing to poor patient care (Biswas, 1994).

Some part of the population prefers indigenous forms of medicine. But a recent study has shown that trainees and doctors of indigenous medicine often lack the clinical expertise for diagnostic and appropriate management of geriatric health issues (Patwardhan et al., 2011).

Geriatric healthcare in India mainly revolves around the tertiary care hospitals as compared to the rehabilitation and daycare centers in western countries. Although in last few years, various new projects have come up like memory clinics, dedicated geriatric day care centers, rehabilitation homes, old age homes and recreational activity centers which have been taking steps forward in India, but are still in their preliminary stages and need a lot of infrastructural consolidation. In spite of some of these facilities being available, the attitude towards utilization of the same is still poor (Krishnaswamy et al., 2008). A substantial proportion of the affected population is kept away from the facilities due to the nonchalant attitude of the caregivers (Goel et al., 2003).

In today's modern world, various factors like urbanization, weakened moral values, and tendency to migrate to modern cities have adversely affected the attitude towards the geriatric population. Lack of bonding amongst family members is further worsening the situation. In the practical era as it is, the elderly members of the family are looked upon as a burden owing to their noncontribution toward the earnings and expenditure on health issues (Bhat & Dhruvarajan, 2001). In terms of training in geriatric medicine, only AIIMS, New Delhi offers a course in India; otherwise, there is no formal training institute. Considering geriatric psychiatry as a super specialty post-MD, two government institutes at Lucknow and Bangalore offer training courses. The geriatric mental health education and training is a part of psychiatry and is covered under the curriculum during postgraduation in psychiatry. The lack of expert and dedicated training institutes for geriatric medicine adds to the burden of existing lack of manpower in handling these issues. Research in different aspects is carried out only by a small number of institutes and professional organizations like Indian Association for Geriatric Mental Health, Geriatric Society of India, Indian Academy of Geriatrics, and the Association of Gerontology. The existing infrastructure for research and training purposes in this stream is clearly scanty and unequipped, and needs a lot of changes and improvement (Gupta, 2009).

Health care utilization is more in urbanized areas as compared to nonurbanized ones. Comparatively, hospitals are sought for communicable diseases more commonly than noncommunicable diseases. Irregular compliance is a major issue in geriatric conditions; reasons for it mostly being drug costs, lack of instructions given to the patients and callous attitude of the caregivers towards the problem (Agrawal & Arokiasamy, 2010).

Although the mental and physical well-being of the elderly has always been mentioned in various government health sector policies, the budget allocation towards health sector, especially towards geriatric and geriatric mental health sector has been negligible (Gokhale, 2003).

BARRIERS TO ACCESSIBILITY OF THE GERIATRIC HEALTH CARE

The need for comprehensive health care of the geriatric population is increasing. But the mental health resources that cater to the needs of this population are estimated to be inadequate (Prakash & Kukreti, 2013). In general, the dearth of the mental health resources in India is a major drawback. This deficiency is echoed more clearly in the unmet mental health care needs of the elderly. For example, the doctor-patient ratio is so huge that only about 5000 psychiatrists are available to address the mental health needs of 21 million of the geriatric population. Moreover, the availability of specialized units for geriatric psychiatry is limited. When available, they are concentrated only at the tertiary level in urban areas. The availability of tertiary hospitals themselves is limited when compared to the size of the population they serve. Especially the tertiary centers run by the Government remain inaccessible and overcrowded. The privately run mental health care tries to compensate for the scarce mental health resources to some extent. But, even these services are concentrated in urban regions and are limited to OPDs. Overall, the healthcare service utilization is estimated to be greater among those from urban background and higher educational status (Thirunavukarasu & Thirunavukarasu, 2010).

More often than not, the geriatric care is provided through a nonfocused and general approach. The scanty resources promote and perpetuate the low level of awareness about mental health and the illnesses of the elderly (Rao & Shaji, 2007). In many cases, the symptoms are attributed to the consequences of normal aging and are often missed by the health care providers. In conclusion, the psychiatric disorders of the geriatric population remain poorly addressed by both the healthcare professionals and the policymakers.

The financial burden of mental illnesses should also be addressed by the State. There are several reasons for the increasing burden due to psychiatric disorders, especially in the geriatric population. Most of their mental illnesses run a chronic course with frequent remissions and relative resistance to treatment. This calls for long-term management and comprehensive care. Presently, more than 80% of Indians do not have any form of health insurance (Prakash & Kukreti, 2014). Moreover, most of the psychiatric disorders are still not covered by the health insurance. Many elderly, especially those from a rural background, seek the traditional and complementary systems of care (Patwardhan et al., 2011).

Community interventions like provisions for day care centers and memory clinics would improve the care for the elderly. But the distribution and utilization of these services are unequally distributed and is limited to a few urban settings only. Even the services from within the community, like that of the non-governmental organizations are still inaccessible to a large proportion of the elderly (Krishnaswamy et al., 2008). On assessing the unmet needs of the rural geriatric population, reportedly 96% of the people never utilize a geriatric welfare service, 46.3% are unaware that there was a geriatric service facility near their homes, though 59% had a government facility just 3 kilometers away (Goel et al, 2003). This highlights the scarce geriatric mental health resources in India and their poor utilization.

These barriers lead to a significant amount of caregiver burden which still remains poorly addressed (Gupta, 2009). Moreover, the ever-increasing globalization, urbanization, and migration has resulted in significant changes in the family structure as well as community support. This transition has led to the predominance of nuclear families and urban residence of the present geriatric population of India. On the other hand, there is no complementary increase in the social security services (Bhat & Dhruvarajan, 2001). The present situation throws light on the unaddressed and unmet needs of the geriatric population.

The training and research in this area are still in their infant stage. The training in the branch of geriatric psychiatry is offered only at very few centers in India. Even the advocacy and research activities are restricted to very few organizations namely, Indian Association for Geriatric Mental Health, Geriatric Society of India, Indian Academy of Geriatrics and the Association of Gerontology (Gupta, 2009).

AN ESTIMATED REQUIREMENT OF MENTAL HEALTH RESOURCES IN INDIA

Mental Health Act, 1987 laid the requirement of mental health resources of the elderly. It was later modified by the Gazette of India no. 252. The latest manpower requirement norms were proposed by Desai (Desai et al., 2004; Tiwari & Pandey, 2012). These estimates have found that there is a huge gap between the available resources and estimated requirements.

The Government is taking steps for the welfare of the elderly by the development of numerous programs like the Maintenance and Welfare of Parents and Senior Citizens Act (2007), National Initiative on Care for the Elderly (2004), and the National Policy for Older Persons (1999). The Ministry of Social Justice and Empowerment established the Integrated Program for Older Persons (2008). When the program was revised, mental healthcare needs of the elderly were addressed more noticeably. There were provisions for specialized geriatric care with an emphasis on providing interventions for geriatric mental health and adequate funding of these facilities (Gokhale, 2003).

The National Programme for the Health Care of the Elderly (NPHCE) is the most recent step taken by the Government. The aims are to increase public awareness regarding the geriatric mental health and to expand the outreach of geriatric mental health services by developing regional geriatric centers at the district level and establishing and promoting community-based clinics for the elderly. It also focuses on research and training of mental health personnel in the field of geriatric psychiatry. The program strives to promote comprehensive care by improving the referral systems and providing support and training to the caregivers. It covers approximately 100 districts in 21 States (Verma & Khanna, 2013).

Despite these efforts, there has been a failure in practical implementation. Presently, most of the welfare programs for the elderly focus on providing social benefits rather than promoting geriatric mental health. It is advisable to focus more on the caregivers by integrating them into the geriatric mental health care system. At the same time, the caregiver burden has to be addressed sufficiently by providing them support and awareness. The community-based approach towards the care of the elderly would be beneficial (Tiwari & Pandey, 2012).

NEED FOR RESEARCH

Because there is a paucity of literature on population-based investigations into geriatric mental health issues, a greater amount of better quality research into the fields of geriatric health services and epidemiology will facilitate the improvement of general health, improve health services, make way for better policies, and increase health awareness. A workshop titled "Research and Health Care Priorities in Geriatric Medicine and Ageing" conducted by the ICMR suggested that more research should be undertaken in the areas dealing with aging, basic sciences, chronic noncommunicable illnesses like depression and cardiovascular disorders, geriatric pharmacology, alternative medicine, health system research, geriatric nutrition, and the functioning of the elderly (Shah, 1999).

CONCLUSION

The rise in geriatric population in India and the world has necessitated a look at the mental health issues in the elderly. There is a need to expand the training in identifying and appropriately managing psychiatric disorders in the elderly. Apart from manpower development, infrastructure development needs to take place. Geriatric mental health care can be delivered through various settings, though services are concentrated in urban areas and have many accessibility barriers including financing. There is a need to expand the geriatric mental health services and to make them available to the population. There is also a need to further the research in geriatric psychiatry and advocate for constructive policy decisions.

REFERENCES

Agrawal A. Disability among the elder population of India: A public health concern. J Med Soc. 2016;30(1):15.

Agrawal G, Arokiasamy P. Morbidity prevalence and health care utilization among older adults in India. J Appl Gerontol. 2010; 29(2):155-79.

Arora VK, Bedi RS. Geriatric tuberculosis in Himachal Pradesh - a clinico-radiological profile. J Assoc Physicians India. 1989;37(3):205-7.

Bhat AK, Dhruvarajan R. Ageing in India: drifting intergenerational relations, challenges and options. Ageing Soc. 2001;21(5):621-40.

Biswas S. Implication of population and aging. In: Ramachandra C, Shah B (Eds). Public Health Implications of Aging in India. Indian Council of Medical Research; 1994. pp. 22-35.

Chandramouli C. Census of India 2011—A story of Innovations. Press Information Bureau, Government of India; 2011.

Conwell Y, Thompson C. Suicidal behavior in elders. Psychiatr Clin North Am. 2008; 31:333-56.

Das SK, Pal S, Ghosal MK. Dementia: Indian scenario. Neurol India. 2012;60:618-24.

Desai NG, Tiwari SC, Nambi S, et al. Urban Mental Health Services in India: How Complete or Incomplete? Indian J Psychiatry. 2004;46(3):195-212.

Fiske A, Wetherell JL, Gatz M. Depression in older adults. Annu Rev Clin Psychol.2009;5:363-89.

Goel PK, Garg SK, Singh JV, et al. Unmet needs of the elderly in a rural population of Meerut. Indian J Comm Med. 2003;28(4):165-6.

Gokhale S. Towards a policy of aging in India. J Aging Soc Policy. 2003;15(2-3):213-34.

Government of India: Morbidity, Health Care and the Condition of the Aged. National Sample Survey Organization, Government of India; 2006.

Government of India: Situation Analysis of the Elderly in India. Central Statistics Office, Ministry of Statistics & Programme Implementation, Government of India; 2011.

Government of India: Situation analysis of the elderly in India. Central Statistics Office, Ministry of Statistics & Programme Implementation, Government of India; 2016.

Goyal A, Kajal KS. Prevalence of depression in elderly population in the southern part of Punjab. J Family Med Prim Care. 2014;3(4):359.

Guha R. Morbidity related epidemiological determinants in Indian aged-An overview. In: Ramachandran CR, Shah B (Eds). Public Health Implications of Ageing in India. New Delhi: Indian Council of Medical Research; 1994.

Gupta R. Systems Perspective: Understanding care giving of the elderly in India. Health Care Women Int. 2009;30(12):1040-54.

Hall RC, Platt DE, Hall RC. Suicide risk assessment: A review of risk factors for suicide in 100 patients who made severe suicide attempts: evaluation of suicide risk in a time of managed care. Psychosomatics. 1999;40:18-27.

Harris T, Cook DG, Victor C, et al. Predictors of depressive symptoms in older people—a survey of two general practice populations. Age Ageing. 2003;32(5):510-8.

Ingle GK, Nath A. Geriatric health in India: Concerns and solutions. Indian J Comm Med. 2008;33(4):214.

Krishnaswamy B, Sein U, Munodawafa D, et al. Ageing in India. Ageing Int 2008;32(4):258-68.

Mathers C. The global burden of disease: 2004 update. World Health Organization: Geneva; 2008.

Murthy P, Manjunatha N, Subodh BN, et al. Substance use and addiction research in India. Indian J Psychiatry. 2010;52(Suppl1):S189.

Nadkarni A, Murthy P, Crome IB, et al. Alcohol use and alcohol-use disorders among older adults in India: A literature review. Aging Ment Health. 2013;17:979-91.

National Institute of Social Defense (NISD). Age Care in India: National Initiative on Care for Elderly. NISD, Ministry of Social Justice and Empowerment, Government of India; 2008.

Nebhinani N, Pareek V, Grover S. Late-life psychosis: An overview. J Geriatric Ment Health. 2014;1:60-70.

Patwardhan K, Gehlot S, Singh G, et al. The Ayurveda education in India: how well are the graduates exposed to basic clinical skills? Evid Based Complement Alternat Med. 2011;2011:21.

Prakash O, Kukreti P. State of geriatric mental health in India. Curr Transl Geriatr Exp Gerontol Rep. 2013;2(1):1-6.

Prakash O, Rajkumar RP. Anxiety disorders in late-life: a clinical overview. Indian J Private Psychiatry. 2009;19.

Premarajan KC, Danabalan M, Chandrasekar R, et al. Prevalence of psychiatry morbidity in an urban community of Pondicherry. Indian J Psychiatry. 1993;35(2):99-102.

Ramchandran V, Menon MS, Murthy BR. Psychiatric disorders in subjects aged over fifty. Indian J Psychiatry. 1979;22:193-8.

Rao TSS, Shaji KS. Demographic aging: Implications for mental health. Indian J Psychiatry. 2007;49(2):78-80.

Reddy PH. The health of the aged in India. Health Transit Rev. 1996;233-44.

Saldanha D, Mani R, Srivastav K, et al. An epidemiological study of dementia under the aegis of mental health program, Maharashtra, Pune Chapter. Indian J Psychiatry. 2010;52:131-9.

Seby K, Chaudhury S, Chakraborty R. Prevalence of psychiatric and physical morbidity in an urban geriatric population. Indian J Psychiatry. 2011;53:121-7.

Sethi BB, Trivedi JK. Drug abuse in rural population. Indian J Psychiatry. 1979;21:211-6.

Shah A. The relationship between suicide rates and age: An analysis of multinational data from the World Health Organization. Int Psychogeriatr. 2007;19:1141-52.

Shah B. Report of the Workshop on Research and Health Care Priorities in Geriatric Medicine and Ageing. New Delhi: Indian Council of Medical Research;1999.

Shaji KS, Jithu VP, Jyothi KS. Indian research on aging and dementia. Indian J Psychiatry. 2010;52:148-52.

Shankardass M: No One Cares about Elder Abuse in India. One World South Asia. 2009.

Thirunavukarasu M, Thirunavukarasu P. Training and national deficit of psychiatrists in India - a critical analysis. Indian J Psychiatry. 2010;52:83-8.

Tiple P, Sharma SN, Srivastava AS. Psychiatric morbidity in geriatric people. Indian J Psychiatry. 2006;48(2):88-94.

Tiwari SC, Pandey NM. Status and requirements of geriatric mental health services in India: An evidence-based commentary. Indian J Psychiatry. 2012;54(1):8-14.

Tiwari SC, Geriatric Psychiatric morbidity in rural northern India: Implications for the future. Int Psychogeriatr. 2000;12(1):35-48.

United Nations. World Population Ageing: 1950–2050. New York: Department of Economic and Social Affairs, Population Division, United Nations; 2002.

Verma R, Khanna P. National program of health-care for the elderly in India: a hope for healthy ageing. Int J Prev Med. 2013;4(10):1103.

Chapter 28

Physical Comorbidity in Psychiatry

R Padmavati

SUMMARY

Recent decades are seeing a gradual rise in the occurrence of physical illnesses in persons suffering from mental illnesses, reaching epidemic proportions in many countries, and this is evolving as a major global challenge in public health. Chronic diseases manifest as comorbid illness in persons with serious mental illnesses. Depression, bipolar disorder, anxiety disorders, and dementia frequently coexist with a myriad of physical illnesses. People suffering from severe mental illnesses (SMIs) generally have a shorter life span than their healthy counterparts. This early mortality has been largely attributed to physical illnesses, especially cardiovascular diseases and metabolic disorders like type 2 diabetes mellitus, or metabolic syndrome. Inequality in the provision and availability of healthcare services continues to grow, leading to poorer outcomes in terms of physical health (Lawrence & Kisley, 2010). A combination of contributory factors has been proposed: mental health services being provided separately from other medical services, the stigma associated with general healthcare provision to persons with psychiatric disorders, and the ramifications of the symptoms and treatment of these psychiatric disorders. Physical illnesses need to be managed adequately along with the mental health condition. Integrated care models have been suggested. Psychosocial intervention strategies may play a vital role in the delivery of lifestyle modifications, dually targeting functional disabilities, resulting from the psychiatric condition and introducing lifestyle changes necessary for chronic disease management.

INTRODUCTION

Recent period is witness to a gradual rise in the occurrence of physical illnesses in persons suffering from mental illnesses, reaching epidemic proportions in many countries (Sartorius, 2007). Protecting and promoting physical health in persons with severe mental illness is emerging as a major global challenge in the areas of ethics and public health (Maj, 2009). Physical illness is also the cause of early mortality in people suffering from SMIs, as compared to their healthy counterparts (DeHert et al., 2011a). Depression, bipolar disorder, anxiety disorders, and dementia frequently coexist with a myriad of physical illnesses, with chronic illnesses forming the major proportion of this comorbidity (Sartorius, 2007).

Mental disorders and physical illnesses are related in multifaceted ways. Psychiatric disorders exacerbate modifiable risk factors for chronic physical illnesses, such as unhealthy eating, tobacco and alcohol use, and physical inactivity. Mental illnesses are also direct risk factors for chronic diseases; risks of having one or more chronic physical illness in an individual with mental illness is higher than a person without it. Also, patients suffering from psychiatric disorders are less likely to seek help for the physical illness, and have poorer adherence to treatment, thereby affecting prognosis (Saxena & Maj, 2017).

Chronic disease groups (cardiovascular, respiratory, metabolic disorders, sensory loss disorders, cancers), often coexist with mental illnesses (substance use, psychoses, and mood disorders), and require similar interventions in terms of healthcare (Patel et al., 2011). Literature of the management of chronic diseases focuses largely on lifestyle modifications which include diet and physical activity (Hartley, 2014). Modifying lifestyle behaviors such as changing poor diet, exercising, stopping smoking and substance abuse significantly improves the quality of life and general health, decreases disease burden, lessens disabilities, and lowers medical costs. In the past 15 years, several models have been developed for the management of chronic illnesses. These models are of high quality and evidence-based (Epping-Jordan et al., 2004). The most noteworthy of all such models, which has been demonstrated to improve health services delivery in developing countries is the Chronic Care Model (CCM) (Bodenheimer et al., 2002). The role of biopsychosocial approach in addressing these interventions has also been addressed (Deter, 2012).

This chapter will provide an overview of physical comorbidity amongst persons with mental illnesses, with emphasis on how psychosocial interventions can incorporate lifestyle modification in the management of mental illnesses. It is not a complete review of all psychiatric conditions, and dementias are not dealt within this chapter.

PHYSICAL COMORBIDITY IN PSYCHIATRIC ILLNESSES

Overview

Physical comorbidities in people suffering from SMIs often remain untreated or inadequately managed, and lead to a worsening of the psychiatric symptoms (Dixon et al., 1999). People with SMIs (specifically bipolar disorder, depression, schizophrenia and schizoaffective disorder) suffer from greater mortality (twice or thrice the risk, as compared to the healthy population), as reported by many researchers (Harris, 1998; Lui et al., 2017). Life-expectancy of patients with SMIs is reduced by 13–30 years, 60% of which is contributed by the comorbid physical illnesses (Holt & Peveler, 2010; DeHert et al., 2011a). Additionally, patients with SMIs, have a higher than the routine rate of undetected and unmanaged physical illnesses (DeHert et al., 2011b). While higher rate ratios have been noted with suicide and homicide, disease burden due to major chronic diseases is much higher in persons with SMIs. Physical illnesses especially DM, cardiovascular disorders, cancer, respiratory disease, and metabolic syndrome are the leading causes of early death in this population (Kisley et al., 2005; Lawrence et al., 2001; Leucht et al. 2007).

Evidence from India also indicates that there is substantial medical comorbidity in patients with mental disorders. In a study investigating, the rate of occurrence of comorbid medical illnesses in people admitted with psychiatric disorders (Manuel et al., 2013), one hundred people with mental illness admitted to general wards of the Department of Psychiatry, were assessed for evidence of concurrent medical comorbidity. The assessment included clinical examination and investigations. Forty-nine percent of inpatients with psychiatric disorders had medical comorbidity (26%—bipolar disorder, 13%—schizophrenia, 8%—depressive disorders) with DM, hypothyroidism, and hypertension being the commonest medical comorbidities.

A hospital-based, retrospective study from a tertiary healthcare facility screened medical case records of 300 patients that visited the psychiatry department (Vaidyanathan et al., 2017). Out of 300 outpatients, 93 (31%) patients had a coexisting physical illness. The predominant system involved was found to be cardiovascular (33.3%) in which hypertension was the most common diagnosis followed by metabolic/endocrine (27%), in which DM and hypothyroidism were the most common diagnoses. About 42% of the patients having disorders due to psychoactive substance use had a comorbid physical illness, with the majority suffering from either gastritis or alcoholic liver disease. The high rates of physical comorbidity in patients with disorders due to psychoactive substance use in India may indicate the reluctance of the Indian population in visiting a psychiatrist until and unless they are forced to do so by underlying physical illness.

Schizophrenia

The literature on medical comorbidity in schizophrenia is abundant (Lambert et al., 2003; DeHert et al., 2011a, 2011b; Suthar & Nebhinani, 2017). Prevalence of obesity, metabolic syndrome, impaired glucose tolerance and diabetes has been reported to be higher in inpatients suffering from schizophrenia as compared to those not having schizophrenia (Subashini et al., 2011). A significant contribution to the premature mortality in patients with schizophrenia is from unrecognized and untreated cardiovascular disease (Smith et al., 2013).

Depression and Anxiety

Depression and anxiety affect many patients with other medical illnesses, and both these disorders result in poorer health and a higher utilization of healthcare services. People suffering from depression present higher health expenditures (Simon, 2003), work disability (Simon, 2003), poorer compliance to treatment (DiMatteo et al., 2006) and a higher mortality postcardiac surgery (Blumenthal et al., 2003). Among people with severe chronic diseases, occurrence of depression is higher than that in general population (Boing et al., 2012).

New onset of coronary events of disease in patients with existing cardiovascular morbidity is associated with anxiety disorders. A higher propensity to develop coronary artery disease is observed in people with phobic anxiety or panic disorder (Coryell et al., 1986). As compared to women with low levels of anxiety, about 60% of women suffering from phobic anxiety had the probability of suffering from a heart attack, and about one-third of these were more likely to die from such a heart attack, according to the Nurses Health Study in women (Albert et al., 2005). The probability of developing a cardiac or cerebrovascular event was increased three-fold in women who suffered from panic attacks, based on Women's Health Initiative data from 3,300 women in the postmenopausal phase (Smoller et al., 2007). Anxiety has also been reported to be an independent risk factor for coronary artery disease and cardiac mortality in a meta-analysis. The association between coronary artery disease and anxiety, especially the mechanisms by which they affect each other, needs to be investigated using better, more valid and reliable measures of anxiety (Roest et al., 2010).

In patients with coronary heart disease suffering from depression, there is a higher risk of cardiac mortality and morbidity. However, underlying mechanisms for this association are still elusive. Carney et al. (2002) proposed explanatory physiological and behavioral mechanisms for this increased risk. These include antidepressant cardiotoxicity, hypertension, cigarette smoking, poor functional capacity, and diabetes (last four being independent cardiac risk factors), higher coronary disease severity in patients with depression, and poor compliance to preventive and treatment regimens for cardiac illness. Further investigation is warranted to ascertain the mechanisms by which depression increases cardiac morbidity and mortality.

Patients with bipolar disorder frequently have co-occurring medical illnesses. More than 80% have at least one current physical ailment, with about one-fifth each having one or two physical co-morbidities each, and about 40% having more than two co-morbidities (Fenn et al., 2005). Patients with bipolar disorder have a greater propensity to suffer type 2 DM, cardiovascular disease, or endocrine disorders, as compared to the general population (McIntyre et al., 2005). In a study from India looking at the case records of 120 bipolar patients for comorbid physical illnesses, 64% of the sample were seen to have a comorbid physical illness, with cardiovascular illnesses being about 20% (Munoli et al., 2014). In a study on bipolar disorder from Brazil, the prevalence of various comorbidities in inpatients with bipolar disorder, Gomes et al. (2013) reported high prevalence of smoking (27%), physical inactivity (64.9%), alcohol use disorders (20.8%), elevated fasting glucose (26.4%), diabetes (13.2%), hypertension (38.4%), hypertriglyceridemia (25.8%), low HDL-cholesterol (27.7%), and abdominal obesity (59.1%). Abdominal obesity was higher in women, while hypertriglyceridemia, diabetes and alcohol use disorders were found to be more in men. Select risk factors for cardiovascular disease included physical inactivity, alcohol abuse, and pattern of medication. The researchers emphasized the need for improving recognition and awareness regarding cardiovascular and metabolic illnesses in these patients.

Patients suffering from SMIs frequently demonstrate poor physical health due to several contributing factors (Lawrence & Kisley, 2010). Psychopharmacological agents, especially second-generation antipsychotics have been well recognised to contribute to the emergence of chronic disease, since the outcome evaluation of the CATIE (Leucht et al., 2009; Daumit et al., 2009). However, lifestyle choices (physical inactivity, poor diet, smoking, etc) play a critical role in the increased prevalence of obesity, diabetes, cardiovascular risk, and several cancers. Psychiatric symptomatology (negative symptoms, depression, disorganized behavior) contribute to increased risk for chronic disease. Adverse effects of medications like sedation, increased appetite and weight gain add to the ill health (DeHert, et al., 2011a).

HEALTHCARE SERVICE UTILIZATION

Patients with SMIs utilize healthcare services for chronic diseases less frequently than those with anxiety and depressive disorders. Poorly diagnosed and managed patients with anxiety or depression demonstrate chronic physical symptoms and frequent access to healthcare. The emergency care is accessed more often by anxious patients while patients with depressive disorders are more often observed in medical units. People suffering from anxiety disorders commonly demonstrate symptoms which are physical in nature, such as irritable bowel, chest pain, unexplained dizziness, breathing difficulties, headache, and chronic fatigue. Although investigations do not often reveal a physical condition, anxiety disorders also do not get identified. There are many reports of patients presenting to the emergency room (ER) with chest pain often demonstrating symptoms of psychiatric disorders, especially of depressive or anxiety disorders (Soares-Filho et al., 2009). Wulsin et al. (1991) investigated the role of psychiatric symptoms in the ER visits for atypical chest pain. In up to 60% of the patients, an initial diagnosis of anxiety (46%), or depression (34%) was made. Multiple diagnoses could be made in 40% of the cases, the most frequent being PD (31%) and major depressive disorder (23%). Another study found that of all the patients presenting to the ER with chest pain, almost one-third could be diagnosed as a PD, and no evidence of coronary artery disease was found in 22.4% of the sample (Lynch & Galbraith, 2003). PD has been shown to contribute to a greater expenditure in the non-psychiatric, general medical services than any other mental illness, and non-diagnosis of PD is the main reason for the continuing use of such services. Demiryoguran et al. (2006) found a greater propensity of anxiety in 31.2% of people with atypical chest pain. In this group, more than three-quarters of patients reported that they had previously received attention in the ER for similar symptoms. Excess utilization of healthcare services has been noted in patients with high depression and anxiety scores with poorer quality of life (Coley et al., 2009).

People suffering from SMIs often do not access healthcare services for the coexisting physical illnesses, which thus remain unrecognised and untreated. Patient-related factors apparently play a significant part in such lack of access. Behavioral and lifestyle risk factors like substance abuse, poor diet, lack of exercise, and being obese (Kendrick, 1996; Brown et al., 1999), psychiatric medicines and their side effects (Mitchell & Malone, 2006) and cognitive impairment, self-neglect, fear/suspiciousness, poor socioeconomic status, motivation, lack of psychosocial support, difficulty communicating needs, social isolation, and low reporting of pain due to either a higher threshold or lowered sensitivity, all related to the chronic mental illness, have been cited as the reason (Dworkin, 1994; Sokal et al., 2004).

Poor physical health outcomes are increasingly being attributed to disparities in healthcare provision. The gap has been ascribed to a combination of factors which include general medical health service settings which do not offer mental healthcare, stigma related to psychiatric illnesses, which precludes proper medical health evaluation by the healthcare providers, consequences of mental illness and the side effects of its treatment. Much of the subsequent excess mortality appears to be explained by the quality of healthcare provided for the SMIs (Druss et al., 2001). Physical comorbidities, especially those that are untreated are observed to occur at a higher rate in patients with SMI, and the mental health is inversely proportional to the occurrence of the physical comorbidities (Dixon et al., 1999). A significant inequality in healthcare service utilization by SMI patients has been seen in most of the studies included in a recent meta-analysis (Mitchell & Malone, 2006). While the cardiovascular disease mortality is the highest in persons with SMI, the chance that they receive specific interventions or medications are low (DeHert et al., 2011a). Nasrallah et al. (2006) provide evidence that screening for hypertension (62% unmanaged) or dyslipidemia (88% unmanaged) is poor in patients diagnosed with schizophrenia. It has also been observed that these patients are poorly monitored for cholesterol levels, and are infrequently prescribed statins. In a report from the UK, patients with schizophrenia were less likely to have their cholesterol levels measured recently, or be treated with a statin (Hippisley-Cox et al., 2007). Patients with SMIs also have fewer cardiac interventions (stenting/bypass grafting etc.) (Druss, 2000; Lawrence et al., 2003; Kisely et al., 2007), and are less likely to receive warfarin or cerebrovascular arteriography after a stroke (Kisely et al., 2009), and adequate care following cardiac failure (Rathore et al., 2008). Ischemic heart disease (IHD) has been found to be the major contributor to mortality in patients with mental illnesses, more so than even suicide, in a study from Australia exploring the correlation between psychiatric disorders and IHD-related hospital admissions, revascularization procedures and deaths. As opposed to the general trend in the healthy population, this mortality rate in patients with mental illnesses did not diminish over time. Although IHD-related rates of hospital admissions were comparable for patients with mental illnesses and the general population, the former group (especially those with psychoses) had fewer revascularization procedures (Lawrence et al., 2003).

Patients with diabetes and comorbid psychiatric disorders have a lower probability of receiving standard levels of care for diabetes (Nasrallah et al., 2006; Lawrence & Kisley, 2010; DeHert et al., 2011b). Depressive disorder and diabetes coexist approximately twice as frequently as chance permits. The clinical outcomes of comorbid diabetes and depression are worsened by each other, posing a major clinical challenge (Holt et al., 2014).

Evidence for inadequate screening or management is noted for other medical conditions as well. Routine cancer screening is done less often for persons with SMIs (Carney & Jones, 2006; Xiong et al., 2008). Cooke et al. (2007) reported that schizophrenia patients with appendicitis present late to the emergency and with more complications like a perforated appendix or gangrene, and the surgical outcomes are worse than subjects without schizophrenia. People with psychoses have a lower chance of receiving treatment for osteoarthritis (Redelmeier et al., 1998). Reviewing data on medical comorbidity, McIntyre et al. (2007) found that in patients with bipolar disorder, chronic health problems were common, under-recognized and suboptimally treated.

Sudden deaths have been reported in people with mental illnesses, especially schizophrenia (Appleby et al., 1998; Chute et al., 1999; Koponen et al., 2008). Sudden deaths may be due to long-standing poor lifestyles, metabolic disorders, and comorbid cardiovascular disease. Some antipsychotic drugs also raise the probability of sudden death due to QT-interval prolongation and serious ventricular arrhythmias. Decreased bioreflex sensitivity and low heart rate variability, both signs of autonomic dysfunction, may also be contributors by causing malignant arrhythmias. However, important questions about sudden death in psychiatric patients remain. How much does the underlying physical illness contribute to sudden death? Does concurrent misuse of illicit drugs, alcohol, or tobacco add to the risk? Do restraint and physiological arousal play a role? Which are the antipsychotic drugs responsible? Does higher dose or polypharmacy play a role?

PSYCHIATRIC COMORBIDITY IN CHRONIC DISEASES

While there is abundant literature and debate on the presence of medical disease comorbidity in psychiatrically ill patients, the opposite remains largely unexplored. Endocrine, cardiac, gastrointestinal, respiratory, trauma-related and, neurological illnesses, and conditions such as HIV are known to present with psychiatric comorbidity. Evidence base pertaining to the prevalence, causal association, and strategies to manage mental illnesses in physical disorders has been highlighted by Gautam (2010).

ADHERENCE TO TREATMENT

While treatment noncompliance is prevalent among all areas in medical sciences, the risk and frequency of such noncompliance in people with psychotic disorders is a huge challenge (Kane et al., 2013; Haddad et al., 2014). Patients who are depressed are thrice more likely to be noncompliant to medical advice as compared to those without depression (DiMatteo et al., 2006). Adherence to treatment by patients suffering from SMIs and comorbid chronic diseases can be very challenging (DeHert, 2011b). Over the past several decades, research has shown that up to 40% patients are noncompliant to medical advice, depending on the illness they suffer from and the complexity of the treatment required. This noncompliance can increase to as high as 70%, if the preventive/treatment regimens require significant lifestyle changes, or are complex (DeHert et al., 2011b).

INTERVENTIONS

Managing anxiety and depression in medically ill patients is contingent upon early recognition by physicians. In patients with chest pain, the symptoms of these mental illnesses often go unrecognized by ER. It is important to thus include these mental illnesses as differentials for atypical chest pain, owing to the high-risk of suicide in such disorders, and the high burden caused due to these diseases (Wulsin et al., 1991).

The management of comorbid chronic disease in the mentally ill needs to follow recommendations made for treating chronic diseases in the general population, as the factors contributing to chronic disease are similar, with the added role of antipsychotic medications. The first line of management of all chronic diseases is centered around pharmacotherapy. Evidence-based practice indicates the effectiveness of pharmacotherapy in improving disease markers such as HbA1c, blood pressure, and serum lipids effectively and rapidly. However, owing to the fact that pharmacotherapy does not always address the etiology of the illness, it may persist and may be exacerbated by stress, poor diet, and lifestyle (Ricanati et al., 2011). Literature frequently reports the implementation of lifestyle improvement in the management of several chronic ailments. In the management of metabolic syndrome and insulin resistance, the American Heart Association and the National Cholesterol Education Program too advise improving lifestyle (including diet and exercise) as the first line (Lerman et al., 2008). The risk of cardiovascular disorders and cancer is effectively reduced by effective lifestyle change. Lifestyle change is seen to cause a reversal of insulin resistance and prevent progression to type 2 DM, decrease hepatic fat (Albu et al., 2010), and resolve metabolic syndrome (Brown et al., 2009). Thus, treating chronic disease with recommended lines of management calls for a model that is patient-centric, and offers coordinated and integrated primary medical and specialty care with a longitudinal delivery program, availability of expert care, and education of both clinicians as well as patients.

Disparities in healthcare provisions for the mentally ill have been widely recognized. Integrated care models have been suggested as a strategy to tackle barriers in the healthcare system which prevent the adequate provision of care, including locating mental and physical healthcare services in the same healthcare system or the coordinated liaison by case managers or other staff between services (Lawrence et al., 2003). Psychosocial intervention strategies may play a vital role in the delivery of lifestyle modifications, dually targeting functional disabilities, resulting from the psychiatric condition and lifestyle changes necessary for chronic disease management. Programs reducing the stigma related to psychiatric disorders are needed within the healthcare system. Psychosocial and cognitive skills training can help address the cognitive impairments and other such consequences of SMIs. A better evidence base is needed to substantiate such ideas because literature available till date comprises of only small-scale trials. Given the evidence of non-pharmacological management of chronic diseases and SMIs, it can be extrapolated to the comorbid mental and chronic disease scenario.

The World Health Organization's Package of Essential Non-Communicable (WHO-PEN) Disease Interventions for Primary Healthcare in Low-Resource Settings (World Health Organization, 2010) includes approaches to effectively reduce the burden of non-communicable diseases in the low-and-middle income countries; such measures including both individual as well as population-based interventions. Such cost-effective interventions are already available and include methods for early detection of non-communicable diseases and their diagnoses using inexpensive technologies, and nonpharmacological and pharmacological approaches. The feasibility of adopting this package in management of the persons with mental illness remains to be tested. While research on testing effectiveness of lifestyle modification in addressing the double-pronged healthcare needs in the mentally ill population can be challenging in view of psychiatric symptomatology (negative symptoms), disability and pharmacological treatment (psychiatric medication), it can be argued that psychosocial intervention methods, which have proven efficacy in the management of psychiatric conditions, can be channelized to lifestyle modification, targeting both the physical and mental health conditions.

CONCLUSION

There is increasing evidence of chronic disease comorbidity amongst the psychiatrically ill population, diagnosed with schizophrenia, bipolar disorder, depression and anxiety disorders. Increased mortality in this group of serious mental disorders has been attributed largely to physical illnesses. Lifestyle factors appear to play a role in the occurrence of chronic cardiovascular and metabolic illnesses, as is also true in the non-psychiatrically ill population. There is a disparity in the care for physical conditions provided to persons with mental illnesses. While persons with anxiety disorders appear to over-utilize emergency services, there is evidence of limited recognition and treatment of the anxiety disorders at these services. Persons with serious mental disorders do not access medical services as needed and often do not receive adequate care for the comorbid chronic diseases. While chronic physical illnesses are mainly treated using medications, the role of non-pharmacological and psychosocial interventions for their management are well documented. Integrated care systems have been strongly recommended.

REFERENCES

Albert CM, Chae CU, Rexrode KM, et al. Phobic anxiety and risk of coronary heart disease and sudden cardiac death among women. Circulation. 2005;111(4):480-7.

Albu JB, Heilbronn LK, Kelley DE, et al. Metabolic changes following a 1-year diet and exercise intervention in patients with type 2 diabetes. Diabetes. 2010;59(3):627-33.

Appleby L, Thomas S, Ferrier N, et al. Sudden unexplained death in psychiatric in-patients. Br J Psychiatry. 1998;176:405-7.

Blumenthal JA, Lett HS, Babyak MA, et al. Depression as a risk factor for mortality after coronary artery bypass surgery. Lancet. 2003;362(9384):604-9.

Bodenheimer T, Wagner E, Grumbach K. Improving primary care for patients with chronic illness: the chronic care model, part 2. JAMA. 2002;288(15):1909-14.

Boing AF, Melo GR, Boing AC, et al. Association between depression and chronic diseases: results from a population-based study. Rev Saude Publica. 2012;46(4):617-23.

Brown S, Birtwistle J, Roe L, et al. The unhealthy lifestyle of people with schizophrenia. Psychol Med. 1999;29(3):697-701.

Brown TM, Sanderson BK, Bittner V. Drugs are not enough: the metabolic syndrome—a call for intensive therapeutic lifestyle change. J Cardiometab Syndr. 2009;4(1):20-5.

Carney CP, Jones LE. The influence of type and severity of mental illness on receipt of screening mammography. J Gen Intern Med. 2006;21(10):1097-104.

Carney RM, Freedland KE, Miller GE, et al. Depression as a risk factor for cardiac mortality and morbidity: a review of potential mechanisms. J Psychosom Res. 2002;53(4):897-902.

Chute D, Grove C, Rajasekhara B, et al. Schizophrenia and sudden death: a medical examiner case study. Am J Forensic Med Pathol. 1999;20(2):131-5.

Coley KC, Saul MI, Seybert AL. Economic burden of not recognizing panic disorder in the emergency department. J Emerg Med. 2009;6(1):3-7.

Cooke BK, Magas LT, Virgo KS, et al. Appendectomy for appendicitis in patients with schizophrenia. Am J Surg. 2007;193(1):41-8.

Coryell W, Noyes R, House JD. Mortality among outpatients with panic disorder. Am J Psychiatry. 1986;143(4):508-10.

Daumit GL, Goff DC, Meyer JM, et al. Antipsychotic effects on estimated 10-year coronary heart disease risk in the CATIE schizophrenia study. Schizophr Res. 2009;105(410):175-87.

DeHert M, Correll CU, Bobes J, et al. Physical illness in patients with severe mental disorders. I. prevalence, impact of medications and disparities in health care. World Psychiatry. 2011a;10(1):52-77.

DeHert M, Cohen D, Bobes J, et al. Physical illness in patients with severe mental disorders. II. barriers to care, monitoring and treatment guidelines, plus recommendations at the system and individual level. World Psychiatry. 2011b;10(2):138-51.

Demiryoguran NS, Karcioglu O, Topacoglu H, et al. Anxiety disorder in patients with non-specific chest pain in the emergency setting. Emerg Med J. 2006;23(2):99-102.

Deter HC. Psychosocial interventions for patients with chronic disease. Biopsychosoc Med. 2012;6(1):2.

DiMatteo MR, Lepper HS, Croghan TW. Depression is a risk factor for noncompliance with medical treatment: meta-analysis of the effects of anxiety and depression on patient adherence. Arch Intern Med. 2006;160(14):2101-7.

Dixon L, Postrado L, Delahanty J, et al. The association of medical comorbidity in schizophrenia with poor physical and mental health. J Nerv Ment Dis. 1999;187(8):496-502.

Druss BG. Mental disorders and use of cardiovascular procedures after myocardial infarction. JAMA. 2000;283(4):506-11.

Druss BG, Bradford WD, Rosenheck RA, et al. Quality of medical care and excess mortality in older patients with mental disorders. Arch Gen Psychiatry. 2001;58(6):565-72.

Dworkin RH. Pain insensitivity in schizophrenia: a neglected phenomenon and some implications. Schizophr Bull. 1994; 20(2):235-48.

Epping-Jordan JE, Pruitt SD, Bengoa R, et al. Improving the quality of health care for chronic conditions. Qual Saf Health Care. 2004;13(4):299-305.

Fenn HH, Bauer MS, Altshuler L, et al. Medical comorbidity and health-related quality of life in bipolar disorder across the adult age span. J Affect Disord. 2005;86(1):47-60.

Gautam S. Fourth revolution in psychiatry—addressing comorbidity with chronic physical disorders. Indian J Psychiatry. 2010;52(3):213-9.

Gomes FA, Almeida KM, Magalhães PV, et al. Cardiovascular risk factors in outpatients with bipolar disorder: a report from the Brazilian research network in bipolar disorder. Rev Bras Psiquiatr. 2013;35(2):126-30.

Haddad P, Brain C, Scott J. Nonadherence with antipsychotic medication in schizophrenia: challenges and management strategies. Patient Relat Outcome Meas. 2014;23(5):43.

Harris EC, Barraclough B. Excess mortality of mental disorder. Br J Psychiatry 1998;173:11-53.

Hartley M. Lifestyle modification as first line of treatment for chronic disease. J Diabetes Metab Disord Control. 2014;1(2):1-5.

Hippisley-Cox J, Parker C, Coupland C, et al. Inequalities in the primary care of patients with coronary heart disease and serious mental health problems: a cross-sectional study. Heart. 2007;93(10): 1256-62.

Holt RIG, Peveler RC. Diabetes and cardiovascular risk in severe mental illness: a missed opportunity and challenge for the future. Pract Diab Int. 2010;27(2):79-84.

Holt RIG, de Groot M, Golden SH. Diabetes and depression. Curr Diab Rep. 2014;14(6):491.

Kane JM, Kishimoto T, Correll CU. Non-adherence to medication in patients with psychotic disorders: epidemiology, contributing factors and management strategies. World Psychiatry. 2013;12(3): 216-26.

Kendrick T. Cardiovascular and respiratory risk factors and symptoms among general practice patients with long-term mental illness. Br J Psychiatry. 1996;169(6):733-9.

Kisely S, Campbell LA, Wang Y. Treatment of ischemic heart disease and stroke in individuals with psychosis under universal healthcare. Br J Psychiatry. 2009;195(6):545-50.

Kisely S, Smith M, Lawrence D, et al. Inequitable access for mentally ill patients to some medically necessary procedures. CMAJ. 2007;176(6):779-84.

Kisely S, Smith M, Lawrence D, Maaten S. Mortality in individuals who have had psychiatric treatment: population-based study in Nova Scotia. Br J Psychiatry. 2005;187:552-8.

Koponen H, Alaräisänen A, Saari K, et al. Schizophrenia and sudden cardiac death—a review. Nord J Psychiatry. 2008;62(5):342-5.

Lambert TJR, Velakoulis D, Pantelis C. Medical comorbidity in schizophrenia. Med J Aust. 2003;178(Suppl):S67-70.

Lawrence DM, Holman CDJ, Jablensky AV, et al. Death rate from ischemic heart disease in western Australian psychiatric patients 1980-1998. Br J Psychiatry. 2003;182(1):31-6.

Lawrence D, Holman CDJ, Jablensky AV. Preventable Physical Illness in People with Mental Illness. The University of Western Australia; 2001.

Lawrence D, Kisely S. Inequalities in healthcare provision for people with severe mental illness. J Psychopharmacol. 2010;24(4 suppl):61-8.

Lerman RH, Minich DM, Darland G, et al. Enhancement of a modified Mediterranean-style, low glycemic load diet with specific phytochemicals improves cardiometabolic risk factors in subjects with metabolic syndrome and hypercholesterolemia in a randomized trial. Nutr Metab. 2008;5(1):29.

Leucht S, Burkhard T, Henderson J, et al. Physical Illness and Schizophrenia: A Review of the Evidence. Cambridge: Cambridge University Press; 2007.

Leucht S, Corves C, Arbter D, et al. Second-generation versus first-generation antipsychotic drugs for schizophrenia: a meta-analysis. Lancet. 2009;373:31-41.

Liu NH, Daumit GL, Dua T, et al: Excess mortality in persons with severe mental disorders: a multilevel intervention framework and priorities for clinical practice, policy and research agendas. World Psychiatry. 2017;16(1):30-40.

Lynch P, Galbraith KM. Panic in the emergency room. Can J Psychiatry. 2003;48(6):361-6.

Maj M. Physical health care in persons with severe mental illness: a public health and ethical priority. World Psychiatry. 2009;8(1):1-2.

Manuel C, Rao P, Rebello P, et al. Medical comorbidity in in-patients with psychiatric disorder. Muller J Med Sci Res. 2013; 4(1):12-17.

McIntyre RS, Konarski JZ, Misener VL, et al. Bipolar disorder and diabetes mellitus: epidemiology, etiology, and treatment implications. Ann Clin Psychiatry. 2005;17(1040-1237):83-93.

McIntyre RS, Soczynska JK, Beyer JL, et al. Medical comorbidity in bipolar disorder: re-prioritizing unmet needs. Curr Opin Psychiatry. 2007;20(4):406-16.

Mitchell AJ, Malone D. Physical health and schizophrenia. Curr Opin Intern Med. 2006;5(5):524-9.

Munoli RN, Praharaj SK, Sharma PS. Co-morbidity in bipolar disorder: a retrospective study. Indian J Psychol Med. 2014;36(3):270-5.

Nasrallah HA, Meyer JM, Goff DC, et al. Low rates of treatment for hypertension, dyslipidemia and diabetes in schizophrenia: data from the CATIE schizophrenia trial sample at baseline. Schizophr Res. 2006;86(1-3):15-22.

Patel V, Chatterji S, Chisholm D, et al. Chronic diseases and injuries in India. Lancet. 2011;377(9763): 413-28.

Rathore SS, Wang Y, Druss BG, et al. Mental disorders, quality of care, and outcomes among older patients hospitalized with heart failure: an analysis of the national heart failure project. Arch Gen Psychiatry. 2008;65(12):1402-8.

Redelmeier DA, Tan SH, Booth GL. The treatment of unrelated disorders in patients with chronic medical diseases. N Engl J Med. 1998;338(21):1516-20.

Ricanati EH, Golubić M, Yang D, et al. Mitigating preventable chronic disease: progress report of the Cleveland clinic's lifestyle 180 program. Nutr Metab. 2011;8(1):83.

Roest AM, Martens EJ, de Jonge P, et al. Anxiety and risk of incident coronary heart disease. J Am Coll Cardiol. 2010;56(1):38-46.

Sartorius N. Physical illness in people with mental disorders. World Psychiatry. 2007;6(1):3-4.

Saxena S, Maj M. Physical health of people with severe mental disorders: leave no one behind. World Psychiatry. 2017;16(1):1-2.

Simon GE. Social and economic burden of mood disorders. Biol Psychiatry. 2003;54(3):208-15.

Smith DJ, Langan J, McLean G, et al. Schizophrenia is associated with excess multiple physical-health comorbidities but low levels of recorded cardiovascular disease in primary care: cross-sectional study. BMJ Open. 2013;3(4):e002808.

Smoller JW, Pollack MH, Wassertheil-Smoller S, et al. Panic attacks and risk of incident cardiovascular events among postmenopausal women in the women's health initiative observational study. Arch Gen Psychiatry. 2007;64(10):1153.

Soares-Filho GLF, Freire RC, Biancha K, et al. Use of the hospital anxiety and depression scale (HADS) in a cardiac emergency room: chest pain unit. Clinics. 2009;64(3):209-14.

Sokal J, Messias E, Dickerson FB, et al. Comorbidity of medical illnesses among adults with serious mental illness who are receiving community psychiatric services. J Nerv Ment Dis. 2004;192(6): 421-7.

Subashini R, Deepa M, Padmavati R, et al. Prevalence of diabetes, obesity, and metabolic syndrome in subjects with and without schizophrenia (cures-104). J Postgrad Med. 2011;57(4):272-7.

Suthar N, Nebhinani N. Cardiovascular disease risk in patients with schizophrenia. Gen Hosp Psychiatry. 2017;45:103.

Vaidyanathan A, Monteiro J, Avinash BL, et al. Physical comorbidities in patients visiting the psychiatric outpatient department in a tertiary hospital in India. Asian J Psychiatry. 2017;25(25):136-7.

World Health Organization. Package of Essential Noncommunicable (PEN) disease interventions for primary health care in low-resource settings. World Health Organization: Geneva; 2010.

Wulsin LR, Arnold LM, Hillard JR. Axis I disorders in ER patients with atypical chest pain. Int J Psychiatry Med. 1991;21(1):37-46.

Xiong G, Bermudes R, Torres S. Use of cancer-screening services among persons with serious mental illness in Sacramento county. Psychiatr Serv. 2008;59(8):929-32.

Social Interventions

Chapter 29

Social Support and Networking

Adarsh Tripathi, Anamika Das, Sujit Kumar Kar

SUMMARY

Social support and network are identified as one of the key factors influencing health and well-being. It can influence physical and mental health through complex inter-related pathways. Research on social relationship and its influence on health started long back and there is a vast literature on the subject available. Social network comprises of the surrounding social relationships of an individual. Social support is a function of these social relationships. Theoretical models conceptualizing various aspects of social network and social support have been developed. Behavioral and psychological processes linking social support and health are delineated. Sociological theories include the main effect hypothesis, i.e. regular positive experiences are related to overall well-being and help avoiding negative experiences, and the buffering hypothesis which states that when any person experience any stressor in life, having enhanced resources via individual or community increases the chances that those stressors will be handled in a better way, thus decreasing the health consequences. Relational Regulation Theory (RRT) explains the main effects of stress on mental health, and it hypothesizes that perceived support is mostly a relative phenomenon, as what and who would be considered as social support is a matter of personal choice. It is evident that the link between social support and mental health comes as a result of ordinary yet effective conversations about day-to-day life or in shared activities rather than in talking about how to cope with stress. Neurobiological underpinning of social support and network have been explored and certain positive findings have been identified. Clinical implications for this research and interventions to enhance social support are discussed. Interventions to enhance social support and interventions improving natural support systems have mainly shown empirical validation.

BACKGROUND

There is a famous saying by philosopher Aristotle that *"man is by nature, a social animal"*. The role of social relationships including social network and social support on health has always been a point of interest for researchers as well as health professionals and it was naturally accepted that the level of an individual's social interconnectedness and embeddedness influences his/her health and well-being. Since long, it was hypothesized that social relationships can maintain or promote psychological and physical health through many different pathways like providing intimacy and companionship, supporting healthy coping, encouraging healthy behavior, and providing information and role models to follow healthy lifestyle, etc. However, it is important to understand that social relationships may not only have positive influence on health, but may also have some negative influences as well. This chapter selectively reviews the vast literature available in this area with a special focus on influence of social factors on mental health.

About a century back, Durkheim (1897–1951), one of the pioneers on sociology, hypothesized that when workers migrated to industrial areas, there was a downfall of psychological well-being due to disruption in the structure of family and community. This break down led to loss of social resources and increased number of suicides in people with fewer social ties.

Interests were rekindled in the 1970s and 1980s to find out the association between social ties and psychological well-being. Several studies were conducted to find the impact of social ties on mental health (Cohen & Wills, 1985) and physical health. Increased longevity was one of the common findings associated with higher social ties across several large studies (e.g. Blazer, 1982; Cerhan & Wallace, 1997; Schoenbach et al., 1986; Vogt et al., 1992). However, controversies persisted about which construct of social relationship has the largest bearing on health, both physical and mental. In the year 1976, physician and epidemiologist, John Cassel and psychiatrist Sidney Cobb studied the relationship between social ties and mental stress. These researches propelled a chain of studies on social integration, network and support, and their role in psychiatry.

Social integration was defined as the existence of social ties. The web that is formed by the surrounding social relationships comprises the social network. Social support is a function of these social relationships. Thus social network refers to a broader term to all the linkages present in the social life of a person, where the linkage may or may not render social support or may play a different role other than providing a support. Social network is thus a more objective concept which includes both the number and frequency of social ties or contacts with support networks whereas social support is a more subjective concept. **Table 1** describes how social support has been conceptualized by different social scientists.

The structure of social network can be described in terms of specific relationship of an individual and other people, i.e. the dyadic characteristics of the network or can also be described as the interplay of the whole network (Heaney & Israel, 2008). The dyadic characteristics comprises of:

a. Reciprocity—Refers to "*how reciprocal is the relation or the extent the support is interchanged*"
b. Intensity—Refers to "*the strength of the relation in measure of emotional closeness*"
c. Complexity—Refers to "*the way it serves different functions in a relationship*"
d. Formality—Refers to "*how formally the relationship operates*"

The characteristics of the whole network comprises of:

a. Density—Refers to "*how much the members know themselves*"
b. Geographic dispersion—Refers to "*how close is one of the members with others*"
c. Homogeneity—Refers to "*how much similar the members are*"
d. Directionality—Refers to "*how equally members share power in the network*"

Social support can be measured in terms of structural or functional support. Structural support refers to—*how integrated a person is within his/her social network*, whereas, functional social support refers to *the specific functions that members of a network generally provide.*

There are also two distinct entities of received and perceived social support. Particular support offered and received during a time of need is known as *received support*. The subjective

Table 1: Social support as conceptualized by different social scientists	
Author	*Concept*
Sidney Cobb (1976)	"Information leading the subject to believe that he (or she) is cared for and loved, esteemed, and a member of a network of mutual obligations"
House (1981)	Conceptualized social support as an interpersonal transaction that involves any number of the following: a. *Emotional support*: Including encouragement, love, care, trust, empathy and understanding b. *Instrumental support*: Directly helping in need by tangible support, like helping people financially c. *Informational support*: Information, advices, and suggestions thus guiding how to adjust to life or any change in it d. *Appraisal support*: Helping in self-evaluation, so that one gets affirmed that one's beliefs and interpretations of circumstances are appropriate
Cohen (1985)	"A social network"'s provision of psychological and material resources intended to benefit an individual's capacity to cope with stress'
Thoits (2010)	"Emotional, informational, or practical assistance from significant others, such as family members, friends, or co-workers; (and that) support actually may be received from others or simply perceived to be available, when needed"

judgement of a recipient whether his social network members will offer help or not during the time of need is *perceived support*. Perceived social support is more strongly linked to mental health than received support, as perceived availability of social support leads to changes in the cognitive appraisal of stress (Uchino, 2009).

RELATIONSHIP OF SOCIAL NETWORK AND SOCIAL SUPPORT WITH MENTAL HEALTH: UNDERLYING THEORIES

Social support is beneficial to promote healthier behaviors like exercises, healthy diet, or even adherence to medications (DiMatteo, 2004). However, increased interactions not only encourage healthy behaviors, but also may endorse risky ones like alcohol intake or smoking (Wills & Yaeger, 2003).

The other major pathway is the psychological process, where social support may be helpful in reducing the perceived stress of the individual about a situation (Gore, 1981), like a person with a good perceived social support may experience less stress, as the person has the faith that people will provide him support. This decreased appraisal of stress influences psychological processes and even the cardiovascular, endocrine, and immune systems. These two pathways are interconnected. Feelings of stress may thus harmfully impact the practice of health behaviors, while health behaviors such as exercise can have beneficial effects on feelings of stress. In addition, psychological and behavioral pathways may have bidirectional influence on social support processes (Barrera, 2000).

Some sociological theories include the *main effect hypothesis* and the *buffering hypothesis*. The main effect hypothesis states that regular positive experiences are related to overall well-being and help avoiding negative experiences. The buffering hypothesis on the other hand states that when any person with enhanced resources of support (via individual or community)

Flowchart 1: Mechanism of impact of social support on mental health

experiences a stressor in life, the chances of handling those stressors in a better way increase; thus decreasing the health consequences (Cassel, 1976).

Flowchart 1 summarizes the mechanisms how social support influences mental health. The *RRT* came up to cover the main effects of stress on mental health as the stress and coping theory does not cover that; this theory was developed to work complementary with the stress and coping social support theory. The theory hypothesizes that perceived support is mostly a relative phenomenon as *what and who would be taken as supportive, is a matter of personal choice*. It is evident that the link between support and mental health comes as a result of ordinary yet effective conversations about day-to-day life or in shared activities rather than in talking about how to cope with stress. So perceived support is not a direct correlate of affect but rather comes from the types of interaction that regulate affect. This regulation is mostly relational as activities are largely a matter of personal taste. This theory also predicts that interventions designed should reflect this influence of relation to make it more successful (Lakey & Orehek, 2011).

The lifespan theory gives a link between social support and health. It says that support is a process grown during the whole lifespan but is concentrated within the childhood because of parent attachment (Uchino, 2009). During the lifespan, this support evolves into various personality traits like low neuroticism, low hostility, high optimism, and social and coping skills.

From the view point of a psychiatrist, the influence of social support and network can be seen in the following ways (Heaney & Israel, 2008).

1. Social support influences health promoting and health damaging behaviors like—increase in physical activity, specific dietary patterns, or sexual practices or even illicit substance use
2. Social support also influences cognitive and emotional states; thus uplifting self-esteem, social competence and self-efficacy
3. Thirdly, there may be direct effects on the outcome of health by a series of physiological responses related to stress.

THE PARADIGM SHIFT

Several crucial changes in the social support system have come through continuous modernization of our society. Rates of migration have increased resulting in separation from family. There is a gradual reduction of extended families and increase in single parent households, which have grossly impaired the conventional social support system. It is well-known that all types and levels of social support are beneficial. It is indeed ironic that as we learn more about the need of these relationships in health, we perceive that their availability is declining.

The image of social support is generally perceived as people sitting and discussing. But with the ongoing trend of urbanization, there is lack of time resources. Presently, online social networks play an important role. Participants are connected through internet to discuss various issues thus rendering social support (Finfgeld, 2000). The major advantages include loose tie relationships thus having no obligation, anonymity and no constraints of space and time. Anonymity gives the freedom of sharing as much information as is comfortable. Individuals can connect with each other irrespective of where they are; which is specially needed for support in unique conditions. The help can be taken at any time during any crisis. The space of internet can be used to extend both emotional and informational support. But it also comes with its disadvantages like lack of tangible support due to lack of proximity or even false identity presentation. The presentation of factitious disorder (Munchausen by internet) can occur where the participant may play a sick role to gain attention of others (Feldman, 2000).

Information and communication technologies (ICT) have now become a part of our life, and it helps in maintaining relationships also. Online communication is closely linked with the number and proportion of strong ties in a person's network (Chen, 2013). Internet use through mobile has enabled connection even on the move, thus making it a time enhancing activity (Ishii, 2004). Social media can reinforce social relationship by having individuals informed of the activities going on in life. It has been seen now that social media can enhance interpersonal relationships and mental health. Popular social media like *Facebook* promote mental well-being by enhancing interpersonal relationships and thus benefitting people suffering from low self-esteem. Perceived social support has been shown to be directly related to the number of friends in Facebook, thus reducing stress (Nabi & Prestin, 2013). As social media makes individuals connected to a wide range of social networks, it can serve as a useful way of sharing and gathering information. If incorporated in daily routine use, social media may help in maintaining interpersonal communications and thus can serve as means for providing and receiving social support (Kim, 2014).

NEUROBIOLOGICAL UNDERPINNINGS

Studies on the neural correlates of social support are limited, but there are some consistent findings. Rejection or any threat to connectedness leads to the activation of neurobiological circuits involving the amygdala, dorsomedial prefrontal cortex, anterior insula, sympathetic nervous system, dorsal anterior cingulate and also the HPA axis (Eisenberger, 2013).

Positive social support leads to inhibition of fear related neurobiological system by activating brain areas such as ventromedial prefrontal cortex, ventral anterior cingulate cortex, right dorsolateral prefrontal cortex, and caudate which are used in the processing of safety cues (Eisenberger, 2013). Thus, it can be seen that social support can decrease threat associated neural and physiological responding by activation of safety-related neural regions and also the associated inhibition of threat-related neural regions. They also show activity when participants think about close others. Positive social support also stimulates the release of oxytocin critical for social functions like identification of facial emotions and understanding the perceptions of trustworthiness. Overall, positive social support by various neurobiological mechanisms has a buffering effect on stress responses, thus having a resultant salutary effect on both mental [e.g. depression and post-traumatic stress disorder (PTSD)] and physical health (e.g. cardiovascular disorders, immune function) (Heinrichs et al., 2003).

CLINICAL IMPLICATIONS OF SOCIAL SUPPORT AND NETWORKING

Social support plays a pivotal role in mental health care. The biopsychosocial model that explains mental illnesses, emphasizes the relevance of social support in mental health care. Routine clinical evaluation need to evaluate the following things regarding social support and networking of the individual:

- Understanding the existing social support and networking of the individual
- Nature of the mental illness of the individual
- Role of social support for the individual with mental illness
- Scopes to strengthen the social support and expand the networking.

Existence of "social support and networking" is not only beneficial for the individuals suffering from mental illness but also a major strength to their caregivers. Existence of social support leads to:

- Sharing of burden
- Better coping
- Early intervention/consultation
- Better quality of life.

Social support is a good prognostic factor in mental illnesses. Patients with major mental illnesses show better response to treatment in presence of adequate social support. Social support is beneficial in patients with depression, anxiety disorders, stress related disorders as well as substance use disorders.

Certain characteristic features of the social support group determine its beneficence, which include:

- Level of education
- Expressed emotion
- Sociocultural beliefs
- Health-related behavior.

Social support group with poor level of education, high expressed emotion, sociocultural myths and negative health-related behavior (e.g. substance users) are rather threat to the process of recovery from mental illness. The clinician needs to address such issues in the management plan. Beneficence of the social support and networking is also determined by its ready availability. The support that is readily available and easily accessible can be potentially more beneficial than other forms of social support.

Social support is also influenced by various sociodemographic variables. Evidence suggests that with increasing age, perceived social support increases, but the relationship is not linear. Adults may perceive little social support. Some studies suggest that perceived and received social support for women is higher in comparison to their male counterparts. Socioeconomic status and employment status have a positive association with social support. Social network also has variations according to some characteristics of network like intensity, density, and geographical proximity.

HOW TO MEASURE SOCIAL SUPPORT?

Social support is itself a wholesome phenomenon whose understanding and measurement needs a complex interplay of various factors. The various scales used for clinical purpose need discussion. **Table 2** summarizes some important instruments to measure social support.

MODES OF INTERVENTION TO ENHANCE SOCIAL SUPPORT AND NETWORKING—CLINICAL WAYS

Interventions can be classified in several ways. Categories of intervention can be:
- Support group interventions
- Interventions to enhance natural networks.

Support Group Interventions

A support group consists of individuals who share a common life stressor and come together to provide mutual support and information. It may include persons having the same disease, disability, loss, relationship challenges or unique life experiences. More similar features make

Table 2: Instruments to measure social support

Instrument	Type	Features
The Berlin Social Support Scales (BSSS) (Schwarzer & Schulz, 2003)	Self-report questionnaire	Assesses perceived emotional support, perceived instrumental support, need for support and support seeking
The Inventory of Socially Supportive Behaviors (ISSB) (Barrera, 1981)	Self-report measure	Assess how often individuals received various forms of assistance during the preceding month. It conceptualizes social support as including tangible forms of assistance such as the provision of goods and services, and intangible forms of assistance, such as guidance and expressions of esteem
Multidimensional Scale of Perceived Social Support (Zimet et al., 1988)	Self-report questionnaire	Measures the extent to which an individual perceives social support from three sources: significant others, family and friends
Social Support Questionnaire (Sarason et al., 1983)	Self-report questionnaire	Measures social support and satisfaction with said social support from the perspective of the interviewee

a better cohesion. A total of 6–12 members can form an effective group and a leader may be chosen among them to organize the group. Some benefits of the support group include normalization of experience, reduction of isolation, sense of belonging and an enhanced self-esteem which together promotes mental health as a whole. There may be upward or downward comparisons in support groups. In upward comparison, any of the members does something positive or acts as a role model for others to look upon, whereas in downward comparison, a participant who is in real difficulty, is talked about and can be impressed for the comparative well-being of others (Knight, 2006).

The most common type of support group beneficial for mental health are self-help groups where participants want to overcome any specific mental illness or at least improve cognitive or social well-being (Humphreys & Rappaport, 1994). It works on the basis that self-help gives the role of helper to a helpee too and this role reversal helps increase self-esteem, decrease stigma, accelerate rehabilitation and enhance decision-making process. The individuals also do not decompensate under stress and thus have a better social functioning. There may be behavior control groups, e.g. alcoholics anonymous or stress coping groups, e.g. mental health support groups, cancer patient groups or groups of single parents. These groups can prove effective in helping people cope with and recover from a wide array of problems thus decreasing psychiatric hospitalizations. It also improves coping skills, acceptance of illness, adherence to medications, decreases worry, and improves satisfaction with health, daily functioning and wholesome illness management. Also, there may be financial benefits by means of reduced hospitalization or short hospital stay (Solomon, 2004). A few disadvantages may result from sharing of inaccurate or misleading information, or perceiving the measure of helping others as a burden. Some famous self-help groups include Alcoholics Anonymous, Emotions Anonymous, GROW, National Alliance on Mental Illness (NAMI), Recovery International, and Neurotics Anonymous.

Interventions to Enhance Natural Networks

Enhancing the social ties, which have already proved to be beneficial, may be helpful. It may extend from family, friends, colleagues, and supervisors (informal network) to health care personnel or service workers like NGOs (formal networks). The amount, type and effectiveness of support differ, according to the network member. Family members are most likely to provide long-term help, whereas neighbors and friends provide short-term help. Evidence shows that it is the perceptions of support recipients rather than specific behaviors which are more involved in well-being. Though, there is a link between the two but research needs to find out factors that make one perceive the behavior to be supportive. Previous preferences, and specific population set are some factors studied. It has been seen that the last social exchange is generally the most effective. This may be increased by mobilizing support, and increasing their receipt. Smoking cessation programs where partners or significant relatives are included are more beneficial. The biggest challenge for the same is faced to find out the network members who are actually committed, thus exploring the existing social ties, ensuring that the commitments remain sustained and also identify behaviors that will increase perceived support. Community members can identify and resolve problems in the community by strengthening the networks that exist in the community.

Various goals are present at the community level:

- Increasing the problem-solving capacity of the community
- Increasing decision-making ability of the community regarding important policies
- Resolving specific issues.

Through these processes, new network ties are formed and strengthened. By participating in groups, there is less social isolation and people can take help of each other (Haber et al., 2007).

CONCLUSION

Social support and networking are essential social pillars. They have a pivotal role in the social existence of the human beings. Existence of social support and networking may have multiple beneficial roles in all domains of life including health. When it comes to the domain of mental health, role of social support and networking is crucial. The clinicians, patients, caregivers and largely every responsible individual of the society need to understand the relevance of social support and networking for their betterment. Researchers have started to identify key components of social support and network, ways for its assessment, clinical strategies to implement them in promotion, prevention, management and rehabilitation of various health conditions including mental health problems. However, theory driven, empirically based interventions to enhance social dimensions need to be developed to improve social functioning and its resultant health benefits.

REFERENCES

Barbara K. Rimer , K. Viswanath (Eds). Health behavior and health education-theory, research, and practice, 4th edition. Jossey-Bass A Wiley Imprint; 2008. pp. 189-210.

Barrera MJ. Social support research in community psychology. In: Rappaport J, Seidman E (Eds). Handbook of Community Psychology. New York: Plenum Publishers; 2000. pp. 215-45.

Blazer DG. Social support and mortality in an elderly community population. Am J Epidemiol. 1982;115:684-94.

Cassel JC. The contribution of the social environment to host resistance. Am J Epidemiol. 1976;104: 107-23.

Cerhan JR, Wallace RB. Change in social ties and subsequent mortality in rural elders. Epidemiology.1997;8:475-81.

Chen W. Internet use, online communication, and ties in Americans' networks. Soc Sci Comput Rev. 2013;31(4):404-23.

Cobb S. Social support as a moderator of life stress. Psychosom Med. 1976;38(5):300-14.

Cohen S, Wills T. Stress, Social Support, and the Buffering Hypothesis. Psychol Bull. 1985;98:310-57.

DiMatteo MR. Social support and patient adherence to medical treatment: a meta-analysis. Health Psychol. 2004;23(2):207-18.

Eisenberger NI. An Empirical Review of the Neural underpinnings of receiving and giving social support: Implications for health. Psychosom Med. 2013;75(6):545-56.

Eisenberger NI, Taylor SE, Gable SL, et al. Neural pathways link social support to attenuated neuroendo-crine stress responses. Neuroimage. 2007:1;35(4):1601-12.

Feldman MD. Munchausen by internet: Detecting factitious illness and crisis on the internet. South Med J. 2000;93:669-72.

Finfgeld DL. Therapeutic groups online: The good, the bad, and the unknown. Issues Ment Health Nurs. 2000;21:241-55.

Gore S. Stress-buffering functions of social supports : An appraisal and clarification of research models. In: Dohrenwend B, Dohrenwend B. Stressful Life Events and Their Context. New York: Prodist;1981. pp. 202-22.

Haber MG, Cohen JL, Lucas T, et al. The relationship between self-reported received and perceived social support: A meta-analytic review. Am J Comm Psychol. 2007;39:133-44.

Heaney CA, Israel BA. Social networks and social support. In: Glanz K, Rimer BK, and Lewis FM, (Eds). Health Behavior and Health Education: Theory, research, and practice. San Francisco: Jossey-Bass, 2001:185-209.

Heinrichs M, Baumgartner T, Kirschbaum C, et al. Social support and oxytocin interact to suppress cortisol and subjective responses to psychosocial stress. Biol Psychiatry. 2003;54(12):1389-98.

Humphreys K, Rappaport Julian. Researching self-help/ mutual aid groups and organizations,Many roads, on journey. Appl Prev Psychol.1994;3(4):217-31.

Ishii K. Internet use via mobile phone in Japan. Telecomm Policy. 2004;28:43-58.

Kim H. Enacted Social support on social media and subjective well-being. Int J Commun. 2014;8:2340-2.

Knight EL. Self help and serious mental illness. MedGenMed. 2006;8(1):68.

Lakey B, Orehek E. Relational Regulation Theory: A new approach to explain the link between perceived support and mental health. Psychol Rev. 2011;118:482-95.

Nabi RL, Prestin A, So J. Facebook friends with (health) benefits? Exploring social network site use and perceptions of social support, stress, and well-being. Cyberpsychol Behav Soc Netw. 2013;16(10):721-7.

Sarason IG, Levine HM, Basham RB, Sarason BR. Assessing social support: The social support questionnaire. J Personality Soc Psychol. 1983;44:127-139.

Schoenbach VJ, Kaplan BH, Fredinan L, et al. Social ties and mortality in Evans County, Georgia. Am J Epidemiol. 1986;123:577-91.

Schwarzer R, Schulz U. Social support in coping with illness: The Berlin Social Support Scales (BSSS). Diagnostica 2003;49:73-82.

Solomon P. Peer support/peer provided services underlying processes, benefits, and critical ingredients: Psychiatr Rehabil J. 2004;27(4):392-401.

Thoits PA. Stress and health: Major findings and policy implications. J Health Soc Behav. 2010;51(Special Issue).

Uchino B. Understanding the links between social support and physical health: A life-span perspective with emphasis on the separability of perceived and received support. Perspect Psychol Sci. 2009;4:236-55.

Vogt TM, Mullooly JP, Ernst D, et al. Social networks as predictors of ischaemic heart disease, cancer, stroke, and hypertension. J Clin Epidemiol. 1992;45:659-66.

Wills TA, Yaeger AM. Family factors and adolescent substance use: models and mechanisms. Curr Dir Psychol Sci. 2003;12(6):222-6.

Zimet GD, Dahlem NW, Zimet SG, Farley GK. The multidimensional scale of perceived social support. J Personality Assess 1988;52(1):30-41.

Chapter 30

Couple Therapies

Adarsh Kohli, Swapnajeet Sahoo

SUMMARY

Couple or marital therapies are included under special type of psychotherapies which have the goal to intervene and bring about the resolution of the problematic interactional patterns of the couple while giving special importance to various emotional and sexual issues as required by the couple in distress. There could be various reasons of distress in a couple which may require couple therapy but the single most common indication is for resolution of their interpersonal conflicts. There are several types of couple therapies namely, feminist therapy, behavioral couple therapy, object relations couple therapy, narrative couple therapy, solution focused brief couple therapy, and couple sex therapy. Each of these types of therapies has its own basis and way of dealing with the couple in distress. The role of the therapist rendering couple therapy is very important as he/she creates a holding environment for the couple, motivates them to express freely and helps them to mend their dysfunctional patterns of communication and problematic behaviors. Evaluation of a couple before starting therapy is an important step and should be done carefully. Steps in couple therapy vary as per the requirements of the couple in distress and nature of their problems. Efficacy of couple therapies have been well-established by several systematic reviews and meta-analysis. However, the situation in India is different because of different family organization as compared to the West. This chapter highlights the basics of couple therapies with special importance to various types of therapies, evaluation of couple for therapy and how to carry on couple therapy.

INTRODUCTION

The word "couple" with regard to relationship has been defined by several authors in several ways. The most commonly understood definition of "couple" is two persons married, engaged, or otherwise romantically paired together/staying together (Merriam Webster, 2017). A couple can present with several relationship and nonrelationship issues leading to significant interpersonal distress to each other. It has been reported by several Western authors that nearly 50% of marriages in their very 1st year and more than 50% of remarriages are being culminated into divorce due to interpersonal intimate distress (Johnson & Lebow, 2000). Thereby, very often a couple seeks the help of a psychiatrist/psychologist to solve their problems which is dealt in a methodological manner of psychotherapy, commonly known as couple therapy. Couple or marital therapy has been defined as a format of intervention involving both members of a dyad in which the main focus of the intervention is resolution of the problematic interactional patterns of couple along with special importance to various emotional and sexual issues as required by the couple in distress (Kay & Tasman, 2006). The nature of intimacy of the relationship, the amount of commitment between the couple and gender issues make couple therapy unique from other types of psychotherapies (Gurman & Fraenkel, 2002).The aim of the couple therapy should be to help the couple transform into a successful dyad from a distressful dyad which is often very challenging and difficult for a therapist, and depends on his/her expertise on working with such couples.

To understand the problems of a couple, we need to understand the life stages of a couple and various problems faced by the couple during these life stages which may cause significant emotional distress. The life stages and the corresponding problems faced by a couple are listed in **Table 1.**

Types of Couple Therapies

The nature of problems faced by a couple in relationship are almost the same all over the world, though there can be several cultural and ethnic variations. There has been a drastic evolution in the area of research on couple therapies over the years. Couple therapies have undergone several modifications and several types of therapies have been developed/theorized (Gurman & Fraenkel, 2002). Some of the important types of couple therapies are described here in brief:

- **Feminist therapy:** It has its roots in the Bowen family systems theory which was developed by Bowen in 1978. It focuses on the gender inequality in power faced by the couples. It was developed with an idea to help the couples in finding a balance between the needs of self and his/her partner, while at the same time remaining emotionally connected with each other (Hare-Mustin, 1978). It tries to explain the importance of gender socialization which prepares men and women to take up functional roles as wife/mother and husband/father in a family. The therapist following this school of thought tries to find out the problems in the role of gender socialization, and how one partner is trying to get the other person change (Lerner, 1988). It encourages the couple to use one another's power properly without hampering each other's roles in the family and at the same time develop both personal plans and family plans to achieve their goals. It suggests that if at least one partner makes efforts to modify self, then the amount of distress and anxiety in the dyad decreases and there occurs a positive change in the relationship (Bevilacqua & Dattilio, 2007)
- **Behavioral Couple Therapy (BCT):** It has been the most researched type of couple therapy with a large number of published controlled trials establishing its efficacy (Epstein & McCrady, 1998; Powers et al., 2008). The therapy is especially tailored to treat alcohol problems, and produce significant reduction in alcohol consumption and improvement in marital functioning. Cognitions and behaviors of a couple impact the various aspects of relationship leading to significant interpersonal acute and chronic stress. Lack of adequate adaptive processes within the dyad during stressful life events, poor communication patterns, and inflexible expectations from one another lead to problems in relationship (Sayers et al., 1998). In BCT, the couples are trained to monitor their partners' behavior, and based on individual assessments, behavioral contingency contracts are made to decrease the unfavorable and increase favorable behaviors within the dyad (Halford, 1998).

Table 1: Life stages of a couple with usual problems faced in each stage

Life stages of a couple	Uniqueness of the stage	Usual problems faced
Initial years of commitment (Johnson & Lebow, 2000)	• There occurs both feelings of love and doubts regarding each other's competency to carry on the relationship in future into marriage • Difference in attitude, beliefs, and behaviors which may or may not be expressed by the couple to each other	• Experiencing challenges to perfectly fit with each other emotionally • Moments of feeling hurt, noting differences, misunderstanding, and feeling each other non-compatible for a long standing relationship
Marriage (Whisman et al., 1997)	• Learning each other more intimately with acceptance of each other's shortcomings • Staying together and spending more time with each other • Consolidating separation from one's family of origin	• Disagreement with one another's perspectives on different socioeconomical matters • Feeling of being powerless and being suppressed in the relationship
Couple with young children (Bradt, 1989)	• Accommodation of a new family member in the family • Shifting of responsibilities and extra amount of work required in upbringing of the child with decline in personal comfort and sexual activities	• Feeling overburdened with responsibilities of upbringing the child • Inability on the part of the young parents to understand the unspoken expectations of each other
Couple with adolescents (Haydee & Alexander, 2005)	• Fundamental shifts in relationships from parents to authority figures • Greater parenting stress related with developmental and emotional issues of the growing adolescent	• Ineffective communication patterns, blaming each other for the problematic behavior of the adolescent • Dysfunction in the family dyad due to the difference of relatedness of the adolescent with a parent with respect to other parent
Aging together (Peake & Steep, 2005)	• Taking care of each other with medical and psychological problems of each other • Knowledge about the universal challenges that every aging adult face • Becoming the caregiver of one another	• Anxiety and fear of losing one another company • Difference in opinions with regard to grown up children and their family matters • Inability to cope up with anger of the aging partner

Improving communication skills and enhancing problem solving skills are two important aspects of BCT. Cognitive restructuring to challenge irrational relationship beliefs is an key aspect of BCT (Baucom & Lester, 1986)

- **Object Relations Couple Therapy (ORCT):** It was developed by Scharff and Scharff in 1987 from the psychoanalytic principles of object relations theory (Scharff & Scharff, 1987).

It focuses on the interaction of the dynamic unconscious in the interpersonal situation of the couple. As per the object relations theory with respect to couples, there occurs a connectedness at both conscious and unconscious level when two partners fall in love with each other, and whether they will remain in love forever, is determined by the aptness of the fit of the unconscious complementariness between the two individuals (Dicks, 1963). As per this theory, in a healthy marriage, the unconscious complementarity of one partner allows for the derepression of the repressed parts of one's object relations so that one can reallocate one's lost parts of the self in relation to his/her partner, but in an unhealthy marriage, there is undoing of the previously used defenses leading to disruption of the internal conflicts (Willi, 1984). The goals of the object relations couple therapy are to recognize and rework on the couple's mutual projective and introjective identifications and to improve couple's contextual holding capacity so that both partners can have a developmental progression (Gurman, 2008)

- **Narrative Couple Therapy (NCT):** It is based on the ideas from the work of White and Epston, who described the narrative way of approaching interpersonal issues (White & Epston, 1990). The therapist tries to help the couple in distress to find out new meaning in their lives by narrating their experiences and retelling stories of various untold aspects of their lives (Freedman & Combs, 1996). The therapist listens to their stories and tries to orient the couple to many other possible narrations from their story. In this way, the therapist is able to find out the power struggle between the couple and their perceptions of one another's responsibilities. The main focus of the therapist is to help the couple to reexplore ways of living by diminishing the effect of problems in the relationships. The therapist's goal is to keep the partners active in the sessions by asking the couple to reimmerse themselves in their problematic stories and trying to find out new directions to solve the same by unfolding new potentials in each other (Gurman, 2008; Monk et al., 1997)

- **Solution Focused Brief Couple Therapy (SFBT) :** It is a brief intervention developed by Shazer, in which the individuals are allowed to find out their solutions in a positive, shared and future-oriented approach (Shazer, 1982). The main aim of the therapy is to resolve the presenting complaint as rapidly and efficiently as possible so that the couple in distress can get back to their usual routine (Hoyt, 2008). Problem solving skills and teaching communication skills are not much emphasized upon and the focus of the therapy is narrowed down to relevant solutions. The therapy begins with the couple's descriptions of how they want their lives to be different if their ongoing problem is solved, i.e. in a way it is the beginning of the end of the story rather than beginning of the problems (Berg & Dolan, 2001). It helps in achieving the solutions to their problems by identifying possible strategies and negotiations with one another. In this type of therapy, the individuals are allowed to be "experts" and are encouraged to find solutions rather than the therapist telling them their maladaptive patterns (Anderson & Goolishian, 1992). By this manner, the couple is made to realize each other's shortcomings and is encouraged to make efforts to reach to a solution which is mutually acceptable to each other without compromising individual abilities (Hoyt & Berg, 2000)

- **Couple Sex Therapy:** Sexual intimacy and adequate sexual functioning are an important aspect of a healthy couple relationship. Sexual dysfunction in a partner can either be secondary to underlying marital discord or primary without any relation with marital discord. Sexual dysfunction can produce or lead to marital dysfunction. There can be problems in each of the sexual stages of intercourse (desire, arousal, orgasm, and resolution) in both males and females. To resolve nonorganic sexual dysfunction in males and females, many types of couple sexual therapies have been developed. Masters and Johnson are regarded as the profounders of couple sex therapy (Masters & Johnson, 1970). Strategies and techniques to treat erectile dysfunction in males and orgasmic dysfunction in females have been very well-established. Most common causes of sexual dysfunction in a couple are lack of proper knowledge about sexual functioning, high anxiety during intimacy, repressive attitudes and assuming rigid sexual roles (Leiblum, 2006). Sex therapy is aimed at learning healthy sexual attitudes and skills, resolving interpersonal anxiety during intimacy and transforming sex to a pleasurable moment with adequate sexual functioning (Lipshultz et al., 2016; McCarthy & Bodnar, 2005).

Evaluation of the Couple for Couple Therapy

Proper evaluation of the couple in distress is the first and foremost step for consideration for couple therapy. Evaluation starts with the presenting complaints which brought the couple for seeking treatment, obtaining information about marital life cycle, sexual functioning, and individual view of the relationship issues and goes with the flow of information provided by the couple. The entire process of detailed evaluation by the therapist may take more than one session with individual partner followed by several conjoint sessions. The therapist would also require interviewing the couple regarding gender roles, power inequalities, financial issues, substance use issues, and any history of intimate partner violence. An attempt should be made as to find out how the conflict originated and the various maintaining factors for the ongoing conflict. In some cases, children can either be the source of conflict or may function as the holding force in the relationship. Assessment regarding any extramarital issues or doubts of infidelity in any one partner warrants special attention. Due attention should also be taken to evaluate individual partners for any psychiatric disorder. The interview pattern should be nondirective and the therapist should take care that none of the partner should feel that the therapist is more concerned with the opposite partner. It is also the responsibility of the therapist to be careful about issues of maintaining strict confidentiality and asking each partner before divulging any information to the other partner. Some therapists also use genograms (generation family tree) as a tool in the evaluation procedure.

Box 1 lists down some of the things to be noted during evaluation of a couple for couple therapy.

Indications and Contraindications of Couple Therapies

The single most important indication of couple therapy is the motivation of both partners for resolving their interpersonal conflicts (Beavers, 1982). Researchers have found that couple therapy is indicated in the following conditions (Wolska, 2011):

- Problems in relationship due to ineffective communication patterns and inefficient problem solving skills in the couple
- Problems in relationship due to previous failed relationships

---

Box 1: Evaluation of couple for couple therapy

- Presenting complaints of the couple
- Current phase of marital life
- Reason for seeking treatment currently
- Past history of treatment attempts
- Expectations of each partner toward each other
- Motivation for treatment
- Precipitating and maintaining factors of the conflict
- Any problems related to upbringing of children
- Role of each partner in the family system and dyad system
- Patterns of communication
- Problems in sexual functioning
- Assessment for any psychiatric disorder in each partner
- Issues related to substance abuse and intimate partner violence
- Extramarital issues

- Partners willing to reintegrate with each other despite having long standing conflicts
- Partners willing to attempt to reach an agreement before taking a final decision of separation/divorce
- Partners experiencing sexual problems.

Similarly, there are a few specific situations in which the therapist cannot decide on starting couple therapy, i.e. contraindications for couple therapy. The therapist should be clear that couple therapy can not be carried out if there is evidence of (1) intimate partner physical violence between the couple, (2) psychiatric illness including ongoing severe addiction problems in any one partner, (3) having extramarital relationship and lack of willingness to continue current relationship, and (4) if the couple has finally agreed upon divorce (Isakson et al., 2006). However, in case of problems related to substance abuse, couple therapy can be indicated only if the partner attains remission or agrees for his/her treatment of addiction. Some authors have also opined that couple therapy is not indicated if the partners want to discuss only their individual problems and do not want to focus on their relationship issues. In such cases, individual therapy rather than couple therapy should be offered.

Characteristics of the Therapist dealing with Couple Therapies

The therapist is the main "holding force" in the couple therapy and he/she is the one who can help in the effective resolution of the conflicts between the couple. The therapist should have basic understanding of how a couple interacts with each other, roles which should be played by the male and female partner in a relationship, and how both of them depend on each other for the smooth functioning of family life. For rendering or carrying out a successful couple therapy, the therapist should have few of the following characteristics as mentioned in **Box 2.**

Steps in Couple Therapy

The decision is to carry out couple therapy after the detail evaluation is made by the treating therapist. The type of couple therapy to be followed depends on the expertise and experience

> **Box 2:** Characteristics of the therapist dealing with couple therapies (Wampold et al., 2011).
>
> The Therapist should:
> - Have good interpersonal skills like a good mastery over verbal fluency, ability to modulate his expressions well, adequate empathy, and ability to listen with warmth and acceptance
> - Make proper nonverbal behaviors in the initial sessions as very often the clients are sensitive to the cues of being understood and being accepted by the therapist in a nonjudgmental way
> - Have the ability to develop a trust and therapeutic alliance between self and the couple
> - Have the potential to provide an acceptable explanation to the distressed couple for their conflicts without hurting each other sentiments
> - Have some qualities that the couple feels him/her to be influential, convincing, and persuasive
> - Be able to monitor the progress of the therapy in a genuine manner
> - Be able to identify resistance during therapy and be able to mend his/her sessions as per the requirements
> - Be able to communicate hope and instigate motivation whenever required
> - Be able to identify the personality features of the male and female partner, and deal with them keeping in view their personalities
> - Be able to identify his/her own psychological conflicts and should not deliberately impose his/her decisions on the couple

of the therapist as well as the time and dedication, the couple is motivated to devote for the therapy. Some therapies (like ORCT and NCT) require a great degree of expertise and many sessions over a long duration, and hence many therapists may not like to go for it. More commonly followed are BCT and SFBT which take nearly 8–25 sessions depending upon the severity of the conflicts and the amount of efforts the couple is putting in to resolve the conflict.

The therapist and the couple are required to establish mutually agreed upon goals of treatment before starting the therapy. The most common goals are helping the partners to negotiate behavior change, to teach effective communication skills and to find out theme of the conflict so as to develop problem solving methods. In this regard, the therapist should make an effort in the initial sessions to find out the expressions of negative behaviors which are commonly known as the four horsemen (Gottman & Silver, 1999). These are (1) criticism (e.g character attacks), (2) contempt (includes sarcasm, mockery, insults etc.), (3) defensiveness (blaming or counterattacking each other for aggressive behavior), and (4) stonewalling (withdrawing from continuing the conversation, leading to further infuriating the opposite partner). These four patterns of negative behaviors in a couple if continued in a relationship have been predicted to culminate into a separation/divorce (Gottman & Silver, 1999).

The next step of the therapist is to conduct sessions so as to make the couple realize how to overcome or stop using the negative behaviors and encourage them to improve communication skills. It is almost equally important to decrease psychologically aggressive behaviors (like name calling, using derogatory statements, personal criticisms, threats, etc.) as well as to decrease disengagement or withdrawal behaviors (like avoiding conservation) so as to improve communication patterns and resolve conflict (Gottman, 1993; Laurent et al., 2008). The therapist should make the couple express their feelings, listen to each other with patience, negotiate with each other's shortcomings and make decisions for further improvement in their relationship. The flow of the sessions in the therapy depends upon the nature of the problems. Both partners are given some homework assignments so as to follow the same principles as discussed in the sessions and to come upon with the difficulties faced outside the sessions in implementing the changes acquired/learnt.

The therapist provides a "holding environment" to the couple in distress and allows them to explore each other in a constructive manner by avoiding dysfunctional patterns of previous behaviors (Scheinkman, 2008). He/she links individual experiences (both past and current) and thoughts with marital relationships, brings to the awareness of the partner the past perceptions of opposite partner, and encourages each other to appreciate the behavior change in them (Kay & Tasman, 2006). Lastly, every couple has unique set of problems and hence, treatment of every couple is different but the goals of therapy are almost the same, i.e. resolution of conflicts/problematic behaviors for continuation of a healthy couple relationship. Ethical issues in couple therapy are similar to any other type of therapy though specific importance is to be given to the issues of confidentiality, limit setting, boundary regulation, and reporting of abuse.

Efficacy and Effectiveness of Couple Therapies

Systematic reviews and meta-analysis of published trials have proved the efficacy and effectiveness of couple therapies (Klann et al., 2011; MacIntosh & Butters, 2014). Most of these studies are clinic based studies and comparison studies (with individual therapy or other types of psychotherapies). Relationship/couple satisfaction has been the primary outcome measure evaluated across all the studies along with several other secondary outcome measures like well-being, aggression, therapeutic alliance, coping, self-regulation, sexual functioning, etc. (Hewison et al., 2016; MacIntosh & Butters, 2014). Meta-analysis are also available suggesting the efficacy of couple therapy in treatment of depression, and have revealed that couple therapies do help in reducing in relationship distress but don't lead to any significant change in depressive symptoms thereby suggesting its efficacy to be inconclusive for the treatment of depression (Barbato & D'Avanzo, 2008). Recent studies have found that there exists an effectiveness gap in couple therapies as most of the randomized controlled trials on couple therapies have found quite significant improvement but in routine practice they have been found to have small to moderate effects (Halford et al., 2016). This suggests that there exists a lacuna in research designs and evaluation of the published trials.

Couple Therapy: Indian Scenario

In India, the family structure is quite different from the family structures of the Western world countries. Traditionally, Indian families are considered as large, joint/extended, and patriarchal (Chadda & Deb, 2013). However, the Indian family has also undergone a significant change with the gradual change in the sociocultural milieu of India. Along with changing time, nowadays, there has been more predominance of nuclear families along with increase in interpersonal and relationship distress in the couples (Thomas, 2012). Difficulties in adjusting work and family, issues with in-laws, lack of trust, etc. are some of the reasons of marital discord commonly encountered in Indian couples coming for therapies (Thomas, 2009).

Due to several interconnected issues in marriage and couple's families, an eclectic framework in couple therapy in Indian scenario has been advised to be the best suited intervention approach. Special importance is given to the family of origin of each partner as the values, beliefs, and behaviors of an individual are governed by his/her family of origin. Identifying common goals with developing effective communication patterns are the basic ingredients of couple therapy. Another problem encountered in Indian couples is lack of proper reporting of sexual problems due to feelings of guilt/shame of not being able to perform and cultural inhibitions of discussing sexual matters with others. The couple should be encouraged to discuss freely about sexual problems encountered by taking into confidence (Manickam, 2010).

"Marriage counseling" is the more popular terminology in the educated Indian populations rather than couple/marital therapy. Only few institutions in India like the National Institute of Mental Health and Neuro Sciences, Bengaluru, and the Schizophrenia Research Foundation, Chennai provide training programs for practicing marital/couple therapies. Other teaching institutions providing certificate courses are the Indira Gandhi National Open University, New Delhi, Christ University, Bengaluru, and the Tata Institute of Social Sciences, Mumbai (Thomas, 2012).

CONCLUSION

Couple therapies are well-established psychotherapeutic interventions for couples in distress. There are several types of couple therapies with a wide range of applications. Proper evaluation of a couple seeking therapy is the deciding factor for carrying out couple therapy. The therapist has to play a very significant role in guiding the couple to transform an unhealthy relationship into a healthy one. However, there exists a lacuna in research and practice in couple therapies as well as lack of proper training centres and experts in this field which are highly essential to improve the current standard of therapies.

REFERENCES

Anderson H, Goolishian H. The client is the expert: A not-knowing approach to therapy. In: McNamee S, Gergen KJ (Eds). Therapy as Social Construction, Inquiries in Social Construction. Thousand Oaks, CA, US: Sage Publications Inc.; 1992. pp. 25-39.

Barbato A, D'Avanzo B. Efficacy of couple therapy as a treatment for depression: a meta-analysis. Psychiatr Q. 2008;79:121-32.

Baucom DH, Lester GW. The usefulness of cognitive restructuring as an adjunct to behavioral marital therapy. Behav Ther. 1986;17:385-403.

Beavers WR. Indications and contraindications for couples therapy. Psychiatr Clin North Am. 1982;5: 469-78.

Berg IK, Dolan YM. Tales of Solutions: A Collection of Hope-inspiring Stories. New York, NY: Norton; 2001.

Bevilacqua LJ, Dattilio FM. Relationship Dysfunction: A Practitioner's Guide to Comparative Treatments. New York: Springer Publishing Company; 2007.

Bradt JO. Becoming parents: Families with young children. In: Carter B, McGoldrick.M (Eds). The Changing Family Life Cycle: A Framework for Family Therapy. Boston: Allyn & Bacon; 1989. pp. 235-54.

Chadda RK, Deb KS. Indian family systems, collectivistic society and psychotherapy. Indian J Psychiatry. 2013;55:S299-309.

Dicks HV. Object relations theory and marital studies. Br J Med Psychol. 1963;36:125-9.

Epstein EE, McCrady BS. Behavioral couples treatment of alcohol and drug use disorders: current status and innovations. Clin Psychol Rev. 1998;18:689-711.

Freedman J, Combs G. Narrative therapy: The social construction of preferred realities. New York, NY: Norton; 1996.

Gottman J, Silver N. The Seven Principles for Making Marriage Work. New York: Crown; 1999.

Gottman JM. The roles of conflict engagement, escalation, and avoidance in marital interaction: a longitudinal view of five types of couples. J Consult Clin Psychol. 1993;61:6-15.

Gurman AS. Clinical Handbook of Couple Therapy, 4th edition. New York, NY: Guilford Press; 2008.

Gurman AS, Fraenkel P. The history of couple therapy: a millennial review. Fam Process. 2002;41:199-260.

Halford WK. The ongoing evolution of behavioral couples therapy: retrospect and prospect. Clin Psychol Rev. 1998;18:613-33.

Halford WK, Pepping CA, Petch J. The gap between couple therapy research efficacy and practice effectiveness. J Marital Fam Ther. 2016;42:32-44.

Hare-Mustin RT. A feminist approach to family therapy. Fam Process. 1978;17:181-94.

Haydee Mas C, Alexander JF. Couples with adolescents. In: Harway M (Ed). Handbook of Couple Therapy. Hoboken,N.J: John Wiley: 2005. pp. 61-79.

Hewison D, Casey P, Mwamba N. The effectiveness of couple therapy: Clinical outcomes in a naturalistic United Kingdom setting. Psychotherapy (Chic). 2016;53:377-87.

Hoyt MF. Solution-focussed couple therapy. In: Gurman Alan S (Ed). Clinical Handbook of Couple Therapy. New York, NY: Guilford Press; 2008. pp. 259-95.

Hoyt MF, Berg IK. Solution-focused couple therapy: helping clients construct self-fulflling realities. In: Hoyt MF (Ed). Some Stories Are Better than Others. Philadelphia: Burnner-Mazel; 2000. pp. 143-66.

Isakson RL, Hawkins EJ, Harmon SC, et al. Assessing couple therapy as a treatment for individual distress: when is referral to couple therapy contraindicated? Contemp Fam Ther. 2006;28: 313-22.

Johnson S, Lebow J. The "coming of age" of couple therapy: a decade review. J Marital Fam Ther. 2000;26:23-38.

Kay J, Tasman A. Essentials of Psychiatry. Chichester,England: Wiley; 2006.

Klann N, Hahlweg K, Baucom DH, et al. The effectiveness of couple therapy in Germany: a replication study. J Marital Fam Ther. 2011;37:200-8.

Laurent HK, Kim HK, Capaldi DM. Interaction and relationship development in stable young couples: effects of positive engagement, psychological aggression, and withdrawal. J Adolesc. 2008;31: 815-35.

Leiblum SR. Principles and Practice of Sex Therapy, 4th edition. New York: Guilford Press; 2006.

Lerner HG. Is family systems theory really systemic? A feminist communication. J Psychother Fam. 1998;3:47-63.

Lipshultz LI, Pastuszak AW, Goldstein AT, et al. Management of Sexual Dysfunction in Men and Women: An Interdisciplinary Approach. New York: Springer; 2016.

MacIntosh HB, Butters M. Measuring outcomes in couple therapy: a systematic review and critical discussion. J Couple Relatsh Ther. 2014;13:44-62.

Manickam LSS. Psychotherapy in India. Indian J Psychiatry. 2010;52:S366-70.

Masters W, Johnson V. Human Sexual Inadequacy. Boston: Little,Brown; 1970.

McCarthy B, Bodnar LE. Sexual dysfunction. In: Freeman A, Felgoise SH, Nezu CM, Nezu AM, Reinecke MA (Eds). Encyclopedia of Cognitive Behavior Therapy. New York: Springer US; 2005. pp. 352-5.

Merriam Webstar (2017). Definition of A COUPLE. [online]. Available from https://www.merriam-webster.com/dictionary/a+couple [accessed December 6, 2017].

Monk G, Winslade J, Croket K, et al. Narrative Therapy in Practice: The Archaeology of Hope. San Francisco: Jossey-Bass; 1997.

Peake TH, Steep AE. Therapy with older couples : Love stories—the good, the bad, and the movies. In: Harway M (Ed). Handbook of Couples Therapy. Hoboken, NJ: John Wiley & Sons; 2005. pp. 80-102.

Powers MB, Vedel E, Emmelkamp PMG. Behavioral couples therapy (BCT) for alcohol and drug use disorders: a meta-analysis. Clin Psychol Rev. 2008;28:952-62.

Sayers SL, Kohn CS, Heavey C. Prevention of marital dysfunction: behavioral approaches and beyond. Clin Psychol Rev. 1998;18:713-44.

Scharff D, Scharff JS. Object Relations Family Therapy. Northvale,NJ: Jason Aronson; 1987.

Scheinkman M. The multi-level approach: a road map for couples therapy. Fam Process. 2008;47: 197-213.

Shazer SD. Patterns of Brief Family Therapy: An Ecosystemic Approach. New York, NY: Guilford Press; 1982.

Thomas B. Treating troubled families: Therapeutic scenario in India. Int Rev Psychiatry. 2012;24:91-8.

Thomas B. Parenting Skills in Families of Adolescents: An Intervention Study. Bangalore: National Institute of Mental Health and Neuro Sciences (NIMHANS); 2009.

Wampold B. In: Carlson J (Ed). Qualities and Actions of Effective Therapists. New York: American Psychological Association; 2011.

Whisman MA, Dixon AE, Johnson B. Therapists' perspectives of couple problems and treatment issues in couple therapy. J Fam Psychol. 1997;11:361-6.

White M, Epston D. Narrative Means to Therapeutic Ends. New York, NY: Norton; 1990.

Willi J. Dynamics of Couples Therapy. New York: Jason Aronson; 1984.

Wolska M. Marital therapy/couples therapy: indications and contraindications. Arch Psychiatry Psychother. 2011;57-64.

Chapter 31

Family Therapy

Ritu Nehra, Swapnajeet Sahoo

SUMMARY

Family therapy is included under special type of psychotherapies, which have the goal to intervene and bring about resolution of the problematic interactional patterns prevailing in the family. There could be many indications for family therapy but the single most common indication is for resolution of interpersonal conflicts. There are several types/models of family therapy namely, psychodynamically oriented family therapy, strategic family therapy, structural family therapy, behavioral and social exchange family therapy, vector therapy, etc. Each of these types has its own basis and way of dealing with the family in distress, and aims at changing/modifying the prevailing disturbed/dysfunctional communication patterns in the family. The role of the therapist rendering family therapy is very important as he/she creates a therapeutic contract with the family, motivates them to express freely, and helps them to mend their dysfunctional patterns of communication and problematic behaviors. Evaluation of the family before starting therapy is an important step and should be done carefully. Efficacy of family therapy has been well-established across the world but there are lacuna in research and practice of family therapy in India. This chapter highlights the basics of family therapy, assessment of family for therapy, and process of family therapy.

INTRODUCTION

The family is the fundamental and smallest unit of a society. Although over the years, the structure of family has undergone significant change, yet it is still the basic unit of human civilization and all human beings give special importance to their families. Family is the closed group of individuals in which one can share his/her joys, sorrows, and problems without any inhibitions. The family not only fulfills an individual's basic needs (like food, shelter, and protection) but also provides an opportunity for personal identity, and shaping social roles and responsibilities. In other words, family helps in determining one's role as husband-wife, mother-father or children, etc. (Ackerman, 1958), and provides the individual a direction for establishing relationship with society. It is also well-known that family relations have a unique power to mold the character of an individual.

Family therapy is a form of psychotherapy, which directly involves the family members along with the concerned subject and takes into account the problematic interactions among the family members (Pinsof & Wynne, 1995). In simpler words, it is a type of therapy in which all the family members are engaged for solving clinical problems related to a single member of the family who may be the sole sufferer of a psychiatric disorder. Since 1950s, after the seminal works by renowned family therapists like Howell, Ackerman and Bowen, family therapy as a means of psychosocial treatment in psychiatric disorders has gained importance. Previously, the studies have focused only on families of patients with schizophrenia, and have identified the link between expressed emotions and relapse in schizophrenia. However, the later studies have also found out the effectiveness of family therapy in a wide range of psychiatric disorders. Currently, there is ample evidence that by educating family members and by modifying the problematic patterns of communication in a family, many clinical situations/disorders like depression, marital issues, substance use disorders, disruptive behaviors, etc. can be resolved (Johnson & Lebow, 2000).

FRAMEWORK OF A FAMILY

A family is just like a system in which every family member plays an assigned role, which is mutually agreed upon by one another. There are certain rules and norms, which are expected to be followed for the healthy functioning of the family. It is only when these rules are not accommodated or followed that the family system gets into conflict and becomes a dysfunctional family. Such dysfunctional families have one or more vulnerable individuals who become symptomatic and present as patients requiring therapy. Some common terminologies used in family therapy are family structure, boundaries, leadership and communication, which are briefly introduced here.

Family structure: It is the repetitive patterns of communication between the family members. As per Minuchin, there are three basic sub-systems in the family, i.e. couple sub-system, parental sub-system and siblings sub-system (Minuchin, 1974). All the sub-systems interact among themselves within defined boundaries. In general, parents have the control of the family if the family is governed by some hierarchical rules and it leads to good understanding and communication in the family. However, if there are no well-set rules prevailing in the family, then parents may not have any control over the family, and other family members (e.g. children) may rule the family (Bentovin, 1989).

Boundaries: The patterns of interactions between the family members are determined by some psychological rules, which are commonly called boundaries. There are mainly three types of boundaries—open, closed, and diffuse. In case of open boundaries, family members carry out their functions without any unnecessary interference from other sub-systems and are considered ideal, as there is always an option to adapt to new change. While in case of closed boundaries, there is limitation of interaction between different sub-systems, and in diffuse boundaries, there is loss of distinction of different sub-systems. There occurs significant interference in the functioning of each other when there are diffuse boundaries leading to enmeshment in relationships.

Leadership: Leadership in a family refers to the ability to decide what should happen in and to the family. It is determined on the bases of age, sex, education, and prevailing cultural patterns in the family. Each family member has a definite role to play, assigned to him by the family and culture. Usually, mother assumes leadership role in matrilineal families and father assumes the same in patrilineal families. In dysfunctional families, the leadership pattern is determined by the conflicts of the individual members. There occurs change in the leadership pattern over the time depending on the nature of conflict.

Communication: Communication pattern in a family is influenced by several psychological and environmental factors. There can be either direct or indirect communication. In direct communication, the words spoken are clear and the message is delivered to the concerned member directly, whereas in indirect communication, the message is mediated through a third person and may be conveyed differently than actually meant. The communication can also be verbal and nonverbal.

PRINCIPLES OF FAMILY THERAPY

The main aim of the family therapy is to ensure proper development of the subject, resolution of interpersonal problems, and improvement in the family interaction patterns. While dealing with a family, the therapist should maintain sufficient degree of flexibility as different members of the family may have different personalities and problems (Avasthi & Khurana, 1999; Chanabasavanna et al., 1987). The therapy can start as a family intervention but later on individual and marital therapies may also be required. Therefore, family therapy can be adjusted to other different forms of psychotherapy depending on the needs of the members and type of problems in the family. The overall purpose of the family therapy is to bring out a positive change in all the members of the family.

Broadly speaking, family therapy can be regarded as an extension of individual psychotherapy techniques. Establishment of an empathetic relationship with different family members is essential in order to identify the existing patterns of communication and interpersonal conflicts. However, there can be extreme resistance in some family members, which may lead to failure to establish empathy. In such cases, therapist should roll with resistance till the resolution of conflicts occurs and should avoid collusion with one/more family members. Counter transference can occur in family therapy which impedes the therapy process but timely identification of the same can be helpful in proper progress of the therapy (Avasthi & Khurana, 1999).

Indications of Family Therapy

There can be many indications of family therapy (Chanabasavanna et al., 1987; Clarkin et al., 1979; Walrond Skinner, 1979). Important indications of family therapy are listed as below:

- Problems in relationship within the family (e.g. marital discord, problems with in-laws, existence of communication gap)
- Interdependence of symptoms (e.g. depression in spouse due to substance abuse in husband)
- Symptomatology in one individual due to a dysfunctional family background (e.g. emotional disorder in children due to parental marital discord)
- Failure of individual psychotherapy because of interpersonal family conflicts
- Separation difficulties
- Severely disorganized family functioning due to poor socioeconomic situations

- Limited resources for individual psychotherapy with more than one family member needing individual therapy
- Psychiatric illness requiring assessment for family therapy (if any of the following indication is met with): neuroses (anxiety and depression), adjustment disorders, conduct and/ or emotional disorder of the childhood, substance abuse (not dependence), sexual dysfunctions (other than sexual deviations).

Contraindications

There can be family or/and therapist factors which may pose contraindication for starting of family therapy (Chanabasavanna et al., 1987; Clarkin et al., 1979; Walrond Skinner, 1979). Some of these are listed below:

Family Factors

- Family in the process of breaking up
- Families with deep-rooted psychopathology
- Presence of multiple family problems (e.g. extra-marital relations, incest, child abuse, homosexual tendencies) not easily accessible to therapy
- Family members staying separately
- Presence of genuine situational constraints (e.g. inability to afford cost or come for therapy as advised, legal issues in the family)
- Nonavailability of the significant family members during therapy sessions
- Unwillingness/uncooperativeness to accept the therapy
- Intensifying physical/self-harm or domestic violence in the family.

Therapist Factors

- Lack of adequate training and commitment
- Inability to develop empathy
- Poor psychological sophistication to understand and analyze the family situations
- Cultural issues (different cultural background of therapist and the family leading to cultural biases)
- Therapist having problems similar to the subjects' problems
- Therapist in social relations or well-known with the family/family member.

ASSESSMENT FOR FAMILY THERAPY

Assessment for family therapy requires a certain degree of clinical experience to set up a balance between disclosure and confidentiality. It should be understood that both insufficient disclosure and lack of adequate confidentiality can lead to ineffective assessment and can pose a sense of having been exposed and dishonored on the part of the individual/family member (Tillet, 1994). Hence, assessment of family should be done under proper supervision from senior therapists. There are several schools of thought on the family assessment methods with few differences in between them.

Usually a four-step decision approach is used during assessment for family therapy (Barker, 1986) which includes:

1. Establishing if there is need for family therapy or not by listening carefully to the patient's complaints as studies have revealed that about 25% of patients presenting for individual psychotherapy actually need family therapy or couple therapy (Tillet, 1994)
2. To decide whether family therapy or marital/couple therapy is required
3. To decide which member of the family should be involved in the therapy, and lastly
4. To evaluate the duration and intensity of therapy.

After analyzing all the family problems, a formulation should be prepared. The formulation so made can have different therapeutic approaches and should be discussed with the family members in order to decide the type of therapy approach needed. The initial step in therapy is often difficult, as it requires the psychological sophistication of the therapist as well as the motivation of the family members to enter into a therapeutic relationship. Usually after deciding the therapy, it is often recommended to give a trial of short-term therapy first, and to reassess the beneficial effects of the therapy. Assessment should include the specific characteristics of the family as mentioned in **Table 1**.

Some assessment techniques are usually employed in family therapy. These are:

1. Circular questioning—i.e. the same question is asked to each family member
2. Family sculpting—is an assessment tool, which examines power and closeness in a family by asking each family member to physically arrange all other family members in order of relationships or in reference to a particular event
3. Reenactment of the situation, which is done by asking the family to act out a situation rather than describe it verbally
4. Reframing—the problem must be put into solvable terms and be referred as a family problem rather than problem of a single family member.

Table 1: Focus of assessment for family therapy

- **Family structure:** Composition of family with all its sub-systems
- **Boundaries:** To examine and draw conclusions regarding the nature of boundaries (closed/open/diffuse) in between the different subsystems. Additionally, look for any alliance, coalition, triangulation, detouring etc.
- Drawing a genogram/family tree with an additional aim to note any influence of any outsider/non-family member on the family sub-systems/individual
- **Leadership patterns:** To determine the power structure (gender/authority figure), level of acceptance by different family members, decision-maker in the family and type of decision-making (autocratic/democratic), etc.
- **Role structure:** Number of roles played by an individual in the family (single/multiple), explicit/implicit role functioning of members, role conflicts, etc.
- **Communication pattern:** Type of communication pattern (direct/indirect; verbal/nonverbal, ambiguous) along with channels of communication and clarity of communication
- **Adaptive patterns:** Coping strategies and problem solving abilities in the family members
- Social support system
- **Values and norms:** This aspect includes the sum total of all those moral, religious and social values, which are and are not acceptable to the family as a whole

Certain assessment instruments have also been developed to help in the assessment procedure. Commonly used tools are:

a. Family Adaptability and Cohesion Evaluation Scale-IV (FACES-IV)—developed to measure the Circumplex Model of Marital and Family Systems, which identifies 16 types of couple and family relationships
b. Family Assessment Measure-III (FAM-III)—assesses family functioning that integrates individual members and collective characteristics of the family
c. Family Environment Scale—examines three dimensions of social climate.

When selecting instruments, one needs to examine family constructs/dynamics to be addressed, and evaluate and understand instrument's limitations.

THERAPY SESSIONS

The therapist and the family members to be enrolled for the family therapy should first of all, sign a psychotherapeutic contract which should be mutually agreeable to both the therapist and all the clients. Starting from the initial interview, there should be proper planning of each session. In the presession planning, the therapist and family should determine in advance who all will be attending the session. In the initial stage, the therapist joins with the family and notes the affective tone and tempo of each member. Then the therapist tries to find out the problem statement, addresses the same and focuses on determining the patterns of interaction sustaining the problem. The therapist may choose to leave the family for few moments during the session and ask the members to think about his (therapist's) conceptualization of the problem (Avasthi & Khurana, 1999). The therapist then should reach an agreement with the family on a solvable problem, state it in behavioral terms so that all the members involved would be able to know the nature of the problem and its possible treatment strategies. The therapist should end the session with a debriefing of the entire session, by setting up an agenda for the next session and fixing up a suitable agreeable appointment date and time, indicating who all to be present for the next session clearly. Gradually as the therapy progresses, change occurs in the family members when they start to gain insight about their dynamics, change repetitive patterns that hinder their family, learn more effective ways of communication and develop more healthy boundaries.

TYPES/MODELS OF FAMILY THERAPY

There are different schools of family therapy, which differ in the method of dealing with the dysfunctional family, but the ultimate goals remain basically the same which is nothing but improving communication styles, accepting one another's problems/incapabilities, and developing ways to avoid clashes. The therapist may select any of the models of family therapy as summarized in **Table 2**.

FAMILY THERAPY: INDIAN SCENARIO

Family therapy in India is still in its preliminary stage. It was Dr Vidya Sagar at Mental Hospital, Amritsar, who was the first to initiate involvement of family in care of persons with mental illness, and asked the family members to stay with their patients during the treatment process.

Table 2: Types of family therapy		
Type of family therapy	*Principle*	*Focus*
Psychodynamically oriented family therapy (Meissner, 1978)	Based on the principles of psychodynamics and object relations	• Listening to the unconscious, maintaining neutral position and creating a psychological space to tolerate and hold anxiety • Handling transference and counter-transference along with interpretation of defenses • To provide insight to the family members rather than motivating them to change
Structural family therapy (von Bertalanffy, 1968)	Based on the systems theory which is a general theory of the organization of parts or subsystems into the whole	• Identification of open (interact with the environment with varying degrees) and closed (no interaction with the environment) systems • Identification of emotional boundaries among the family members, communication and feedback mechanisms • Handling of interaction patterns, redefining roles and modifying interpersonal boundaries
Strategic family therapy (Hayes, 1991)	• Views the patient's symptoms as the representation of failed attempts to solve the prevailing problems that have become self-reinforcing • One unsuccessful attempt generates a series of problems further leading to severe interpersonal problems	• Using the complaints as an entry point and correct the sequence of dysfunctional behavior • Paradoxically suggesting a behavior that is to be eliminated which the family can only defeat by giving up the symptoms
Behavioral social exchange therapy	• Based on the principle of behavioral conditioning • Views family as an organization that promotes adaptive behaviors through reward and disregard any maladaptive behavior by not giving any reinforcement	• Communication training • Structured problem solving with appropriate rewarding strategy
Vector therapy (Howells, 1969)	• Views the individual as being influenced upon by emotional forces within the family in the space of life • Visualizes that the individual's actions are the sum total of emotional forces acting on him; if the total forces is positive then it can be utilized in the therapy but if negative then it should be removed	• Readjusting the pattern of emotional forces in the family as well as in the individual (e.g. self-directed anger) • May allow the family to disrupt and result in new better working families from the fragments

This was the first family psychiatry approach in India and it was noted that there occurred significant improvement in the functioning of the patients along with reduction in stigma associated with mental illness. Following this, family psychiatric center was established at NIMHANS, Bengaluru in 1976 in which entire family stayed with their patient in family wards for a period of 2–3 weeks during which proper guidance, psychoeducation, and resolution of family conflicts were conducted through an eclectic approach (Avasthi & Khurana, 1999). Till date, NIMHANS, Bengaluru has the only structured family therapy unit set up in India which offers training and certificate courses to trainees and mental health professionals. Additionally, there are universities and colleges such as the Indira Gandhi National Open University, New Delhi; Christ University and Sampurna Montfort College, Bangalore; the Tata Institute of Social Sciences, Mumbai; and Total Response to Alcohol and Drug Abuse in Kerala, which provide postgraduate programs in social work, psychology and counseling, and training students in family counseling (Thomas, 2012). Currently, in general hospital psychiatry units also, patients are admitted along with their family members, who are involved in the entire treatment procedure and formal structured family therapy is also conducted but this has not been systematically studied. There is also an association named the Indian Association for Family therapy (IAFT) which periodically conducts training programs and conferences on marital and family therapy (Rastogi et al., 2005).

Therapists in India face a multitude of problems while dealing with Indian families during family therapy. These are mainly because of rural-urban differences, linguistic diversity, cultural variations, family power structure, and members in different stages of family life cycle. There is also lack of promotion of family therapy, nonacceptance of family therapy as one of the methods of treatment and lack of research publications in this area (Thomas, 2012).

CONCLUSION

Family therapy is a well-established psychotherapeutic intervention for dysfunctional and disturbed families. There are several models/schools of family therapies with almost similar aims and objectives of treatment. Proper evaluation of a family seeking therapy is the deciding factor for carrying out family therapy. The therapist has to play a very significant role in guiding the family members to transform unhealthy relationships and problematic interaction patterns into a healthy one. However, there exists a lacuna in research and practice in family therapy, which makes it highly essential to improve the current standard of therapies.

REFERENCES

Ackerman N. The Psychodynamics of Family Life: Diagnosis and Treatment of Family Relationships. New York: Basic Books;1958.

Avasthi A, Khurana H. Family therapy and marital therapy. In: Vyas JN, Ahuja N (Eds). Textbook of Postgraduate Psychiatry. New Delhi: Jaypee Brothers Medical Publishers (P) Ltd; 1999. pp. 842–54.

Bentovin A. Applications of Systemic Family Therapy: The Milan Approach. London: Grune & Stratton, 1985.

Chanabasavanna SM, Andrade C, Rasquinha LP, et al. Family therapy at NIMHANS. Indian J Soc Psychiatry. 1987;3:368–78.

Clarkin JE, Frances AJ, Moodie JL. Selection criteria for family therapy. Fam Process.1979;18:391-403.

Hayes HA reintroduction to family therapy. Classification of three schools. Aus NZ J Fam Ther .1991;12: 27-43.

Howells J. Vector therapy in family therapy. Soc. Psychiatry Psychiatr. Epidemiol.1969;4(4):169-72.

Johnson S, Lebow J. The "coming of age" of couple therapy: A decade review. J Marital Fam Ther. 2000;26:23-38.

Meissner W. The conceptualization of marriage and family dynamics from psychoanalytic perspective. In: Paolino TJ, McCardy BS (Eds). Marriage and Marital Therapy.New York: Brunner/Mazel;1978.

Minuchin S. Families and Family Therapy. Cambridge: Harvard University Press;1974.

Pinsof WM, Wynne LC. The efficacy of marital and family therapy: an empirical overview, conclusions, and recommendations. J Marital Fam Ther. 1995;21(4):585-613.

Rastogi M, Natarajan R, Thomas V. On becoming a profession: the growth of marriage and family therapy in India. Contemp Fam Ther. 2005;27(4):453-71.

Thomas B. Treating troubled families: therapeutic scenario in India. Int Rev Psychiatry. 2012;24(2):91-98.

Tillett R. Activity in a district psychotherapy service. Psychiatr Bull. 1994;18:544-7.

Von Bertalanffy L. General Systems Theory: Foundations, Development, and Application. New York: George Braziller; 1968.

Walrond Skinner S. Indications and contraindications for the use of family therapy. J Child Psychol Psychiatr. 1979;19:57-62.

Chapter 32

Group Therapy

Alafia Jeelani, Shyam Sundar Arumugham

SUMMARY

Group therapies utilize group dynamics and interpersonal interactions during therapy sessions for therapeutic benefit. Group therapies range from process oriented dynamic therapies to structured time-limited therapies, which focus on psychoeducation and skill building. The therapist plays the role of a leader/conductor and should be competent in handling group interactions and processes during therapy sessions. The role of the therapist begins from careful selection and composition of group members. Process variables, and client and therapist factors influence the outcome of therapy. Group therapies have been evaluated in diverse treatment populations across various diagnostic categories. The level of intervention should be varied based on the diagnosis, stage of treatment, and the theoretical model of therapy. While the available evidence supports the efficacy of group interventions, the relative contribution of nonspecific factors versus specific treatment techniques towards the outcome has to be evaluated.

INTRODUCTION

Group therapy involves provision of psychotherapy in small groups. In addition to the logistic advantage of combining multiple clients in the same therapy session, group therapy utilizes group dynamics and interpersonal interactions during sessions for therapeutic benefits. Despite its origins in the psychodynamic context, other schools of therapy including cognitive-behavioral, gestalt, interpersonal therapy, etc. have also utilized the group format. Certain modes of therapy such as psychodrama are preferentially administered in group format. Current day usage of the term group therapy includes a heterogeneous set of treatments each with its own goals and techniques.

BASIC PRINCIPLES

History

Long before the advent of mental health professionals, religious, and tribal healers used social aggregates such as early shamanic séances, ancient Greek drama and medieval morality plays to promote healing and behavioral change. Group therapy in the sense of a professionally guided and planned enterprise to treat psychopathology is an American intervention of the

20th century (Anthony, 1971; Sadock & Sadock, 2008). Among its predecessors was Joseph Pratt, an internist who as early as in 1905 offered lectures to patients with tuberculosis involving information combined with inspirational exhortations and accrued psychological gains. Edward Lazell (1921) adopted Pratt's approach to patients with schizophrenia using supportive lectures along psychoanalytic lines. In mid-1920s, Trigant Burrow, a psychoanalyst, discarded the couch in favor of small, al fresco discussion groups including patients, their families, and colleagues, which he called group analysis (Burrow, 1927).

Group interventions were developed further by Louis Wender, Paul Schilder, Jacob L Moreno, Samuel R Slavson, Fritz Redl, and Alexander Wolf in the mid 20th century. Many of these therapists worked with a psychodynamic orientation. Group therapy was extended to children and adolescents with the involvement of parents and teachers in the group. In the background of World War II, there was a surge in psychiatric morbidity which led to increased use of group therapy due to the limited manpower. Group therapy was gradually adapted to varied settings including outpatient/inpatient treatment facilities as well as long-term rehabilitation programs (Scheidlinger, 2000).

Theoretical Basis

Group therapy can be understood on the basis of general systems theory. The individuals undergoing therapy can be considered as subsystems, which have an effect on each other as well on the group as a whole. The self versus other relationship is an important process across group therapies (Holmes & Kivlighan, 2000). Group therapy differs from individual therapy in the presence of a host of interpersonal relationships over a single relationship. Over the course of therapy, the group develops recognizable patterns of interactions called group dynamics. Systems result from group dynamics and their interaction to give rise to group cohesion (the perception that group therapy is beneficial and supportive), adoption of group norms (based on guidance from the therapist) and group roles for enhancing one's learning experiences. Building group cohesion is crucial in therapy as it aids other therapeutic factors and determines a healthy therapeutic relationship (Burlingame et al., 2002; Leszez & Malat, 2012). Some authors claim that common factors such as therapeutic relationship may be more crucial for treatment outcome compared to specific treatment techniques (Wampold, 2001). Group experiences provide a powerful change environment, and a wholesome learning experience. A sense of hope develops with the universality that others have had similar experiences, fostering acceptance and altruism. Improvement in symptoms is a result of both self-disclosures that aid catharsis and feedback that perpetuates an interpersonal learning cycle (Budman et al., 1989).

Selection and Composition of Group

Current guidelines are more liberal with regards to selection of patients for group therapy. However, there are certain factors, which predict better response to group therapy. Individuals with manifest interpersonal problems and poor self-other awareness may benefit from group therapy. Client characteristics such as psychological mindedness, capacity for self-reflection/empathy, and motivation for self-disclosure in group settings are ideally preferred (AGPA, 2007;

Spitz, 2009). Those in concurrent individual therapy or with a successful history of previous therapy are likely to do better in group therapy (Stone & Rutan, 1984).

Certain psychological instruments may be used for objective screening of client characteristics that influence participation in group therapy (AGPA, 2007). The Group Therapy Questionnaire (Burlingame et al., 2006) and Group Selection Questionnaire (Burlingame et al., 2011) are specific self-report questionnaires used for this purpose. The NEO – Five Factor Inventory (NEO-FFI) (Costa & McCrae, 1992; Ogrodniczuk & Piper, 2003) has also been suggested for screening for personality traits such as neuroticism, extraversion, and conscientiousness which influence participation in group therapy. The above recommendations should be treated as broad guidelines and clients may be accommodated in groups with appropriate composition.

The composition of group may vary based on the school of therapy and diagnosis. Homogeneity with respect to diagnosis is preferred for cognitive-behavioral group therapies. While heterogeneity in psychopathology is preferred for psychodynamic group therapies, the group should be preferably homogeneous in terms of ego functioning (Knauss, 2005; AGPA, 2007). Homogeneous groups are also recommended for clients with deviance and antisocial personality disorders irrespective of the model of therapy.

Group Development

Models of group development explain the stages, which the groups pass through. The therapist may have to vary his interventions based on the stage of development. The American Group Psychotherapy Association guidelines (2007) describe a five-stage sequence based on established models (Tuckman, 1965; Garland et al., 1973; Wheelan et al., 2003). A brief description of commonly described stages follows:

Preaffiliation/Forming

The first stage is characterized by anxiety related to therapy, tentative interactions, and high level of dependence on therapist. The therapist plays an active role in setting norms, highlighting commonalities, building trust and creating a safe atmosphere for discussion. Pretherapy preparation improves treatment retention and meaningful engagement in therapy (Burlingame et al., 2006; Piper & Perrault, 1989). Preparation involves education regarding therapy process, clarification of roles, explaining norms, and issues related to confidentiality and initiating the process of informed consent (Burlingame et al., 2006; AGPA, 2007).

Storming

After successful formation of the group, members enter a "storming" stage (Tuckman, 1965). Issues related to "power and control" emerge (Garland et al., 1973). Members may challenge the authority of the group leader and subgroups may arise. The therapist should be prepared to engage with negative feelings arising from the group. The therapist encourages group cohesion and provides a safe atmosphere to facilitate interpersonal learning. Conflicts and power struggles within the group have to be handled; and the discussions should be streamlined keeping the treatment in focus with firm limit setting.

Norming/Intimacy

In this stage, the group becomes more cohesive and engages constructively in discussion. The members develop a sense of belonging and trust in the group. Members feel more comfortable in discussing sensitive issues. As members become more active, the therapist may assume a more peripheral role. The therapist encourages sharing of experiences, highlights commonalities in experience, and steers discussion to a problem-solving mode. The therapist facilitates working process, and interventions reflect a balance of support and confrontation.

Performing/Differentiation

The fourth stage involves interpersonal and productive work. The focus shifts to self-other differentiation. Differences between the members become apparent. Power struggles and conflicts may resurface in the process. The therapist should be aware of the developments and should communicate to the members that such differentiation themes denote progress in therapy. The therapist keeps the group motivated to reach the decided goals, serves as a role model and also prevents the group from diverting into maladaptive interpersonal patterns.

Termination

The final stage of termination calls for a review of progress and consolidation of gains. Negative emotions associated with separation and loss may arise which may sometimes lead to regression and relapse of symptoms. These emotions and the process of separation have to be worked through. The therapist encourages members to express feelings associated with separation and prepares them to face future challenges with the gains acquired during the therapy (Joyce et al., 2010).

During the process of therapy, each member can be periodically assessed for group processes and outcomes, with such instruments as the Clinical Outcome Results Evaluation-Revised Battery (Burlingame et al., 2006).

Role of the Group Therapist

The role of therapist is 2-fold—to monitor each member of the group as well as the group interactions. The role of the therapist begins from selection/preparation of the group through successful execution and termination of therapy. Regardless of the therapeutic orientation, the therapist provides structure to therapy, and channels and utilizes group interactions for therapeutic benefits. The therapist functions as the group leader who executes and supervises the group processes. Building a working alliance, conveying genuine care/concern for members, ability to coordinate and manage group boundaries are some of the principal functions of the therapist. Self-disclosure may be helpful, when employed judiciously. In certain cases, utilizing a cotherapist of the opposite gender may be beneficial to serve as role model for healthy heterosexual relationships.

Duration of Therapy and Frequency of Sessions

Duration of group therapy can differ based on the purpose and goals of therapy. On an average, time-limited groups are conducted for 6-12 sessions. Typically, groups are conducted not more than twice a week, unless it is in a residential setting. Sessions may range between 1 ½ and 2 hours depending on the context and group composition (SAMHSA/CSAT, 2005).

SPECIALIZED GROUP PSYCHOTHERAPY TECHNIQUES

As with individual therapy, multiple models exist for group therapy as well. Some of the important models of group therapy are briefly discussed below:

Psychodynamic Models

As with individual therapies, different models of psychodynamic group therapies exist which have different theoretical foundations. Traditional psychoanalytic groups are based on the Freudian theory of the unconscious and resolution of intrapsychic conflict managed through defense mechanisms. The ultimate goal is to build insight by resolving "fixation" from early stages of development by observing repetitive patterns; overcoming resistance; recalling, reliving, and re-experiencing the emotions correctively in the transference with the group and the therapist. Groups using object relations approaches assume that behaviors are driven towards gaining relationships and attachments, while self and ego psychology aim to strengthen the integrity of self; with both approaches emphasizing the role of interpersonal factors in cure (Rutan, 1993).

Interpersonal Models

Interpersonal Psychotherapy for Groups (IPT-G) emphasizes on social relations in psychopathology. The basic assumption is that problems arise as a result of maladaptive interpersonal beliefs and behaviors, and groups serve as a feedback mechanism for mastering healthy behaviors within the group, ultimately leading to enhanced skills to build healthy relationships in the real world (Yalom & Vinogradov, 1993). Behavioral patterns that are maladaptive become much more evident in the "here-and-now" interactions and therapy aims to enhance the quality of relationships, discuss about interpersonal dynamics as they occur in the group and resolution of issues through direct feedback (Rothke, 1986).

Group Cognitive-behavioral Therapy

Cognitive Behavioral Therapy Groups (CBT-G) evolved through emerging literature on populations requiring group assertive training (Fensterheim, 1972), using principles of social learning theory. Components of traditional CBT are employed in a group format. Techniques such as relaxation, problem solving, and cognitive restructuring are used. Group members are required to provide feedback to other members, learn skills for leadership, and are a source of peer reinforcement. Application of intragroup learning can be facilitated through behavioral rehearsal and extra-group socializing (Rose, 1993; Rose, 2002).

Psychodrama

Psychodrama focuses on resolution of issues through action. The "protagonist" or the index client acts out the presenting issues along with other members in the session with the help of the "director" or group leader. Action oriented techniques such as mirroring, self-presentation, soliloquy, role reversal, doubling, etc. are used (Sacks, 1993).

Short-term Psychotherapy Groups

These are highly focused therapies targeting specific therapeutic goals. Treatment typically lasts for less than 6 sessions (Garfield, 1986), sometimes 12–15 sessions with each session ranging between 45 and 90 minutes. It emerged due to limited availability of service providers, need for interventions to be cost-effective, and increased demand for short-term intervention (Klein, 1993).

Self-help Groups

Self-help groups are formed within the community when people facing a common problem come together to share their difficulties and learn from each other. Compassionate Friends (for grief work) and Alcoholics Anonymous (AA) are some of the well-known self-help groups. The role of a mental health professional in such groups includes referral, disseminating knowledge through training, and providing consultation (Lieberman, 1993).

SPECIAL PRACTICES IN GROUP PSYCHOTHERAPIES

Group therapy may sometimes have to be combined with individual therapy. In such cases, it may be helpful to have an interpersonal framework for group and an intrapsychic or behavioral framework for individual therapy. If the two formats are handled by different therapists, a collaborative relationship between the therapists is necessary. The client should be clear about the goals of each modality to prevent confusion and competition. It is fairly common to have combined therapy, where a single therapist provides individual and group therapy to the group members. In such cases, the client should be prepared about the issues that would be discussed in each format. Further, issues related to confidentiality and envy in the group setting should be handled appropriately (AGPA, 2007). Pharmacotherapy may be prescribed to patients undergoing group therapy. A close coordination of the therapist with the prescriber would be helpful in such instances. If the therapist is involved in prescription of medications, a separate time may be allocated to discuss medication related issues. Psychological issues related to medication intake may be discussed in the group sessions.

GROUP PSYCHOTHERAPY WITH SPECIAL POPULATIONS

Children and Adolescents

Children and adolescents have been treated in the group format for around a century (Thienemann, 2009). Earlier approaches took the form of activity therapy, an adaptation of psychodynamic therapy for children, which focused on activity rather than interpretation (Reid & Kolvin, 1993). Later, other schools of therapy started utilizing the group format for this population. For instance, psychodynamic, client-centerd and cognitive behavioral approaches, skill building and support groups have been employed for children and adolescents. Often groups comprise of children at the same level of development. However, a wider age range may sometimes be employed based on the needs of the group (Thienemann, 2009). Similarly, therapeutic techniques may be tailored to the developmental stage of children. For example, activity and play-related interventions may be more suitable for younger children, while adolescents may be more amenable to verbal interactions. Parents may have to be involved in certain groups. Although meta-analysis has shown that group therapy is effective in this population, the literature is plagued with methodological shortcomings (Hoag & Burlingame, 1997).

Physical Illness

Availability of social support may enhance coping with existing physical illness (Lipowski, 1989). Consultation liaison settings employ brief supportive work to influence interpersonal process. Short-term structured groups have been conducted for people with diabetes (Deakin et al., 2005) and sexually transmitted diseases (Weinhardt et al., 1999). Active techniques (Marcovitz & Smith, 1983), such as structuring, focusing on the here and now, coping tasks and homework are commonly employed. Group contracts are made and the therapist uses educational component and structured discussion. Some clinicians recommend only structured educationally oriented groups (Jacobs & Goodman, 1989) for the concern that interpretive interventions may break down defenses and stir up anxiety (Tattersall et al., 1985). All support groups may have some common goals such as sharing experiences, enhancing coping skills, psychosocial functioning, and improving adherence. Goals may also have to be tailored to the particular disorder. For example, support groups for HIV-infected persons may focus on issues such as encouraging disclosures, reducing stigma and discrimination, improving self-esteem, etc. (Bateganya et al., 2015). Confidentiality issues may be especially pertinent. Often, groups are also held with families and friends to facilitate acceptance and support.

Substance use Disorders

Group therapy is commonly used in the management of substance use disorders. The group format may be helpful in this population as it provides a positive peer support, reduces sense of isolation, facilitates vicarious learning, functions as a source of encouragement, offers family-like learning experiences and provides for structure and hope (SAMHSA/CSAT, 2005). Many rehabilitation centers utilize group activities towards the same end. Self-help groups such as AA are also commonly sought out by this population. Therapy groups may also address interpersonal issues by involving family members. The client's prognosis is found to be better with greater duration and quality of treatment (Project MATCH Research Group, 1998; Leshner, 1997).

Elderly

Group therapy with the elderly ranges from the traditional psychodynamic to group CBT and support groups. Cognitive stimulation, reality orientation groups (Woods et al., 2012) and validation therapy (Feil, 2014) are geared to people with dementia. Reminiscence group therapy involving recollection, re-evaluation and review of past events has been used in people with dementia and geriatric depression (Gaggioli et al., 2014). In addition, activity-based groups such as exercise and music therapy are also designed for elderly population. Whatever the orientation and focus, specific adaptations may have to be made to accommodate issues such as cognitive impairment, medical needs, hearing and visual impairment, hydration, transportation, etc. The groups may have to be flexible for delays and absences for medical needs and consultations. Certain themes commonly addressed in the elderly population include loss of independence, shame, low self-esteem, memory impairment, existential crisis and loss of purpose (Agronin, 2009). Some degree of homogeneity in group selections with respect to cognitive functioning may be helpful.

Severe Mental Illness

Group therapy for psychotic disorders including schizophrenia usually encompasses educative and supportive interventions. The goals of treatment may vary based on the treatment setting. Inpatient groups have less ambitious goals compared to outpatient groups which tend to focus on relapse prevention and improving socio-occupational functioning. Therapeutic groups based on psychoanalytic principles and exploration of delusions, anger, hostility, etc. may be overwhelming to the patient and are sometimes discouraged (Spitz, 2009). Commonly employed techniques include education, problem solving, and improving coping skills. Evidence from controlled trials exists for CBT-G, group social skills training, group music therapy, and group psychoeducation. A recent meta-analysis including 34 trials found that group therapy was more effective than treatment as usual for negative symptoms and not for positive symptoms of schizophrenia. While the above results are encouraging, group interventions were not superior to active sham groups. This finding underscores the need for quality research in evaluating group therapy. An important predictor of outcome was treatment intensity. Therapeutic orientation was not found to be associated with outcome, further reinforcing that nonspecific factors may play a role (Orfanos et al., 2015).

TRAINING AND RESEARCH

Training

Professional organizations such as the AGPA have issued guidelines to help therapists focus on the quality of training and maintain professional standards. Therapists trained in an individual format may have some reservations with respect to therapeutic distance and loss of control over therapy in the group format (Mackenzie, 2002). Training often involves multiple components including didactic learning, supervision, observation, and experiential learning (Salvendy, 1985). Experiential learning in a group therapy as a member is often included as a component of training. The goal of such training is to understand how the group process works. As the primary goal of such training is not for personal therapy as such, trainees may be given some choice on the extent of disclosure (Herlihy et al., 2015).

Research

Group interventions, particularly the structured time-limited therapies, have been studied in controlled trials. However, group analytic therapies are not always amenable to randomized controlled trials as they are not strictly manualized, not time-limited and do not focus on a particular diagnosis (Knauss, 2005). Available evidence suggests that group interventions are significantly more effective than nonactive control groups (Thimm & Antonsen, 2014). Systematic reviews emphasize the need for better quality studies to firmly establish the efficacy of group therapies, especially in comparison with active control groups (Okumura & Ichikura, 2014). Comparative studies have shown that group therapy is at least as effective as individual therapy (McRoberts et al., 1998; Burlingame et al., 2004). Group therapy has been evaluated for multiple indications including depression, anxiety disorders, schizophrenia, addiction disorders, etc. Group processes such as group cohesion and a positive therapeutic alliance have an impact on therapeutic outcomes (Budman et al., 1989; MacKenzie, 1996; MacKenzie, 2001). The role of specific treatment techniques as opposed to group processes as a mediator of efficacy has to be evaluated.

ETHICAL ISSUES

Like any other clinical endeavor, group therapists should be well aware of professional guidelines such as the one by the AGPA, 2007 and local laws related to practice. Therapeutic competence is an important aspect of ethical practice. Like any other therapeutic endeavor, group therapy may not be helpful for everyone. Group work may also have detrimental effects, such as worsening of symptoms, emergence of new symptoms, verbal abuse, unhealthy interactions among group members, etc. The group leader may not have complete control over the interactions of group members in and out of therapy. Factors such as inappropriate selection of members, leadership style of the therapist, personality of the therapist and countertransference may lead to negative outcomes (Roback, 2000). Group processes such as highly critical interpersonal feedback, inappropriate interactions, and breaches of confidentiality may also be relevant. The role of the therapist begins from selection of patients to preventing adverse outcomes. A written informed consent and a group confidentiality agreement are inherent procedures to ensure ethical conduct of group therapy.

CONCLUSION

Group therapies are an important format for provision of psychotherapy to the clients. The advantages of group therapies are cost effectiveness and utilization of group processes in the therapeutic endeavor. Group therapies can be conducted with various theoretical underpinnings, and the conduct may differ across centers and therapists. Group therapies can also be conducted for special populations like children and adolescents, those with physical illnesses, those with substance use disorders, and others. The group therapist needs to consider several ethical issues that may crop up during the therapy process. Further training and expansion of group therapy services may help to deliver competent services to a larger population.

REFERENCES

AGPA Practice Guidelines for Group Psychotherapy. (2017). Available from http://www.agpa.org/home/practice-resources/practice-guidelines-for-group-psychotherapy.

Agronin M. Group therapy in older adults. Curr Psychiatry Rep. 2009;11(1):27-32.

Anthony EJ The history of group psychotherapy. In: Kaplan HI, Sadock BJ (Eds). Comprehensive Group Psychotherapy. Baltimore: Williams & Wilkins; 1971. pp. 4-31.

Bateganya M, Amanyeiwe U, Roxo U, et al. The impact of support groups for people living with HIV on clinical outcomes: a systematic review of the literature. J Acquir Immune Defic Syndr. 2015;68: S368-74.

Budman SH, Soldz S, Demby A, et al. Cohesion, alliance and outcome in group psychotherapy. Psychiatry. 1989;52(3):339-50.

Burlingame GM, Fuhriman A, Johnson JE. Cohesion in group psychotherapy. In: Norcross JC (Ed). Psychotherapy Relationships that Work: Therapist Contributions and Responsiveness to Patients. New York: Oxford University Press; 2002. pp. 71-87.

Burlingame GM, MacKenzie KR, Strauss B, et al. Small group treatment: evidence for effectiveness and mechanisms of change. In: Lambert MJ (Ed) Handbook of Psychotherapy and Behavior Change, 5th edition, 2004; pp. 647-96.

Burlingame GM, Strauss B, Joyce A, et al. CORE Battery-Revised: An assessment tool kit for promoting optimal group selection, process, and outcome. New York: American Group Psychotherapy Association; 2006.

Burlingame GM, Cox JC, Davies DR, et al. The Group Selection Questionnaire: further refinements in group member selection. Group Dyn. 2011;15(1):60-74.

Burrow T. The problem of the transference. Psychol Psychother: Theory Res Prac. 1927;7(2):193-202.

Costa PT, McCrae RR. Normal personality assessment in clinical practice: The NEO Personality Inventory. Psychol Assess. 1992;4(1):5.

Deakin T, McShane CE, Cade JE, et al. Group based training for self-management strategies in people with type 2 diabetes mellitus. Cochrane Database Syst Rev. 2005;2(2).

Feil N. Validation therapy with late-onset dementia populations. Caregiving Dementia Res Appl. 2014;1:199-218.

Fensterheim H. Behavior therapy: Assertive training in groups. In: Sager CJ, Kaplan HS (Eds). Progress in group and family therapy. New York: Brunner/Mazel; 1972.

Gaggioli A, Scaratti C, Morganti L, et al. Effectiveness of group reminiscence for improving wellbeing of institutionalized elderly adults: study protocol for a randomized controlled trial. Trials. 2014;15:408.

Garfield SL. Research on client variables in psychotherapy. In: Garfield SL, Bergin AE (Eds). Handbook of Psychotherapy and Behavior Change, 3rd edition. New York: Wiley; 1986. pp. 213-56.

Garland J, Jones H, Kolodny R. A model for stages of development in social work groups. In: Bernstein S (Ed). Exploration in Group Work: Essays in Theory and Practice Boston: Milford House; 1973. pp. 17-71.

Herlihy B, Corey G. Education and Training of Group Counselors. Boundary Issues in Counseling. American Counseling Association; 2015. pp. 161-85.

Hoag MJ, Burlingame GM. Evaluating the effectiveness of child and adolescent group treatment: a meta-analytic review. J Clin Child Psychol. 1997;26(3): 234-46.

Holmes SE, Kivlighan Jr DM. Comparison of therapeutic factors in group and individual treatment processes. J Counsel Psychol. 2000;47(4):478-84.

Jacobs MK., Goodman G. Psychology and self-help groups: predictions on a partnership. Am Psychol. 1989;44(3):536.

Joyce PR, McKenzie JM, Carter JD, et al. Temperament, character and personality disorders as predictors of response to interpersonal psychotherapy and cognitive-behavioural therapy for depression. Focus. 2010;8(2):261-8.

Klein. Short term group therapy. In: Kaplan HI, Sadock BJ (Eds). Comprehensive Group Psychotherapy, 3rd edition. Baltimore: Williams and Wilkins; 1993. pp. 256-70.

Knauss W. Group psychotherapy. In: Gabbard GO, Beck JS, Holmes J (Eds). Oxford Textbook of Psychotherapy, 1st edition. Oxford University Press; 2005. pp. 35-43.

Lazell EW. The group treatment of dementia praecox. Psychoanalytic Rev. 1921;8:168.

Leshner AI. Introduction to the special issue: The National Institute on Drug Abuse's (NIDA's) Drug Abuse Treatment Outcome Study (DATOS). Psychol Addic Behav. 1997;11(4):211.

Leszcz M, Malat J. The Interpersonal Model of Group Psychotherapy. In: Kleinberg JL (Ed). The Wiley-Blackwell Handbook of Group Psychotherapy. West Sussex, UK: John Wiley & Sons Ltd; 2012. pp. 33-58.

Lieberman: Self help groups. In: Kaplan HI, Sadock BJ (Eds). Comprehensive Group Psychotherapy, 3rd edition. Baltimore: Williams and Wilkins; 1993. pp. 292-304.

Lipowski ZJ. Delirium in the elderly patient. N Engl J Med. 1989;320(9):578-82.

MacKenzie KR. Group psychotherapy. In: Livesley JW (Ed). Handbook of Personality Disorders. New York: Guilford Press; 2001. pp. 497-526.

MacKenzie KR. Time-limited group psychotherapy. Int J of Group Psychother. 1996;46(1):41-60.

Mackenzie RK. Group psychotherapy. Encyclopedia of Psychotherapy. Academic Press; 2002. pp. 891-906.

Marcovitz RJ, Smith JE. An approach to time-limited dynamic inpatient group psychotherapy. Small Group Res 1983;14(3):369-76.

McRoberts C, Burlingame GM, Hoag MJ. Comparative efficacy of individual and group psychotherapy: a meta-analytic perspective. Group Dyn. 1998;2(2):101-17.

Ogrodniczuk JS, Piper WE. The effect of group climate on outcome in two forms of short-term group therapy. Group Dyn. 2003;7(1):64-76.

Okumura Y, Ichikura K. Efficacy and acceptability of group cognitive behavioral therapy for depression: a systematic review and meta-analysis. J Affect Disord. 2014;164:155-64.

Orfanos S, Banks C, Priebe S. Are group psychotherapeutic treatments effective for patients with schizophrenia? a systematic review and meta-analysis. Psychother Psychosoma. 2015;84(4):241-9.

Piper WE, Perrault EL. Pretherapy preparation for group members. Int J Group Psychother. 1989;39(1): 17-34.

Project Match Research Group. Matching patients with alcohol disorders to treatments: Clinical implications from Project MATCH. J Mental Health. 1998;7(6):589-602.

Reid S, Kolvin I. Group psychotherapy for children and adolescents. Arch D is Child. 1993;69(2):244-50.

Roback HB. Adverse outcomes in group psychotherapy. J Psychother Prac and Res. 2000;9(3):113-22.

Rose SD. Cognitive behavioral group therapy. In: Hersen M, Sledge WH (Eds). Encyclopedia of Psychotherapy. Cambridge Academic Press; 2002. pp. 435-50.

Rose SD. Group cognitive behavioral therapy. In: Kaplan HI, Sadock BJ (Eds). Comprehensive Group Psychotherapy, 3rd edition. Baltimore: Williams and Wilkins; 1993. pp. 205-14.

Rothke S. The role of interpersonal feedback in group psychotherapy. Inter J Group Psychother. 1986;36(2):225-40.

Rutan JS. Psychoanalytically group therapy. In: Kaplan HI, Sadock BJ (Eds). Comprehensive Group Psychotherapy, 3rd edition. Baltimore: Williams and Wilkins; 1993. pp. 138-46.

Sacks JM. Psychodrama. in comprehensive group psychotherapy. In: Kaplan HI, Sadock BJ (Eds). Maryland, USA: Williams & Wilkins, 1993. pp. 214-28.

Sadock BJ, Sadock VA. Kaplan and Sadock's Synopsis of Psychiatry: Behavioral Sciences/Clinical Psychiatry, 10th Edition. Philadelphia: Lippincott Williams & Wilkins; 2007.

Salvendy JT. The making of the group therapist: the role of experiential learning. Group.1985;9(4):35-44.

SAMHSA/CSAT: Groups and Substance Abuse Treatment, Treatment Improvement protocols. Center for Substance Abuse Treatment 2005. Rockville (MD).

Scheidlinger S. The group psychotherapy movement at the millennium: some historical perspectives. Int J Group Psychother. 2000;50(3):315-39.

Spitz HI. Group psychotherapy. In: Sadock BJ, Sadock VA, Ruiz P (Eds). Kaplan & Sadock's Comprehensive Textbook of Psychiatry. Philadelphia, PA: Lippincott Williams & Wilkins; 2009. pp. 2833-45.

Stone WN, Rutan JS. Duration of treatment in group psychotherapy. Int J Group Psychother. 1984;34(1): 93-109.

Tattersall RB, McCulloch DK, Aveline M. Group therapy in the treatment of diabetes. Diab Care. 1985;8(2):180-8.

Thienemann ML. Group psychotherapy. Child psychiatry: Psychiatric treatment. In: Kaplan & Sadock's Comprehensive Textbook of Psychiatry, 9th edition. Lippincott Williams & Wilkins; 2009. pp. 3732-41.

Thimm JC, Antonsen L. Effectiveness of cognitive behavioral group therapy for depression in routine practice. BMC Psychiatry. 2014;14:292.

Tuckman BW. Developmental sequence in small groups. Psychol Bull. 1965;63(6):384-99.

Wampold BE. Contextualizing psychotherapy as a healing practice: Culture, history, and methods. Appl Prev Psychol. 2001;10(2):69–86.

Weinhardt LS, Carey MP, Johnson BT, et al. Effects of HIV counseling and testing on sexual risk behavior: a meta-analytic review of published research, 1985-1997. Am J Public Health.1999;89(9):1397-405.

Wheelan SA, Davidson B, Tilin F. Group development across time: Reality or illusion? Small Group Research. 2003;34(2):223-45.

Woods B, Aguirre E, Spector AE, et al. Cognitive stimulation to improve cognitive functioning in people with dementia. Cochrane Database Syst Rev. 2012;(2):CD005562.

Yalom, Vinogradov. Interpersonal group psychotherapy. In: Kaplan HI, Sadock BJ (Eds). Comprehensive Group Psychotherapy, 3rd edition. Baltimore: Williams and Wilkins; 1993. pp. 185-95.

Chapter 33

Community Models of Care

BS Chavan, Ajeet Sidana

SUMMARY

Mental, neurological, and substance use disorders (MNS) are leading cause of global burden of disease (GBD). About 35–50% of the serious cases from the developed countries and 76–85% in the less developed countries receive no treatment in previous 12 months (Demyttenaere et al., 2004). The World Health Organization (WHO) has targeted eight common conditions (epilepsy, dementia, suicide, depression, schizophrenia, and other psychotic disorders, alcohol use disorders, disorders due to use of illicit substances and childhood mental illnesses) in its Mental Health Gap Action Program (mhGAP) in low and middle-income (LAMIC) countries, (WHO, 2008). The need of the hour is to reach out to the patients in the community through innovative and easy to implement community care models. A community mental health model needs to be comprehensive enough to meet all the needs of persons with mental disorders and their families in the community. Large number of community mental health models have been tried including integration of mental health into primary health care, community outreach clinics (COCs), community camps, crisis resolution and home based treatment (CRHT), self-help groups (SHGs), therapeutic community (TC), tele-counseling, halfway home (HWH), day care center, and residential home for mentally challenged and mentally ill destitute. The chapter provides brief review on these models of community mental health care along with research cum clinical evidence on their effectiveness. There is a possibility that many more models operating in the country might have been left out due to lack of access to such models.

INTRODUCTION

According to the GBD Study 2010, a significant section of the total burden of disease worldwide was contributed by MNS disorders. MNS disorders contributed to 28.5% of the total YLDs (years lived with disability), 10.4% of the total DALYs (disability-adjusted life years), and 2.3% of the YLLs (years of life lost due to premature mortality), making the group as the leading cause of YLDs. Between these three, mental illnesses contributed the most to the DALYs, i.e. 56.7%, followed by neurological and substance use disorders (SUDs) (28.6% and 14.7% respectively). When these rates are compared to those found in the first GBD study conducted in 1990, a 37.6% increase in the burden due to mental illnesses and SUDs is observed. This is primarily explained by the growth and aging of the general population (Whiteford et al., 2013). It is estimated that the classical maladies such as infections and malnutrition shall be replaced by depression, cardiovascular illnesses, and other noncommunicable diseases (NCDs) as the leading causes of morbidity, mortality, and disability in the next two decades. It is also expected that by the year 2020, seven out of every ten deaths will be attributable to NCDs in the developing regions of the world. Depression, which currently holds the fourth place from the top in the leading causes of DALYs, is expected to move up to the second position at the same time (World Health Organization, 2001).

Prevalence of mental disorders in India, as estimated in meta-analysis and reviews varies from 58.2 per thousand population (Reddy & Chandrashekar, 1998) to 73 per thousand (Ganguly, 2000). In the recently conducted National Mental Health Survey (National Mental Health Survey, 2016) of India, the current prevalence of mental morbidity, excluding tobacco use disorders, among individuals above the age of 18 years was 10.6% and the lifetime prevalence was 13.7%.

Although almost a third of the total burden caused due to MNS disorders is accounted for by cases originating from India and China, yet a majority of these patients do not receive the treatment that they require (Charlson et al., 2016). This is substantiated by a large-scale multi-country survey, which was supported by the WHO. This survey demonstrated that 76–85% and 35–50% of the severely mentally ill people from less-developed and developed countries respectively had received no form of psychiatric treatment in the year preceding assessment (Demyttenaere et al., 2004). The situation in India is similar, with one study reporting that the mental health service gap in the metropolitan cities of our country being in the range of 82–96% (Desai et al., 2004). In the most recent National Mental Health Survey (Gururaj et al., 2016), average treatment gap across various disorders except epilepsy was more than 60%, highest (86.3%) being for alcohol use disorders. The likely reasons for huge treatment include chronic nature of disorders, which often require regular and long-term care, lack of availability and under-utilization of mental healthcare services, limited affordability, lack of education about mental illness, and stigma. Almost 15% of the population of India above the age of 18 years warrants psychiatric interventions for at least one psychiatric disorder. These disorders, which may be severe mental illnesses, common mental disorders (CMDs) or SUDs are not only prevalent, but also often occur together. These maladies affect all age groups, including the elderly and the adolescent population. The existing mental health facilities and resources are inadequate, poorly coordinated and fragmented, and deficient in all components at the state level.

WHAT IS TO BE DONE?

In order to bridge the gap, *first* and foremost task is to find out what's needed and what's available. The *second* task should be to know the reasons for not seeking treatment among persons with mental health problems. The *third* effort should be to improve utilization and access to mental health care, *fourth* should be identifying cost-effective interventions, and the *fifth* task should be to decide priorities in mental health. For example, World Health Organization (WHO, 2008), in its mhGAP for low and middle income countries targeted eight common conditions—depression, schizophrenia and other psychotic disorders, suicide, epilepsy, dementia, disorders due to the use of alcohol, those due to the use of illicit drugs, and mental disorders in children (WHO, 2008).

Thus, in order to address the issue of huge treatment gap and burden due to MNS, the above-mentioned factors need to be considered for making the interventions acceptable and cost-effective. Since the local conditions in each country will be different, one model may not be suitable for every country. In addition to considering local needs and resources, all the stake-holders including mental health professionals, consumers, care providers, and community leaders must be on board for preparing an intervention model. The model should be simple, replicable, and sustainable.

WHAT IS COMMUNITY MENTAL HEALTH MODEL?

The essence of community psychiatry is the provision of universal, need-based mental health services, irrespective of whether a person is able to pay for them (Chavan et al., 2012). In the 1960s, the then US President, John F Kennedy, while introducing the Community Mental Health Centers Act of 1963, started what was the first community mental health movement, the US government's first such initiative. In the following two decades (the 1960s and 1970s), USA's community mental health services included community-based treatment as well as prevention and consultation at several community institutions and agencies such as churches and schools (Stephen et al., 2009). The idea behind initiating community services was that the community was a better treatment setting than the hospitals, which restricted the patient's activity level and their access to the outside world.

The community mental health services were primarily started with the idea that it is cost-effective to treat individuals suffering from mental illness in the community than to treat them in hospital settings, where they remain inactive with limited access to outside world.

Although, there is no agreed definition of community mental health model, there is a general agreement that the purpose of community mental health model is to shift from the traditional healthcare practice to provide care in the settings where the person with mental illness resides or spends a significant amount of time. Caplan and Caplan (1967) gave following principles of community services:
- Responsibility to a defined population
- Treatment close to the patient's home
- Multidisciplinary team approach
- Continuity of care
- Consumer participation
- Comprehensive services.

Thus, a community mental health model should be comprehensive enough so as to meet all the needs of persons with mental disorders and their families in the community, using community resources (Caplan & Caplan, 1967). Community mental health model should have following components:
- Focus on awareness regarding mental health and substance abuse problems
- Promotion of positive mental health across the different sections of the community with specific focus on vulnerable and marginalized population. Psychoeducation of various groups, where persons with mental health problems visit, i.e. religious organizations, self-help groups, faith healers, and local bodies, etc.
- Focus on stigma reduction
- Rehabilitation services should be the integral component
- Services should be located at a site, which is easily accessible

- Linkages with primary health care as well as tertiary care hospitals, social welfare, and state legal services authority
- Protection of the human rights of mentally ill persons.

It may not possible to ensure all the facilities in the beginning. However, the expansion should be a part of the initial planning so that additional resources are projected in the future planning. In fact, the addition of additional services should be need-based, as the needs would vary from community to community. It is important to carry out a brief survey for collecting information on felt need of community mental health services in the community, the existing general as well as community mental health service, community's willingness to start or strengthen the existing community mental health services, prevailing knowledge and attitude of community regarding the mental disorders, availability of local community resources, and current treatment seeking pattern in the community (Chavan et al., 2012).

A paradigm shift from the existing approach of segregation to inclusive care is required if community mental health services are to be effectively implemented. Also, instead of the existing biomedical model, the biopsychosocial model needs to be embraced, if mental health services are to be taken from the hospital bed to the patient's doorstep. The shift of care from hospitals to the community, along with the focus shifting from short-term treatment to long-term rehabilitation, based on teamwork rather than individual management, are steps which will help mental health care changing from treatment to service (WHO, 2008).

In contrast to the developed countries, the developing countries including India have many limitations in setting-up community-based mental health services (Chavan et al., 2012), which include shortage of funds and manpower, lack of priority to mental health, lack of awareness about the mental illness in the community, poor accessibility due to physical and psychological barriers, lack of infrastructure, faith in indigenous system of care including faith healing, stigma in seeking treatment, and negative attitude towards regular medicine use.

Regular monitoring and review of community mental health services should be an inbuilt component of the services from the inception. Although each service can design its own monitoring mechanism, the following impact indicators can be used to assess the impact of the services in meeting the mental health needs of the community (Chavan et al., 2012).

- Reduction of the treatment gap
- Reduction in stigma
- Reduction in suicide rates
- Reduction in deaths due to overdose of substance
- Reduction in violence due to mental illness and substance use
- Rehabilitation of person with chronic mental illnesses
- Reduction of violence in the community and schools.

COMMUNITY MENTAL HEALTH MODELS IN INDIA

Integration of Mental Health into Primary Health Care

Initiation and early experience: The two landmark Indian studies conducted at Sakalwara in Karnataka (Chandrashekar et al., 1981) and Raipur Rani in Haryana (Wig et al., 1981) demonstrated that mental health can be integrated with primary health care. These two successful studies were the launching pad for the National Mental Health Programme (NMHP) of India in 1982. The envisioned integration of mental health care into primary health services was one of the objectives of this program. Following this, a district mental health program was tested at Bellary, and the success of this model made way for the District Mental Health Program (DMHP), which was initially implemented in four districts in 1996-97. In the 12th 5-year plan, this number increased to 123, and now the government of India aims to expand the DMHP to all districts (Gangadhar & Kishorekumar, 2012).

In April 2011, Ministry of Health and Family Welfare appointed a Mental Health Policy Group to frame the National Mental Health Policy and also to take up the task of reviewing and redesigning the DMHP (Policy Group DMHP, 2012). The policy group pointed out that DMHP had many limitations including poor community involvement, lack of monitoring and evaluation, lack of clarity about the objectives, lack of Hospital Management Information System, inconsistent fund flow, inadequate human resources and training, nonavailability of drugs, lack of technical support for information, education, and communication (IEC) activities, inadequate provision of care for full range of mental illness, nonavailability of crisis management and inpatient services, lack of continuity of care in the community, and lack of involvement of users, caregivers, Nongovernmental Organizations (NGOs) and private sector. The policy group gave recommendations to redraft the DMHP so that above-mentioned shortcomings are removed. There is a need to have another review of DMHP to see the impact of these recommendations.

Composition of the Team

The DMHP team consists of a psychiatrist, psychiatric nurse, psychiatric social worker, clinical psychologist and ancillary staff. The objectives of the team is to identify patients with mental illnesses and treat them, and also provide training to the medical officers working in primary health care, to identify and treat common mental and SUDs, and also to impart training to the nonmedical staff to identify the CMDs and bring them into treatment to reduce treatment lag. Since the medical officers are already overloaded in providing the general health care, it is practically not feasible for them to provide the mental health care.

Treatment Offered

After they are trained under the DMHP, the medical officers at primary health centers (PHCs) can provide essential drugs such as antidepressants, oral and parenteral antipsychotics, minor tranquilizers, and antiepileptics to patients presenting with CMDs such as depression, psychosis, neuroses, intellectual disability, SUDs, and epilepsy. They are also expected to provide brief psychosocial intervention for minor mental health problems.

Linkages with the Community

Although there is a provision for the training of community leaders under the DMHP, community participation in the program is minimal. There is a need for linkages with the community through the training of auxiliary nurse midwifes (ANMs), accredited social health activists (ASHAs) and PHC level paramedical staff—for diagnosis, treatment, and ensuring the involvement of family members and community. The services at Subcentre, PHC, community health center level also need to be strengthened and made more accessible to the patients.

Services Beyond Hospital

Community Outreach Clinics

Community outreach clinics are useful and effective to provide treatment at the doorsteps of patients within the community by using the community infrastructure. These clinics are not only effective in providing treatment of mental disorders and alcohol and drug abuse but also open the possibility of incorporating the mental health care into general health care, as these clinics can be located in the PHC, and the medical officer and other paramedical staff can get a hand on training. Since mentally ill patients are treated along with patients of general medical problems, there will be a minimum perceived stigma. Also, the locations of COCs in the community provide an opportunity to understand the local factors which might be important in causation, maintenance, and treatment seeking pattern. Since such clinics are being run primarily by academic institutes, the undergraduate and postgraduate students get an opportunity to learn community mental health services.

Recently, Patra et al. (2016) studied the pattern of service users from four COCs being run by the Department of Psychiatry, Government Medical College and Hospital (GMCH), Chandigarh. The results showed that service users were mainly daily wagers from lower socioeconomic strata, and the majority had the diagnosis of CMDs including substance use. The findings showed that it is possible to manage CMDs and substance abuse in the COCs as there was no referral to tertiary care hospital. This could be one strategy to reduce treatment gap.

However, most of the COCs in India are running out of the hospital-based resources without any extra manpower or financial resources, and thus there is always a risk of discontinuation of such services. Also, the services are generally available on a weekly basis and there are no backup facilities for crisis situations. Since there is good evidence about their utility, COCs should be included in the government program with separate manpower and budget.

Community Camps

The camp approach has been a popular method in India and other developing countries to reach out to patients in the community. In India, camps were initially organized for issues pertaining to immunization, ophthalmologic care, and family planning (Ranganathan, 1994). Over time, when it was observed that such camps are successfully addressing pertinent issues, it prompted the use of the "camp approach" in the delivery of mental health care. This was implemented probably for the first time by Purohit and Razdan (1988). Since then, this approach has been tested by several professionals (Datta et al., 1991; Ranganathan, 1994; Chavan and Priti, 1999). It was concluded that the camp approach for mental illnesses is feasible, acceptable, and cost-effective. Hence, it was adopted as a potential management approach for various disorders, including SUDs. Recently Sidana et al. (2014) carried out 10-year outcome of patients with substance use who were treated in the community camps and concluded that community camps for treatment of substance abuse are cheaper, less stigmatizing, and patients maintain higher rates of abstinence with lower rates of relapse.

However, similar to COCs, community camps, despite the evidence of their acceptability, cost-effectiveness and better outcome, are being organized sporadically by certain public institutions, NGOs, and private clinicians as there is no regular support from the government.

Crisis Resolution and Home-based Treatment

Community care in the West is being delivered through multidisciplinary community mental health teams, and crisis resolution and home treatment (CRHT) team. CRHT is one of the alternatives to hospital-based care (Johnson, 2013). However, similar models in India are almost nonexistent despite the felt need by the caregivers. In the routine psychiatry practice, mental health professionals are frequently visited by the caregivers of mentally ill patients who refuse to come to the hospital for treatment and caregivers ask for urgent intervention. Without seeing the patient, such requests of caregivers are declined by the mental health professionals, and caregivers are advised to bring the patient either forcefully with assistance from relatives and friends or with the help of local police. Although, under the Mental Health Act (1987), local police is supposed to provide assistance in such cases, but due to limited awareness among the police, the majority of such requests are turned down. Unlike the rural areas where still there is good social support and social cohesiveness, the urban areas with huge treatment gap (Desai et al., 2004), breaking down of joint family system, migration, and limited social support from the friends and neighbors, the need of CRHT is much higher. Also, in addition to the objectives of NMHP, the majority of community-based models in India have been targeted towards rural population, and community models for the urban population are almost nonexistent.

Need for CRHT: The family and caregivers of patients with mental illnesses face difficulties, when patients refuse to seek treatment from hospital-based facilities. The patient might have long-standing illness and family had been managing the patient with or without hospital-based treatment. However, certain situations like aggression and violence, suicidal threats or attempts, drug-induced adverse reaction or drug overdose, life threat to others, and damage to property might require immediate intervention. Similarly, cases like wandering and homeless mentally ill, elderly patients with mental illness and patients with chronic mental illness having gross personal neglect need urgent attention.

Since CRHT model of community care was not available anywhere in India, Department of Psychiatry, GMCH, envisaged development and delivery of a mental health service using CRHT model available in the West after local adaptation. The larger purpose of Chandigarh model of CRHT was to reduce treatment gap and hospitalization through providing evidence-based clinical services at home to patients who are either unmanageable or indulge in aggression and violence with risk to self or others. In last 2 years, the department has developed SOPs for the CRHT and has covered more than 250 families. The initial review (unpublished) shows that CRHT is feasible, cost-effective, and replicable.

Self-help Groups

Self-help groups are groups of people who share mutual concerns and come together for providing support to each other. Members of SHG share a common problem and get connected to each other to search for solution to a problem which bothers each of them. Although, family, friends, and relatives are available for help whenever any family faces any problem, the traditional support is gradually diminishing due to break-down in joint family system and industrialization. Since the members of SHG have been dealing with the problem for long period, they acquire better coping skills to handle the problem and thus they are better skilled than the friends and relatives. The experience and coping skills of individual members of SHG are shared with each other and thus the whole group gets benefited.

Self-help groups may either operate informally or get themselves registered under a common umbrella. These groups usually meet locally, in members' homes or at a common place in the community like schools, churches, temples, or other community centers. During the meetings, members share their personal stories, concerns, worries, and their experience of dealing with these issues. When they meet other members facing a similar problem, they learn that they are not alone; there are many others who are facing the same problem. SHG can have professionals on its panel as their leader to provide them information and training (Gartner and Riessman, 1977). Some of the SHGs use "peer participatory" model and do not allow the professionals to attend meetings unless they are willing to share the group problem and attend either as members or as invited speakers. Members of SHGs have reported that rather than objective and specialized knowledge imparted by professionals, they were helped to a much greater degree by experiential knowledge. Equality among peers is an important feature of such groups, and information dispersal is from peer-to-peer, rather than in a top-down direction. Both the old as well as new members get the benefit. The older and experienced members extend help to new members, and in turn, they also get the benefit as they feel good by supporting other members who require their help.

One of the possible outcomes of peer model of SHG is empowerment. The SHG members become dependent on each other and perhaps also get spiritual power. Since they all are experiencing a similar problem, together they learn to handle the problem in a better way. Since they all share a common shame and stigma, a common platform of the meeting provides them emotional, social, and practical support enhancing their self-esteem and self-efficacy. The members of the SHG can enhance their social skills and promote their social rehabilitation (Katz, 1979). The members can also learn to deal with stress, loss, and personal change (Silverman, 1992).

The evaluation of the effectiveness of SHGs is, however, a daunting task and, at present, the evidence at best is equivocal. AA membership has often been claimed to maintain significant abstinence. One- and five-year sobriety rates of an Indian cohort of 187 AA attendees were found to be 33.3% and 16.5% respectively (Kuruvilla et al., 2004; Kuruvilla & Jacob, 2007). Though a few authors have argued in favor of a greater efficacy of such SHGs (Groh et al., 2008), it has also been observed that evidence pertaining to such claims is in general qualitatively poor, being based on volunteering patients leading to self-inclusion as opposed to random selection, inflating the effectiveness figures falsely. Elsewhere, proponents of SHGs question the premise of basing such groups on evidence, claiming that it goes away from a holistic understanding of health (Nayar et al., 2004). In a recent review (Kaskutas, 2009), using the "6 criteria to establish causation" approach, the author found that AA effectiveness lacked specificity.

Many SHGs have been established in India by parents/guardians of those with mental illness. *Prayatan* is one such SHG formed by parents/guardians of individuals with chronic mental illness in Chandigarh. With about 200 members in its fold, the SHG is actively involved in policy matters/advocacy and support to families with mental illness. *Prayatan*, a registered body, has an executive committee which is elected for two years and meets on the last Saturday of every month at the premises of Disability Assessment, Rehabilitation and Triage (DART). The meeting is open to all members. It invites experts from the Department of Psychiatry, GMCH to give talks on relevant issues decided by the members. The most important item on the agenda is an "open discussion" on issues related to mental health which are not generally addressed during treatment at a tertiary care hospital. Common issues discussed are: (i) vocational and social rehabilitation of persons with chronic mental disorders, (ii) rights of persons with disability due to mental disorders, (iii) problems faced by caregivers in obtaining disability and guardianship certificates, (iv) financial support to persons with mental disorders without any support, (v) campaign against stigma, and (vi) arranging free legal aid for the persons and caregivers of mentally ill. The group works on the philosophy of "give and take help". The group has adopted few families who have landed in difficult life situation due to the burden of mental illness and arrange for their medication and other needs.

Another SHG in Chandigarh, named Umeed, working for the persons with intellectual disability, autism, and cerebral palsy and their family members, is well known for its innovative approach in the field of job placement and social integration of mentally challenged persons in a congenial and protected environment within the community. Umeed, with the approval of Chandigarh Administration, has set up kiosks for sale of snacks, juice bar, ice-cream parlors, STD/PCO, and photostat. The kiosks are managed by the mentally challenged children and their parents. Each kiosk provides rehabilitation to three families. The parent and the child of the same family are not recruited for the same kiosk so as to avert misuse. Profits from these kiosks are then pooled and divided in the ratio of 40% for the salary of children, 40% for parents and 20% is retained for future expansion. Salary of the children is directly deposited in their joint bank account, and no cash is handed over to them. This secures the child income from being used by their parents for meeting out the present needs, and the money is saved for the future use. Thus, Umeed not only provides employment to these children but also secures their future, makes them more competent and at the same time does not cause any burden on the government. Umeed has been instrumental in changing the perception of the society for those with a mental handicap. For its work, Umeed has received the Presidential Award as the best placement agency in the field of mental retardation in 2003. After 20 years of experience, the authors feel that unlike the West, the SHG in India needs constant support and guidance from the professionals who work as a catalyst for promoting and giving direction to their efforts. Since the professionals work in the government sector, their close association with SHG creates a conflict of interest as the SHG on many occasions has to protest against the government.

Therapeutic Community

Therapeutic communities were initially started as residential facility for treatment of SUD and later extended to other disorders including mental disorders. TCs began in 1950s as a part of self-help recovery movement. Some of the SHGs started residential program to support abstinence from substance abuse. Such residential facilities were democratically run and self-supported by the group. The first TC was the "Synanon" residential rehabilitation community, which was founded in 1958 in California.

Historically, TCs came up as an alternative to medically oriented treatment strategies for the treatment of drug dependence and the persons staying in TCs were not allowed to use medicines. The TC believes that people can change, and that learning occurs through challenge and action, and understanding and sharing common human experiences. However, over the years, the philosophy of TCs has changed, and a large number of TCs now practice comprehensive medical treatment.

The efficacy of this approach has been well studied for substance use problem. It appears that the approach is notorious for its high attrition rates (only about 14–25% complete the prescribed treatment) and frequent readmission (3–7 times in 5 years). Although the mortality rate is a crude indicator, at 3 years it is about 2.2% (Berg, 2003). Studies have shown that after being enrolled and completing a 12-month TC program, clients are likely to have lower levels of cocaine, heroin, and alcohol use, less likely to indulge in criminal behavior, less likely to be unemployed, and less likely to be depressed (NIDA Research Report Series, 2002). Based on data from 3,271 patients distributed across 61 TCs, a recent review found that though substance use rates decrease while the patient is in the TC, they frequently relapse once they leave (Malivert et al., 2012). Completion of treatment at the TC was found to be the strongest predictor of remaining abstinent on follow-up.

Tele-counseling

Helpline services (tele-counseling services or crisis hotlines) have been available all over the world for at least five decades. Initially started in the UK by the Samaritans in 1953, similar services spread fast all over the Western world. Though several such helpline services are now available in most cities of the world, published research in relation to such services is for drug cessation programs, most commonly smoking cessation (Sood et al., 2009). Other helpline programs relevant to psychiatry include suicide prevention helpline and child helpline. Unlike telepsychiatry, calls to helplines are initiated by the client and are available around the clock.

Helpline services usually offer counseling (Psychological First Aid) provided either by volunteers or by trained professionals, usually psychotherapists, in crisis situations. Some helpline centers also follow-up clients that have called (call-back) to know if further help is required or direct them to appropriate services. Helpline agencies may also provide face-to-face counseling as an option. In noncrisis situations, services provided can range from individual psychotherapy, couple therapy, and family therapy, although such services are provided more commonly in the Western world. Recently, internet-based counseling services are also being offered for substance cessation and mental illness.

Effectiveness: Despite the availability of suicide helplines; there is no evidence of an actual decrease in the incidence of suicide in the community. Still, a reduction in suicidality was observed during the course of the call session, accompanied by a reduction in pathologic pain and feelings of hopelessness in the weeks following the telephone call (Gould et al., 2007). The caller's intent to die at the end of the call was the most potent predictor of subsequent suicidal behavior. Other than crisis/suicide helplines, services for smoking (or drugs and alcohol) cessation have also developed in Western countries. Such helplines provide not only counseling and information related to smoking cessation but also self-help materials (Pizzi et al., 2009). When followed-up for about 12 months, 27–34% of individuals maintained abstinence. The important factors which are associated with increased chances for abstinence are: proactive calling (i.e. regularly following up individuals), no nicotine use at baseline, additional support from a healthcare professional, additional social support, stress or depressive mood, nicotine replacement therapy for 5 weeks or more, and exposure to second-hand smoke (Helgason et al., 2004).

Limitations: There are numerous reasons cited for limited effectiveness of helpline services. One criticism of suicide hotlines is that those who were determined to kill themselves and those who have social anxiety would be unlikely to call anyone. Another problem in the functioning of crisis hotlines is that, they often contact local police authorities, which can further worsen the problem at home. One of the deterrents of calling these hotlines is the fear and embarrassment of having the police visit one's home. Also, tracing the caller's identity and retrieving personal details such as his address can be perceived as a serious breach of privacy and trust, pushing the person further towards hopelessness and isolation. Thus, such hotlines avoid such practices and offer help only when asked for, allaying the callers' fear of potential embarrassment.

Most suicide helplines in India are run by NGOs. To name a few: Sneha (Chennai), Aasra (Navi Mumbai), Samaritans Sahara (Kolkata), Maitreya (Pondicherry), Roshni (Secunderabad), and Aasha Helpline (Chandigarh). Though there are no systemic data for the utility of helpline services in India, they are known to provide significant help to adolescents at the times of crisis (like the declaration of examination results).

Between 2004 and 2008, the Department of Psychiatry, GMCH, Chandigarh operated AASHA helpline services consisting of two arms: (a) a 24 × 7 suicide prevention helpline and (b) a crisis intervention team (CIT). The helpline team consisted of counselors, a medical social worker, and a nurse. Callers included those with active suicidal thoughts, those in emotional turmoil, family members of those with mental illness, individuals with adverse effects of psychoactive drugs and general public inquiry for the need for psychiatric services for their near and dear ones. Telephone calls were attended by counselors, and appropriate psychological intervention/referral/advice was provided. When needed, conference calling with a psychiatrist was arranged. Callers, who were referred to OPD or were given simple advice, would be followed-up and motivated to seek treatment if required. The number of callers to the helpline increased in subsequent years with a maximum of 1,800 calls in 2008. Around 62% of the callers were males, the mean age was 26 years, and most calls (66%) originated from Chandigarh. Common problems (60%) were related to academic, interpersonal, and sexual issues. Helpline staff also received some missed calls, and despite best efforts, only 50% of such callers chose to elaborate their problem. In case involuntary admission was required, the crisis intervention team would be involved. The family members (if available) would be asked to send a requisition, following which the patient would be taken to the hospital. The team was involved in a number of situations where no immediate information about the client was available, e.g. aimless wanderers, agitated individuals on the street (intoxicated/psychotic), individuals with mental illness who refused any entry into their home, etc. Among patients seen by our team, 60% of individuals were less than 40 years of age, 59% were male, and only 35% had a diagnosis of schizophrenia. Sixty-six percent of those seen by the CIT needed admission while the rest were provided with counseling. After brief treatment, the majority showed improvement, and it was possible to obtain additional information about their family. It was possible to restore the person to their families in about half of the cases, and the rest were sent to the residential facility provided by the NGO and the Department agreed to provide technical support for long-term care.

Half Way Home and Day Care Center

A half way home is a transient home for a person with mental illnesses who do not require specialized care at tertiary care hospital but at the same time patient has not recovered adequately to go back to the society to work independently. The patient stays at the HWH for a period of 3–6 months, depending upon the clinical need. The aim of HWH is to regain the skills which the patient was having before the onset of illness. It provides social, vocational, and cognitive skills to the members of the home till he/she achieves it at a maximum level.

Day care centers are similar to HWH except not having a residential facility. Patients come in the morning to learn skills and go back home by the evening. There are several NGOrun halfway homes in India. Amongst others, some of the notable ones are Richmond Fellowship Society (Bengaluru and Delhi), Paripurnata (Kolkata), Roshni (Guwahati), and Banyan (Chennai).

Home for Mentally Challenged and Mentally Ill Destitute

These are almost permanent types of home for mentally ill patients. The residents are provided with social, vocational, and cognitive skills. One of them named "Samarth" is funded by the National Trust for short-term and long-term stay of persons suffering from intellectual disability, autism, cerebral palsy, and multiple disabilities. Details are available at *www. thenationaltrust.gov.in*, and such facilities are available throughout India.

Recently, "Parivartan" has set-up short stay residential facility called "Aavas" for homeless mentally ill persons who have recovered from acute care but do not have a place to stay. The facility is free and is linked to rehabilitation facility being run by the Department of Psychiatry, GMCH, Chandigarh. Further details can be accessed from *www.parivartan.in.net*

CONCLUSION

One of the main reasons for significant burden due to MNS is huge treatment gap. The purpose of community mental health services is to bridge this gap by developing community mental health model(s), which is acceptable to the community, feasible, replicable, cost-effective, and sustainable. Majority of the community mental health models have been found effective; however, their sustainability remains questionable. Thus, there is a need to have designated staff and regular inflow of funds to continue and sustain various community mental health services. The bottlenecks in integration of mental health care into general health care through

DMHP need to be identified and corrected. Regular monitoring and review of community mental health services is required to see the overall impact of these services on various impact indictors in the long run.

REFERENCES

Berg JE. Mortality and return to work of drug abusers from therapeutic community treatment 3 years after entry. Prim Care Companion J Clin Psychiatry. 2003;5:164-7.

Caplan G, Caplan, RB. Development of community psychiatry concepts in the United States. In: Freedman AM, Kaplan HI (Eds). Comprehensive Textbook of Psychiatry. Baltimore: Williams & Wilkins; 1967. pp.1499-516.

Charlson FJ, Baxter AJ, Cheng HG, et al. The burden of mental, neurological, and substance use disorders in China and India: a systematic analysis of community representative epidemiological studies. Lancet. 2016;388(10042):376-89.

Chandrashekar CR, Isaac MK, Kapur RL, et al. Management of priority mental disorders in the community. Indian J Psychiatry.1981;23:174-8.

Chavan BS, Priti A. Treatment of alcohol and drug abuse in camp settings. Indian J Psychiatry. 1999;41(2):140-4.

Chavan BS, Rozatakar A, Sidana A. Models of community mental health. In: Chavan BS, Gupta N, Arun P, et al (Eds). Community Mental Health in India, 1st edition. New Delhi: Jaypee Brothers Medical Publishers (P) Ltd; 2012. pp. 269-80.

Datta S, Prasantham BJ, Kuruvilla K. Community treatment for alcoholism. Indian J Psychiatry 1991;33:305-6.

Desai NG, Tiwari SC, Nambi S, et al. Urban mental health services in India: How complete or incomplete? Indian J Psychiatry. 2004;46:195-212.

Demyttenaere K, Bruffaerts R, Posada-Villa J, et al. Prevalence, severity and unmet need for treatment of mental disorders in the World Health Organization World Mental Health Surveys. JAMA. 2004;291(21):2581-90.

Gartner A, Riessman F. Self-help in the human services. San Francisco: Jossey Bass; 1977.

Gangadhar BN, Kishorekumar KV. District mental health programme. In: Chavan BS, Gupta N, Arun P, Sidana A, Jadhav S (Eds). Community Mental Health in India, 1st edition. New Delhi: Jaypee Brothers Medical Publishers (P) Ltd; 2012. pp. 65-73.

Ganguli HC. Epidemiological findings on prevalence of mental disorders in India. Indian J Psychiatry. 2000;42(1):14-20.

Gould MS, Kalafat J, Munfakh JLH, et al. An evaluation of crisis hotline outcomes. Part 2: Suicidal Callers. Suicide Life Threat Behav. 2007;37(3):338-52.

Groh DR, Jason LA, Keys CB. Social network variables in alcoholics anonymous: a literature review. Clin Psychol Rev. 2008;28:430-50.

Helgason AR, Tomson T, Lund KE, et al. Factors related to abstinence in a telephone helpline for smoking cessation. Eur J Public Health. 2004;14:306-10.

Johnson S. Crisis resolution and home treatment teams: an evolving model. Adv Psychiatr Treat. 2013;19(2):115-23.

Kaskutas LA. Alcoholics anonymous effectiveness: faith meets science. J Addict Dis. 2009; 28(2):145-57.

Katz AH. Self-help health groups: some clarifications. Soc Sci Med. 1979;13:491-4.

Kuruvilla PK, Jacob KS. Five-year follow up for sobriety in a cohort of men who had attended an alcoholics anonymous programme in India. Nat Med J India. 2007;20(5):234-6.

Kuruvilla PK, Vijayakumar N, Jacob KS. A cohort study of male subjects attending an alcoholics anonymous program in India: one-year follow-up for sobriety. J Stud Alcohol. 2004;65: 546-9.

Malivert M, Fatséas M, Denis C, et al. Effectiveness of therapeutic communities: a systematic review. Eur Addict Res. 2012;18(1):1-11.

Gururaj G, Varghese M, Benegal V, and NMHS collaborators group. National Mental Health Survey of India, 2015-16: Prevalence, patterns and outcomes. Bengaluru, National Institute of Mental Health and Neuro Sciences, NIMHANS Publication No. 129, 2016.

Nayar KR, Kyobutungi C, Razum O. Self-help: What future role in healthcare for low and middle-income countries? Int J Equity Health. 2004;3:1.

NIDA Research Report Series. Therapeutic Community. National Institute on Drug Abuse, 2002.

Patra S, Chavan BS, Gupta N, et al. Clinical profile of patients seeking services at urban community psychiatric services in Chandigarh. Indian J Psychiatry. 2016;58(4):410-6.

Pizzi E, Di Pucchio A, Mastrobattista L, et al. A helpline telephone service for tobacco related issues: the Italian experience. Int J Environ Res Public Health. 2009;6:900–14.

Policy Group District Mental Health Programme. (2012). Available from-https://mhpolicy.files.word-press.com/2012/07/final-dmhp-design-xii-plan2.pdf.

Purohit DR, Razdan VK. Evolution and appraisal of com-munity camp-approach to opium detoxification in North India. Indian J Soc Psychiatry. 1988;4:15-21.

Ranganthan S. The Manjakkudi experience: A camp approach towards treating alcoholics. Addiction 1994;89:1071-5.

Reddy MV, Chandrashekar CR. Prevalence of mental and behavioural disorders in India: a meta-analysis. Indian J Psychiatry. 1998;40:149-57.

Sidana A, Chavan BS, Garg R, et al. Long term outcome of substance abuse treatment through integrated camp approach. Indian J Soc Psychiatry. 2014;30(3-4):94-101.

Silverman PR. Critical aspects of the mutual help experience. In: Katz AH, Hedrick HL, Isenberg DH, Thompson LM, Goodrich T, Kutscher AH (Eds). Self-help: Concepts and Applications. Philadelphia: Charles Press; 1992.

Sood A, Andoh J, Verhulst S, et al. "Real-world" effectiveness of reactive telephone counseling for smoking cessation: a randomized controlled trial. Chest. 2009;136:1229-36.

Stephen P, Kliewer P, McNally M, et al. Deinstitutionalization: its impact on community mental health centers and the seriously Mentally Ill. Alabama Counsel Assoc J. 2009;35(1):40-5.

Whiteford HA, Degenhardt L, Rehm J, et al. Global burden of disease attributable to mental and substance use disorders: findings from the Global Burden of Disease Study 2010. Lancet. 2013;382(9904):1575-86.

World Health Organization. Mental Health: A Call for Action by World Health Ministers. Geneva: World Health Organization, 2008.

World Health Organization. mhGAP - Mental Health Action Programme: Scaling Up Care for Mental, Neurological and Substance Use Disorders. Geneva: World Health Organization, 2008.

Wig NN, Murthy RS, Harding TW: A model for rural psychiatric services- Raipur Rani experience. Indian J Psychiatry. 1981;23(4):275-90.

Chapter 34

Psychosocial Rehabilitation

Hemendra Singh, Murali Thyloth

SUMMARY

Though medications are available for most of psychiatric illnesses, a significant proportion of patients does not recover and live with longstanding disabilities. These patients need psychosocial rehabilitation (PSR) programs which may include simple measures like daily household routines, and complex interventions, such as skills training, vocational training, etc. Some patients might be helped by community based nonresidential and residential rehabilitation facilities like day care centers, half way homes, etc. Simple intervention strategies at community level play a major role in psychiatric rehabilitation. It is important to create its awareness in the community, develop resources, and encourage community participation and social network with various stakeholders. Its implementation through personnel working in existing community-based rehabilitation programs make rehabilitation cost-effective. In other words, PSR supports the goals that psychiatry holds for patients: to "live, love, and work meaningfully and productively in the world" (Creasey & McCarthy, 1981). As per the famous statement by Gittelman and Freedman (1988), "if psychiatrists fail to support rehabilitative interventions, they will find themselves treating only half the illness."

INTRODUCTION

Chronic mental illness is a severe and persisting emotional disorder that interferes with the functional capacities in relation to many primary aspects of daily life, such as self-care, interpersonal relationship, and work or school that may often necessitate prolonged mental health care (Talbott, 1978). Three criteria have been used uniformly to define the chronic mental illness, i.e. duration of 2 years and associated disability which requires continuous care (Bachrach, 1988). The individual views it as a disability and loss of function, whereas the community and the family perceive it as loss of productivity and burden respectively. Mental, neurological, and substance abuse disorders constitute nearly 13% of the global burden of disease, surpassing both cardiovascular disease (CVD) and cancer (World Health Organization, 2008). Mental illnesses are viewed to be more disabling than infectious diseases and CVD put together. PSR is a recent development in India and has various challenges, such as limited medical management, ineffective psychosocial therapies, poor awareness, inadequate facilities, and inadequate manpower. In India, there is a huge disparity between available mental health resources and mental illnesses, where on an average one psychiatrist serves 200,000 or more people. There is a large mental health gap both in psychiatric treatment as well as in rehabilitation.

The goal of psychiatric rehabilitation is to help individuals with persistent and serious mental illness to develop emotional, social, and intellectual skills needed to live, learn, and work in the community with the least amount of professional support (Anthony et al., 2002). Since most of patients suffering from chronic mental illness require social integration, it is important to develop individualized cultural specific rehabilitation formulation as well as PSR interventions based on the rehabilitation formulation.

The International Classification of Impairment, Disability, and Handicaps (ICIDH), published by the World Health Organization (World Health Organization, 1980), covers various long-term consequences of the major mental illnesses. The adverse effects of the presumptive, pathological abnormalities of the brain on the functions of the central nervous system are defined as impairments, such as symptoms of mental illnesses or neurocognitions. For example, delusions, hallucinations, negative symptoms, dysfunction of learning, concentration, inaccurate perception of social and emotional cues, problem in decision making, poorly sustained attention, judgement and memory impairment. These symptoms of illness and impairment of neurocognitions lead to disability. Disability is an inability to perform as expected in the socioeconomic and cultural context. For example, self-care, activity of daily living, social role, family role, vocational competence, interpersonal relationships. Handicap is a disadvantage in competitions along with others, e.g. job interviews, transport, money management, etc. (Liberman, 2008). The ICIDH has been recently revised. The revised International Classification of Functioning, Disability and Health (ICF) includes a change from negative descriptions of impairments, disabilities, and handicaps to neutral descriptions of body structure and function, activities and participation. ICF has included the role of the environmental factors as a facilitator or a barrier for the disability (World Health Organization, 2001). There is a paradigm shift to focus more on the psychological intervention rather than focusing on irreversible risk factors as these interventions can be made cost-effective and socially acceptable to overcome the consequences of a mental illness. It is important to focus on the psychological interventions based on the rehabilitation formulation plan according to the type and stage of illness.

INDIVIDUALIZATION OF REHABILITATION FORMULATION

Treatment should be individualized as per nature and stage of illness along with the cultural values and goals of an individual. There is a recently published case regarding psychological formulation as a means of psychosocial intervention in psychiatric rehabilitation setting (Hewitt, 2008). However, we have hypothesized PSR formulation based on disease process and environmental factors (**Figure 1**).

Getting to Know Mr A

Mr A is a 40 years old, unmarried male, educated up to 12th, belonging to socioeconomic status, from Bengaluru with good premorbid functioning. He has family history of poor social support and good understanding about warning signs and nature of illness. He has been brought by old

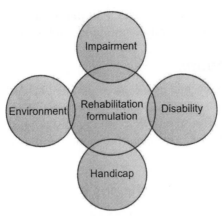

Figure 1: Model of the psychosocial rehabilitation formulation.

parents with insidious onset progressive illness of 20 years duration, characterized delusion of persecution, 2nd and 3rd person auditory hallucinations, lack of socialization, poor attention, lack of motivation, and poor self care with occupational dysfunction. He has been treated with multiple antipsychotics along with electroconvulsive therapy at different hospitals and had developed extrapyramidal symptoms (EPS). He has never been able to work for more than 3 months and left jobs due to psychotic symptoms and EPS. Rehabilitation issues with Mr A can be described as:

Impairments: Impairment in Mr A is due to negative symptoms in form of social withdrawal, lack of attention, and poor motivation, and positive symptoms like presence of auditory hallucination and delusions.

Disabilities: Mr A has disabilities in form of poor self-care, impairment in interpersonal as well as family relationship, inability to come for follow-up without help of his old parents, inability to utilize other resources like transportation, and occupational dysfunction.

Handicap: Mr A was unable to utilize disability and pension benefits, transportation, and various rehabilitation benefits.

Environmental factors: Both protective and risk factors were present in this case, such as good understanding of the illness by parents, poor family support, presence of the expressed emotions, poor access to the job, and social integration.

All these issues are important for the process, form, and content of psychiatric rehabilitation. The rehabilitation process begins with a comprehensive elicitation of the individual's short and long-term goals for functioning.

PSYCHOSOCIAL REHABILITATION INTERVENTION

There are yet no clear cut guidelines on how to develop family intervention programs in India. However, The Schizophrenia Research Foundation at Chennai has started offering rehabilitation programs for the chronic mentally ill in a day care setting employing three modules: medication management, vocational rehabilitation, and family management

(Nagaswami, 1990; Shankar & Sarada, 1991). PSR interventions need to be implemented at various levels, such as individual, family, community, and professional level.

Individual Interventions

Interventions at individual level focus on the assessment of various factors which are target for the rehabilitation. Steps include assessment of various dimensions of PSR, prioritization of psychosocial interventions, program planning, meeting short- and long-term goals with implementation of the psychosocial intervention and assertive regular follow-up and reassessment of the goals.

Assessments of Various Dimensions of PSR

It is important to have initial assessment of various issues of PSR formulation such as impairment, disability, handicap, and role of environmental protective and risk factors.

- *Impairment*: It can be assessed by a mental health professional by performing the serial mental status examination
- *Disability*: It can be assessed by using structural interviews and scales, such as modified Disability Assessment Schedule (WHO DAS–II) (Thara et al., 1988), IDEAS (Indian Psychiatric Society, 2002), etc.
- *Handicap*: It can be assessed by clinical interview
- *Environmental factors*: It is important to know both protective as well as risk factors related to social environment by using patient's history and collateral information from the family, and bystanders of the patients.

Prioritization of Intervention Plans

Intervention plans are prioritized as per the needs of the individual and the family, and assessed needs.

Program Planning

It should be individualized, based on family's needs and to be realistic, and domiciliary or center based. It needs professional and family inputs. Planning always depends on availability of facilities and logistic issues.

Short-term and Long-term Goals with Implementation of Rehabilitation Interventions

It is important to plan both short-term and long-term goals to facilitate the social and instrumental role functioning.

Short-term goals: These include management of disruptive behavior, work behavior, active symptoms, medication management, negative symptoms, interpersonal relationships skills, and social skills training for the individual.

Social skills training consists of learning activities, utilizing behavioral techniques that enable persons with schizophrenia and other disabling mental disorders to acquire interpersonal disease management and independent living skills for improved functioning in their communities (Kopelowicz1 et al., 2006). Various studies have found that these behavioral techniques could produce significant improvements in memory, attention, and executive functions (Krabbendam & Aleman, 2003). There is also normalization of selected impairments in cognitive functioning (Wykes, 2004). When the type and frequency of training is linked to the phase of the disorder, patients can learn and retain a wide variety of social and independent living skills (Kopelowiczl et al, 2006). Skills deficit are seen during all phases of the illness, such as nonacquisition of skills due to early onset illness, disuse atrophy of skills during prolonged illness or hospitalization, institutional neuroses during prolonged inpatient care, and person developing sick role. Starting with efficacy and effectiveness, various studies have critically evaluated the evidence of effects of skills training on individuals with serious mental disorders (Liberman et al., 2005; Pilling et al., 2002). Studies have found significant and substantial improvements in participants' knowledge and behaviors with skill training. Furthermore, participants are able to retain their improvements for up to 2 years during maximum follow-up (Kopelowiczl, 2006).

Training of skills is needed for individuals with deficits in various skills due to disability. Deficits in skills may be due to failure to acquire the skills as it happens with persons with mental retardation or early onset schizophrenia or skills lost after acquisition because these were not used. The deficits could be in social skills, cognition, daily living skills, occupational skills, social networking skills, and community participation skills. Teaching skills for persons with disability has been very effective in bringing them back to the community. We have given an example of structured daily activities **(Table 1)**.

Techniques to teach various skills include coaching, modeling, prompting, shaping overcorrection, video feedback, classroom teaching, buddy training program, cognitive

Table 1: Sample of activity scheduling for Mr A	
6.00–7.00 AM	Waking up, making bed and attending to personal hygiene
7.00–8.00 AM	Physical exercises
8.00–9.00 AM	Breakfast and medication administration
9.00–9.30 AM	Prayers
9.30–10.30 AM	Reading newspaper, watching television, group discussions, etc.
10.30–12.00 noon	Activity therapy program
12.30–1.00 PM	Lunch and wash own plate
1.00–2.00 PM	Medication administration and post lunch rest
2.00–3.00 PM	Activity program
3.00–3.30 PM	Coffee or tea
3:30–4:00 PM	Creative activity program
4.00–5.00 PM	Outdoor games, singing, dancing, walking, meeting visitors, etc.
5:00–6:00 PM	Gardening
6.00–8.00 PM	Watching television, group activity
8.00–9.00 PM	Dinner
9.00–10.00 PM	Watching television, sleep

training, grain sorting, letter cancellation, computer based cognitive tasks, etc. Various therapies have been used for skill training, such as activity scheduling, behavior modification, buddy training, token economy, and group therapies. Most of these techniques use behavioral methods.

We mentioned in detail how to train a patient in basic living skills. Basic living skills are those skills, which help patients to take care of themselves without depending on others for maintaining their activities of daily living. These include skills for brushing teeth, bathing, dressing, grooming, and eating habits which are important to maintain personal cleanliness. For example, brushing the teeth requires various steps. The entire task has to be split into small steps and each step needs to be demonstrated. The steps involved are: picking up toothbrush and paste, holding the brush in the right hand, applying toothpaste on the brush, placing the brush in the mouth, brushing the teeth in a uniform "up and down", circular motion for few minutes, rinsing the mouth thoroughly with water, cleaning the tongue properly, washing the face with water, taking the soap and applying on the face with closed eyes, washing the face thoroughly, wiping the face with a clean towel, etc.

Various simple steps are required for structured daily activity, such as identifying reinforcement, and mixing of material and social reinforcement. Each step needs to be reinforced with praise, criticizing mistakes or sometimes punishment for the mistakes, and spacing reinforcement over a period of time to improve generalization.

Long-term goals: The main long-term goal for most of patients in PSR are vocational training and job placement. The person and the family member may be helped in finding a suitable job in the community. This can be achieved by using the community network and different organizations. It is equally important to have vigilant observation of the work performance of the patient and to maintain regular contact with employer to monitor the patient's work, performance. Other long-term goals are related to supply of medication, residence, finances, follow-up arrangement, family arrangement, and community reintegration.

Assertive Regular Follow-up and Reassessment of the Goals

Success of rehabilitation depends on regular follow-up. But due to lack of resources or due to distance, the patient may not be able to come for regular follow-up. Hence it is important to have assertive follow-up and documentation regarding, who brings the patient? What frequency? Functional aspects, earnings, evaluation of coping strategies, crisis management as and when it occurs? During intervention program, it is essential to monitor change in targeted behavior, change in functioning, individuals' appraisal and his/her family's perspective. Sometimes, persons with mental illness are at increased risk of a relapse or recurrence. Regular follow-up will also help to detect long-term side effects of medications. The place and frequency of follow-up may be decided depending on the convenience of patient and family.

Family Level Psychosocial Interventions

It is important to involve the family in PSR. Brown described five components of expressed emotions, such as emotional over involvement, critical comments, hostility, positive remarks, and warmth (Brown, 1985). Sometimes, over involvement, hostility, and criticism within family may worsen patients. Hence, it is important to know expectation of the families, their coping strategies, expressed emotions, interpersonal aspects, resource utilization, family burden, and social position. Intervention, such as family psychoeducation, strategies to reduce expressed emotions, and enhancing social skills and coping strategies in the family are important aspects.

Community Level Psychosocial Intervention

Community-based rehabilitation services are provided in close collaboration between specialists and locally available personnel within an explicit human rights and developmental framework (World Health Organization, 2008). There are various reasons to have the community level rehabilitation in lower- and middle-income countries. One of the most important barriers to appropriate service provision to people with chronic psychotic disorders is the scarcity of adequately trained mental health personnel (Saxena et al., 2007). Hence, nonspecialist, cost-effective human resources are important to implement public health oriented services in low- and middle-income countries, since it is difficult to have specialist resource (Patel et al., 2007). Community-based interventions, such as psychotropic medications, psychoeducation, adherence management, PSR and support for livelihoods have been found to be effective for disability in persons with psychotic disorders in low-resource settings (Chatterjee et al., 2003; Chatterjee et al., 2009). However, in community setting there are various hurdles, such as dealing with medication maintenance, continuous structured activity, interpersonal relationships, social and vocational adequacy, crisis intervention, and immediate attention during relapse.

Community-Based Rehabilitation Settings

Depending on needs of persons with mental illness, a particular type of rehabilitation facility needs to be selected. Pattern of usage of these facilities depend on availability, accessibility, and acceptability. Currently most of these facilities are limited to a few cities. It is necessary to make these facilities available to all people who need them. These can be divided into nonresidential and residential settings.

Nonresidential Settings

Day care center is a nonresidential care which provides structural daily activities, support, and supervision for the patients in transition between hospitalization and home. Day care forms a vital component of any good quality community-oriented psychiatric service (Holloway, 1988). Day care settings have the tough task of balancing adequate work oriented care and a nonthreatening social environment (Gopinath & Rao, 1994). The first day care center in the country was started at the National Institute of Mental Health and Neurosciences, Bengaluru with vocational training. The day care center with vocational training "Chetana" was started by the Richmond Fellowship Society, Bengaluru during September, 1997. PSR program included, individual and group based family-oriented interventions along with training in prevocational and vocational skills and job placements. Users were offered training in various trades, such as tailoring, embroidery, hand block printing, paper cover-making, greeting card-making, handicraft work, book binding, screen printing, basic computers, and plastic welding and moulding. The users and their families have perceived or reported widespread benefits that have accrued either directly or indirectly by the center through the wide-ranging PSR services offered to them (Sahu et al., 2014). Various interventions at these day care centers are aimed to improve self-esteem, and are easy to manage, feasible at most places, and need low investments. Most of these are provided by trained and vocationally oriented supervisors.

Residential Settings

Residential settings are meant for the patients of various needs who are symptomatically stable but also need various rehabilitation interventions to get integrated into the society. These setting are:

Hospitals: The focus of hospitalization is medical treatment. Here a person with an illness is evaluated and appropriate treatment is initiated. The aim of the hospital care is control of his symptoms. An assessment of the need for rehabilitation interventions and initiation of the program are done. Here the patients are given individual attention and care by mental health professionals. The stay in the hospital should be brief and once the acute symptoms are controlled, the patient should be discharged from the hospital and advised for a regular outpatient follow-up.

Halfway homes: The first halfway home in our country was started by the Medico-Pastoral Association at Bengaluru in1974. Here patients are kept for a limited period with homogeneity of diagnosis and often managed by nonmedical staff. There are frequent family visits and patients follow structured programs and psychosocial therapies. Residential settings like halfway homes have important role in fulfilling the needs of the persons with severe mental illness.

Hostels: It is like any other regular hostel in structure and administration. It is meant for a person with mental illness who can lead an independent life, but does not have any family support to live with the family. It is best for those who are employed and have good financial resources. Here the persons are provided with boarding and lodging which is shared with other inmates.

Long-stay homes: These are meant for patients, who are not able to live independently in the community and require care for a longer periods of time. These is mainly custodial in nature with some therapeutic inputs. Most of the long-stay facilities are run by nongovernmental organizations. The duration of stay may be for life. The family needs to make a substantial amount of money as deposit to take care of the person. In government sector, the mental institutes or mental hospitals provide long-term care. It is often reported that more than 50% of the mental hospital beds are occupied by the long-stay patients. Long stay homes are recent concepts based on lump sum payments. However, there is dearth of published studies from our region regarding the kind of programs followed by them. Most of these facilities probably are based on commercial interest and many times people dump the patients at such centers. There are no systematic studies regarding the type of staff which manages the patients for the long-stay.

CONCLUSION

Psychosocial rehabilitation is an essential component of comprehensive psychiatric management. In our country, though we have feasible, cost-effective rehabilitation interventions, there is lack of training programs, and specialized trained health professional in the field of psychiatric rehabilitation. Knowing the magnitude of the problem, it is the responsibility of all stakeholders to come forward to help the patients to integrate into the main stream of their life. There is a need to create formal psychiatric rehabilitation programs in various psychiatric facilities.

REFERENCES

American Psychiatric Association. Practice guideline for the treatment of persons with schizophrenia. Am J Psychiatry. 2004;161(2 suppl):1-56.

Anthony W, Cohen M, Farkas M, et al. Psychiatric Rehabilitation , 2nd edition. Boston: Center for Psychiatric Rehabilitation, Boston University, 2002.

Bachrach LL. Defining chronic mental illness: a concept paper. Hosp Community Psychiatry. 1988;39(4):383-8.

Bellack A. Skills training for people with severe mental illness. Psychiatr Rehabil J. 2004;7:375-91.

Brown G. The discovery of expressed emotion: induction or deduction? In Expressed Emotion in Families. J Leff, C Vaughn (Eds), New York: Guilford Press, 1985, pp, 7-25.

Chatterjee S, Patel V, Chatterjee A, et al. Evaluation of a community based rehabilitation model for chronic schizophrenia in rural India. Br J Psychiatry. 2003;182:57-62.

Chatterjee S, Pillai A, Jain S, et al. Outcomes of people with psychotic disorders in a community-based rehabilitation programme in rural India. Br J Psychiatry. 2009;195(5):433-9.

Creasey DE, McCarthy TP. Training vocational rehabilitation counselors who work with chronic mental patients. Am J Psychiatry. 1981;138(8):1102-6.

Gittelman M, Freedman AM. Treating half the illness. Hosp Community Psychiatry. 1988;39:347.

Gopinath PS, Rao K. Rehabilitation in psychiatry: an overview. Indian J Psychiatry. 1994;36:49-60.

Heinssen RK, Liberman RP, Kopelowicz A. Psychosocial skills training for schizophrenia: lessons from the laboratory. Schizophr Bull. 2000;26:21-46.

Hewitt M. Using psychological formulation as a means of intervention in a psychiatric rehabilitation setting. Int J Psychosoc Rehabil. 2008;12:1.

Holloway F. Day care and community support. In: Lavender A, Holloway F (Eds). Community Care in Practice: Services for the Continuing Care User. Chichester: John Wiley & Sons; 1988. pp. 161-85.

Kopelowicz1 A, Liberman RP, Zarate R. Recent advances in social skills training for schizophrenia. Schizophr Bull. 2006;32:S12-23.

Krabbendam L, Aleman A. Cognitive rehabilitation in schizophrenia: a quantitative analysis of controlled studies. Psychopharmacol. 2003;169(3-4):376-82.

Lehman AF, Kreyenbuhl J, Buchanan RW, et al. The schizophrenia patient outcomes research team: updated treatment recommendations 2003. Schizophr Bull. 2004;30:193-217.

Liberman RP, Kopelowicz A, Silverstein SM. Psychiatric rehabilitation. In: Sadock BJ, Sadock VA (Eds). Comprehensive Textbook of Psychiatry. Baltimore, Md: Lippincott Williams & Wilkins; 2005. pp. 3884-930.

Libermann RP. Recovery from Disability: Manual of Psychiatric Rehabilitation. Washington, DC: American Psychiatric Publishing; 2008.

Nagaswami V. Integration of psychosocial rehabilitation in national health care programs. Psychosocial Rehabil J. 1990;14(1):53-65.

Patel V, Farooq S, Thara R. What is the best approach to treating schizophrenia in developing countries? PLoS Medicine. 2007;4(6):e159.

Pilling S, Bebbington P, Kuipers E, et al. Psychological treatments in schizophrenia: II. Meta-analyses of randomized controlled trials of social skills training and cognitive remediation. Psychol Med. 2002;32:783-91.

Sahu KK, Niveditha S, Dharitri R, et al. A decade and half of day care service for persons with psychiatric disabilities. RFS (I) Experience. Int J Psychosoc Rehabil. 2014;18(2):37-47.

Saxena S, Thornicroft G, Knapp M, et al. Resources for mental health: scarcity, inequity, and inefficiency. Lancet. 2007;370(9590):878-89.

Shankar R, Sarada M. Interventions with families of people with schizophrenia: the issues facing a community-based rehabilitation center in India. Psychosoc Rehabil J 1991;15:85-90.

Talbott JA (Ed): The Chronic Mental Patient: Problems, Solutions, and Recommendations for a Public Policy. Washington, DC, American Psychiatric Association, 1978.

Thara R, Rajkumar S, Valecha V. The schedule for assessment of psychiatric disability-A Modification of the Das-II. Indian J Psychiatry. 1988;30(1):47-53.

The Rehabilitation Committee of the Indian Psychiatry Society. Indian Disability Evaluation Assessment Scale (IDEAS). A scale for measuring and quantifying disability in mental disorders. Indian Psychiatric Society. 2002.

World Health Organization. The Global Burden of Disease: 2004. Update. Geneva: World Health Organization, 2008.

World Health Organization. International Classification of Impairments, Disabilities and Handicaps. Geneva: World Health Organization, 1980.

World Health Organization. International Classification of Functioning, Disability and Health (ICF). Geneva: WHO, 2001.

World Health Organization. A Strategy for Rehabilitation, Equalization of Opportunities, Poverty Reduction and Social Inclusion of People with Disabilities International Labour Office, United Nations Educational, Scientific and Cultural Organization, Geneva: World Health Organization. 2004.

Wykes T. Cognitive remediation is better than cognitive behavior therapy. In: McDonald C, Schulze K, Murray RM, Wright P (Eds). Schizophrenia: Challenging the Orthodox. London, England: Taylor & Francis; 2004. pp. 163-172.

Chapter 35

Preventive Psychiatry

Mamta Sood, Vijay Krishnan

SUMMARY

Preventive psychiatry is a public health approach that aims at the prevention of mental illnesses in the framework of primary, secondary, and tertiary prevention, and promotion of mental health. A report by the committee on prevention of mental disorders from the Institute of Medicine of USA in 1994 and two reports by the World Health Organization (WHO) in 2002 and 2004 provided direction for preventive and promotive efforts in mental disorders and mental health respectively. Preventive psychiatry can help in narrowing the treatment gap and burden due to mental and substance use disorders (SUDs). Mental health and mental disorders have multiple determinants. Therefore, preventive strategies need to act on multiple inter-related determinants and strategies need to be multipronged. Evidence-based interventions for promotion of well-being and prevention of mental disorders exist but most of the implemented strategies have focused on mental health literacy and stigma reduction. Evaluation of preventive interventions needs to be carried out to make these effective in real world situations. It is also important to integrate prevention into clinical practice.

INTRODUCTION

Mental and substance use disorders (MSUDs) are common and result in significant morbidity, dysfunction and poor quality of life. In the Global Burden of Disease Studies, 13% of the disability adjusted life years have been attributed to the MSUDs (Vigo et al., 2016). Only 30% of the burden due to MSUDs can be tackled with available interventions (Jacka & Reavley, 2014) and treatment gap for these conditions remains at 60–80%. In the last few decades, it has been recognized that preventive psychiatry can play an important role in narrowing this gap, and there is need to shift focus from treatment to prevention and to implement evidence-based and disorder-specific preventive strategies for mental disorders, where they exist.

In this chapter, we refer to preventive psychiatry as a public health approach that aims at prevention of mental illnesses and promotion of mental health. Preventive approaches aim to decrease prevalence, morbidity, and dysfunction due to mental illnesses. Mental health promotion is a related concept. It aims at enhancing favorable psychological traits such as resilience or assertiveness. For promotive interventions, mental health is considered to be a resource, and positive mental health is conceptualized as a human right, with effects upon social inequalities, human capital, and an overall health gain. By contrast, prevention is more narrowly focused on known risk factors and deficits, whose influence increases the incidence or prevalence of mental illness. Thus, mental health promotion might be a useful strategy for prevention, as positive mental health is a strong protective factor for mental illness risk; however, a reduction in mental illness is only one amongst many objectives of mental health promotion interventions (World Health Organization, 2002; World Health Organization, 2004).

HISTORY OF PREVENTION IN PSYCHIATRY

The roots of preventive psychiatry can be traced to prevention practices in medicine that were developed for infectious diseases. Early preventive interventions included sanitation, vaccination, and quarantining, whose primary aim was limiting the spread of contagious illnesses. Preventive medicine later came to be included in all processes involved in "mobilizing... resources to solve the major health problems affecting communities" (Detels & Breslow, 2002), and interventions that curtailed the illness period or prevented relapse and complications were also considered preventive as they reduced the illness burden in the community.

The report by Institute of Medicine (IOM) Committee on Prevention of Mental Disorders organized these interventions as primary, secondary, and tertiary prevention in the practice of medicine. These principles could also be applied to chronic noncommunicable diseases with etiology related to complex genetic and lifestyle factors (Institute of Medicine, 1994). Prevention in psychiatry was viewed with skepticism arising from a lack of etiological information about the causes of mental illnesses.

Beginning in the early part of the 20th century, many ideas were influential in bringing prevention in psychiatry to the mainstream. Foremost of these was the "mental hygiene" movement' that aimed at the prevention of mental illnesses and the promotion of sound mental health in communities. In part, this was driven by a need to tackle mental health issues outside the institutional settings where most patients were managed at that time. The pioneers of the movement included Adolf Meyer, a psychiatrist famous for his work on social milieu as a causative agent in mental illness; and Clifford Beers, an activist whose early experiences as an inmate in an "asylum" made him aware of the perils of institutionalized care (Koplan et al., 2007). The aims of this movement, as stated by Meyer, remain relevant even today: "more extensive training of the average physician in the timely understanding of mental difficulties; provision for early study and treatment within the means and taste of the patient; and a more sympathetic and hopeful attitude on the part of the public"(Meyer, 1918).

Later factors were the community mental health movement of the 1960s with aims of ensuring early treatment and improved reintegration of those with mental illness. Simultaneously, accounts of early childhood experiences preceding mental illness by the psychodynamic psychiatrists; and work in psychiatric epidemiology, such as the Stirling County study, suggested that environmental factors such as education, employment, and economic class were associated with psychiatric illness (Leighton et al., 1963). In 1994, a report by the committee on prevention of mental disorders from IOM highlighted that the principles of prevention in medicine could be applied to prevention in psychiatry even in absence of clear etiology (Institute of Medicine, 1994). The WHO brought out two reports in 2002 and 2004 on prevention of mental disorders and promotion of mental health (World Health Organization, 2002, World Health Organization, 2004).

Thus various factors have influenced the growth of preventive psychiatry, which continues to be focused on early recognition, extension of services, and the use of epidemiological information to guide specific interventions. Psychiatric prevention approaches make use of biological, psychological, and social interventions. There is a strong need for emphasis and formal inclusion of preventive psychiatry in undergraduate and postgraduate curriculum of psychiatry.

In India, preventive elements in the National Mental Health Programme include information, education, and communication activities to improve mental health literacy and health awareness, to reduce stigma, to improve access to mental healthcare services via the district mental health programmes, provisions for out-patient treatment of mental illness in general hospitals; and capacity expansions by training of medical practitioners to recognize, assess, treat or refer patients with mental illness.

KEY CONCEPTS IN PREVENTIVE PSYCHIATRY

Types of Prevention

Preventive interventions have traditionally been divided into primary, secondary, or tertiary prevention (Leavell & Clark, 1958; Institute of Medicine, 1994; World Health Organization, 2002), based upon the population that is addressed and the intended outcome **(Table 1)**.

Primary prevention: It refers to interventions aimed at those who are presently not suffering from any illness. The focus of such an intervention is to prevent the onset of illness, and the effect of successful intervention is reduction in the incidence of illness. For example, the rubella vaccine is routinely administered to healthy antenatal women to prevent intrauterine rubella, as it is known to cause intellectual disability.

Table 1: Concept of prevention in psychiatry

	Primary prevention	Secondary prevention	Tertiary prevention
Population	Healthy	Overtly symptomatic or in early stages of illness	Established illness
Target	Prevent onset of illness	Reduce time spent in illness; prevent recurrence	Reduce functional deficit
Possible outcome measure	Incidence of illness	Prevalence, duration of illness	Functioning and disability, cost of illness
Focus of intervention	Mental health promotion Risk factor reduction Education	Improved access to services Effective treatment (medication and psychosocial)	Rehabilitation Reintegration Social support
Mode of effectiveness at the population level	Alters the risk factor profile of the entire population	Reduces the burden of illness upon the community	

Secondary prevention: Intervention targets persons with known illness, early in its course (ideally before symptoms come to clinical prominence). The aim is to reduce the time spent with illness, which in turn has effects upon morbidity and the occurrence of complications. Effective intervention is associated with a reduced prevalence of symptomatic illness. Most treatment interventions, especially those for initial episodes of illness used early in the course of illness, can be considered secondary prevention interventions. For example, interventions to reduce duration of untreated psychosis or maintenance treatment after a first episode of schizophrenia.

Tertiary prevention: As the illness is established, it may not be possible to fully eliminate symptomatic illness. At this stage, the focus is on managing the consequences of illness, in order to provide the best possible functional outcome for the individual patient. For example, psychiatric rehabilitation interventions like social skills training or supported employment can be considered as tertiary prevention interventions.

Classification of Psychiatric Prevention

The IOM report (Munoz et al., 1996) categorizes primary prevention interventions by the method of targeting populations for intervention into universal, selective, and indicated; universal intervention strategies focus at the general population, selective ones target at the risk groups, and the indicated act on the high risk persons with minimal but detectable signs or symptoms of mental disorder.

Universal interventions can be applied to entire populations without any attempt to select candidates on the basis of risk. These are usually the least intensive and have the lowest cost. As they do not involve any selection process, they avoid problems both relating to false positives and negatives; moreover, in the realm of mental health, selection procedures might be stigmatizing. They can be conveniently delivered to a cohort of subjects, e.g. school-based interventions can be delivered to entire class. Similarly, teachers or parents can be trained to identify mental illness among students. However, as universal interventions are developed for delivery to a large group, these are typically general in their approach and are not flexible to the needs of the specific group. Many of those who receive the intervention are not at risk; thus these interventions are not very efficient either in terms of resources or cost.

Selective interventions are those that are delivered to persons who belong to a high-risk group, but do not themselves suffer from symptoms of the illness. The selection of high-risk groups for intervention improves the power and efficiency of intervention, and this makes more intensive intervention possible. The primary problems are due to the method of risk stratification, which is usually based on epidemiological considerations or statistical associations (Rose et al., 2008). Selection on these basis risks false positive identification, which could also be stigmatizing in psychiatry. Moreover, it has frequently been found that in most diseases, only a small minority of the cases who present with a clinical condition belong to the high-risk group for the same condition (e.g. although increasing maternal age is a very strong predictor for Down's syndrome in the offspring, the majority of children with the syndrome are born to younger mothers who would not be targeted by a high-risk strategy). The implication is that strategies targeted at the population but causing a small change for everyone, may be more effective for the community than a strategy that aims to cause a large change in identified high-risk populations (Rose et al., 2008).

Indicated interventions are those that are directed at patients who already suffer from either subsyndromal symptoms, or conditions that predispose to the condition of interest. Indicated interventions are attractive as the subjects for such an intervention are supposed to have early forms of the illness, and thus the biological process of illness is thought to have begun definitely. Thus, all intervention in this group should theoretically lead to a reduction in illness incidence. However, in the field of mental health, the chain of events leading up to the onset of mental illness cannot be reliably assessed, and thus the current mental state cannot be reliably related to future events. For example, the relationship between subsyndromal symptoms and syndromal disorder is unclear—transition rates between psychotic prodromal states and full-blown psychotic episodes are widely variable, ranging from 1–70% in various studies. It is difficult to establish whether the "prodrome" represents an early form of the illness (which warrants preventive action), a naturally occurring abortive form (which is likely to be stable or self-limiting), a precursor condition (a vulnerability that requires management independently), or a proxy for help-seeking rather than a true biological precursor to illness (van Os and Guloksuz, 2017). Moreover, mental disorders and vulnerabilities are known to be "pleomorphic"(Kraemer et al., 2001), i.e. the same vulnerability may lead to different outcomes, with alterations in other factors.

Intervention Types

Primary prevention is aimed at the individuals without recognized illness, decreasing the incidence of disease by reduction of risk factors and enhancement of protective factors. The risk and the protective factors in psychiatry include individual, family related, and social and environmental determinants of mental health. Social, environmental, and economic determinants of mental health are related to macro-level issues. The risk factors are poverty, poor housing, war, lack of basic facilities like education, poor work conditions, etc. Protective factors include social support, social services, empowerment, etc. Micro-level risk and protective factors work on individuals, small groups like families, or social networks. The risk factors can be malleable and nonmalleable. Another useful way of assessing these factors relates to their location with respect to the client: these factors may be within the person (biological or psychological factors), interpersonal (relationships), or present in the broader environment (World Health Organization, 2002; 2004).

Risk factors for mental illness are those factors that are associated with an increased probability of onset, longer duration or increased severity of an illness; or some combination of the above. Protective factors refer to the conditions that improve a person's resistance to risk factors and disorders. Protective factors are similar to positive mental health, and include self-esteem, emotional resilience, positive thinking, problem solving, and stress management skills (World Health Organization 2002; 2004).

Risk and protective factors may be generic or specific. Generic factors like poverty and child abuse have been associated with many mental disorders like depression, anxiety disorders, psychosis, substance use, and personality disorders. Interventions addressing the generic factors will have effect on the occurrence or consequences of all these disorders. Many of the risk factors for mental illness fall into this category. Others are specific and are clearly associated with a disorder, e.g. major depression is a specific risk factor for suicide.

PREVENTIVE INTERVENTIONS

Evidence-based interventions for promotion of well-being and prevention of mental disorders exist. Mental health and mental disorders have multiple determinants. Therefore, preventive strategies need to act on multiple inter-related determinants and strategies need to be multipronged.

The mechanisms, whereby preventive interventions exercise their functions, may be complex and inter-related. In a review of multiple interventions, Coie et al., 1993 suggested that these interventions may have direct effects on the disease process or may interact with risk factors to buffer their effects or may disrupt mediational chain by which risk factor leads to disorder or may prevent initial occurrence of risk factors. By and large, preventive interventions are delivered in combination with each other, and with treatment services. Each intervention may focus on a particular domain of vulnerability. The combination may be for reasons of convenience, or in order to ensure that it covers a number of vulnerabilities leading up to the same final outcome.

A number of these interventions aim at altering social determinants of illness. For example, improved access to housing has been shown to be associated with improvements in markers for both physical and mental health, and to reduce mental strain. Independent housing is also associated with improved mental health outcomes in severe mental illness, even after accounting for potential confounding factors such as medication adherence and other measures of social support. Similarly, interventions to improve access to education, reduce poverty and improve nutritional outcomes have potential benefits for mental health. Other policy interventions could also have wide-ranging effects. Taxation, and restrictions on sale of alcohol and tobacco are useful policy tools that have been used to reduce rates of substance abuse and complications related to their use. Studies of price elasticity have shown that increasing the cost of purchasing tobacco or alcohol products is more effective in preventing youth from starting use than prohibition-based approaches.

Apart from considerations as to whether the interventions are aimed at a selected high-risk population, useful classifications must also include considerations of setting, expertise and life stage, which would influence the implementation. A comprehensive classification of interventions published by the WHO in 2004 is tabulated in **Table 2** (World Health Organization, 2004).

Prevention of Mental Disorders (World Health Organization, 2004)

In this section, we focus on a few interventions as examples of potential strategies for preventive psychiatry. More comprehensive reviews are available in the WHO reports on this topic (World Health Organization, 2004; Bhui & Dinos, 2011).

Conduct disorders: The prevalence of conduct disorders ranges from 2–10% and have high social and economic costs. The risk factors that can be modified are: maternal smoking during pregnancy, impulsivity, poor parenting, antisocial behavior and substance use in parents,

Table 2: Classification of preventive interventions (based on World Health Organization, 2004)

Focus/Setting	Action	Examples
Policy and government	Framing rules, laws, policy; funding support	• Alcohol/tobacco price regulations and taxation • Nutritional supplementation, complementary feeding • Improved access to education,healthcare services • Housing and poverty alleviation programs • Framing mental health policy and legislation that supports preventive principles
Educational institutions	Improved recognition; school-based interventions	• Teachers' training to improve recognition of Attention-deficit/hyperactivity disorder, conduct disorders, depression, specific learning disorders • School-based interventions to combat childhood abuse
Home visit based interventions	Healthcare worker or nurse visits to provide support to high-risk persons	• Parenting assistance to adolescent mothers • Health visitors
Media	Radio, television, internet-based public health infomercials	• Improve mental health literacy • Reduce stigma • Inform about availability of services • Public attitudes towards body image, stress
Workplace/educational institution-based interventions	Screening by mental health professionals; training of trainers	• Workplace mental health screening • Stress management skills training
Helplines	Suicide and mental health helplines	• Evidence to show that suicide helplines are not effective in preventing attempts

child abuse, early onset of aggression and substance use, poor peer relationships and residing in poor and crime prone localities. The preventive interventions, that focus on improving the social competence and prosocial behavior of children, parents, peers and teachers, can reduce the risk of developing these problems.

Depressive disorders: These are the most common mental disorders. The risk factors for development of depression are inadequate parenting, child neglect and abuse, stressful life events, bullying and parental depression. The protective factors for depression are sense of mastery, self-esteem, self-efficacy, stress resistance and social support. School-based interventions aimed at enhancing cognitive, problem-solving and social skills of children and adolescents, exercise programs for the elderly, interventions to reduce child abuse and neglect and bullying are some of the universal interventions. Parenting interventions for parents of children with conduct problems, interventions for children of depressed parents, children with parental death or divorce, interventions for unemployed and chronically ill elderly, provision of adequate social and economic support to those exposed to war, conflicts, and natural disasters are some of the examples for selective interventions. Indicated interventions using elements of cognitive behavior therapy given in group format have been found useful for those with high depressive symptoms but have not yet developed depressive disorders.

Anxiety disorders: These are common and are of different types. Most of these disorders appear in childhood and adolescence. The risk factors for anxiety disorders are traumatic events, learning anxiety from anxious parents by modeling, considering oneself to have low self-efficacy, poor control and inadequate social support. The interventions to reduce anxiety should focus on reducing traumatizing events or exposure, enhancing emotional resilience, anticipatory education, and post-trauma interventions.

Psychotic disorders: These have onset in early adulthood and may result in disruption of skills needed to complete education, choose vocation, and relationships. The risk factors for schizophrenia include obstetric complications, childhood trauma, migration, socioeconomic disadvantage, urban birth and use of cannabis. Improving mental health literacy, early recognition, help seeking and treatment are some of the strategies for prevention of psychotic disorders.

Substance use disorders: It result in significant disability and burden. Taxation, restrictions on availability and total ban on direct and indirect advertising are some of the effective regulatory interventions. School-based prevention programs are helpful in improving knowledge and attitudes towards the addictive substances. Brief interventions in form of advice from a general practitioner routinely given to all patients who smoke and drink are effective.

Evaluation of Preventive Interventions

Although the number of evidence-based preventive interventions available worldwide have expanded over the past few decades, the most recent mental health atlas (World Health Organization, 2014) found that only 41 out of 194 member states had implemented these at a population level. Most of these have been focused on mental health literacy and stigma reduction.

Psychiatric prevention has to contend with problems that are specific to this field, i.e. etiology of mental illness is unknown for almost all disorders. Models of causation are mostly speculative, and most suggest that mental illness is the final outcome of complex interactions between a plethora of factors (Coie et al., 1993). The influence of many such factors are plastic and reversible, and thus preventionists must choose intervention targets that offer the greatest benefit at the least cost at the population level. For selective and targeted interventions, an important consideration is the method of selection of candidates based upon the risk stratification. For the screening method to be effective, it must be used in an appropriate population for which it has been validated, and care must be taken to ensure that it is culturally appropriate (Sharan & Singh, 2017).

While designing interventions for preventive psychiatry, it is important to consider following points:

- The outcome of preventive intervention is measured at an aggregate level as a reduction in the rate in a naturally occurring event. Therefore, any evaluation must be based on adequate knowledge of the natural history of the event in question, and of expected fluctuations

- Understanding the effectiveness of an intervention depends on an adequate comparison group. Ideally, the comparison group should be comparable on all characteristics except the absence of intervention and interventions are best evaluated by a randomized controlled design. However, such trials are difficult to implement in practice, and much of the evidence comes from quasiexperimental and observational designs
- It is important that the interventions must be effective in the real world, where it is difficult to control for confounding factors. In the field of preventive medicine, many interventions with initial efficacy in clinical trials have failed to translate to improvements when implemented at a larger scale. Thus, evaluation must continue beyond the pilot phase, and the intervention program may require modification to be effective in each setting
- Preventive interventions may not have immediate effects. For many psychiatric illnesses, vulnerabilities may extend from early childhood risk exposure, with a long period when vulnerable individuals cannot be differentiated from those who are not at risk. For example, many of the neurodevelopmental risks for schizophrenia have been hypothesized to be due to antenatal, perinatal and early developmental insults, but their manifestations typically occur decades later during adolescence. With such long timeframes, intervention may require very long follow-up periods to establish their effectiveness. As an alternative, proxy predictors may need to be developed, that would make study easier, but could be measured at a more proximal time point
- The effect of a preventive intervention may be direct. But more frequently, the effect is to modify a factor with further effects upon the manifest outcome. The choice of outcome measures becomes very important in this context, and must include both the proximate psychological factor that is modified (in order to ensure that the intervention is effective as a process) but also the distal outcome that is desired. For example, a relapse prevention intervention may include psychoeducation as a component. The evaluation of such an intervention would require measurement of both improved knowledge of illness, as also a change in attitude towards medication (i.e. improved compliance). These intermediate outcomes must be compared with the final desired outcome, i.e. a decrease in the actual relapse rate. A failure to measure any one of these could lead to faulty inferences.

CLINICAL PRACTICE AND PREVENTIVE PSYCHIATRY

As a relatively new concept in social psychiatry, the scope of preventive psychiatry is still being defined. Every clinical intervention may be seen to have a preventive intent, as the final measure of outcome is of clinical importance: the nonoccurrence of phenomena such as illness relapse or recurrence, adverse drug reactions, complications such as suicide; or functional deficits. However, preventive psychiatry is seen to be broader than clinical psychiatry, as it encompasses interventions aimed at individuals who may be overtly normal but at high risk; or to be focused on outcomes that are outside the ambit of clinical care. It is important to integrate prevention into clinical practice (Compton, 2009).

How does Preventive Psychiatry Differ from Clinical Practice?

- *Clinical outcomes are short-term oriented*: The immediate outcome is often the first consideration for a clinician attending to a patient. Such immediate outcomes may be the curtailing of an illness episode or the amelioration of specific symptoms by means of a set of defined interventions. While this has a preventive function by preventing known complications of the illness, these considerations are secondary. The "lag" between intervention and outcome is on average longer for preventive interventions and may sometimes be measured in decades

- *Focus on individuals*: Despite the growth of the evidence-based medicine movement, individual clinical decisions are largely taken by doctors in consultation with patients, and do not rely entirely on epidemiological data. This is borne out by the repeated finding that clinical guideline adherence remains low at all levels of care around the world, and in almost all settings (Bauer, 2002; Howes et al., 2014). A preventive approach, being oriented towards the nonoccurrence of an adverse outcome, is much more dependent on statistical reductions in risk or prevalence rates assessed at an aggregate level. Thus, in order to be a preventionist, clinicians must integrate evidence into their practice at all times

- Another important consideration is the *prevention paradox*, initially described by Geoffrey Rose in the 1950s. This is the observation that a preventive intervention that is most effective at the population level may not be one that provides a large benefit to individual patients; conversely, a highly effective clinical intervention for individuals may not be effective at the population level. The implications of this much-replicated observation are two-fold: the scaling up of clinical interventions to a population level may be inefficient as a means of achieving population level prevention, and interventions for prevention must be piloted at a population level, and not devised merely on the basis of their intuitive appeal (Rose, 2008)

- *Clients' involvement in defining outcomes*: Clinical practice relies on the doctor-patient dyad. As professionals, clinicians interpret the findings and give them a coherent explanation and context, but the starting point is usually a problem perceived by the individual patient (or significant others). On the other hand, preventive approaches would demand that professionals be proactive in identifying difficulties before they arise, either in individuals without overt problems at high risk, or within clinical populations (Mrazek & Ritchie, 2007)

- *Setting*: Medical interventions are usually implemented in a hospital or outpatient clinic, or sometimes as a part of defined outreach activity. Prevention encompasses a variety of interventions that may occur at social or educational institutions or within the family. In order to be a preventionist, medical professionals must thus engage with a number of social institutions that are outside the ambit of routine clinical care. For example, the SOLVE program developed by the International Labour Organization and piloted in a number of developing countries, involves integrating health (including mental health) prevention education using a training of trainers approach. This program demonstrates the need to involve a number of stakeholders (employers, administrators, employees' groups and trade unions, health professionals) in order to implement such a program (SOLVE, 2012)

- *Personnel delivering the interventions*: Clinical interventions are delivered by medical professionals, and are recognized as medical. Preventive interventions for psychiatry include a host of interventions directed at the so-called "social determinants of health" such as empowerment, poverty alleviation or education. These may be delivered by change in government policy, by teachers or social workers, etc.

Clinicians and Preventive Psychiatry

A preventive approach in clinical practice is helpful to clarify one's objectives and establish a framework for thinking about longer-term care. In psychiatry, this is important as many of the disorders are chronic and have significant effects upon functioning. Clinicians can implement preventive strategies in various ways (**Boxes 1 and 2**):

- *Case formulation*: Biopsychosocial case formulation may be a practical approach for psychiatrists to practice prevention in their daily routine. This requires the clinician to consider predisposing, precipitating, perpetuating, and protective factors in the individual, and further divide them into biological, psychological, and social factors. The aim of this process is to go beyond merely considering presenting symptoms as the targets of care, and to identify risk factors that may be modifiable by intervention. Another potential strategy is the routine use of multidisciplinary teams of doctors, nurses, psychologists, occupational therapists, and social workers, who can work together to identify targets and take relevant responsibilities to achieve the outcome that is most appropriate to the patient

---

Box 1: A template for integrating preventive psychiatry in clinical practice*

- What is the problem that can occur (nature of the problem)?
- What are the chances of developing the problem (prevalence)?
- How to reduce chances of developing the problem (reducing incidence—primary prevention)?
- What increases the chance of having the problem (risk factors)?
- What decreases the chance of having the problem (protective factors)?
- What are the early signs for identification of the problem (early detection—secondary prevention)?
- What to do once the problem has occurred (early intervention—secondary prevention)?
- How to minimize the impact of the problem (prevention of complications/further deterioration—tertiary prevention)?
- If problem persists despite treatment, how to modify biopsychosocial factors so that there is improvement in quality of life and functioning (tertiary prevention)?

*(From Sood M, Krishnan V. Preventive psychiatry in clinical practice. Indian Journal of Social Psychiatry 2017 with permission).

- *Medical comorbidity*: Patients with mental illness are subject to a number of preventable conditions including infections such as HIV or tuberculosis, as well as noncommunicable conditions like cardiovascular and cerebrovascular insult. These factors contribute to the repeated finding of mortality at an earlier age even after excluding deaths due to suicide or other unnatural causes (Walker et al., 2015) with all-cause mortality comparable to heavy smoking (Chesney et al., 2014). Important factors such as substance use including smoking, obesity, and metabolic syndrome are all potentially preventable with early recognition and interventions like awareness and patient education
- *Outreach activities*: A variety of outreach activities have been attempted, in order to make sure that patients who do not routinely attend psychiatric clinics, also receive care. These include mental health camps for rapid screening and referral, telepsychiatry interventions, and consultation-liaison services in the outpatient, inpatient, or community settings.

These are important tools for secondary and tertiary prevention, as they expand psychiatric services into the community, and into general medical care. The availability of consultation and referral services has been shown to improve general practitioners' comfort in dealing with mental health conditions

- *Advocacy*: Clinicians can lead the advocacy efforts to increase awareness amongst mental health patients of their rights, and to counter societal stigma and systematic discrimination towards patients. These are barriers to treatment seeking amongst both patients with currently undiagnosed illness, and those with established mental health diagnoses
- *Policy interventions*: Clinicians can also help in designing and testing preventive interventions, which require expertise in their formulation and delivery
- *Interventions for families and caregivers*: Informal caregivers provide support and care for most patients with mental disorders, often far more than provided by the healthcare or social service sector. In addition, biological relatives of those with mental disorder are at a higher risk of developing mental disorders, and may experience "courtesy stigma" by virtue of their relationship with a person with mental illness. These factors contribute to higher rates of distress and mental disorders in this group. Clinicians can provide support to caregivers to prevent stress and identify early signs of mental illness. Measures such as respite admission or day care, which reduce the burden upon caregivers, may also reduce stress. Other factors such as financial burden and time taken away from work may be reduced by changes in the health system that ensure that care is made available as conveniently as possible.

Box 2: Points to consider for integrating preventive psychiatry in clinical practice*

Prevention in mental health is practiced at primary, secondary, and tertiary prevention. Mental health promotion is related concept. Preventive efforts in clinical practice can be guided by following points:
- Knowledge about the epidemiological data related to a specific mental illnesses
- Knowledge about the evidence-based preventive efforts available for specific mental illness
- Directed towards all the persons (patients, caregivers accompanying and at home, teachers, employers) during the clinical encounter
- Age, gender, and culture sensitivity
- Sociodemographic characteristics of a person seeking relief from a problem in the clinical encounter
- Whether the patient has first episode or established or treatment refractory mental illness
- Whether the illness is of short or long duration
- Good communication skills

*(From Sood M, Krishnan V. Preventive psychiatry in clinical practice. Indian Journal of Social Psychiatry 2017; 33:79-85 with permission).

CONCLUSION

Preventive psychiatry is public health approach to prevention of mental illness and promotion of mental health. Similar to prevention medicine, in mental health also, concepts of primary, secondary, and tertiary prevention have been used to study, design, and implement preventive interventions aimed at reducing risk factors and enhancing protective factors. For various psychiatric disorders, evidence-based preventive strategies exist. However, most of the implemented strategies have focused on mental health literacy and stigma reduction. Psychiatrists must incorporate preventive strategies in their clinical practice.

REFERENCES

Bauer MS. A review of quantitative studies of adherence to mental health clinical practice guidelines. Harv Rev Psychiatry.2002;10(3):138-53.

Bhui K, Dinos S. Preventive psychiatry: a paradigm to improve population mental health and well-being. Br J Psychiatry. 2011;198:417-9.

Chesney E, Goodwin GM, Fazel S. Risks of all—cause and suicide mortality in mental disorders: a meta-review. World Psychiatry. 2014; 13:153-60.

Coie JD, Watt NF, West SG, et al. The science of prevention: a conceptual framework and some directions for a national research program. Am Psychol.1993;48:1013.

Compton MT(Ed). Clinical Manual of Prevention in Mental Health. Washington, DC: American Psychiatric Publishing, Inc.; 2009.

Detels R, Breslow L. Current scope and concerns in public health. In: Oxford Textbook of Public Health. Detels R, McEwen J, Beaglehole R, Tanaka H (Eds.) 4th Ed, Vol 1. pp.3-20, Oxford University Press, UK, 2006.

Howes OD, Vergunst F, Gee S, et al. Adherence to treatment guidelines in clinical practice: study of antipsychotic treatment prior to clozapine initiation. Br J Psychiatry. 2012;201(6):481-5.

Institute of Medicine. Reducing Risks for Mental Disorders: Frontiers for Preventive Intervention Research. Washington, DC: The National Academies Press; 1994.

Jacka FN, Reavley NJ. Prevention of mental disorders: Evidence, challenges and opportunities. BMC Medicine. 2014;12:75.

Koplan C, Charuvastra A, Compton MT, et al. Prevention Psychiatry. Psychiatric Annals. 2007;37:319-328.

Kraemer HC, Stice E, Kazdin A, Offord D, Kupfer D. How do risk factors work together? Mediators, moderators, and independent, overlapping, and proxy risk factors. Am J Psychiatry 2001;158:848-56.

Leavell HR, Clark EG. Preventive Medicine for the Doctor in his Community. An Epidemiologic Approach. Prev Med Dr His Community Epidemiol Approach.1958.

Leighton DC, Harding JS, Macklin DB, et al. Psychiatric findings of the Stirling County study. Am J Psychiatry. 1963;119:1021-6.

Meyer A. The Mental Hygiene Movement. Can Med Assoc J. 1918;8:632-4.

Mrazek PJ, Ritchie GF. Becoming a preventionist. Psychiatric Annals. 2007;37(5):365-60.

Muñoz RF, Mrazek PJ, Haggerty RJ. Institute of Medicine report on prevention of mental disorders: Summary and commentary. Am Psychol. 1996;51(11):1116-22.

National Mental Health Programme of India. Ministry of Health and Family Welfare,Government of India: New Delhi, 1982.

Rose G, Khaw KT, Marmot M. Rose's Strategy of Preventive Medicine. Revised Edition. Oxford, New York: Oxford University Press; 2008.p.192.

SOLVE : integrating health promotion into workplace OSH policies : trainer's guide/International Labour Office. -Geneva: ILO, 2012.

Sood M, Krishnan V. Preventive psychiatry in clinical practice. Indian J Soc Psychiatry 2017;33(2):79-85.

van Os J, Guloksuz S. A critique of the "ultra-high risk" and "transition" paradigm. World Psychiatry 2017;16(2):200–6.

Vigo D, Thornicroft G, Atun R. Estimating the true global burden of mental illness. Lancet Psychiatry. 2016;3(2):171-8.

Walker ER, McGee RE, Druss BG. Mortality in mental disorders and global disease burden implications. JAMA Psychiatry 2015; 72:334–41.

World Health Organization. Prevention of Mental Disorders: Effective Interventions and Policy Options - Summary Report. 2004.

World Health Organization. Mental Health Atlas. Geneva: WHO, 2014.

Chapter 36

Cultural Interventions

Vinod K Sinha, KL Vidya

SUMMARY

Practices intervening in various kinds of indispositions have been transmitted across generations and are diverse in different cultures. The World Health Organization (WHO) also considers those people, who are recognized by their communities as competent to provide health care services using range of substances and methods based on community's social, cultural, and religious systems, as traditional healers, who cater to huge population, decreasing the treatment gap, especially for mental illness. Apart from magic, mystic, ceremonies and rituals, herbal medicines are prevalent in cultures from all over the world. Owing to its cultural diversity, interventions are countless too in India; few of them are enumerated in this chapter. Like any other form of treatment, cultural interventions are also not immune to adverse effects. However, in conditions both physical and mental, which remain chronic, relapsing with enigmatic etiology, where "cure" is illusory, going back to the roots of various cultural interventions might help in discovering the missing links.

INTRODUCTION

Psychopharmacology has revolutionized the way in which mentally ill persons are treated. Since the advent of chlorpromazine, several antipsychotics and other psychotropic medications have significantly decreased morbidity associated with mental illness. Electroconvulsive therapy and other newer somatic treatments have further added to the therapeutics. Various psychotherapeutic methods have enhanced the outcome in depression, anxiety, and even personality disorders. However, despite all these developments, still we mental health professionals feel intimidated while dealing with dissociation, conversion, trance and possession states, somatization, and so on. It also reminds us of various cultural interventions which continue to rule when it comes to treating these conditions. From patient point of view, "desperation of cure" is one of the main reasons, which takes majority to cultural interventions even in cases of severe mental illnesses across the world.

CULTURE AND PSYCHOPATHOLOGY INTERPLAY

Influence of culture both on mental health and malady is unquestionable. Though it can be a source of resilience, it can also lead to conflicts and psychopathology. Owing to the dynamic nature and consequential effect, culture has on a mentally ill person seeking help, the concept of cultural formulation continues even in the newer diagnostic systems, incorporation of which helps in avoiding misdiagnosing, improving rapport and therapeutic efficacy, and clarifying the cultural epidemiology (American Psychiatric Association, 2013).

Culture influences mental illness starting premorbid personality, onset, and clinical presentation to course and outcome. Cultural influences on psychiatric syndromes can occur in at least six distinct ways (Tseng, 2006):

1. *Pathogenic effect*: Cultural influence on formation of a disorder
2. *Psychoselective effect*: Culture selecting certain coping patterns to deal with stress
3. *Psychoplastic effect*: Culture modifying the clinical manifestation
4. *Pathoelaborating effect*: Culture elaborating mental conditions into a unique nature
5. *Psychofacilitating effect*: Culture promoting the frequency of occurrence
6. *Psychoreactive effect*: Culture shaping folk responses to the clinical condition.

TRADITIONAL HEALING AND INTERVENTIONS ACROSS THE GLOBE

The one, who is ill, seeks solace. Interventions for ailments both physical and mental, have been there since time immemorial. These practices have been transmitted across generations and are diverse in different cultures. The WHO considers those people, who are recognized by their communities as competent to provide health care services using range of substances and methods based on community's social, cultural, and religious systems, as traditional healers (Bojuwoye, 2005).

In most societies of the earlier periods, religion, magic, and supernatural healing were integral parts of life. When a state of disequilibrium in the form of disease, illness, or discomfort was experienced, help was sought through one of these methods (Rosman & Rubel, 1992).

Traditional African Practices

Consulting traditional healers after hospitalization continues in majority of native Africans despite strong Western cultural influences. Traditional healing remains integral part of the culture and is holistic. Physical and mental ailments are not differentiated and rather both are dealt together from the root cause (Bojuwoye, 2005). Various healers in the community include herbalists, called Iyanga and diviners, known as Sangoma, Ngaka, Nanga, etc. It is believed that ancestral spirits are responsible for the selection of these healers (Mafamdi & Sodi, 1999).

The healing process involves divination, in which healer goes into trance and communicates with ancestral spirits who help in the diagnosis which is a dynamic process in terms of ill feelings, rivalry, inner chaos, negative powers of unconscious factors and so on. Treatment includes prescription of herbs along with rituals to restore harmony (Bojuwoye, 2005).

Views of Aboriginals from North America

Fundamental cultural difference between the aboriginal people from North America and western thought is in the perception of one's relationship with universe and its creator. The aboriginals believe that they are the least important creatures of the universe and completely dependent upon the four basic elements namely fire, water, earth, and air. Society is granted with sacred ceremonies, traditional healers, and sacred teachings, such as medicine wheel to help in maintaining good health, harmony, and life. The medicine wheel philosophy connects stages of human life with that of cosmos. Understanding of medicine wheel is the beginning of healing (Poonwassie & Charter, 2001). Though there are auxiliary cultural groupings, which identify their own healers and processes, it predominantly involves storytelling, teaching and sharing circles, participation in ceremonies, the sweat lodge (a ritual steam bath in North America), and role modeling (Rowan et al., 2014).

Caribbean Cultural Healing

Following emancipation, Caribbean culture has been influenced by various religious groups including Christians, Hindus, Muslims, Seventh day Adventists, Jehovah's witnesses and so on. Acculturation has further resulted in practices like Shango and Vodoun (Marshall, 2001).

Illnesses are believed to be associated with evil spirits, which have to be cast out by traditional medicines, which include herbs and oils given by Shango healers. The practice of Vodoun resulted from mixture of African and French culture in which rituals take the form of dancing, offering gifts, and making animal sacrifices to pacify the spirits (Blom et al., 2015).

Traditional Interventions among Chinese

Chinese still continue to have disinclination towards modern intervention and prefer to cope within the family as far as possible. Similar to their South east Asian neighbors, Chinese too deny and suppress emotions at the same time and somatize distress (Tseng et al., 1995). According to traditional Chinese medicine, mental illness is said to result from imbalance of Yin and Yang forces, a stagnation of qi, which is vital energy and blood in various organs. Qigong or "exercise of vital energy" is a highly popular Chinese life style, which is believed to be helpful in maintaining overall wellbeing. It involves series of physical movements, regulated breathing and consciously regulating the flow of qi to balance Yin and Yang. A typical consultation session involves four techniques: observation, questioning, smelling, and pulse taking. After this a formal diagnosis is given based on the traditional theory, and treatment would involve herbs, acupuncture and dietary advice. Similar to other South Asian cultures, position of the healer is august and patient expects healer to be directive, edifying, and authoritarian (So, 2005).

Off late, there have been efforts to generate evidence for the efficacy of Traditional Chinese Medicine through clinical trials in cases of schizophrenia, depression, bipolar disorder, anxiety, and obsessive compulsive disorders (So, 2005). A double blind randomized controlled trial on acupuncture in depression showed results, which were comparable with other, established forms of medications and psychotherapy (Schnyer, 2001). Wendan decoction is one of the traditional Chinese herbal formulas used for psychosis, and has gained lot of scientific scrutiny by randomized trials (Deng & Xu, 2017). Research on herbs like ginkgo biloba, kava, and valerian is continuing (So, 2005).

Other Indigenous Practices

Ayahuasca is one thing which demands special mention. It is a decoctum made of admixture of plants containing dimethyltryptamine and harmine. For millennia, it has been used as a central element of spiritual, religious, healing ritual originally by indigenous groups of the Amazon basin and later by the mestizo populations of that region (Frecska et al., 2016).

In the context of Mexican traditional healing, diagnosis of mental illness is made using magico-religious processes, such as reading arrangements of kernels of corn that are dropped in a gourd filled with water or reading of an egg with which patient undergoes a ritual called Limpia. Healing starts with a physical maneuver to gather pulse to the naval center. This follows series of prayers, Limpia rituals, rubbings, bath, and fomentations with medicinal plants (Chevez, 2005).

INDIAN CULTURAL INTERVENTIONS

Mental disorders contribute about 14% of the global burden of disease. In 2010, mental and substance use disorders accounted for 7.4% of all DALYs worldwide (Campion & Bhugra, 1996). Despite the staggering burden of mental illness, the treatment gap remains wide. A large proportion of people with mental health problems do not receive treatment from a western/ modern health facility (Whiteford et al., 2013). A multicenter survey by WHO showed that 76–85% of people with serious mental illnesses had received no treatment in the previous 12 months and that for those who received, it was inadequate (Chisholm et al., 2007). A survey conducted in 1993-94, reported that 45% of psychiatric patients in India, consult a religious healer before attending hospital (Kumar et al., 2005).

Traditional healers constitute a major provider of care considering the huge patient-psychiatrist ratio in India. A study said that besides the modern doctors there are mainly three types of traditional healers: Vaids, practising an empirical system of indigenous medicine; Mantarwadis, curing through astrology and charms; and Patris, who acted as mediums for spirits and demons. It was found that a large majority, i.e. 59% of those with symptoms had consulted some form of cultural intervention (Kapur, 1975).

Considering the cultural diversity of the Indian subcontinent, traditional healing interventions are countless too. However, the major Indian systems of medicine have been grouped together under the acronym AYUSH, which stands for Ayurveda, Yoga, Unani, Siddha, and Homeopathy. Apart from these, people in distress also consult various palmists, horoscope specialists, herbalists, diviners, sorcerers, and shamans (Kakar, 1982).

Ayurveda

Ayurveda is one of the oldest healing traditions in the world, which dates back to early Vedic civilizations. It is rather integral part of the Indian culture. Graha chikitsa or Bhut vidya is one of the eight branches of Ayurveda, which deals with factors affecting mind. According to Ayurvedic principles, health can be achieved only when there is harmony between body, mind, and soul along with Mother Nature. Mental equilibrium is considered as the balance between three qualities of mind namely, Sattva, Rajas and Tamas (Abhyankar, 2015).

A traditional Ayurvedic therapist is called Vaidya, who makes diagnosis based on history of symptoms, lifestyle, and examination of pulse called Nadi. Therapeutic techniques involve purification, pacification and efforts to remove the root cause. Purification includes purging, emesis, controlled bleeding or blood-letting, and emphasizing on personal hygiene.

Pacification consists of topical applications of oils, herbs, massages, and ingestion of decoctions from plants and metals. Lifestyle modification including dietary changes, sleep, abstinence from alcohol, are all intended towards removing the root cause (Kumar et al., 2005).

Herbal Medicines

Herbalists are one of the most sought after traditional healers in India. Culturally herbal medicines are believed to be having no or minimal side effects and are accepted by majority. There are two category of people who dispense herbal medicines, one who has studied herbalism as part of training in Ayurveda and others who inherit the knowledge of herbs from his ancestors as legacy.

Indian system of herbal medicines uses innumerable herbs in its armamentarium. However to name a few, Ashwagandha-*Withania somnifera* is traditionally used to restore sleep rhythms as well as a rejuvenator for stress (Andrade, 2009). Sarpagandha plant, *Rauwolfia serpentina*, is valued in Ayurveda for the treatment of insomnia and insanity. Shankhapushpi, is consumed for mental peace and tranquility (Dev, 1999). Brahmi-*Bacopa monnieri* is believed to be enhancer of memory and concentration. It has also been studied as an add-on therapy in schizophrenia, giving promising results (Sarkar et al., 2012; Singh, 2013). Mandookaparni is another herb believed to be having antiamnestic properties (Andrade & Chandra, 2006). However all these are coming under the scrutiny of scientific trials only from last few decades.

Practice of Yoga

Yoga has developed in India and has its foundations in the ancient Indian civilization. It is a process of uniting one's finite, microscopic, individual self with the infinite, macroscopic, pure consciousness (Pankhania, 2005). Patanjali gave this tradition its classical format by compiling it in his "YogaSutras", a text on Yoga theory and practice. He outlined eight limbs or steps of Yoga: Yama, abstention; Niyama, observances; Asana, postures; Pranayama, controlled breathing; Pratyahara, weaning from food; Dharana, focus; Dhyana, meditation; and Samadhi, highest state of consciousness (Abhyankar, 2015). Yoga offers a holistic framework for physical, mental, and spiritual wellbeing and helps the individual become balanced and integrated. Yoga helps the ego surrender its authority and embrace universal love and wisdom (Gangadhar & Porandla, 2015). At the basic level itself, it promotes "asceticism", a healthy ego defense mechanism, which further adds to resilience. Millions of people throughout the world today practice Yoga on regular basis.

Clinical trials on Yoga as a therapy for physical as well as psychological problems have started emerging in last two-three decades. In randomized comparisons, Yoga was nearly as effective as tricyclic antidepressant imipramine (Janakiramaiah et al., 2010). Yogasana-based therapy alone too reduced depression to the level of remission (Gangadhar et al., 2013). In depressed patients, Yoga therapy increased the levels of brain derived neurotrophic factor in serum, which was correlated with the antidepressant effects of Yoga (Naveen et al., 2013). Results of studies on effectiveness of Yoga in anxiety and OCD symptomatology have been encouraging (Kirkwood et al., 2005; Shannahoff-Khalsa, 2004). Clinical trials have confirmed the benefits of Yoga as an adjunct to antipsychotic therapy in schizophrenia. Interestingly, the benefits were noted in the negative as well as cognitive symptoms which are difficult to treat by antipsychotics alone (Gangadhar & Varambally, 2012).

Religious/Faith Healings

In India, many people troubled by emotional distress or more serious mental illnesses go to Hindu, Muslim, Christian, and other religious centers. There are few temples which are known for healing powers, where patients with severe mental illnesses are brought for healing. The healing power identified with these institutions is believed to reside in the site itself, rather than in the religious leader or any medicines provided at the site (Sood, 2016). Here, the patients are encouraged to take part in the daily routines of the temple, such as cleaning the compound, watering the plants, and so forth. One study published in 2002, observed a reduction of nearly 20% in brief psychiatric rating scale scores in about 31 patients of severe mental illnesses, with 5 weeks mean duration of stay, which the authors attributed to strong cultural belief, nonthreatening, reassuring setting, and supportive milieu (Raghuram et al., 2002).

Muslims approach Dargahs for social and mental health issues especially marital and family problems. The main role of Imam in this context is to provide counseling in accordance with Quranic principles and teachings of Prophet Muhammad. This form of intervention is proved to be effective in improving marital adjustments (Esmat, 2016).

Christians in India when faced with any kind of mental agony, distress or disequilibrium, tend to approach the priest in local church and usually are directed to Charismatic Prayer. Here the condition is understood either as a psychosomatic or as a spirito- somatic phenomenon. The collective healing process takes place on a weekly basis and the client has to stay in the accommodation provided by the Church during the period. To start with, there is a cleansing and disengagement through confession and counseling. Thereafter, comes a phase of personal emptying, transition and reorientation. The procedure is finally completed with the person being spiritually "refilled" by the Holy Spirit. The dominant recurring element in the whole process is the continuous statement of healing "testimonies" (Jansen & Lang, 2012).

Mindfulness and Buddhist Healing

Mindfulness is a process of learning to pay attention moment by moment, intentionally, and with curiosity and compassion. Traditionally in Buddhism, it has been used as a way for enlightenment and to become free of suffering. In West, it has been popularized by Jon Kabat Zinn as Mindfulness Based Stress Reduction. It has been studied and has given promising results in depression, anxiety disorders, eating disorders, OCD hypochondriasis, somatization, and the search for evidence is on (Groves, 2016).

Shamanism and Exorcism

Shaman is an individual who is believed to have the power to heal the sick through his ability of communicating with the world of spirits. It goes well with the Indian cultural belief that mental illness results due to possession by spirits or as a result of witchcrafts. Shamanism involves ceremonial rituals, which include chanting, singing, rhythmic sounds, dancing, inflicting physical pains, use of herbs, vermilions, and holy waters, etc (Sadock et al., 2015).

Exorcism is a religious practice specifically intended to evict the demons and/or spirits from a person who is believed to be possessed. Among Hindus, Atharvaveda is said to contain the secrets related to exorcism, magic, and alchemy. The means used here are the Mantras and Yajna, used in tantric traditions (Narayana, 1995).

In Islam, exorcism is called Ruqya. It is used to repair the damage caused by Sihr or black magic. Usually performed in Dargahs, by Imams or Peers, this includes reciting verses from Quran, sprinkling of holy water, beating spirits called Jinn out of one's body, which is believed to free him/her from misery (Sabry & Vohra, 2013).

In Christianity, exorcist is usually a member of the Christian church who may use prayers and religious material such as set formulas, gestures, symbols, icons, amulets etc. They often invoke Jesus and several other angels and archangels to intervene with the exorcism (Jansen & Lang, 2012).

Miscellaneous Cultural Remedies

India is a culturally diverse country with more than 1.3 billion population belonging to different regions, religions, castes, creeds, and tribes. Practices, people follow also vary accordingly. Aum chanting, use of Mudras, wearing different gems, "Rudraksha", amulets, and use of crystals, tying holy threads, horse shoe metal rings, etc. are common culturally accepted remedies for various stressors and illnesses (Gopichandran, 2015). Skin branding (Patra, 2016), drinking or taking dip in holy water, applying black mark on face to divert the evil eye, observing different kinds of fasts, fasts by proxy, "Nazar utarna", different forms of exorcism like "Phookna", "Jhadna" etc. are practiced extensively all over India; However, these have rarely come under scientific scrutiny and it is hard to find literature on the same.

CULTURAL ADAPTATIONS OF CONTEMPORARY THERAPIES

Though the cultures all over the world are distinct, all of them are familiar with the concept of talking to the person in need, be it from a family member, friend, community figure, Shaman, religious leader, healer or a modern mental health professional. This basic resemblance needs to be capitalized while dealing with needy from distinct background.

While adapting an established therapeutic intervention, clinicians may have to make a range of technical, theoretical, and conceptual adjustments to the treatment planning. These may include (Jhonson & Sandhu, 2010):

- Translating the treatment manual into language understandable to the client
- Incorporating cultural and religious beliefs into the existing approach so as to make the client understand the concepts better. Folklores, stories and proverbs can be made use of
- Outcome goals should be made culturally congruent and relevant, especially in developing realistic expectations
- Cultural rituals like prayers, chanting and confessions can be integrated and used as adjuncts to the standard treatments. In these cases, clinician should be aware of culturally based coping response
- Working with religion is crucial especially for clients with strong religious beliefs. Spiritual and religious conceptualization of their problem can be way more important to them than the preset understanding of the therapist
- Collaborating with traditional and indigenous healers may go a long way.

LIMITATIONS AND CHALLENGES

As with any other form of treatment, cultural interventions are not free of flaws. Apart from lacking sound scientific evidence, idiosyncrasies with respect to each method, procedure, duration, outcome, etc. are rules rather than exceptions in these mediations. This also reflects in difficulty developing guidelines for the same. Further research also demands significant funds for which sponsors are hard to find.

Due to the lack of quality check, misuse of these methods cannot be prevented. The line between authentic cultural intervention and quackery remains contentious subject. It further adds to exploitation of the needy in terms of health, wealth, and sex. Certain folk interventions also include oral ingestions, inhalations, and topical applications, adverse effects of which are inevitable (Wasti et al., 2015). Unless the folk healer is competent enough to handle the situation, it becomes difficult as the present health care professionals lack the expertise in these and find it difficult even to know the causative agent. Many patients continue to take modern medicines as well as culturally accepted oral preparations, which eventually cause interactions between the constituents, affecting the outcome.

Posing these methods for experimentation or research in native followers is a major challenge. Considering the number of ethnic groups, cultural adaptations of existing psychotherapies for various societies is a mammoth task.

CONCLUSION

Having served for millennia of years all over the world, ignoring cultural interventions can be detrimental. Further, despite advancements in therapeutics, cure remains elusive in psychiatric disorders. Perhaps, going back to the roots of various cultural interventions might bring out the missing dimension of modern psychiatry.

REFERENCES

Abhyankar R. Psychiatric thoughts in ancient India. Mens Sana Monogr. 2015;13(1):59-69.

American Psychiatric Association. Diagnostic and Statistical Manual of Mental Disorders. 5th Edition. Washington DC: American Psychiatric Press; 2013.

Andrade C. Ashwagandha for anxiety disorders. World J Biol Psychiatry. 2009;10(4 Pt 2):686-7.

Andrade C, Chandra JS. Anti-amnestic properties of Brahmi and Mandookaparni in a rat model. Indian J Psychiatry.2006;48(4):232-7.

Blom JD, Poulina IT, van Gellecum TL, et al. Traditional healing practices originating in Aruba, Bonaire, and Curaçao: A review of the literature on psychiatry and Brua. Transcult Psychiatry. 2015;52(6):840-60.

Bojuwoye O. Traditional healing practices in southern Africa: Ancestral spirits, ritual ceremonies and holistic healing. In: Moodley R, West W (Eds). Integrating Traditional Healing Practices into Counseling and Psychotherapy. California: Sage Publications; 2005.

Campion J, Bhugra R. Experiences of religious healing in psychiatric patients in South India. Soc Psychiatry Psychiatr Epidemiol. 1997;32:215-21.

Chevez LG. Latin American healers and healing: Healing as a redefinition process. In: Moodley R, West W (Eds). Integrating Traditional Healing Practices into Counseling and Psychotherapy. California: Sage Publications; 2005.

Chisholm D, Flisher A, Lund C, et al. Scaling up services for mental health disorders. Lancet. 2007;370:1241-52.

Deng H, Xu J. Wendan decoction (Traditional Chinese medicine) for schizophrenia. Cochrane Database Syst Rev. 2017;6.

Dev S. Ancient-modern concordance in Ayurvedic plants: some examples. Environ Health Perspect. 1999;107(10):783-9.

Esmat D. Improving marital adjustment levels of incompatible couples with islamic counseling. Psychol Stud. 2010;6:167-86.

Frecska E, Bokor P, Andrassy G, et al. The potential use of Ayahuasca in psychiatry. Neuropsychopharmacol Hung. 2016;18(2):79-86.

Gangadhar BN, Porandla K. Yoga and mental health services. Indian J Psychiatry. 2015;57(4):338-40.

Gangadhar BN, Naveen GH, Rao MG, et al. Positive antidepressant effects of generic yoga in depressive out-patients: A comparative study. Indian J Psychiatry.2013;55(Suppl 3):369-73.

Gangadhar BN, Varambally S. Yoga therapy for schizophrenia. Int J Yoga. 2012;5(2) :85-91.

Gopichandran V. Faith healing and faith in healing. Indian J Med Ethics. 2015;12(4):238-40.

Groves P. Mindfulness in psychiatry—where are we now? BJ Psych Bull. 2016;40(6):289-92.

Janakiramaiah N, Gangadhar BN, Naga Venkatesha Murthy PJ, et al. Antidepressant efficacy of Sudarshan Kriya Yoga (SKY) in melancholia: A randomized comparison with electroconvulsive therapy (ECT) and imipramine. J Affect Disord. 2000;57(1-3):255-9.

Jansen E, Lang C. Transforming the self and healing the body through the use of testimonies in a divine retreat center, Kerala. J Relig Health. 2012;51(2):542-51.

Johnson LR, Sandhu DS. Treatment planning in a multicultural context. In: Leach MM, Aten JD (Eds). Culture and the Therapeutic Process. NewYork: Routledge; 2010.

Kakar S. Shamans, Mystics and Doctors. Oxford, UK: Oxford University Press; 1982.

Kapur RL. Mental health care in rural India: a study of existing patterns and their implications for future policy. Br J Psychiatry. 1975;127:286-93.

Kumar M, Bhugra D, Singh J. South asian (Indian) traditional healing. In: Moodley R, West W, editors. Integrating Traditional Healing Practices into Counseling and Psychotherapy. California: Sage Publications; 2005.

Kirkwood G, Rampes H, Tuffrey V, et al. Yoga for anxiety: A systematic review of the research evidence. Br J Sports Med. 2005;39:884-91.

Mafamdi J, Sodi T. The process of becoming an indigenous healer among venda speaking people of South Africa. In: Madu SN, Baguma PK, Pritz A (Eds). Cross Cultural Dialogue on Psychotherapy in Africa. Pietersburg: UNN Press; 1999.

Marshall R. Caribbean healers and healing: Awakening spiritual and cultural healing powers. In: Moodley R, West W (Eds). Integrating Traditional Healing Practices into Counseling and Psychotherapy. California: Sage Publications; 2005.

Narayana A. Medical science in ancient Indian culture with special reference to Atharvaveda. Bull Indian Inst Hist Med Hyderabad. 1995;25(1-2):100-10.

Naveen GH, Thirthalli J, Rao MG, et al. Positive therapeutic and neurotropic effects of yoga in depression: A comparative study. Indian J Psychiatry. 2013;55(Suppl 3):400-4.

Pankhania J. Yoga and its practice in psychological healing. In: Moodley R, West W (Eds). Integrating Traditional Healing Practices into Counseling and Psychotherapy. California: Sage publications; 2005.

Patra PK. Branding in children: a barbaric practice still exists in India. Pan Afr Med J. 2016;23:62.

Poonwassie A, Charter A. Aboriginal world view of helping: Empowering approaches. Can J Counsel. 2001;56(1):63-74.

Raghuram R, Venkateswaran A, Ramakrishna J, et al. Traditional community resources for mental health: A report of temple healing from India. BMJ. 2002;325:38-40.

Rosman A, Rubel PG. The Tapestry of Culture: An Introduction to Cultural Anthropology. 4th edition. New York: McGraw-Hill; 1992.

Rowan M, Poole N, Shea B, et al. Cultural interventions to treat addictions in Indigenous populations: findings from a scoping study. Subst Abuse Treat Prev Policy. 2014;9:34.

Sabry WM, Vohra A. Role of Islam in the management of psychiatric disorders. Indian J psychiatry. 2013;55(suppl 2):205-14.

Sadock BJ, Sadock VA, Ruiz PR. Synopsis of Psychiatry Behavioural Sciences/Clinical Psychiatry. 11th edition. Philedelphia: Wolters Kluwer; 2015.

Sarkar S, Mishra BR, Praharaj SK, et al. Add-on effect of Brahmi in the management of schizophrenia. J Ayurveda Integr Med. 2012;3(4):223-5.

Schnyer R. Acupuncture in the Treatment of Depression: A Manual for Practice and Research. Edinburgh: Academic Press; 2001.

Shannahoff-Khalsa DS. An introduction to Kundalini yoga meditation techniques that are specific for the treatment of psychiatric disorders. J Altern Complement Med. 2004;10(1):91–101.

Singh HK. Brain enhancing ingredients from Ayurvedic medicine: quintessential example of Bacopa monniera, a narrative review. Nutrients. 2013;5(2):478-97.

So JK. Traditional and cultural healing among the chinese. In: Moodley R, West W (Eds). Integrating traditional healing practices into counseling and psychotherapy. California: Sage Publications; 2005.

Sood A. The global mental health movement and its impact on traditional healing in India: A case study of the Balaji temple in Rajastan. Transcult Psychiatry. 2016;53(6):766-82.

Tseng WS. From peculiar psychiatric disorders through culture-bound syndromes to culture-related specific syndromes. Transcult Psychiatry. 2006;43:554.

Tseng WS, Lu QY, Yin PY. Psychotherapy for the chinese: cultural considerations. In: Tseng WS, Yeh EK (Eds). Chinese Societies and Mental Health. Hongkong: Oxford University Press; 1995.

Wasti H, Kanchan T, Acharya J. Faith healers, myths and deaths. Med Leg J. 2015;83(3):136-8.

Whiteford HA, Degenhardt L, Rehm J, et al. Global burden of disease attributable to mental and substance use disorders: findings from the Global Burden of Disease Study 2010. Lancet.2013;382(9904):1575-86.

Social Issues and Mental Health

Chapter 37

Stigma of Mental Illness

Priti Arun, Rohit Garg

SUMMARY

Patients with psychiatric disorders suffer from stigma and discrimination. Stigma is also one of the major reasons for treatment gap in psychiatry. Stigma toward persons with psychiatric disorders is seen throughout the world. Public believes that mentally ill are dangerous and violent, and desires social distance from the mentally ill. Longitudinal time trends have shown that public stigma has not changed much in the past few decades. Stigma is universal among patients with psychiatric disorders irrespective of the disorder, they are suffering from. Age, gender, educational achievement, employment level, socioeconomic status, and other variables are no bar to stigma. Family members of persons with psychiatric disorders also feel stigmatized and suffer from guilt, shame, blame, embarrassment, fear, disrespect, anxiety, social isolation and exclusion, and increased burden of care. Education and contact leads to reduction in stigmatizing attitudes among the public. Future research should focus on longitudinal assessment of strategies to reduce stigma using sound methodology.

INTRODUCTION

Persons suffering from mental disorders face stigma and discrimination along with signs and symptoms of the disorders, and the resulting disabilities (Corrigan & Watson, 2002). Stigma is a major barrier to seeking help causing a huge treatment gap (Kohn et al., 2004). Stigma leads to reduced confidence and self-esteem, reduced participation in the family and society, social isolation, guilt, embarrassment and shame, and limits opportunities for education, employment, and housing (Ping Tsao et al., 2008). Stigma and its consequences are faced by caregivers also.

Stigma related to various minority groups has been an area of interest for social psychologists and sociologists for quite some time. However, the need to study stigma among persons with mental disorders has been recognized recently. There is now a huge amount of literature on stigma of mental disorders, its causative and correlating factors , and its impact on the sufferers (Corrigan & Watson, 2002). There has been a very encouraging surge toward understanding and developing strategies to reduce stigma of mental disorders with the World Psychiatric Association leading the way with its "Open The Doors" program. Researchers have conceptualized that stigma should be understood, identified and targeted as a potential clinical risk factor among patients with mental disorders in view of its deleterious consequences (Shrivastava et al., 2013).

DEFINITIONS OF STIGMA

Stigma as defined by Goffman (1963) had attributes that make a person unworthy, incomplete and defiled. Other researchers have defined and described stigma in various ways. Link and Phelan (2001) have given components that co-occur in context with power, which include labeling, stereotyping, separation, status loss, and discrimination. According to Thornicroft (2007), stigma has three elements of knowledge, attitude, and behavior reflected in ignorance and misinformation, prejudice, and discrimination respectively. The World Health Organization (WHO) defines stigma as *"a mark of shame, disgrace or disapproval which results in an individual being rejected, discriminated against, and excluded from participating in a number of different areas of society"* (World Health Organization, 2001). Pescosolido and Martin (2015) have defined stigma in terms of how stigma is experienced by person or action related to it.

Types of Stigma

Public Stigma: *"Public stigma is the stigma held by public against persons with mental disorders due to which public fears, rejects, and avoids them."*

Interpersonal Stigma: *"Stigma which happens during interactions between the stigmatized and the stigmatizing groups".*

Self-stigma: Self-stigma is defined as *"subjective negative feelings and behavior, stereotype endorsement regarding self which results from experiences, perceptions, or anticipation of negative social reactions"* (Livingston & Boyd, 2010). It results from internalization of shame, blame, hopelessness, guilt, and fear of discrimination. It also contains elements of felt stigma.

Experienced Stigma (Enacted Stigma): *"Actual discrimination or participation restrictions suffered by the persons suffering from mental illness"* (Van Brakel, 2006).

Perceived Stigma (Felt Stigma): *"Stigma that persons with mental illness fear or perceive to be present in public regarding them or their group".* According to Brohan et al. (2010), some researchers differentiate felt stigma from perceived stigma and claim that felt stigma encompasses perceived stigma and elements of shame. Thus, felt stigma can be understood to have components of both perceived and self-stigma. Others consider felt stigma same as perceived stigma.

Courtesy/Associative/Family Stigma: Stigma perceived or experienced because of being associated or related to a person with a stigmatized condition.

Structural Stigma: This is the broader, macrosocial form of stigma. The term was given by Link and Phelan (2001) and further defined by Corrigan et al. (2004). It refers to institutional policies, cultural, and societal norms that intentionally restrict the opportunities for stigmatized individuals or unintentionally result in consequences for them. Examples of structural stigma are the criminalization of suicide attempters and inequitable distribution of resources for mental health.

EVOLUTION OF THE CONCEPT OF STIGMA

The word "stigma" originated in ancient Greek Society, where slaves were identified by marks on their body. In his classic description, Goffman (1963) described that stigmatization is manifested in three different ways: abomination of the body (negative attributions toward appearance), blemishing of individual personal character, and tribal stigma which could be related to one's race, ethnicity, or religion. Subsequent formulations have described psychosocial processes that cause stigmatization. According to Florez, stigma identifies and devalues others by mark of social disgrace (Arboleda Florez, 2002).

According to Corrigan and Watson (2002) social cognitive model of stigma, stigma has three components: stereotypes, prejudice, and discrimination. Stereotypes are efficient, social knowledge structures learned by members of a social group that predetermine their attitudes. People who are prejudiced endorse learned negative stereotypes and generate negative emotional reactions. Discrimination is caused by prejudice. This behavior may be not helping even when able to do so like avoiding the person, oppressive treatment and segregated places of treatment. Stigma is further perpetuated when stigmatizing mark is visible, and appears to be in control of bearer (Arboleda Florez, 2002). Other themes that describe stigma toward mental illness, affect the public behavior toward persons with mental illness, i.e. fear and exclusion, authoritarianism and benevolence (Corrigan & Watson, 2002).

Link et al. (2001) have given a slightly different model of stigma. According to them, "stigma exists when elements of labeling, stereotyping, separation, status loss, and discrimination co-occur in a power situation that allows these processes to unfold".

These models also describe development of self-stigma. According to the modified labeling theory, persons have internalized stereotypes regarding mental disorders before they suffer from mental illness (Corrigan et al., 2003). These stereotypes become relevant to self and lead to self-stigma at the onset of psychiatric disorders.

Blame, shame, and contamination are the major stereotypes in family stigma. Family can be blamed for poor household environment leading to or maintaining mental illness in a family member (Larson & Corrigan, 2008), which can result in shame. Shame further causes avoidance and social isolation. Contamination is the process in which diminished worth is attributed to a family member because of association with a mentally ill person (Larson & Corrigan, 2008).

Why does Stigma have Different Impact on Different Persons?

Stigma affects different persons in different ways. Some perceive it as more stressful, while others remain relatively unaffected. Rusch et al. (2009) have explained this on the basis of "stress and coping model" by Lazarus and Folkman (1984). Four elements are included in this model. These are how a person cognitively evaluates stress of stigma, how the person evaluates personal and public factors, how the person emotionally responds to stigma stress, and how the outcome is affected by stress.

Corrigan et al. (2003) have given a model of the personal response to stigma. Persons with mental illness perceive and interpret their own condition and others' negative responses. Persons who do not identify with the stigmatized group, are less likely to be affected by stigma.

However, those who identify with the group, feel stigmatized. Further, perceived legitimacy of public stigma moderates reactions to stigma. If the stigmatizing attitudes are considered to be legitimate, self-esteem, and self-efficacy are affected and vice-versa.

PUBLIC STIGMA

People with mental illness are feared, rejected, and avoided by public due to the beliefs and attitudes held (Corrigan & Penn, 1999). Factor analytic studies have revealed that stigma has multiple constructs and each construct has multiple correlates (Jorm et al., 2012). Most important and common are desire for social distance from the mentally ill, and beliefs in dangerousness apart from desire for social control, perception of mental disorders due to personal weakness, etc. Beliefs in dangerousness of people with mental disorders (Jorm et al., 2012) and desire for social distance (Jorm & Oh, 2009) are higher against persons with mental disorders than average persons and persons with physical disorders. These attributes are highest against persons with substance dependence, followed by schizophrenia/psychosis, depression, anxiety, and eating disorders. Males are perceived to be more dangerous than females. The perception of dangerousness is generally not based on personal experience of behavior and exceeds the research evidence. The most common source of these beliefs is media. Contact with persons with mental disorders reduces the desire for social distance and beliefs in dangerousness.

Research on Public Stigma

Research shows that majority of people in United States and Europe have stigma against persons with mental illness. Stigma is lesser in Asia and Africa, though it remains unclear if it is due to lack of research or actual cultural influences (Corrigan & Watson, 2002).

Stigma in Global Context—Mental Health Study (Pescosolido et al., 2013) done in 16 countries (Argentina, Bangladesh, Brazil, Bulgaria, China, Cyprus, Finland, Germany, Great Britain, Hungary, Iceland, Japan, New Zealand, Philippines, South Africa, Spain, and America) provides a global analysis of public stigma. Initial data from Bulgaria, Germany, Iceland, Hungary, and Spain found that 56.4% respondents were unwilling to have a person with depression or schizophrenia marry into his or her family, and 33.7% believed that persons with depression or schizophrenia do not get accepted in the community. Almost one-fourth believed that a person with mental health problem should not be given a job. Public is more rejective of a person with schizophrenia as compared to a person with depression regardless of the country. Public is unwilling to see individuals with mental disorder in positions of authority or power fearing violence (Pescosolido et al., 2013).

Various reviews on public stigma against mental disorders have been conducted in United States (Parcesepe & Cabassa, 2013), Latin America and Caribbean (Mascayano et al., 2016), Greece (Tzouvara et al., 2016) and Japan (Ando et al., 2013). These reviews have found that public holds beliefs about dangerousness, and violence (Parcesepe & Cabassa, 2013; Mascayano et al., 2016), and desire for social distance from persons with mental disorders (Parcesepe & Cabassa, 2013; Tzouvara et al., 2016; Ando et al., 2013). Social distance was greatest for those with drug abuse disorders, followed by alcohol abuse, schizophrenia and depression (Parcesepe & Cabassa, 2013). People do not want to share rooms or work environment with the mentally ill or employing them (Tzouvara et al., 2016). The reviews also found positive attitudes toward seeking professional help by mentally ill persons (Parcesepe & Cabassa, 2013), benevolence and compassion toward the mentally ill (Mascayano et al., 2016; Tzouvara et al., 2016), and some positivity toward social care (Tzouvara et al., 2016).

Has Public Stigma has Changed over the Years?

Recent research has focused on time trends in public stigma (Schomerus et al., 2012; Pescosolido et al., 2013; Evans Lacko et al., 2013), and found that mental health literacy, correct recognition of mental disorders and attitudes toward psychiatric medications increased over time. Though there was insignificant decline in personal blame for schizophrenia and depression, social rejection of mentally ill persons remained disturbingly stable over 20 years. There was decline in willingness to accept a person with schizophrenia as a neighbor or coworker, whereas the acceptance for a person with depression remains the same. Acceptance of a more intimate relationship like a friend or someone with mental disorder marrying into one's family did not change for any disorder (Schomerus et al., 2012). However, desire for social distance and perceived danger associated with people with these disorders did not decrease significantly (Pescosolido et al., 2013).

Indian Research on Public Stigma

Indian studies have reported that public fears and rejects mentally ill (Neki, 1966), has misconceptions and ignorance (Dube, 1970), and pessimistic attitudes (Wig, 1980) toward mental disorders. Verghese and Baig (1974) found that public had positive attitudes but did not want a marriage alliance with a family having a person with mental disorder. A recent Indian study on 291 persons concluded (Jadhav et al., 2007) that rural persons had higher stigma and deploy a punitive model toward the severely mentally ill, while the urban group expressed a liberal view. Zieger et al. (2016) found that public stigma toward the mentally ill was higher in Kolkata (n = 158) than Chennai (n = 166). Lower education was associated with higher stigma while stronger religious devotion was associated with lower stigma in both cities.

SELF-STIGMA

It is estimated that 41.7% persons with severe mental disorder have self-stigma (Gerlinger et al., 2013) and nearly one-third patients with severe mental disorder have high self-stigma (Brohan et al., 2010; West et al., 2011). An Indian study (Garg et al., 2012) assessed self-stigma among 218 patients suffering from schizophrenia, depression, substance dependence and obsessive compulsive disorder (OCD), and found that stigma was highest among patients with substance dependence, younger age, and in those with symptomatic illness.

Stigma of Schizophrenia

Recent studies on persons with schizophrenia have found that self-stigma was pervasive during treatment (Ren et al., 2016), as well as during convalescence (Ritsher & Phelan, 2004;

Sartorius, 1998). Patients with schizophrenia experienced unfair treatment at jobs (Gao et al., 2005), experienced discrimination during social activities (Schulze et al., 2003), and had moderate impact of stigma on their lives (Phillips et al., 2002). In a cross national survey in 27 countries with 732 patients with schizophrenia, Thornicroft et al. (2009) found that discrimination from friends and family was experienced by more than 40% participants, and nearly 30% reported discrimination while finding and keeping a job or maintaining intimate or sexual relationships. Over one-third of participants anticipated discrimination in absence of actual experienced discrimination.

An Indian study found that urban patients with schizophrenia hide their disorder and avoided disorder histories while applying for a job, whereas rural patients experienced higher shame, ridicule, and discrimination (Loganathan & Murthy, 2008). Acute phase of disorder and socially unacceptable behavior were highly related to stigma. Patients also experienced being ridiculed by their family members and spouses. Singh et al. (2016) have found that significant proportion of patients with schizophrenia experience stigma and it leads to lower functioning.

Stigma of Bipolar Disorder

A number of reviews are available on stigma due to mental disorder (Hawke et al., 2013; Ellison et al., 2013; Latalova et al., 2013). Stigma due to bipolar disorder has been found to be comparable to schizophrenia but lesser than depression (Latalova et al., 2013). Patients experience stigma internally, within social circles, healthcare, workplace, and school. Stigma restricts professional growth, limits life opportunities, leads to social isolation and withdrawal, reduces functioning, social esteem and self-esteem, and reduced quality of life (QoL). A recent Indian study (Grover et al., 2016) has found that 28% remitted patients with bipolar disorder experience moderate to high stigma and more than 40% report restriction in activities.

Stigma of Personality Disorders

A recent review (Sheehan et al., 2016) found that personality disorders might be more stigmatizing than psychiatric disorders, with fear and frustration among the public. The patients are commonly perceived as manipulative, difficult, annoying, undeserving, and misbehaving. Stigma of borderline personality disorder is high and most researched. There is lesser stigma associated with obsessive compulsive personality disorder. Patients with borderline personality disorder have been shown to endorse more shame than patients with anxiety and depression.

Stigma of Mental Disorders in Children and Adolescents

In a review, Kaushik et al. (2016) found that public stigma is higher against young people with mental health difficulties as compared to unaffected peers and peers with learning disabilities and physical disorders. Alcohol misuse was less stigmatizing than mental health difficulties. Self-stigma increases with age but decreases in externalizing disorders, e.g. conduct disorder. Adolescents, who perceived less control over their mental health difficulties and believed their problems to be life-long, showed higher stigma. Parental secrecy increases while parental optimism reduces self-stigma.

Stigma Related to Alcohol Dependence

Schomerus et al. (2011) reviewed population surveys comparing public stigma related to alcohol dependence with other mental disorders and found that alcohol-dependent persons are less frequently regarded as mentally ill, held more responsible for their condition (as lacking willpower and having a bad character), provoke more social rejection (higher for alcoholism, schizophrenia, and depression in that order), and more negative emotions like (more anger, irritation, and repulsion), but less empathy, pity, and desire for help, and are at particular risk for structural discrimination. Addiction to illegal drugs is more stigmatizing than alcohol addiction. A recent Indian (Garg et al., 2012) study found higher self-stigma among patients with substance dependence as compared to patients with psychiatric disorders.

Stigma and Suicide

In a review, Carpiniello and Pinna (2017) found that public considers suicidal people as weak, cowardly, senseless, thoughtless, irresponsible, and attention seeking. Individuals who attempt suicide are subjected to stigmatization and "social distancing". Those who have attempted suicide face stigma from society. They are often ashamed and embarrassed by their behavior and tend to hide the occurrence. Caregivers of subjects who have committed or attempted suicide also face stigms, since they are blamed for suicide and feel guilt and shame. Stigma causes distress, reduces self-esteem, acts as a barrier to help seeking, and increase the chances of suicide.

Raguram and Weiss (1996) have reported that persons presenting with a somatic form of depression are less stigmatized than those with psychological symptoms. This is a possible reason for somatizing the psychic distress, seen all over the world, though more often in non-Western settings.

ASSOCIATIVE/COURTESY/CAREGIVER STIGMA

Forty-three to ninety-two percent caregivers of people with mental disorders report feeling stigmatized (Van Brakel, 2006). Courtesy stigma has been found among families of patients with bipolar disorder (Hawke et al., 2013; Ellison et al., 2013; Latalova et al., 2013) and schizophrenia (Gao et al., 2005). Family members of people with mental disorders experience stigma during social interactions, feel isolated, ignored, blamed, and criticized by the family, friends, neighbors, colleagues, and even mental health providers (Shamsaei et al., 2013).They face stigma in mental healthcare settings, employment for their ill relative and in contact with police (Krupchanka et al., 2017). Caregivers also experience stigma with patients' hospitalization (Weller et al., 2015). Family members suffer from emotional consequences like disregard, disrespect, fear, anxiety, guilt, shame, desperation, worry, intense concern; social consequences like discrimination, losing job, reputation, and housing and interpersonal consequences like social isolation, trying to hide the disorder from others, etc. All these factors result in increased burden of care and reduced QoL (Park & Park, 2014).

A recent multicentric nationwide Indian study (Grover et al., 2017) among more than 1,000 caregivers of patients with schizophrenia, bipolar disorder, and depression found higher stigma among caregivers of patients with schizophrenia, bipolar disorder and depression in that order. Koschorke et al. (2017) found that 21% caregivers of patients with schizophrenia had high caregiver stigma and 45% felt uncomfortable to disclose their family member's condition. Severity of positive symptoms of schizophrenia, higher levels of disability and younger age of patient increased stigma. Another Indian study (Thara & Srinivasan, 2000) found that female sex of the patient, and a younger age of both patient and caregiver were associated with greater caregiver stigma. Marriage and fear of rejection by neighbors were some of the more stigmatizing aspects.

IMPACT OF STIGMA

Stigma causes discrimination in interpersonal interactions, employment, housing, criminal justice system, and marital prospects (Rusch et al., 2005). Public stigma results in allocation of comparatively fewer financial resources into the mental health system.

Impact on Treatment

Patients with mental disorders are aware of the prejudices against them and do not want to be seen as part of the mentally ill minority. They avoid stigma by not pursuing psychiatric treatment and medications, and do not disclose their illness to others. Stigma is ranked 4th among barriers to help seeking (Clement et al., 2015; Schnyder et al., 2017). Stigma also hampers compliance to treatment, leads to premature treatment discontinuation and results in increased rehospitalizations. It inhibits recovery, and worsens course and outcome of mental disorders.

Impact on Self-esteem, Hope, and Quality of Life

Self-stigma reduces hope, QoL, self-esteem, self-efficacy, and empowerment of persons with mental disorder (Livingston & Boyd, 2010). Impact of internalized stigma on hope and QoL has been found to be related to levels of self-esteem (Mashiach-Eizenberg et al., 2013). According to Yanos et al. (2008), hopelessness and low self-esteem due to stigma causes depression and increases suicidal risk. Internalized stigma is also linked to impaired social functioning (Lysaker et al., 2007; Lysaker et al., 2010).

MEASUREMENT OF STIGMA

Many measures have been designed to assess different types of stigma in different groups. The commonly used measures for public stigma, self-stigma, courtesy stigma, and stigma among adolescents are briefly discussed.

Measures of Community/Public Stigma and Attitudes

"Reported and Intended Behavior Scale" measures social distance in context to living with, working with, working nearby, and continuing a relationship with someone with a mental disorder (Evans Lacko et al., 2011). "Attribution Questionnaire" (Corrigan et al., 2003) assesses blame, anger, pity, help, dangerousness, fear, avoidance, segregation, and coercion against persons with mental illness. "Emotional Reactions to Mental Disorder

Scale" (Angermeyer & Matschinger, 1996) is a 12-item five-point Likert-scale, with each item assessing an emotional response. "Opinions about Mental Disorder" is a 51-item instrument assessing authoritarianism, benevolence, mental hygiene ideology, social restrictiveness, and interpersonal etiology. "Community Attitudes toward Mentally Ill" (Taylor & Dear, 1981) is a 40-item questionnaire on acceptance of community mental health care. "Dangerousness Scale" (Penn et al., 1994) assesses beliefs about dangerousness of a persons with mental illness using eight questions. "Semantic Differential" (Nunnally, 1961) rates opinion about mentally ill on a series of bipolar adjectives, including "dangerous-safe".

Measures of Personal Stigma

"Discrimination and Stigma Scale" (Thornicroft et al., 2009) is a 36-item scale developed and adapted in 27 countries. Thirty two items assess discrimination in key areas of everyday life and social participation (e.g. work, marriage, housing, and leisure activities). Four items assess participants' self-limitation in key aspects of everyday life. "Perceived Devaluation and Discrimination Scale" measures perceived stigma with 12-likert type items. There are six items each for perceived devaluation and perceived discrimination. It is unique in that it can also be used for public stigma. "Internalized Stigma of Mental Illness Scale" is a 29-item self-complete measure. It does not measure perceived stigma but measures experienced stigma, self-stigma (alienation, stereotype endorsement, and social withdrawal) and stigma resistance. "Self-stigma of Mental Disorder Scale" is a 40-item self-complete measure. There are ten-items for perceived stigma and 30-item for self-stigma (ten each for stereotype agreement, stereotype self-concurrence, and self-esteem decrement). "Consumer Experiences of Stigma Questionnaire", a 21-item self-complete survey, measures experienced stigma and discrimination. "Depression Self-stigma Scale" is a 32-item self-complete measure of personal stigma. "Stigma Scale" is a 28-item self-complete measure. The 28-items are further divided into three domains namely discrimination (13 items), disclosure (ten items), and positive aspects of stigma (five items). The Stigma Scale has been translated and standardized in India on 218 patients suffering from depression, OCD, substance use disorders (SUDs) and schizophrenia and other psychotic disorders. The Indian Hindi version has good reliability (Garg et al., 2013).

Measures for Adolescents

Two scales measure public stigma against adolescents with mental disorders. "Peer Mental Health Stigmatization Scale" assesses older children and adolescent's attitudes toward peers with mental disorder. "Stigma Scale for Receiving Psychological Help" measures anticipated community stigma toward adolescents.

Moses (2009) has developed two measures to assess stigma among adolescents with mental disorders. The first assesses self-stigma using 5-items. The second assesses secrecy as a coping strategy using 7-items.

Associative Stigma

"Devaluation of Consumers' Families Scale" (Struening et al., 2001) has 7-items which measure caregivers' perception of the views of general public regarding caregivers of patients with mental disorders. "Stigma by Association Scale" (Pryor et al., 2012) assesses caregiver's cognitive, emotional, and behavioral reactions to being related to someone with a stigmatized condition. This scale has 28 items. "The Affiliate Stigma Scale" (Mak & Cheung, 2008) assesses caregivers' stress, burden, and positive perceptions of caring using 22 items. "Experience of Caregiving Inventory" (Szmukler et al., 1996) has eight-items to assess effects on family due to caring for a person with mental disorder. In India, the Hindi Stigma Scale for patients (Garg et al., 2013) has been modified and adapted for caregivers and has good reliability.

STRATEGIES TO REDUCE AND OVERCOME STIGMA

Over the last decade, organizations like WHO, World Psychiatric Association (WPA) and World Association of Social Psychiatry have recognized stigma reduction as a major goal and support for stigma reduction, as also evident in many government declarations and action plans (Stuart, 2008). Programs to diminish stigma have been started at many places in recent years. Some examples are "Changing Minds" (Royal College of Psychiatrists of the UK), "Like Minds Like Mine" (New Zealand), "Opening Minds" (Canada), "Beyond Blue" (Australia), "See Me" (Scotland), "Time To Change" (England), "Anti Stigma Programme European Network" (European Union).

In 1996, WPA launched a global program (Open The Doors) against stigma of schizophrenia. The main principles guiding the "Open The Doors" program are to work with patients and relatives, health professionals, health authorities, media, and general public. By 2005, "Open The Doors" included 18 countries including India.

Strategies to Reduce Public Stigma

Three major strategies have been used to reduce public stigma: education, contact, and protest.

1. *Education*: Educational approaches challenge negative stereotypes and replace them with factual information using group discussions, public announcements, books, flyers, movies, videos, web pages, podcasts, virtual reality, and other audiovisual aids. Educational programs are cost effective and reach a wider target audience. An example is the Elimination of Barriers Initiative, a 3 years program in United States, which involved education or social marketing to reduce stigma and discrimination, reduce barriers to treatment and build public support for recovery. It involved meetings in public, using print and electronic media (Corrigan & Gelb, 2006). California Mental Health Services Authority developed and distributed a 1 hour documentary, narrated by actor Glenn Close, "A New State of Mind: Ending the Stigma of Mental Illness", to raise awareness of stigma and its negative effects, and to promote a message of hope, resilience, and recovery. The program uses education along with contact. Public is educated about mental illness using profiles and stories of people who have personally experienced mental health challenges and recovered from them (Cerully et al., 2016).

   In Scotland, "rights-based" program (See Me) educates public about rights of persons with mental disorders. "Defeat Depression" campaign in United Kingdom in 1990s aimed to reduce stigma by providing information on depression to public and professionals. In

Australia, "Beyond Blue" program has been associated with improved public attitude and knowledge regarding depression, with greater effects associated with greater exposure to the program. In Germany, BASTA (meaning STOP)—The alliance for Mentally Ill People (previously called "Bavarian Anti-stigma Action"), is active in various fields like in education programs in schools and police academies with active participation of mental health consumers, education of the media, and exhibitions of art by people with mental illness, and other cultural activities. Another German initiative is Irrsinnig Menschlich (Madly Human). It also involves educational antistigma activities. Sane Australia is a nationwide antistigma effort successful in educating journalists.

2. *Contact:* It involves contact of general public with members of the stigmatized group. Persons with mental illness describe their experiences of living with and overcoming mental health challenges. Contact can be face-to-face (one-to-one or with a group) or via a video or a movie depicting mental disorder. An example is the "In Our Own Voice" program, developed by the National Alliance of Mental Disorder in US. It is a 90-minute standardized contact program in which people with mental disorder interact with an audience, particularly about recovery from mental disorder (Corrigan & Gelb, 2006). The contact-based strategy of the "Hjärnkoll" program in Sweden achieved a positive impact on mental health literacy, attitudes, and intended social contact with people with mental illness. The "Time To Change" program in England used contact-based education and found it useful at the population level to reduce stigma. "Opening Minds" in Canada also used contact-based education and found it to be useful, though at a regional level. "Like Minds Like Mine" program in New Zealand includes involvement of mentally ill persons at all levels (local, regional, and national).

3. *Protest:* Social activism or protest is used to highlight various forms of injustices due to stigma, and reprimand offenders for their stereotypes and discrimination. Protest might include public rallies, boycotts and withholding benefits from people or organizations who discriminate. In the US, Stigma Busters, a form of protest, was developed to challenge stigmatizing images in the media by the National Alliance of Mental Disorder. Members contact newspaper editors, radio, and TV station managers and people of authority whenever a stigmatizing event happens in the media. Stigma Busters also reinforces antistigma actions by media by praising them publicly and sending them personal letters (Corrigan & Gelb, 2006). In the year 2000, Stigma Busters persuaded a channel to cancel a program "Wonderland," which portrayed persons with mental illness as dangerous and unpredictable. However, there is a concern that while protest may change stigmatizing behaviors, it might not change or even worsen the attitudes of people. BASTA in Germany also uses protest through email alerts. Sane Australia also fights stigmatizing media messages.

Corrigan et al. (2012) conducted a meta-analysis to evaluate the outcome of these strategies and identified 72 studies involving more than 38,000 participants. Majority of studies used contact or education. Both strategies led to significant change in attitudes and behaviors of public. However, the effect size was 2-fold stronger for contact than education. Education was more effective for adolescents (Corrigan et al., 2012). Face-to-face contact was found to be better than video contact.

Strategies to Reduce Self-stigma

Self-stigma reduction interventions target three areas: "stereotype endorsement", "alienation", and "social withdrawal". Interventions that focus on self-stigma aim to increase self-esteem, hope, and self-efficacy and decrease social avoidance which have all been consistently found to be inversely associated with self-stigma.

Research on self-stigma reduction has been less extensive than public stigma. Recent reviews describe various strategies and interventions used to counteract self-stigma among persons with mental illnesses (Mittal et al., 2012; Yanos et al., 2015; Tsang et al., 2016; Wood et al., 2016). Almost all the interventions have psychoeducation as the major component. Many strategies combine cognitive restructuring, cognitive behavior therapy (CBT), narrative enhancement, social skills training, and other approaches. All the strategies use groups-based approaches except self-stigma reduction program which uses group as well as individual sessions.

The most common method is psychoeducation or psychoeducation combined with cognitive restructuring. In these programs, participants learn facts that counter stereotypes of disorder. These strategies use participants' personal experience with prejudice and discuss the implications of its internalization. Healthy self-concept is a group-based psychoeducation program, whereas Ending Self-stigma uses psychoeducation combined with cognitive restructuring (Yanos et al., 2015).

A second approach is CBT, in which individuals are taught to challenge negative statements about self through feedback from others. The aim of CBT is to develop skills in correcting participant's own negative self-directed cognitions (Mittal et al., 2012).

A third group-based approach called "Acceptance and Commitment Therapy" utilizes mindfulness strategies to promote self-esteem.

A fourth intervention is the "Narrative Enhancement and Cognitive Therapy". It is a CBT based, structured, group-based intervention. Participants share personal stories and experiences with mental disorder, focusing on themes to counter negative self-stereotypes. It also combines psychoeducation, cognitive restructuring, and narrative enhancement to counter the impact of stigma on identity. The Antistigma Photo-voice Intervention requires participants to take pictures and record narratives related to their personal experiences with stigma along with psychoeducation and narrative enhancement.

Corrigan et al. (2013) have given the strategy of "Coming Out Proud" or "Disclosure" for reducing self-stigma. Disclosure offers benefits like enhanced self-esteem and self-efficacy, which promotes emotional and mental health. There is no need to worry about hiding disorder; the person may receive approval for disclosing and being honest thus improving relationships and may learn of similar experiences from other people. Disclosure has potential costs as well, including physical and emotional harm (hate crimes), discrimination, disapproval from others, self-consciousness, and doubts about competence. The balance of costs and benefits depends on the individual and the setting. Social avoidance, secrecy, selective disclosure, indiscriminant disclosure and broadcast experience are hierarchies of disclosure.

Meta-analyses (Tsang et al., 2016; Wood et al., 2016) has found that there is a small to moderate significant effect of psychoeducational therapeutic intervention on self-efficacy and insight. Internalized stigma, self-esteem, and empowerment improve but not significantly. Inconsistent effects have been found for "Coming Out Proud and Narrative Enhancement and Cognitive Therapy" while no significant effects have been found for CBT and social skills training.

Livingston et al. (2012) reviewed interventions to reduce stigma of SUDs and found positive effect of interventions on at least one outcome measure of stigma. A review of antistigma interventions at workplace (Hanisch et al., 2016) showed improved knowledge and supportive behavior toward people with mental health problems.

In India, Dharitri et al. (2015) tested an intervention to reduce stigma among caregivers (n = 213), patients (schizophrenia, bipolar disorder, depression and chronic anxiety disorder (n = 223) and community (n = 899). Ten psycho-education session in groups of 80–120 persons through slide shows and discussions, ten exhibitions through posters and explanations, ten shows of street play, and printed educational materials were used. Assessments were done at 1 and 3 months after interventions. The percentage of respondents expressing stigmatizing views in caregivers and community groups reduced significantly. However, people maintained concern about disclosure of mental disorder.

Criticism of the Interventions

The interventions to reduce stigma have been criticized on certain aspects:
1. Most studies assess change in knowledge and attitudes of participants and ignore whether there is a change in their actual behavior toward mentally ill
2. Majority of the studies assess immediate post intervention changes in stigma. There are negligible studies carrying out interventions in the long-term to assess if the impact of interventions persists or not
3. Majority of stigma research has come from high income countries. There is a need to carry out research in low-and-middle income countries since majority of world population resides in these countries
4. There is negligible research on stigma by the family members against patients with mental illness
5. Varying methodology of the studies conducted, reliability and validity of the measures used, and lack of randomized controlled trials are some other limitations.

CONCLUSION

Patients with mental disorders and their caregivers are stigmatized by the public. Self-stigma among persons with mental disorders leads to shame, reduced hope, reduced self-esteem, and self-efficacy. Stigma leads to severe limitation in life opportunities and participation restriction for persons suffering from mental disorders. Various strategies to reduce public and self-stigma have been described, tested, and found to have efficacy in reducing stigma. However, much still needs to be done to reduce the impact of stigma and discrimination related to mental disorders.

REFERENCES

Ando S, Yamaguchi S, Aoki Y, et al. Review of mental-health-related stigma in Japan. Psychiatry and Clin Neurosc. 2013;67(7):471-82.

Angermeyer MC, Matschinger H. The effect of personal experience with mental illness on the attitude towards individuals suffering from mental disorders. Soc Psychiatry Psychiatr Epidemiol. 1996;31(6):321-6.

Arboleda-Flórez J. What causes stigma? World Psychiatry. 2002;1(1):25-6.

Brohan E, Slade M, Clement S. Experiences of mental illness stigma, prejudice and discrimination: a review of measures. BMC Health Services Research. 2010;10:80.

Carpiniello B, Pinna F. The Reciprocal relationship between suicidality and stigma. Frontiers in Psychiatry. 2017;8:35.

Cerully JL, Collins RL, Wong EC, et al. Effects of stigma and discrimination reduction programs conducted under the California Mental Health Services Authority: An evaluation of Runyon Saltzman Einhorn, Inc., Documentary Screening Events. Rand Health Quarterly. 2016;5(4):8.

Clement S, Schauman O, Graham T, et al. What is the impact of mental health-related stigma on help-seeking?A systematic review of quantitative and qualitative studies. Psychological Medicine. 2015;45(1):11-27.

Corrigan P, Gelb B. Three programs that use mass approaches to challenge the stigma of mental illness. Psychiatr Serv. 2006;57(3):393-8.

Corrigan P, Markowitz FE, Watson A, et al. An attribution model of public discrimination towards persons with mental illness. J Health Soc Behavior. 2003;44:162-79.

Corrigan PW, Penn DL. Lessons from social psychology on discrediting psychiatric stigma. Am Psychol. 1999;54(9):765-76.

Corrigan PW, Watson AC. Understanding the impact of stigma on people with mental illness. World Psychiatry. 2002;1(1):16-20.

Corrigan PW, Markowitz FE, Watson AC. Structural levels of mental illness stigma and discrimination. Schizophr Bull. 2004;30(3):481-91.

Corrigan PW, Morris SB, Michaels PJ, et al. Challenging the public stigma of mental illness: a meta-analysis of outcome studies. Psychiatr Serv. 2012;63(10):963-73.

Corrigan PW, Kosyluk KA, Rüsch N. Reducing self-stigma by coming out proud. Am J Public Health. 2013;103(5):794-800.

Corrigan PW, Watson AC, Ottati V. From whence comes mental illness stigma? Int J Soc Psychiatry. 2003;49(2):142-57.

Dharitri R, Rao SN, Kalyanasundaram S. Stigma of mental illness: An interventional study to reduce its impact in the community. Indian J Psychiatry. 2015;57(2):165-73.

Dube KC. A study of prevalence and biosocial variables in mental illness in a rural and urban community in Uttar Pradesh, India. Acta Psychiatr Scand. 1970;46:327-59.

Ellison N, Mason O, Scior K. Bipolar disorder and stigma: a systematic review of the literature. J Affect Disord. 2013;151(3):805-20.

Evans-Lacko S, Henderson C, Thornicroft G. Public knowledge, attitudes and behaviour regarding people with mental illness in England 2009-2012.Br J Psychiatry. 2013;55:51-7.

Evans-Lacko S, Rose D, Little K, et al. Development and psychometric properties of the reported and intended behaviour scale (RIBS): a stigma-related behaviour measure. Epidemiol Psychiatr Sci. 2011;20(3):263-71.

Folkman S. Personal control and stress and coping processes: a theoretical analysis. J Pers and Soc Psychol.1984;46(4):839-52.

Gao SY, Fei LP, Wang XQ, et al. Discrimination in schizophrenia patients and their families. Chinese Mental Health Journal. 2005;19(2):82-5.

Garg R, Arun P, Chavan BS. Reliability of the stigma scale in the Indian setting. Indian J Soc Research. 2013;54:267-76.

Garg R, Chavan BS, Arun P. Stigma and discrimination: how do persons with psychiatric disorders and substance dependence view themselves? Indian J Soc Psychiatry. 2012;28(3-4):121-30.

Gerlinger G, Hauser M, De Hert M, et al. Personal stigma in schizophrenia spectrum disorders: a systematic review of prevalence rates, correlates, impact and interventions. World Psychiatry. 2013;12(2):155-64.

Goffman E: Stigma: Notes on the Management of Spoiled Identity. New York: Prentice Hall; 1963.

Grover S, Avasthi A, Singh A, et al. Stigma experienced by caregivers of patients with severe mental disorders: A nationwide multicentric study. Int J Soc Psychiatry. 2017;63(5):407-17.

Grover S, Hazari N, Aneja J. Stigma and its correlates among patients with bipolar disorder: A study from a tertiary care hospital of North India. Psychiatry Res. 2016;244:109-16.

Hanisch SE, Twomey CD, Szeto AC, et al. The effectiveness of interventions targeting the stigma of mental illness at the workplace: a systematic review. BMC Psychiatry. 2016;16:1.

Hawke LD, Parikh SV, Michalak EE. Stigma and bipolar disorder: a review of the literature. J Affect Disord. 2013;150(2):181-91.

Jadhav S, Littlewood R, Ryder AG, et al. Stigmatization of severe mental illness in India: Against the simple industrialization hypothesis. Indian J Psychiatry 2007;49(3):189-94.

Jorm AF, Reavley NJ, Ross AM. Belief in the dangerousness of people with mental disorders: a review. Aust N Z J Psychiatry. 2012;46(11):1029-45.

Jorm AF, Oh E. Desire for social distance from people with mental disorders. Aust N Z J Psychiatry 2009;43(3):183-200.

Kaushik A, Kostaki E, Kyriakopoulos M. The stigma of mental illness in children and adolescents: A systematic review. Psychiatry Res. 2016;243:469-94.

Kohn R, Saxena S, Levav I, et al. The treatment gap in mental health care. Bull World Health Organ. 2004;82(11):858-66.

Koschorke M, Padmavati R, Kumar S, et al. Experiences of stigma and discrimination faced by family caregivers of people with schizophrenia in India. Social Science & Medicine. 2017;178:66-77.

Krupchanka D, Kruk N, Sartorius N, et al. Experience of stigma in the public life of relatives of people diagnosed with schizophrenia in the Republic of Belarus. Soc Psychiatry Psychiatr Epidemiol. 2017;52(4):493-501.

Larson JE, Corrigan P. The stigma of families with mental illness. Acad Psychiatry. 2008;32(2):87-91.

Latalova K, Ociskova M, Prasko J, et al. Self-stigmatization in patients with bipolar disorder. Neuro Endocrinol Letters. 2013;34(4):265-72.

Link BG, Phelan JC. Conceptualizing stigma. Annual Review of Sociology. 2001;27:363-85.

Livingston JD, Milne T, Fang ML, et al. The effectiveness of interventions for reducing stigma related to substance use disorders: a systematic review. Addiction. 2012;107(1):39-50.

Livingston JD, Boyd JE. Correlates and consequences of internalized stigma for people living with mental illness: a systematic review and meta-analysis. Soc Sci Medicine. 2010;71(12):2150-61.

Loganathan S, Murthy SR. Experiences of stigma and discrimination endured by people suffering from schizophrenia. Indian J Psychiatry. 2008;50(1):39-46.

Lysaker PH, Roe D, Yanos PT. Toward understanding the insight paradox: internalized stigma moderates the association between insight and social functioning, hope, and self-esteem among people with schizophrenia spectrum disorders. Schizophr Bull. 2007;33(1):192-9.

Lysaker PH, Yanos PT, Outcalt J, et al. Association of stigma, self-esteem, and symptoms with concurrent and prospective assessment of social anxiety in schizophrenia. Clin. Schizophr Relat Psychoses 2010;4(1):41-8.

Mak WS, Cheung RM. Affiliate stigma among caregivers of people with intellectual disability or mental illness. J Applied Res Intellect Disabil. 2008;21(6):532-45.

Mascayano F, Tapia T, Schilling S, et al. Stigma toward mental illness in Latin America and the Caribbean: a systematic review. Revista Brasileira de Psiquiatria. 2016;38(1):73-85.

Mashiach-Eizenberg M, Hasson-Ohayon I, Yanos PT, et al. Internalized stigma and quality of life among persons with severe mental illness: the mediating roles of self-esteem and hope. Psychiatry Res. 2013;208(1):15-20.

Mittal D, Sullivan G, Chekuri L, et al. Empirical studies of self-stigma reduction strategies: A critical review of the literature. Psychiatr Serv. 2012;63(10):974-81.

Moses T. Self-labeling and its effects among adolescents diagnosed with mental disorders. Social Sci Med. 2009;68(3):570-8.

Neki JS. Problems of motivation affecting the psychiatrist, the general practitioner and the public in their interactions in the field of mental health. Indian J Psychiatry. 1966;8:117-24.

Nunnally JC. Popular Conceptions of Mental Health. New York: Holt, Rinchart, Winston;1961.

Parcesepe AM, Cabassa LJ. Public stigma of mental illness in the United States: a systematic literature review. Adm Policy Ment Health. 2013;40(5):384-99.

Park S, Park KS. Family stigma: a concept analysis. Asian Nursing Research. 2014;8(3):165-71.

Penn DL, Kommana S, Mansfield M, et al. Dispelling the stigma of schizophrenia: II. The impact of information on dangerousness. Schizophr Bull. 1999;25(3):437-46.

Pescosolido BA, Martin JK. The Stigma Complex. Annu Rev Sociology. 2015;41:87-116.

Pescosolido BA, Medina TR, Martin JK, et al. The "backbone" of stigma: identifying the global core of public prejudice associated with mental illness. Am J Public Health 2013;103(5):853-60.

Phillips MR, Pearson V, Li F, et al. Stigma and expressed emotion: A study of people with schizophrenia and their family members in China. Br J Psychiatry. 2002;181(4):488-93.

Ping Tsao CI, Tummala A, Roberts LW. Stigma in mental health care. Acad Psychiatry. 2008;32(2): 70-2.

Pryor JB, Reeder GD, Monroe AE. The infection of bad company: Stigma by association. J Pers Soc Psychol. 2012;102(2):224-41.

Raguram R, Weiss MG, Channabasavanna SM, et al. Stigma, depression, and somatization in South India. Am J Psychiatry. 1996;153(8):1043-9.

Ren Z, Wang H, Feng B, et al. An exploratory cross-sectional study on the impact of education on perception of stigma by Chinese patients with schizophrenia. BMC Health Serv Res. 2016;16:210.

Ritsher JB, Phelan JC. Internalized stigma predicts erosion of morale among psychiatric outpatients. Psychiatry Res. 2004;30(129):257–65.

Rüsch N, Angermeyer MC, Corrigan PW. Mental illness stigma: concepts, consequences, and initiatives to reduce stigma. Eur Psychiatry. 2005;20(8):529-39.

Rüsch N, Corrigan PW, Powell K, et al. A stress-coping model of mental illness stigma: II. Emotional stress responses, coping behavior and outcome. Schizophr Res. 2009;110(1-3):65-71.

Rüsch N, Corrigan PW, Wassel A, et al. A stress-coping model of mental illness stigma: I. Predictors of cognitive stress appraisal. Schizophr Res. 2009;110(1-3):59-64.

Sartorius N. Stigma: what can psychiatrists do about it? Lancet. 1998;26(352):1058-9.

Schnyder N, Panczak R, Groth N, Schultze-Lutter F. Association between mental health-related stigma and active help-seeking: systematic review and meta-analysis. Br J Psychiatry. 2017;210: 261-8.

Schomerus G, Lucht M, Holzinger A, et al. The stigma of alcohol dependence compared with other mental disorders: a review of population studies. Alcohol Alcohol 2011;46(2):105-12.

Schomerus G, Schwahn C, Holzinger A, et al. Evolution of public attitudes about mental illness: a systematic review and meta-analysis. Acta Psychiatr Scand. 2012;125(6):440-52.

Schulze B, Angermeyer MC. Subjective experiences of stigma: A focus group study of schizophrenic patients, their relatives and mental health professionals. Soc Sci Med. 2003;56:299–312.

Shamsaei F, Kermanshahi SM K, Vanaki Z, et al. Family care giving in bipolar disorder: Experiences of Stigma. Iran J Psychiatry. 2013;8(4):188-94.

Sheehan L, Nieweglowski K, Corrigan P. The stigma of personality disorders. Curr Psychiatry Rep. 2016;18(1):11.

Shrivastava A, Bureau Y, Rewari N, et al. Clinical risk of stigma and discrimination of mental illnesses: Need for objective assessment and quantification. Indian J Psychiatry. 2013;55(2):178-82.

Singh A, Mattoo SK, Grover S. Stigma and its correlates in patients with schizophrenia attending a general hospital psychiatric unit. Indian J Psychiatry. 2016;58(3):291-300.

Struening EL, Perlick DA, Link BG, et al. Stigma as a barrier to recovery: The extent to which caregivers believe most people devalue consumers and their families. Psychiatr Serv. 2001;52(12): 1633-8.

Stuart H. Fighting the stigma caused by mental disorders: past perspectives, present activities, and future directions. World Psychiatry. 2008;7(3):185-8.

Szmukler GI, Burgess P, Herman H, et al. Caring for relatives with serious mental illness—the development of the Experience of Caregiving Inventory. Soc Psychiatr Psychiatric Epidemiol. 1996;31: 134-48.

Taylor SM, Dear MJ. Scaling community attitudes toward the mentally ill. Schizophr Bull. 1981;7(2): 225-40.

Thara R, Srinivasan TN. How stigmatizing is schizophrenia in India. Int J Soc Psychiatry. 2000;46:135-41.

Thornicroft G, Brohan E, Rose D, et al. Global pattern of experienced and anticipated discrimination against people with schizophrenia: a cross-sectional survey. Lancet. 2009;373(9661):408-15.

Thornicroft G, Rose D, Kassam A, et al. Stigma: ignorance, prejudice or discrimination? Br J Psychiatry. 2007;190:192-3.

Tsang HW, Ching SC, Tang KH, et al. Therapeutic intervention for internalized stigma of severe mental illness: A systematic review and meta-analysis. Schizophr Res. 2016;173(1-2):45-53.

Tzouvara V, Papadopoulos C, Randhawa G. Systematic review of the prevalence of mental illness stigma within the Greek culture. Int J Soc Psychiatry. 2016;62(3):292-305.

Van Brakel WH. Measuring—health-related stigma—a literature review. Psychol Health Med. 2006;11(3):307-34.

Verghese A, Baig A. Public attitudes towards mental illness: The Vellore Study. Indian J Psychiatry. 1974;16:8-18.

Weller BE, Faulkner M, Doyle O, et al. Impact of patients' psychiatric hospitalization on caregivers: a systematic review. Psychiatr Serv. 2015;66(5):527-35.

West ML, Yanos PT, Smith SM, et al. Prevalence of internalized stigma among persons with severe mental illness. Stigma Res Action. 2011;1(1):3-10.

Wig N, Sulliman A, Routledge R, et al. Community reaction to mental disorders: A key informant study in 3 different developing countries. Acta Psychiatr Scand. 1980;61:111-26.

Wood L, Byrne R, Varese F, et al. Psychosocial interventions for internalized stigma in people with a schizophrenia-spectrum diagnosis: A systematic narrative synthesis and meta-analysis. Schizophr Res. 2016;176(2-3):291-303.

World Health Organisation. Mental Health Action Plan. 2013-2020. Geneva: WHO, 2013.

World Health Organisation. Mental Health: New Understanding, New Hope. The World Health Report. Geneva: WHO, 2001.

Yanos PT, Lucksted A, Drapalski AL, et al. Interventions targeting mental health self-stigma: A review and comparison. Psychiatr Rehabil J. 2015;38(2):171-8.

Yanos PT, Roe D, Markus K, et al. Pathways between internalized stigma and outcomes related to recovery in schizophrenia spectrum disorders. Psychiatr Serv. 2008;59(12):1437-42.

Zieger A, Mungee A, Schomerus G, et al. Perceived stigma of mental illness: A comparison between two metropolitan cities in India. Indian J Psychiatry. 2016;58(4):432-7.

Chapter 38

Migration and Mental Health

Sumeet Gupta, Baxi Sinha

SUMMARY

Migration is a phenomenon which is present in all places and since all ages. It is becoming widespread with increasing interconnectivity within the globe. Migrants are considered as highly vulnerable population group for all sorts of psychological and social problems and hence there is a need to study the connection between mental health and migration. This chapter discusses briefly the reasons and types of migration, and the associated psychosocial issues. Phases through which a migrant passes through during the process of migration are also touched upon. Various psychiatric disorders associated with migration have been described in detail followed by their management. Migration in special population like children, women, and elderly has also been briefly touched upon.

MIGRATION AND MENTAL HEALTH

Migration is a ubiquitous phenomenon. The history of human migration goes as far back as the history of humankind. The 20th century witnessed an unprecedented level of human migration. A United Nations report (Migration Report, 2015) estimated that that there were about 244 million migrants worldwide accounting for about 3% of the world's population. About two-thirds of international migrants are living in only 20 countries. The last decade also witnessed a significant increase in the refugee population, which reached 19.5 million in 2014. The countries currently hosting the largest refugee populations are Turkey, Pakistan, and Iran. India currently hosts about 5 million migrants, mainly from the neighboring countries such as Nepal, Tibet, and Bangladesh. Conversely, India also has the largest "diaspora" in the world at about 16 million.

In today's increasingly interconnected world, human migration touches nearly all corners of the globe. Migrants are one of the most vulnerable members of the society despite many benefits of migration. In addition to overcoming the challenges of adjusting to an alien environment and navigating the complex process of acculturation, migrants frequently face economic hardship and discrimination. Therefore, it is not surprising that their health including mental health has been a concern for some time.

There is no uniform definition of migrants. The United Nations Convention on the Rights of Migrants defines a migrant worker as a "person who is to be engaged, is engaged or has been engaged in a remunerated activity in a State of which he/she is not a national".

Alternatively, migration is defined as "the movement of people across a specified boundary, national (i.e. internal) or international to establish a new permanent place of residence" (United Nations Convention on Migrants' Rights 2003). As specified in the latter definition, migration is not always restricted to crossing international boundaries. Internally displaced persons and rural–urban migration have become major issues for large countries such as India and China. Migration is not a homogeneous phenomenon; hence, migrants comprise of a very heterogeneous group with different reasons for migration, ethnicity, source and host countries, and legal status. Moreover, migration is not always a voluntary process; examples of involuntary migration include asylum seekers (who move across international border in search for protection) and refugees (who have already been granted protection by another country). In this review, we have used a broad definition for migrants (that includes both voluntary and forced migrants).

The health of migrants especially mental health has become a prominent issue over the past few decades. In particular, findings that migrants might be more predisposed to psychotic disorders than nonmigrant groups (Harrison, 1988; Cantor-Graae & Selten, 2005, Fearon et al., 2006), offers a unique opportunity to study the role of social and psychological factors in the aetiology of psychosis. However, due to heterogeneity of the problem and involvement of many contributory factors, so far results have been inconsistent and often contradictory.

Reasons for Migration

The migrant population is increasing rapidly in line with globalization. Ease of travel and access to information has facilitated the process, and migration is likely to continue to rise. The reasons for the migration can be classified as "pull or push factors". Pull factors include better employment opportunities, political freedom, and a better living environment, whereas common push factors include war, natural disaster, and political persecution. **Table 1** shows different types of migrants along with common reasons for migration.

Phases of Migration

The migratory process can be divided into three phases: premigratory, migratory, and post-migratory phases. Each of these has its own challenges and opportunities. Moreover, every

Table 1: Type of migrants and reasons for migration	
Voluntary migration	*Involuntary (forced) migration*
Economic migrants—Indian information technology workers to the USA	War—Tamil migrants from Sri Lanka, Syrian migrants to Europe
Resettlement—Jews to Israel	Slaves or forced labor—Africans to Southeast USA
Rural–urban migration in India is due to better employment opportunities	Lack of food/famine—Ethiopians to Sudan
–	Political persecution—Iraqis to Europe/other Persian Gulf states during Saddam Hussein's regime
–	Natural disaster—Chernobyl nuclear disaster in Ukraine

Flowchart 1: Phases of migration: Risk and resilience factors.

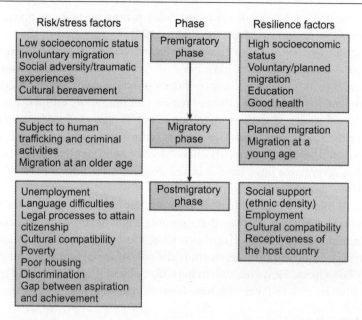

Risk/stress factors	Phase	Resilience factors
Low socioeconomic status Involuntary migration Social adversity/traumatic experiences Cultural bereavement	Premigratory phase	High socioeconomic status Voluntary/planned migration Education Good health
Subject to human trafficking and criminal activities Migration at an older age	Migratory phase	Planned migration Migration at a young age
Unemployment Language difficulties Legal processes to attain citizenship Cultural compatibility Poverty Poor housing Discrimination Gap between aspiration and achievement	Postmigratory phase	Social support (ethnic density) Employment Cultural compatibility Receptiveness of the host country

individual follows unique trajectories when settling in a new society or country. The outcome and success of migration is determined by a combination of risk and resilience factors related to the individual and to the environment (of both source and host countries). **Flowchart 1** summarizes common risk and resilience factors.

The process of adaptation to a new culture (i.e. acculturation) is also complex. Many authors have used terms such as cultural shock, cultural bereavement and cultural congruity to describe the process of adjusting to a change in culture (Eisenburch, 1990; Bhugra, 2005). The process of acculturation varies from person-to-person and can cause major internal conflict. Berry (1980) proposed a theory to explain how individuals from a cultural background react when in contact with another culture. The theory states that individual migrants can fall into one of four categories depending on how they react to the host culture and how much of the source culture is retained (**Figure 1**):

1. Integration (biculturalism)—The migrant retains some aspects of the original cultural values, but adapts to the host culture by learning the necessary skills and values
2. Assimilation—The migrant seeks to become a part of the host culture to the exclusion of the original culture
3. Separation (rejection)—The migrant identifies exclusively with the original culture
4. Marginalization—The migrant perceives the original culture as negative, but is unable to adapt to the host culture.

If acculturation is not a successful and positive experience, then it can predispose individuals to mental health problems. Children of migrants (the second generation) can also experience problems associated with cultural identity and conflict with their migrant parents (Islam, 2012).

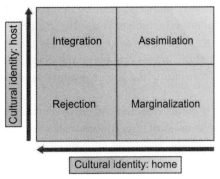

Figure 1: Cultural adaptation (Berry 1980).

Migration and Mental Health Problems

Studying migrants and their experiences in migration offers a unique insight to the human response to changes. Amongst all of the changes humans face during their lives, the extent of change involved in migration is unparalleled because apart from losing their social support and native environment, migrants also have to adjust to an alien culture and a different language, usually with loss of the social support network. Therefore, the relationship between migration and mental health has generated interest among researchers and clinicians alike. So far, evidence for a relationship between migration and mental health remains unclear.

On one hand, it has been suggested that migrants are a vulnerable group who are more likely to have mental health problems; on the other hand, migrants with better health compared with the host population has been described (Dhadda & Greene, 2017). The best way to fully understand the effect of migration on mental health would be to compare the mental health of migrants with their probable mental health status if they had stayed in the home country. However, this type of investigation is not feasible.

There are many difficulties in assessing mental health of migrants. Firstly, migrants are not a homogeneous group—there are many individual and environmental variables (related to home and host societies). Secondly, most studies have a cross-sectional or retrospective design, compare the prevalence of mental illness in migrants with that of matched host or source populations, and lack methodological rigor. Lastly, there is a lack of culturally sensitive instruments for identifying suitable cases. A general finding is that the poorer the host country, the higher the prevalence of mental disorder (Carballo et al., 1998; Lindert et al., 2009). Furthermore, the quality of the study especially the sampling method seems to affect the magnitude of the difference in prevalence of mental illness between migrant and host populations. Studies with high methodological rigor tend to report a greater similarity between these populations (Bhugra, 2004; Fazel et al., 2005). However, despite these shortcomings, the growing number of migrants means that studying this relationship is more important now than ever before.

The risk of developing mental illness depends on many person-related (e.g. genetic predisposition to mental disorder, coping skills) and environment-related (exposure to racism, ethnic density, social support, and receptivity of host country) factors. The effect of environmental factors was clearly demonstrated by Bogic et al. (2012) who studied refuges from former Yugoslavia 9 year after the Balkan Wars. These authors compared refugees hosted by the Germany, Italy, and the UK. After adjusting for various confounding variables, they found that refugees in Italy had the lowest rate of mental disorders which was related to being in employment, having appropriate living arrangements and feeling accepted in the host country.

Although most research addresses the negative consequences of migration, many migrants not only survive the stresses of migration but also benefit from their experiences and opportunities in the host countries, emerging with more resilience against mental disorder (Papadopoulos, 2006).

Migration and Psychotic Disorders

Interest in a possible relationship between migration and psychotic disorders started in 1932, when Odegaard (1932) reported higher incidence of schizophrenia among Norwegian migrants to the USA as compared with native Americans or Norwegians. By their histories of poor social adaptation in Norway, he argued that this could be attributed to the selective migration of people at a high-risk of developing schizophrenia. Presumably, these persons would have developed schizophrenia, had they stayed in Norway. A re-emergence of interest in the topic has been fuelled by the findings of increased schizophrenia risk in the first- and second-generation Afro-Caribbean populations in the UK (King et al., 1994; Bhugra et al., 1997; Harrison et al., 1988).

Cantor-Graae and Selten (2005) conducted a systematic review and meta-analysis of incidence studies published between 1970 and 2003. A consistent finding of this review was a higher incidence of schizophrenia amongst immigrants compared to native populations. There was a significant heterogeneity which confirmed that migrants are not a homogeneous group. The most prominent finding was higher incidence rate amongst first-generation black migrants, although incidence rate was also high in the second-generation population. Moreover, a UK study showed that the increased incidence of mental disorder was not restricted to schizophrenia. The migrant population in the UK was also at an increased risk of psychosis (including affective psychosis). However, regarding incidence rate for schizophrenia, there were significant differences amongst those of different ethnic backgrounds. The highest risk was experienced by Afro-Caribbean and black African migrants (risk ratios 6.6 and 4.1 respectively, compared with the white British population). Although South Asian migrant community also had a higher risk ratio, this was not statistically significant (Fearon et al., 2006).

Recently, Kirkbride et al. (2012) conducted a systematic review and meta-analysis of studies in England between 1950 and 2009. They have suggested an increased risk of psychotic illness (both affective and nonaffective psychoses) in black African and Caribbean populations compared with the native white population. The analysis also suggested a higher incidence of psychotic illness in the South Asian population, but the risk was lower than for black African and Caribbean migrants. There was some suggestion that the difference could be due to socioeconomic factors; however, the difference persisted even after the adjustment for socioeconomic status.

Many hypotheses have been proposed to explain the differences in risk between migrant and host populations. The self-selection hypothesis suggests that people who are predisposed to psychotic illness are more likely to migrate. However, findings that incidence rates are 5-fold higher amongst Surinamese migrants to the Netherlands compared with the native population and an increased risk in second-generation migrants point against the selection hypothesis (Selten et al., 2002). Source countries have higher incident rates of psychosis. However, international comparative studies have failed to show any corresponding increased incidence in the country of origin (Bhugra et al., 1996; Jablensky et al., 1992). Another suggestion is that migration stress might predispose people to developing psychotic illnesses. Hollander et al. (2016) compared the risk of nonaffective psychosis in the native Swedish population with that of refugee and nonrefugee migrants. The incidence rate for nonaffective psychotic disorders was 66% higher in refugees than in nonrefugee migrants from similar regions of origin, and nearly three times greater than in the native-born Swedish population. Hence, authors suggested that exposure to social adversity prior to migration might contribute to increased risk. However, this does not explain the increased risk in second-generation migrants. Another possible explanation could be misdiagnosis. Migrants are more likely to be diagnosed with schizophrenia due to language difficulty and cross-cultural differences. However, this is unlikely to explain the different incidence rates in migrants as compared with their home countries.

So far, a consistent finding is that migrants (especially black African and Caribbean migrants in the UK and Surinamese migrants in the Netherlands) are at a high-risk of developing nonaffective psychosis including schizophrenia. There are two possible explanations for this: (1) social selection (i.e. downward social mobility of predisposed persons) and (2) social causation (adversity and stress). Selten and Cantor-Graae, (2007) proposed that the chronic experience of social defeat described as having a subordinate position or outsider status, leads to sensitisation of the mesolimbic dopamine system. The findings that schizophrenia risks are highest for the least successful immigrant groups, e.g. Moroccan men in the Netherlands, the Inuit in Denmark and Afro-Caribbean migrants in the UK (Selten et al., 2007), as well as the increased risk for second-generation migrants support this hypothesis. Supportive evidence is also available for the protective effect of high ethnic density (i.e. number of the people of same ethnicity living in the same vicinity), especially regarding nonaffective psychotic illness (Shaw, 2012).

Migration and Post-traumatic Stress Disorder

Political refugees and those escaping war or serious natural disasters are more likely to suffer from post-traumatic stress disorder (PTSD). Chen et al. (2017) assessed 2,239 humanitarian migrants arriving in Australia and found that 31% suffered from PTSD. Postmigratory predictors of PTSD include poor social integration, economic problems, anxiety about family or friends overseas, and loneliness. There is some suggestion that PTSD presentation might be different in migrants and may be influenced by their cultural background. For example, Jenkins, (1991) reported that Salvadoran refugee women in North America explained their suffering as "nervios", a culturally accepted way of responding to abnormal stressors with the presentation of dysphoria, aches and pains, and subjective bouts of feeling intense heat.

Migration and other Common Mental Health Problems

In general, the health of newly arrived immigrants is better than that of source and host country populations. This is because migrants have overcome many obstacles to reach to the new country and so have to be mentally and physically strong. However, the advantage of the so-called healthy migrant effect gradually weakens over time such that risks for migrants match those of the host population (Kirmayer, 2011). A US study found that rates of anxiety, depression, impulse control, and substance abuse disorder were lower for new immigrants (OR = 0.7, 95% CI = 0.5–0.9), but gradually increased to the levels of the local population. Incidence rates in migrants who arrived before the age of 12 years and for the children of immigrants were similar to those in the host population (Breslau et al., 2007). A systematic review of refugees who had been living in the host country for more than 5 years reported that the prevalence of depression and anxiety disorder were higher than in the native population. Commonly reported predictors were premigratory traumatic experience and postmigratory stress (Bogic et al., 2012). However, most studies have failed to show a consistent and significant difference in the prevalence or incidence of common psychiatric disorders between migrant and native populations.

Mental Health Problems in Special Populations: Children, Women, and the Elderly

In the past, most children, women, and elderly migrants would have accompanied primary male migrants. However, this situation is changing especially for women. There is some evidence that children tend to adjust to a new society better than the adults (Bhugra et al., 2011). However, they have to deal with stresses related to friction between the source and host cultures. Children tend to identify more with the culture of the host country, unlike their parents who are more likely to identify more with the culture of origin. This type of family stress is commonly reported. On the other hand, women have to adjust to different gender role expectations in different societies. In the UK, the attempted suicide rate is higher in women of South Asian origin than in white women and South Asian men (Bhugra et al., 1999). In addition to a history of mental disorder, inter-racial relationships and cultural alienation (alienation from both the original and host culture) are reported risk factors for migrant women (Bhugra & Hicks, 2004). Elderly people who migrated earlier in life as primary migrants or later in life with family members are reported to have a similar prevalence of dementia and depression compared with the host population. However, studies in UK found elderly migrants access specialist mental health services less often compared with the native population (Shah, 2011).

Migrants and Access to Health Services

Migrants' access to mental health services depends on a variety of factors, such as legal status in the host country, language problems, awareness, and accessibility of mental health services, migrants' concepts about mental illness, stigma of mental illness, and institutional discrimination (Ingelby, 2011; Singh & Burns, 2006). Therefore, it is not surprising that migrants either do not have access to mental health services or face many obstacles in accessing these services especially during the initial part of their stay. However, service utilization improves with the length of time, a migrant has stayed in the host country due to reduced language barriers and increased acculturation. However, there is an evidence that migrants accessing mental health services are treated differently from the host population. Studies in Europe suggest that migrants are more likely to be detained and/or restrained and treated with older generation antipsychotic drugs (Singh & Burns, 2006; Lay et al., 2005). Lastly, a lack of awareness of cross-cultural issues in clinicians especially differences in the presentation of psychiatric problems can lead to misdiagnosis.

Pharmacological and Psychological Treatments

The pharmacokinetic and pharmacodynamic properties of psychotropic drugs differ amongst different ethnic groups. For example, Asians are more sensitive to the extrapyramidal adverse effects of haloperidol and Hispanics are more likely to respond to a lower dosage of tricyclic antidepressant drugs. Similarly, attitudes towards pharmacological treatments, herbal medications or complimentary therapies differ amongst different cultural groups (Poole, 2011). These cultural differences become more important when treating psychological illnesses. For example, Indian patients are reported to feel more at ease in being dependent on therapist, in sharp contrast to Western patients. Therefore, it is essential for psychotherapists to adapt their approach to the cultural background of migrants.

Recommendations for Policymakers

The following recommendations are made for policymakers (Bhugra et al., 2011; Bhugra et al., 2014; Priebe et al., 2016):

1. *Promote social integration*: This appears to be a key strategy to reduce the incidence of mental disorders amongst migrants. It requires close collaboration amongst different services such as the health care, social care, and voluntary services. Strategies include providing easy access to school and employment opportunities, and fostering relationships within the same ethnic group and with the wider community

2. *Improve the availability and accessibility of mental health services*: As previously mentioned, migrants usually find it difficult to access mental health services for a variety of reasons. Therefore, it is extremely important that provision should be made to cater for their mental health needs. Two ways to improve availability are to either start up new services for migrants or strengthen existing services. The latter option is usually preferable, unless there is large-scale migration. Legal entitlement and provision of mental health services vary amongst different host countries; therefore, it is important to inform migrants about local service provision (preferably in their own language) at the earliest opportunity

3. *Use interpreter services and new technologies to overcome language barriers*: Language problems represent one of the biggest hurdles in assessing a patient's mental health. Therefore, policymakers should ensure adequate provision of professional interpreters. A few European countries have also used cultural mediators or consultants, i.e. members of migrant and ethnic communities who are usually responsible for outreach services and informing clinicians about cultural issues. Use of telepsychiatry can also ensure that

migrants are assessed by clinicians who speak their own language and are aware of cultural issues and local service provisions. Lastly, emphasis should be given to improving the language skills of migrants to foster their inclusion in the host society

4. *Provide culturally sensitive services*: The attitude of clinicians towards migrants and their awareness of cross-cultural issues can greatly affect their ability to correctly diagnose and effectively manage mental disorders. Therefore, many experts advocate that clinicians should be regularly provided with effective training on cross-cultural issues, such as the use of different idioms for distress and beliefs, and expectations about mental health problems and treatment.

Recommendations for Clinicians

Clinicians should be aware of the risk and resilience factors commonly associated with mental health in migrants (Bhugra and Jones, 2001; Ingleby, 2011). The mental health assessment of migrants should include a comprehensive assessment of their adjustment to the host culture, their current beliefs and attitudes towards treatment, and their social support. Exploration of postmigratory stressors (including in second-generation migrants) should include cultural bereavement and conflict, racial discrimination, employment, and the gap between aspiration and achievement. There is an emerging evidence for the protective effect of ethnic density; therefore, assessing the level of social support available within the relevant ethnic group should also form an important aspect of the assessment. Refugees and asylum seekers require sensitive handling during assessment because they might be suspicious owing to previous negative experiences with authorities. Clinicians also need to use and develop culturally valid assessment tools and interventions.

CONCLUSION

Migration is a very stressful process even when voluntary. Moreover, refugees can undergo horrific ordeals involving persecution, trauma, and economic hardship. So far, evidence suggests that migrants are more likely to develop nonaffective psychotic illnesses and PTSD, with PTSD being more common in refugees and asylum seekers. Evidence for other mental disorders is unequivocal. Migrants constitute 3% of the world's population, but they do not have equal access to mental health services. Additionally, they are a vulnerable population group. Dealing with postmigration factors (such as poor acceptance by the host country, racial discrimination, poor employment opportunities, and little social support) and adequate provision of mental health services can significantly improve the well-being of migrants. Overcoming these problems needs collaborative efforts at all levels. Further research is necessary to understand the risk and resilience factors for different migrant groups and to develop evidence-based therapies for these vulnerable populations.

REFERENCES

Berry JW. Acculturation as varieties of adaptation. In: Padilla AM (Ed). Acculturation: Theory, Models and Some New Findings. Boulder: Westview; 1980. pp. 9-25.

Bhugra D. Migration and mental health. Acta Psychiatr Scand. 2004;109:243–58.

Bhugra D. Cultural identities and cultural congruency: a new model for evaluating mental distress in immigrants. Acta Psychiatr Scand. 2005:111(2):84–93.

Bhugra D, Baldwin D, Desai M, et al. Attempted suicide in West London. II: Social and cultural factors. Psychiatr Med. 1999;29:1131–9.

Bhugra D, Gupta S, Bhui K, et al. WPA guidance on mental health and mental health care in migrants. World Psychiatry. 2011;10(1):2-10.

Bhugra D, Gupta S, Schouler-Ocak M, et al. EPA guidance mental health care of migrants. Eur Psychiatry. 2014;29(2):107-15.

Bhugra D, Hicks MH. Effect of an educational pamphlet on help-seeking attitudes for depression among British South Asian Women. Psychiatr Serv. 2004;55:827-34.

Bhugra D, Hilwig M, Hossein B. First-contact incidence rates of schizophrenia in Trinidad and one-year follow-up. Br J Psychiatry. 1996;169:587–92.

Bhugra D. Jones P. Migration and mental illness. Advances in Psychiatric Treatment. 2001;7:216–23.

Bhugra D, Leff J, Mallett R, et al. Incidence and outcome of schizophrenia in whites, African-Caribbeans and Asians in London. Psychol Med. 1997;27:791-8.

Bogic M, Ajdukovic D, Bremner S, et al. Factors associated with mental disorders in long-settled war refugees: refugees from the former Yugoslavia in Germany, Italy and the UK. Br J Psychiatry. 2012;200:216-23.

Breslau J, Aguilar-Gaxiola S, Borges G, et al. Risk for psychiatric disorder among immigrants and their US-born descendants: evidence from the National Comorbidity Survey Replication. J Nerv Ment Dis. 2007;195:189–95.

Cantor-Graae E, Selten JP. Schizophrenia and migration: a meta-analysis and review. Am J Psychiatry. 2005;162:12–24.

Carballo M, Divino JJ, Zeric, D. Migration and health in the European Union. Trop Med Int Health. 1998;3:936–44.

Chen W, Hall BJ, Ling L, et al. Pre-migration and post-migration factors associated with mental health in humanitarian migrants in Australia and the moderation effect of post-migration stressors: findings from the first wave data of the BNLA cohort study. Lancet Psychiatry. 2017;4(3):218–29.

Dhadda A, Greene G. The healthy migrant effect for mental health in England: Propensity-score Matched Analysis Using the EMPIRIC Survey. J Imm Minority Health. 2017;1:1-10.

Eisenbruch M. The cultural bereavement interview: a new clinical research approach for refugees. Psychiatr Clin N Am. 1990;13:715–35.

Fazel M, Wheeler J, Danesh J. Prevalence of serious mental disorder in 7000 refugees resettled in western countries: a systematic review. Lancet. 2005;365:1309-14.

Fearon P, Kirkbride JB, Morgan C, et al. Incidence of schizophrenia and other psychoses in ethnic minority groups: results from the MRC AESOP Study. Psychol Med. 2006;36:1541–50.

Harrison G, Owens D, Holton A, et al. A prospective study of severe mental disorder in Afro-Caribbean patients. Psychol Med. 1988;18:643–57.

Hollander AC, Dal H, Lewis G, et al. Refugee migration and risk of schizophrenia and other non-affective psychoses: cohort study of 1.3 million people in Sweden. Br Med J. 2016;352:i1030.

Ingelby D. Adapting mental health services to the needs of migrants and ethnic minorities. In: Bhugra D, Gupta S (Eds). Migration and mental health. London: Cambridge University Press; 2011. pp. 231-44.

Islam F. Health equity for South Asian communities: health services & health policy report. Canada, Council of Agencies Serving South Asians (CASSA); 2012.

Jablensky A, Sartorius N, Ernberg G, et al. Schizophrenia: manifestations, incidence and course in different cultures: A World Health Organization ten-country study. Psychol Med. 1992;20:1-97.

Jenkins JH. The state construction of affect: political ethos and mental health among Salvadoran refugees. Cult Med Psychiatry. 1991;15:139-65.

King MB, Cole E, Leavy G, et al. Incidence of psychotic illness in London. Br Med J. 1994;309:1115–9.

Kirkbride JB, Errazuriz A, Croudace TJ, et al. Incidence of schizophrenia and other psychoses in England,1950–2009: A Systematic Review and Meta-Analyses. PLoS One. 2012;7(3):e31660.

Kirmayer LJ, Narasiah L, Munoz M, et al. Common mental health problems in immigrants and refugees: general approach in primary care.CMAJ. 2011;183(12):E959-67.

Lay B, Lauber C, Rössler W. Are immigrants at a disadvantage in psychiatric in-patient care? Acta Psychiatr Scand. 2005;111(5):358-66.

Lindert J, Ehrenstein OS, Priebe S, et al. Depression and anxiety in labor migrants and refugees—a systematic review and meta-analysis. Soc Sci Med. 2009;69:246-57.

Migration Report: United Nations, Department of Economic and Social Affairs, Population Division (2016). International Migration Report; 2015.

Odegaard O. Emigration and insanity. Acta Psychiatr Scand (Suppl). 1932;4:1–206.

Papadopoulos RK. Refugees and psychological trauma: psychosocial perspectives. Cambridge: Harvard University Press; 2006.

Poole N. Ethno-psychopharmacology. In: Bhugra D, Gupta S (Eds). Migration and mental health. London: Cambridge University Press; 2011. pp. 299-312.

Priebe S, Giacco D, El-Nagib R. Public health aspects of mental health among migrants and refugees: a review of the evidence on mental health care for refugees, asylum seekers and irregular migrants in the WHO European Region. Copenhagen: WHO Regional Office for Europe; 2016.

Selten JP, Cantor-Graae E, Kahn R. Migration and schizophrenia. Curr Opin Psychiatry. 2007;20(2):111-5.

Selten JP, Cantor-Graae E, Slaets J, et al. Ødegaard's selection hypothesis revisited: schizophrenia in Surinamese immigrants to the Netherlands. Am J Psychiatry. 2002;159:669-71.

Shah A. Migration and mental health of older people. In: Bhugra D, Gupta S (Eds). Migration and mental health. London: Cambridge University Press; 2011. pp. 173-95.

Shaw, RJ, Atkin, K, Bécares, L, et al. Impact of ethnic density on adult mental disorders: narrative review. Br J Psychiatry. 2012;201(1):11-9.

Singh SP, Burns T. Race and mental health: there is more to race than racism. Br Med J. 2006;333:648-51.

United Nations Convention on Migrants' Rights 2003: Paris, United Nations Educational, Scientific and Cultural Organisation; 2005.

Chapter 39

Psychiatry in Armed Forces

MSVK Raju

SUMMARY

Wars and armed forces have contributed a lot to the development of the discipline of psychiatry. Psychiatric casualties of war have been described in historical and scriptural descriptions of battle field scenarios. Arjuna's deployment distress is vividly described in the Bhagavad Gita (1986). One can say perhaps that military psychiatry originated in India from that point. Psychiatry in the armed forces can be called a forerunner of community and social psychiatry in the world. Social psychiatry is that branch of psychiatry which focuses on the interpersonal and cultural context of mental disorder and mental well-being. Armed forces of a country offer a unique milieu and invaluable opportunity to study mental health and unhealth in trained men and women as well as their family members. This chapter discusses evolution and growth of mental health services in armed forces in the background of specific stressors faced by the forces in wars and peace keeping, and managing the countries' internal turmoil, and also managing their personal issues while working in a highly disciplined sector.

INTRODUCTION

The armed forces of a democratic country like India take into account the fundamental tenets of democracy in laying down its rules to meet its primary responsibility of protecting the nation from external aggression and quelling internal strife which might threaten its integrity. These basic rules together may be called "military ethos" which includes an obligation to kill and get killed (Mahalingam, 2013). Soldiers are not born; they are made into a fighting machine by rigorous physical training and mental toughening. Development of traditions and culture of armed forces is a part of the military ethos. All the three branches, called "Services" in this context, of the armed forces, i.e. Army, Navy, and Air Force have their own unique cultures. Within the overall system of cultures, each regiment and corps of the army or ship and squadron of navy and air force has its own subculture which binds officers, men and women into an effective fighting unit. This enduring bond and pride in one's regiment, ship or squadron is called *esprit-de-corps* or "esprit" in short. This *esprit* is inculcated into soldiers, sailors, and airmen constantly by educating them of the unit's heritage of exploits, heroes, battle honours and unit traditions. Actually, it is a well-known fact that individual soldiers do not have the nation in mind when they are fighting and or even when getting prepared to make the supreme sacrifice (Boring, 1979; Menninger, 1979; Mahalingam, 2013). It is their self-esteem as a soldier and *esprit w*hich makes them function with a single-minded dedication to the military task at hand. It is the commander's responsibility to develop and sustain these qualities by personal example of leadership, skill, integrity, fair play, and justice. In psychiatric terms, one may say commanders entrench themselves in the soldier's mind as another superego of adult life!

MILITARY STRESS AND ADJUSTMENT

India has the third largest armed force in the world and is the largest voluntary armed force of the world. Future officers undergo training in the officer academies whereas persons below officer rank (PBOR) get trained in the respective regimental centers. A raw young recruit becomes a "trained soldier" after taking oath on completion of military training and becomes a "seasoned soldier" after taking part in actual active operations. The aim of military training is to make him physically tough, adept at using arms and the equipment of his trade, and most importantly, to loosen his personal identity and direct his emotional investment in the group; he wears a number (chest number) during training and finds that his individual choices are curtailed—everything has to be done in the prescribed way, everybody has to wear same clothes at same time, everybody has to get up at the same time, go to bed at same time and so on. Strenuous physical exercise and restrictions on freedom test the young prospective soldier but enable him to fit into the group which will give him self-esteem and ensure security in battle field conditions (Boring, 1979; Menninger, 1979).

The general demand for adjustment on a soldier is called military stress. Besides the regimentation, the fact that every request has to be routed through a chain of command and everybody is required to receive orders also down the line through the same chain, could be quite frustrating even for a seasoned soldier. Isolation, long separation from family, exposure to extreme climatic conditions, tough and variable terrain, lack of communication, health risks, and the ever-present risk to life and limb are some of the stressors of military life. A loner is a misfit in the military milieu. Air force and navy bring to bear different kind of stressors on officers and men. Flying is a hazardous and strange occupation as human body is not designed to fly. Aircrew are routinely subjected to the stress of situational awareness (SA), spatial disorientation (SD), gravitational stress (G stress), high cognitive demands, complex ergonomics, and fatigue (Shrinagesh, 1960; Navathe & Singh, 1994; Kumar & Malik, 2003; Baijal et al., 2006). Fear of flying occurs both in peace and war time during tactical missions, strategic missions as well as in air lift operations for various reasons (Jones, 1995). The Navy is unique among the services in that it operates on land, sea, air, and under water. Naval officers and men are required to sail at short notice and obliged to remain out of communication for long periods while afloat. Submariners work in cramped spaces closed to atmosphere. Their privacy gets severely restricted as they are obliged to share bed (Hot Bunking) and even carry ablutions in the direct vision of others. Breathing vitiated air, restriction on water usage with no opportunity to stretch limbs or exercise have to be endured over prolonged periods. Nuclear submarines can stay under water for months! Besides the stressors which the air-crew of air force face, naval air-crew have to contend with the additional stress of landing and taking off aircraft on a small deck area with the ship rolling and pitching in turbulent sea (Pawar, 2001).

COMBAT STRESS

The stress that a soldier is subjected to while engaged in actual operations against an adversary is called combat stress which is deliberately created by the adversary to kill, wound or to demoralise the soldiers in many ways. Combat situation is characterized by sudden and often unpredictable extremes—swinging climatic conditions; cognitive stressors like unpredictability; intense noise or extreme silence; difficult choices or no choice; too little information or too much information; thick darkness or blinding dazzle; too little time or long waiting and, sleeplessness and rumour together in various degree take their toll. A soldier in combat is obliged to handle fear of losing life, limb, or comrades. Seeing killed, wounded, or mutilated comrade may make a soldier feel guilty, intensely angry, anxious, sad, or frustrated. Soldiers are also obliged to endure boredom in isolated outposts (Boring, 1979; Menninger, 1979; Campise et al., 2006; Raju, 2013). Raju et al. (2001) devised an instrument to quantify stressors experienced by soldiers in general. Soldiers gave higher weightage to items related to homefront matters and personal issues except court martial which was ranked number 2. They gave a rank of 7 to combat (weighted 68 on a maximum of 100) and 16th rank to fighting terrorists (weighted 60). Right form independence, the Indian soldier is obliged to participate in counter insurgency operations or low-intensity conflicts (LIC) almost on a continuous basis (Badrinath, 2003; Bhat et al., 2003; Chaudhary et al., 2006; Raju, 2013), interspersed with full scale wars on Eastern, Western, and Northern fronts. Even in the "Peace Keeping Operations" conducted by Indian forces in other countries, more than 2000 officers and men of India laid down their lives (Raju, 2014). Perhaps it is a measure of training of Indian soldier and their battle-hardened minds which makes them perceive actual operations as only moderately stressful. But combat stress gets compounded by home-front concerns which are known to prey on soldiers' minds all over the world. A soldier learns to maintain reasonable equanimity while coping with overwhelming stress of various kinds by living, training and fighting together with his comrades. The regimental system in the fighting arms of India, where a soldier enters a unit and retires from the same unit, has stood the test of times as a good system that fosters effective vertical and horizontal bonding (Mahalingam, 2013).

Morale is a good indicator of mental health in soldiers. It is defined in many ways by various authorities (Boring, 1979; Campise et al., 2006). Fundamentally, it is the capacity to stay on the allotted job with determination and zest. In other words, one can say that it is the wanting to want to do what one has to do. It is often the determining factor in the successful completion of a task and depends on group characteristics more than on individual personalities of soldiers. Physical fitness, high standard of training, confidence in leaders, confidence in the equipment, cohesion and conviction that one's cause of fighting is right, are some of the factors which contribute to keep the morale high (Boring, 1979; Menninger, 1979; Mahalingam, 2013). Soldiers dread injury more than death. The confidence that he will be well taken care of, if injured, by timely and skilled medical and surgical intervention, is an important morale booster for soldier in the battle field (Carver, 1989). Medical men are therefore called as "morale builders" (Thapar, 1965). Morale is a big bulwark against psychotrauma in war.

NATURE OF WAR

An estimated 14,500 wars have been fought accounting for the loss of 3.5 billion lives since the beginning of recorded history 4,000 years ago (Raju, 2013). Currently 60 armed conflicts and wars are being fought in various parts of the globe. Sadly, most of the wars are fought in low- and middle-income countries, where mental health resources are much less than desired. In fact, war is a big mental health problem in the world.

Six generations of war are currently described (Kumar, 2014; Fedyk, 2016). War was like a game till the beginning of the last century. It was fought between massed troops of adversaries in a limited area—Kurukshetra, Panipat, Waterloo for example. Soldiers were arranged closely in file and column, and fought from dawn (reveille) to dusk (retreat). First World War-WWI (1909–1914) changed it all: battle lines stretched for miles and miles, and science entered the battle field in a big way in the form of machine gun, battle tank, chemicals and nascent air power (Crocq & Crocq, 2000; Raju, 2013). Thousands died to gain a foot of ground in the unforgiving soggy trenches of Europe and scorching sands of Middle East. It was "Total War" in the Second World War-WWII (1939-1946); factories, communication hubs, airfields, and railways were systematically bombed to destroy the war making capability of the adversary (Gabriel & Metz, 1992; Crocq and Crocq, 2000; Raju, 2013). Fighting was no more confined to a limited area or a border. Civilians also became casualties in a big way; after the dropping of nuclear bomb on 6th August 1945, the world has not remained the same. The angst of instant incineration has come to stay in the penumbra of the consciousness of everybody now; Vietnam War (1965-1971) with its spurts of high intensity engagements, interspersed with periods of liull, brought the concept of "LIC" which is enthusiastically copied by insurgent groups all over the world (Raju, 2013). The armed forces of India have been relentlessly engaged in quelling insurgencies since independence in various parts of the country. After the collapse of the Soviet Union and end of "cold war", intranational ethnic strife and large-scale migration of people within and across boundaries of nations made operational scenario for armed forces immensely complex. Armed forces of nation states are getting deployed as "Peace Keeping Forces" largely under the UN umbrella to bring the warring factions to the negotiating table, and restore administration and public service in strife torn countries (Raju, 2014). The 11th September 2001 bombing of World Trade Centre and 26th Nov 2008 terrorist attack on Mumbai, London subway bombing, recent bombing of a mosque in Sinai in Egypt and many similar such incidents in many countries added another chapter to the history of war—terrorism brought war to the door step. Unarmed people are targeted in stealthy wars that are being waged to create fear and to make legitimate states impotent. The looming threat of "cyber war" or "information war" (Kumar, 2014), that aims to paralyse functioning of forces, to put economies in disarray, and to make life generally difficult for people, has the potential to turn out to be as another kind of total war that is silent but could be as deadly, added another dimension to the anxieties and sadness of today. The latest is the so called "No contact war" where adversaries are killed from afar by means of "drones" (Kumar, 2014; Fedyk, 2016). Battle fields have become diffuse, national boundaries are becoming somewhat notional; the implications of these developments in war-making for the armed forces and society are yet to be grasped fully.

As instrument of state, armed forces of a nation are obliged to continuously reorient and re-engineer themselves to achieve their mission. There is always a cost to pay. Soldiering had never been easy but for the present-day armed forces, particularly that of a developing country like India, it has become enormously demanding and intensely stressful in various ways. Moreover, scarce resources have to be diverted to maintain large standing armed forces. It costs lives and money to wage war or enforce peace.

PSYCHIATRIC CASUALTIES

Combat stress behaviors cover the full range of behaviors, both positive and negative, that are seen in combat situations. The positives, which emerge in battle, are heroic acts of valour and high morale. Combat fatigue and misconduct behaviors are the negative outcomes of fighting. Combat fatigue was referred earlier on as "War Neurosis", "Shell Shock", and "Exhaustion" in various wars. Mild combat fatigue manifests in form of symptoms and signs of anxiety. In addition to the predominant anxiety, overactivity or underactivity occur in moderate combat fatigue. Psychotic symptoms characterize severe combat fatigue. Combat fatigue is not considered as a psychiatric disorder in battle. All psychological symptoms arising in battle field are considered as combat fatigue and treated as close to the battle field as possible on the time-honoured principles of Proximity, Immediacy, Expectancy, and Simplicity (PIES), enunciated initially by Thomas Salmon in WWI. Such behaviors as rape, stealing, ill-treating unarmed people and assaulting comrades or superior officers are considered misconduct behaviors and are handled appropriately as per military law. Nuclear, chemical, and biological warfare produce specific kinds of manifestations in a disaster like scenario (Raju, 2013). Detailed descriptions of management are deliberately avoided here.

Psychiatric casualties of war have been described since the beginning of recorded history (Crocq & Crocq, 2000; Raju, 2013; Jones & Wessely, 2014). It was found that they bear a definite relationship to the intensity of battle. One million and 2.5 million Indian soldiers fought under the British flag in WWI and WWII respectively. Psychiatric casualties in respect of armed forces personnel of India are not available but a most conservative estimate of 25,000 in WWI and 50,000 in WWII can be made from the figures available for physical casualties (Raju, 2013). Forward psychiatric facilities, called "Exhaustion Centres" manned by psychiatrists were available close to the battle field in the Eastern theatre in India during WWII (Raju, 2013). Kirpal Singh reported "a large number" of severe combat fatigue cases from Burma front. For unknown reason, psychiatrists were not made available to fighting formations after independence. One study each from the wars of 1965 and 1971 was reported but not much information about combat fatigue could be gathered from these studies (Raju, 2013). No information about psychiatric casualties of peace keeping operations also is available (Raju, 2014). Significantly high levels of anxiety, depression and alcohol abuse were reported in soldiers operating in LIC areas (Bhat et al., 2003; Chaudhary et al., 2006). High incidence (75.7%) of PTSD in poly trauma cases in LIC soldiers has been reported. At the end of one year, only about 5% of these cases were found to be symptomatic (Saldanha et al., 1996). Raju (2013, 2014) reviewed the psychiatric issues related to nuclear, chemical and biological warfare situations, and in the context of prisoners of war, terrorism and peace keeping operations.

SELECTION AND SCREENING

Screening to reject persons for military service on account of mental illnesses or unsuitable personality who are unlikely to fit into a team and selecting an appropriate person for a particular job became important during WWI, when science entered the battle field in a big way and men in hitherto unimaginable numbers had to be selected in a short period (Menninger, 1979). Advances in communications, arms, support services, medical services, transport, mobility, management, advances in navy and air force—all made war-making a highly complex science which demanded individuals with special skills, aptitudes, and capacity. Screening became controversial when it was found that in spite of large scale rejections on grounds of "weak personalities". Soldiers continued to breakdown under stress of combat. It was realized that the validity of tests that would predict a future breakdown was indeed limited (Jones et al., 2003; Rona et al., 2006; Mukherjee et al., 2009). However, the fact remains that a modern soldier will be required to have at least average intelligence and an aptitude for a given job to effectively function as a soldier, and perform trade specific task and multitasking in times of need. In India, cadets and recruits get rejected even after a certain period of training when they are assessed as "unlikely to be efficient soldiers" after assessment of their performance while still undergoing training. Norms for various jobs are created afterwards thorough job analysis and are regularly updated in our country by the Defence Institute of Psychological Research. Screening tests for PBOR are in the process of implementation. Prospective officer cadets are put through a screening test at first. Persons so selected are subjected to a rigorous process of psychological testing, group testing, and interview over a period of 5 days. Predictive validity of the selection process is tested by the post selection performance of cadets in training (Mukherjee et al., 2009).

MENTAL HEALTH WORKFORCE AND FUNCTIONING

In India, the earliest mental hospitals were constructed to take care of the British soldiers. During WWII, psychiatric services rapidly expanded, and 42 psychiatric centers came up at various locations in India by 1945. At present, the Indian Armed Forces are served by a network of 32 psychiatric centers in military hospitals (MHs) of army, navy and air force, dispersed across the country. There are about 60 psychiatrists in the armed forces. Depending on the bed strength, each center may have 1–5 psychiatrists (Bhat, 2017). In the great expansion of the medical corps in WWII, medical officers (MOs) were given training for six months and allowed to function as "Graded Specialists in Psychiatry". This practice is long discarded. The armed forces select candidates, train them for three years and conduct their own university level examination to get graded specialists. Before the final examination, a screening examination and mid-course examination are conducted. Failure at any of the examination may disqualify a person to continue further training. The lowest level specialist is called a "Graded Specialist". A graded specialist can become a "Classified Specialist" after 5 years of service, after successfully undergoing a minimum period of 1-month observation under a "Senior Adviser in Psychiatry" to become a classified specialist. A postgraduate degree in psychiatry from a recognized university is mandatory for becoming a classified specialist. Most of the armed forces psychiatrists undergo postgraduate training at the Armed Forces Medical College located in Pune. The military and professional qualities of classified specialist are assessed every year in the chain of command of medical services. Selected persons on attaining the rank of Colonel are appointed as "Senior Advisers". The highest appointment for a psychiatrist is "Consultant", which is tenable by a psychiatrist holding the rank of Brigadier.

Psychiatric centers are located at big MHs. Their bed strength may vary anywhere between 20 and 65 beds (Bhat, 2017). Besides the psychiatrists, each of the centers are staffed by psychiatric nurses as per requirement and by a category of specialized paramedical men called "Psychiatric Nursing Assistants". They are usually referred as "PNAs". Depending on their level of knowledge and skill, the PNAs are grouped into Class 3 to Class 1 grades. Each psychiatric center is provided with PNAs in the ratio of 2 per 5 patients. PNAs are trained at AFMC and other designated MHs. They observe patients round the clock and submit observational reports in writing to the psychiatrist twice in a day. They also offer diversional, occupational and group therapy to the patients and look after their personal hygiene, nutritional care, security, and general welfare in various ways as well. A clinical psychologist is also posted at each psychiatric center. At present, the armed forces are deficient in clinical psychologists.

The commanding officer (CO) of a MH is responsible for the efficient functioning of the psychiatric center. Senior advisers monitor the professional aspect of functioning of psychiatric centers under their jurisdiction regularly through various reports and carry out personal inspection of each psychiatric center at least once in a year. Fatal case medical documents are scrutinized at various levels, right up to the service headquarters. Lapses in management of cases are dealt with as per procedures. In certain cases, a psychiatrist may lose his specialist status in the medical services. Each psychiatric center submits an annual "Specialist Return" on a prescribed format to the Senior Adviser who puts his remarks and transmits it further up through the channel to the Director General Medical Services of the respective service headquarters.

MENTAL HEALTH MORBIDITY

Governments in some countries are keeping the information about mental health morbidity in public domain, but the incidence and prevalence of mental illnesses in the armed forces of India is classified information and therefore cannot be quoted here, but it can be stated that it is much less than the prevalence figures in the general population. Because of the closed society and constant supervision, behavioral abnormalities and symptoms are detected quite early in the armed forces. Suspected cases of mental illnesses are referred to the nearest psychiatric center by regimental medical officer (RMO) or authorized medical attendant along with a note on prescribed form from the CO of the unit to which the soldier belongs. The note from the CO describes the suspected patient's premorbid behavior, his work record and such other information which came to his knowledge. In the armed forces, the fitness of officers and men is assessed on a scale of five by a medical board based on the recommendations of the specialist. Full medical documents including a detailed handwritten summary and opinion of the specialist is submitted to the medical board. In certain cases, a specialist's opinion has to be concurred by a senior adviser. All efforts are made to retain in service even the seriously ill, till the person is eligible to earn minimum pension. Consumption of alcohol is a part of military culture and when consumed in moderation could be a great motivator (Raju et al., 2002). There are divergent views in medical community about alcohol in the armed forces. A rising trend of alcohol consumption in PBOR was observed in a hospital based study (Raju et al., 2002). Most of the alcohol dependent subjects were not able to hold jobs beyond three years (Raju et al., 2002). However, after the deterrent new army order in 2001, retention rates increased four times (Saldanha et al., 2007).

Suicide is a major concern for the armed forces. Contrary to what is reported in the lay press, the prevalence of suicides in the armed forces is less than that of general population. The figures are in the public domain. During the period 2003-2007 a total of 635 suicides occurred; from 2007 to 2010, the number came down to 533 which further came down to 413 during the period 2012- 2015 (Bhat, 2017; Kaur, 2017). This improvement can be attributed to various preventive measures taken at individual, unit and administrative levels over the past 10 years.

STRESS MANAGEMENT IN ARMED FORCES

Stress is inevitable in any war or war like situation. Stress management in any armed forces should ideally involve a gamut of activities, starting from the homes of soldiers to the regimental centers, academies, before deployment, during deployment and after deployment in combat and back at home to complete the cycle of stress management. The present author along with a team of psychologists from Defence Institute of Psychological Research (DIPR) conducted "Combat Stress Management" camps for officers, for the first time in free India, to create awareness in them to combat stress, to identify symptoms of combat stress and manage stress at individual level by various methods (Raju, 2013). A series of measures at organizational levels to reduce stress, which included more liberally spaced leave, opportunities to live with families, grievance redressal mechanisms, enhanced field service pay and so on, were also suggested and incrementally implemented as well (Ryali et al., 2011). Stress management course for instructors of various army, navy and air force training establishments were also conducted. Middle ranked officers were made to undergo a short course in military psychology. Subsequent to these initiatives, a mental health program for the army was chalked out to train military mental health mentors, religious teachers and officers, junior commissioned officers (JCOs) and non-commissioned officers (NCOs) at various levels in a mission mode. A small manual on combat stress management in Hindi and English was published by DIPR (Raju & Singh, 2004) to further enhance awareness levels in mental health. Non-specialist medical officers are given lectures and demonstrations on mental health issues at various "*in service*" courses of armed forces medical services.

MILITARY FAMILIES

Family relationships are particularly important for military personnel. On a rough estimate, India has 5.5 million family members of armed forces personnel. In many cases, military runs in the families. For the soldier, family is a big support as well as source of concern. Family concerns are among the top of the presumptive life stress scale (Raju et al., 2001). The lot of families has much improved over the years with improved housing, health care, and education facilities. Welfare activities are run through Wives Welfare Associations of the army, navy and air force. Family concerns are cited as precipitating factors in 66% of cases of suicide (Bhat, 2017). Easy communication could be a big support as well as a source of stress for the soldier who is far away. Professional counseling services are made available at some garrisons. Perhaps there is a case for nodal officer with a small team at every garrison who can liaise with civil authorities to solve disputes related to property issues and so on. The Army Welfare Education Society runs a chain 130 army public schools, 249 pre-primary schools and 11 technical colleges. Air Force and Navy run their own public schools. Children of armed forces personnel learn to be self-reliant because of long absences of a parent on field postings, courses and operational duties. Families of armed forces personnel are not eligible for indoor admission to psychiatric centres, but outpatient services are offered free of cost. Jyoti et al reviewed issues related to army wives (Prakash et al., 2011). No significant differences in behavior problems between children of armed forces personnel and children of civilian population was found (Prakash et al., 2006). The issue of "Secondary Traumatisation" in wives of homecoming soldier is recognized around the world (Prakash et al., 2011; Raju, 2014).

CONCLUSION

India has a long heritage of organized armed forces. Battle field psychology is highlighted eons ago in the Gita. Modern combat psychiatrist exactly does what Krishna did exhorting the reluctant warrior to fight right in the battle field. Psychological issues in the armed forces became subject of serious study in the WWI but hardly any information is available on the mental health of Indian soldier. The interregnum too was devoid of any significant literature on military psychiatry. Psychiatric services expanded rapidly during the WWII in India and laid down the frame work for mental health services in the armed forces. Over the past decade, significant strides have been made in developing a mental health infrastructure at various levels. Modern war is a mind game. The Indian Armed Forces have a group of enthusiastic, highly talented and skilled psychiatrists with operational experience and a responsive command structure which is very much alive to the psychological issues relevant to the armed forces; given the prevailing positives, one would hope to see the emergence of embedded mental health teams at formation level, psychological support, and counseling centers at every garrison for families of armed forces personnel, and a director of armed forces psychiatry at Delhi to oversee mental health efforts and to apprise regularly the same to highest medical authority of armed forces. The subject of social psychiatry in armed forces is vast. The issues related to women in armed forces and ex-servicemen are not covered in the present article. Only a glimpse of various issues could be described here for the sake of brevity and limitations of space.

REFERENCES

Badrinath P. Psychological impact of protracted service in low intensity conflict. Operations in armed forces personnel. USI Journal. 2003;xxxiii:38-58.

Baijal R, Jha N, Sinha A, et al. Stimulation based SD training in Indian Air Force, Indian J Aerospace Med. 2006;50(2):1-6.

Bhagavad Gita 1.2. Mumbai: Bhaktivedanta Book Trust; 1986.

Bhat PS, Mehta VK, Chaudhary S. Evaluation of Psychological effects of counter Insurgency operations on Soldiers. Armed Forces Research Committee Project No. 3164. 2003.

Bhat PS. Combat Psychiatry: Indian perspective. Med J Armed Forces India. 2017;73(4):404-6.

Boring EG. Psychology for the Armed Forces. Dehradun: Natraj Publishers; 1979.

Campise RA, Geller SK, Campise ME. Combat Stress. In: Hand KC, Zilmer EA (Eds).Military Psychology. New York: Guilford Press; 2006.

Carver. Morale in battle—the medical and the military. J R Soc Med. 1989;82(2):67-71.

Chaudhary S, Singh H, Goel DS. Psychological effects of low intensity conflict operations. Indian J Psychiatry. 2006;48(4):223-31.

Crocq MA, Crocq L. From shell shock and war neurosis to posttraumatic stress disorder: a history of psychotraumatology. Dialogues Clin Neurosci. 2000;2(1):47-55.

Fedyk N. Russian "New Generation Warfare". Theory, Practice, and Lessons for US Strategists. Small War. 2016;25(7):45.

Gabriel RA, Metz KS. A short history of war: The evolution of warfare and weapons. Strategic Studies Institute, US Army War College; 1992.

Jones DR. US Air Force Comabat Psychiatry. In: Bones FD, Sparaceno U, Wilcox V, Rosenberg JM, Stokes JW (Eds).War Psychiatry. Washinton DC: TMM Publication, Borden Institute, Walter Reed Army Medical Centre; 1995.

Jones E, Hyams KC, Wessely S. Screening for vulnerability to psychological disorders in the Military: A historical survey. J Med Screening. 2003;10(1):40-6.

Jones E, Wessely S. Battle for the mind: World War I and the birth of military Psychiatry. Lancet. 2014;384:1708-14.

Kaur R. Mental illness in India. Defence Life Science Journal. 2017;73:404-6.

Kumar BKU, Malik H. An analysis of fatal human error in aircraft accidents in Indian Air Force. Indian J Aerospace Med. 2003;47(1):30-5.

Kumar D. No contact war and the China factor. Scholar Warrior Spring; 2014;pp.77-84.

Mahalingam V. Role of military culture and traditions in building ethics, morale and combat effectiveness in fighting units. J Defence Studies. 2013;7:95-108.

Menninger WC. Psychiatry in troubled world—yesterday's war and today's challenge. New York: The Macmillan Company; 1979.

Mukherjee S, Kumar U, Mandal MK. Status of military psychology in India. J Indian Acad App Psychol. 2009;35(2):181-94.

Navathe PA, Singh B. Prevention of spatial disorientation in Indian air force crew. Aviation, space, and environmental medicine. 1994;65(2):1082-5.

Pawar AA. Psychiatry at Sea (Souvenir). Armed Forces Medical College, Pune, ANCIPS; 2001.

Prakash J, Bavdekar RD, Joshi SB. The war of waiting wives; psychosocial battle in home front. Med J Armed Forces India. 2011;67:58-63.

Prakash J, Sudarsanan S, Pardal PK, et al. Study of behavioural problems in a paediatric outpatient department. Med J Armed Forces India. 2006;62(4):339-41.

Raju MSVK, Chaudhary S, Sudarsanan S, et al. Trends and issues in relation to alcohol dependence in armed forces. Med J Armed Forces India. 2002;58(2):143-8.

Raju MSVK, Singh NP. Combat Stress behaviours in LIC operations. Delhi Defence Institute of Psychological Research; 2004.

Raju MSVK, Srivastava K, Chaudhary S, et al. Quantification of stressful life events in soldiers. Indian J Psychiatry. 2001;43:213-8.

Raju MSVK. Looking back and ahead—some perspectives of military psychiatry. AP J Psychol Med. 2013;14(2):85-94.

Raju MSVK. Psychological aspects of peacekeeping operations. Indust Psychiatry J. 2014;23: 149-56.

Rona RJ, Hooper R, Jones M, et al. Mental health screening in the armed forces before Iraq war. Br Med J. 2006;333(7576):991.

Ryali VSSR, Bhat PS, Srivastava K. Stress in the armed forces how true and what to do. Med J Armed Forces India. 2011;67:209-11.

Saldanha D, Chaudhary S, Pawar AA, et al. Changing pattern of alcohol abuse in the army before and after 2001. Med J Armed Forces India. 2007;63:160-2.

Saldanha D, Goel DS, Kapoor S. Posttraumatic stress disorder in poly trauma cases. Med J Armed Forces India. 1996;52(1):35-9.

Shrinagesh SM. Psychophysiological Mechanisms in Flying. PRW Note 203, Psychological Research wing, DRDO, Ministry of Defence; 1960.

Thapar DR.The Morale builders. Bombay: Asia Publishing House; 1965.

Chapter 40

Legislation and Mental Health

RC Jiloha, Deeksha Elwadhi

SUMMARY

The current judicial system of India is still largely influenced by years of the British rule. The advancement in our understanding of health and diseases has brought forth a new understanding regarding mental illnesses as well. The earlier legislations were mainly focused on the protection of the society from the "deviant behaviors" of such individuals. With remarkable progress in treatment of mental illnesses, the focus has shifted on to treatment and welfare of such patients. The world today is also ushering in a dawn of equality and justice with the legislations moving toward rights-based paradigm.

The United Nations Convention on the Rights of Persons with Disabilities (UNCRPD) recommended major changes in law and policy concerning disability in 2006 with the premise of protecting legal capacity, equality, and dignity of persons with mental illness. As a consequence, in India, the Mental Health Act (MHA), 1987 and the Rights of Persons with Disabilities Act, 1995 were revised as the Mental Healthcare Act, 2017 and the Rights of Persons with Disabilities Act, 2016 to protect the rights of persons with mental illness and also to protect them from injustice and discrimination. The Indian laws concerned with determination of competency, criminal, and civil responsibility of persons with mental illness are also discussed in this chapter.

INTRODUCTION

Scientific progress in the cure and treatment of medical disorders and diseases has paralleled with the strengthening of the legal framework pertaining to the issues related to these disorders and diseases. Mental illness brings in a unique vulnerability to its afflicted, which predisposes the patients to become victims of neglect and abuse (Jiloha, 2015). Only 63% of the countries are reported to have dedicated mental health legislation (World Health Organization, 2014). Legislation serves to regulate, authorize, sanction, outlaw, grant, declare , restrict or facilitate the smooth functioning and existence of the modern society.

Since time immemorial, segregation and custodial care of mentally ill persons into asylums away from the main-stream society has been governed by certain laws. Legislation has often represented the mind set and attitude of the society toward mental illness and the mentally ill. In view of the recent developments, worldwide mental health legislation is focusing on the quality of mental healthcare, rights of the mentally ill, administrative measures, community participation, budget and involvement of stakeholders in provision of services.

There can be two kinds of approaches toward mental health legislation: specific and generalized. In the former, specific issues pertaining to the uniqueness of mental illnesses are dealt within a consolidated single law, whereas in the latter, provisions are made in the existing laws to include legislation related to mental health (Freeman & Pathare, 2005).

The understanding of mental health legislation is of paramount importance for a psychiatrist because of the various underpinnings it carries, with service provision and treatment being governed by the laws. In addition, the psychiatrist has to deal with the patients who come in conflict with the common law of land. With psychiatry gradually moving toward rights-based approach, it becomes essential for all mental health professionals to have a clear understanding of the dynamic interplay of mental illness and law.

LEGAL DEFINITION OF MENTAL ILLNESS

The Indian Lunacy Act (ILA) 1912 used the term lunatic, which included idiots (mentally subnormal) and the persons with "unsound mind". The term "unsound mind" has also been used in the Indian Penal Code (IPC) and is equated to mean insanity. Legal insanity is different from medical insanity. The MHA, 1987 defined a mentally ill person as, "a person who is in need of treatment by reason of any mental disorder other than mental retardation". This definition did not describe what mental illness is. The Mental Healthcare Act (MHCA), 2017, defines mental illness as, "a substantial disorder of thinking, mood, perception, orientation or memory that grossly impairs judgment, behavior, capacity to recognize reality or ability to meet the ordinary demands of life, mental conditions associated with the abuse of alcohol and drugs, but does not include mental retardation which is a condition of arrested or incomplete development of mind of a person, specially characterized by subnormality of intelligence".

NEED FOR LEGISLATION IN MENTAL HEALTH: CHALLENGES AND SPECIAL ISSUES CONCERNING THE MENTALLY ILL

Persons with mental illness are often victims of abuse and their rights are violated. Legislation therefore comes to their rescue and provides a safeguard against such atrocities. However, legislation, if not in accordance with the riding principles of equal rights and dignity, can worsen the stigma associated with such illnesses, giving them a judicial fervor rather than a medical one. Mental disorders contribute significantly to the disability-adjusted life years, thus increasing the socioeconomic burden. The trends indicate a further increase in the burden in the coming future. With the widespread stigma and discrimination accompanying mental illnesses, the felt burden increases significantly in these patients (Sayers, 2001).

Mental health legislation can thus contribute significantly in dealing with certain critical issues in a legal framework including community integration, better access to treatment, and quality of care for persons with mental illness along with protection and promotion of their civil rights including provision for housing, education and employment (Freeman & Pathare, 2005).

In 1996, the World Health Organization (WHO), gave ten basic principles to assist countries in developing laws related to mental health (World Health Organization, 1996). These included:

1. Promotion of mental health and prevention of mental disorders
2. Access to basic mental health care
3. Mental health assessments in accordance with internationally accepted principles
4. Provision of least restrictive type of mental health care
5. Self-determination
6. Right to be assisted in the exercise of self-determination
7. Availability of review procedure
8. Automatic periodic review mechanism
9. Qualified decision-maker
10. Respect of the rule of law.

SPECIFIC LAWS GOVERNING MENTAL HEALTH

History of Mental Health Laws in India

The first Lunacy Act (ILA) (Act 36), drafted in 1858, laid down the guidelines for the establishment of mental asylums and procedures for admitting patients, which was replaced by the ILA (Act 4) in 1912. The postindependence period saw tremendous growth in health services and a paradigm shift in the management of the mentally ill, moving from captivity to community integration. The main focus of concern remained the lack of infrastructure and manpower. Considering the limited resources, integration of mental health with primary health care has generally been considered to deal with the increasing burden of mental and substance use disorders.

Replacement of the ILA, 1912 by the MHA, 1987, and the enactment of the Persons with Disabilities Act, 1995 heralded the dawn of a new era, which brought the concept of equal opportunities, rights and full participation of persons with disability, and also included mental illness under the ambit of disability. Another key development that has affected the growth of legislation in psychiatry has been the development of private psychiatry in a big way and problems associated with the regulation of provision of services.

It is of crucial interest to understand the salient features of the previous legislation and their shortcomings for understanding the culmination to the MHCA, 2017.

Indian Lunacy Act, 1912

The purpose of the ILA was to ensure custodial care and preventing the lunatics from harming society, which reflected the general perception of mental illness at that time. There was no provision of treatment, rights or welfare, and there was no time limit specified for involuntary admission. The draconian law prevailed for more than 70 years and could not keep pace with the fast occurring developments in the field of psychiatry.

The Mental Health Act, 1987

The MHA, 1987, spread in 10 chapters and 98 sections came as a result of mammoth efforts of India's mental health professionals. It was a step toward the treatment-centric paradigm of psychiatry and laid emphasis on psychiatric hospitals/nursing homes, and tried to bring mental illnesses at par with physical illnesses by replacing offensive terms like lunatic and mental hospital with mentally ill and psychiatric hospital/nursing homes respectively.

Creation of mental health authorities and provision of judicial safeguard for human rights and property were the important milestones of the Act. However, it did not promote community mental health care or integration with primary health care, and neither made provisions of rehabilitation or choice and consent for treatment (Trivedi, 2009).

UN Convention on the Rights of Persons with Disabilities

Adopted on December 13, 2006 and implemented on May 3, 2008, the UNCRPD includes mental illness into disabilities. India is one of the signatories and ratified it in October, 2007. The convention is a flag bearer for the movement of rights-based legislation and policies concerning persons with disabilities. It held the state responsible for ensuring that appropriate measures are in place for full inclusion and participation of the disabled individuals. The convention is based on the presumption of legal capacity, equality and dignity for persons with disability. India, being a signatory, was obliged to modify the existing laws in accordance with the principles suggested by the UNCRPD (Choudhary et al., 2011).

Mental Healthcare Act, 2017

The MHCA, 2017 provides for mental health care and services for persons with mental illness, and protect, promote and fulfill the rights of such persons during delivery of mental health care and services and for matters connected. It is divided into 16 chapters and 126 sections. **Table 1** lists the chapters and their salient features.

The MHCA, 2017 takes precedence in defining mental health care including rehabilitation of persons with mental illness. It covers all health establishments (general hospitals/nursing homes owned by others), where persons with mental illness are admitted for care, treatment, convalescence, or rehabilitation, designated as mental health establishments. The Mental Health Professional as per the MHCA can be a psychiatrist, or AYUSH (Ayurveda, Yoga, Unani, Siddha, Homeopathy) practitioner having a degree in "Manas Rog".

The Act emphasizes on diagnosing mental disorders in accordance with the nationally or internationally recognized criteria, and denies any conformity with moral, social, cultural, work or political values, or religious beliefs to make a diagnosis of mental illness. It establishes soundness of mind to be a legal concept to be decided by a competent court.

Advance directive and nominated representative are fairly new concepts and their understanding becomes pertinent for the health professionals for adequate provision of care.

Every person, who is not a minor, can make an advance directive in writing, specifying the way the person wishes/not wishes to be cared for and treated for a mental illness; and appoint a nominated representative, who will be responsible for making the above decisions in cases when the person is unable to do so. The legal guardian will be the nominated representative for a minor.

As per the MHCA, 2017, an advance directive shall be invoked only when the person ceases to have capacity to make mental health care decisions and can be revoked, amended or cancelled by the person. Medical professionals are bound to follow the advance directive

Chapter number	Heading	Salient features
Table 1: Salient features of the Mental Healthcare Act, 2017		
I	Preliminary	Definitions of various terminologies used in the Act
II	Mental illness and capacity to make mental healthcare and treatment decisions	Directions regarding the diagnosis of mental illness; capacity to make decisions
III	Advance directive	Description of advance directive, its making, and provision of online registration for recordkeeping
IV	Nominated representative	Description of the appointment, revocation, and duties of the nominated representative
V	Rights of persons with mental illness	Enlists the basic rights of persons with mental illness and directs the government to make provisions regarding their fulfillment
VI	Duties of appropriate government	Entails the duties of the appropriate government
VII	Central Mental Health Authority	Describes the composition and functions of the Central Mental Health Authority
VIII	State Mental Health Authority	Describes the composition and functions of the State Mental Health Authority
IX	Finance, accounts, and audit	Describes the grants by the central government and use of funds by the central authority
X	Mental health establishments	Procedure for registration of mental health establishments, inspection and inquiry, and provisions of their adequate functioning
XI	Mental health review boards	Composition and functions of the mental health review board and judiciary powers
XII	Admission, treatment, and discharge	Describes the admission procedures, emergency, and prohibitory treatment modalities
XIII	Responsibilities of other agencies	Outlines the duties of police officers in regard to the wandering persons with mental illness and suspected neglect of such persons; prisoners with mental illness
XIV	Restriction to discharge functions by professionals not covered by profession	Limitations of the professionals to work under the Act and principles of ethical evidence-based treatments
XV	Offences and penalties	Describes the offenses and penalties in contravention to the Act
XVI	Miscellaneous	Deals with locus of power, special provision for neglected areas, decriminalizing suicide and laying of rules and regulations

and the Act absolves the medical practitioner from the liability of unforeseen consequences of a valid advanced directive. The advance directive does not apply to emergency treatment.

Rights of persons with mental illness and duties of the government: MHCA has been envisaged with the underlying principles of protection, promotion, and fulfillment of the rights of persons with mental illness The principles are outlined as below:

- Right to access mental health care
- Right to community living
- Right to protection from cruel, inhuman and degrading treatment
- Right to equality and nondiscrimination
- Right to information
- Right to confidentiality
- Right to free legal aid
- Right to make complaints about deficiencies in provision of services.

The government has to ensure provision of services needed for the fulfillment of the above rights to ensure that persons with mental illness achieve their full potential. It directs the government to launch programs for awareness and promotion of mental health, eradication of stigma, and suicide reduction with provisions for human resource development and training. A significant breakthrough is that the Act tries to ensure parity in mental health services by directing every insurer to make provision for medical insurance for treatment of mental illness.

Central and State Mental Health Authority: The Act directs the central government to form a Central Mental Health Authority, chaired by the Secretary/Additional Secretary (Department of Health and Family Welfare, Government of India), and having bureaucrats, Director General of Health Services, directors of central institutes of mental health and mental health professionals from different disciplines as its members. In addition, the authority will have representation from the main stakeholders with two representatives of persons with mental illness, caregivers and nongovernmental organizations (NGOs).

Functions of the central authority are as follows:

1. Registration of all mental health establishments under control of central government
2. Developing quality and service provision norms
3. Supervise the mental health establishments and address complaints
4. Maintenance of a national register of clinical psychologists, mental health nurses, and psychiatric social workers
5. Training about provisions and implementation of the act
6. Advisory role to the central government relating to matters of mental health care.

On the similar lines, the state government will establish the State Mental Health Authority, with the influence being limited to the concerned state and its government.

Mental Health Review Board: The Act directs the formation of a Mental Health Review Board (MHRB), which will be a quasijudicial body consisting of District Judge as the chairperson with a representative of the District Collector/Magistrate/Deputy Commissioner of the concerned district along with two members from the medical fraternity (a psychiatrist and a medical practitioner). In addition, two representatives from persons with mental illness/caregivers/ NGOs working in the field of mental health will also be members of the board. The proceedings will be judicial in nature and include:

1. Registering, reviewing, altering, modifying, or cancelling advance directives
2. Appointing a nominated representative
3. Addressing grievances against the decisions of medical officer or mental health professionals in-charge of mental health establishments
4. Taking decisions regarding nondisclosure of information
5. Addressing complaints pertaining to shortcomings in care and services specified
6. Inspection of prisons or jails.

Admission, Treatment, and Discharge

Independent admission (Sections 85–86): Any person requesting admission for his mental illness can be admitted under Sections 85-86. The patient cannot be given treatment without his informed consent and the patient's discharge request cannot be refused by the medical health practitioner. Discharge can only be prevented for 24 hours to allow assessment for supported admission.

Admission of a minor (Section 87): In exceptional circumstances, the nominated representative can apply for admission. An independent examination by two psychiatrists in preceding 7 days should confirm the necessity of admission. The minor will be admitted separately with an accompanying attendant (nominated representative) throughout admission. Information regarding the admission of a minor has to be given to the concerned board within 72 hours.

Supported admission (admission on request of a nominated representative, Section 89): An independent examination by two psychiatrists should confirm the risk of bodily harm or violence to self or to others, or lack of capacity to care for self. In these cases the patient will need very high support from nominated representative and the treatment is as per advance directives or consent from the nominated representative. Admission under this section is valid for 30 days, following which the patient can be discharged or continue as an independent patient as in the above section. The review board has to be informed of all supported admissions within a week, and in case of women and minors within 3 days.

Supported admission beyond 30 days (Section 90): Section 90 is meant for patients already admitted for 30 days under Section 89, with criteria of admission still valid or requiring admission within 7 days of discharge under Section 89. The stay is extended after independent examination by two psychiatrists. The MHRB has to be informed and approval sought within 21 days. The admission of a person with mental illness to a mental health establishment under this section is limited to a period up to 90 days in the first instance, which can be extended for a period of 120 days and thereafter for a period of 180 days.

Emergency treatment (Section 94): Any medical practitioner can offer emergency treatment in cases where it is immediately necessary to prevent death or irreversible harm with consent of nominated representative at any health establishment or in community, limited to 72 hours.

Prohibited procedures, seclusion and restraint: Unmodified electroconvulsive therapy (ECT), sterilization, chaining, solitary confinement, and ECT for minors is prohibited. When ECT is deemed necessary for a minor, a prior consent of the nominated representative and permission from the concerned board is needed. Psychosurgery as a treatment can be performed only after informed consent from the patient and prior approval of the review board. Physical restraints are permitted only in situation of great imminent danger for limited time after authorization from the medical officer in charge, with the board being informed regarding all instances of physical restraints.

Decriminalizing suicide: Section 115 of the MHCA states that, "notwithstanding anything contained in Section 309 of the IPC, any person who attempts to commit suicide shall be presumed, unless proved otherwise, to have severe stress and shall not be tried and punished under the said Code". It puts the responsibility to provide care, treatment, and rehabilitation to the person having severe stress who attempted to commit suicide on the appropriate government.

Other Significant Acts in Mental Health

The Narcotic Drugs and Psychotropic Substances Act, 1985

The Narcotic Drugs and Psychotropic Substances Act, 1985, was enacted, consolidating, and amending the provisions for the control and regulation of operation relating to narcotic drugs and psychotropic substances under the Opium Act, 1878 and the Dangerous Drugs Act, 1930. This Act was amended in 1989, 2001, and 2014. The last amendment was aimed at ensuring essential opioid medicines for medical use, which was tragically difficult in the previous Acts. Spread in eight chapters, the Act enlists punishments for production, possession, transportation, trading, purchase and use of any of the listed substances.

National Trust for the Welfare of Persons with Autism, Cerebral Palsy, Mental Retardation, and Multiple Disabilities Act, 1999

This Act seeks to provide for the constitution of a body at the National level for the Welfare of Persons with Autism, Cerebral Palsy, Mental Retardation and Multiple Disabilities, and for matters connected, to enable and empower persons with disability to live as independently and as fully as possible within and as close to the community to which they belong and to facilitate the realization of equal opportunities, protection of rights, and full participation of persons with disability.

The Rights of Persons with Disabilities Act, 2016

In 1992, India signed the Proclamation on the Full Participation and Equality of People with Disabilities and thereafter, came Persons with Disabilities (Equal Opportunities, Protection of Rights, and Full Participation) Act, 1995, recognizing mental illness as a disability. This brought a new era in the disability-related legislation, however it had lot of shortcomings including poor implementation, lack of awareness, and limited state participation (Bhargava et al., 2012).

With the ratification of the UNCRPD on October 1, 2007, the Persons with Disabilities Act of 1995 was amended and The Rights of Persons with Disabilities Act was passed by the Indian Parliament in December, 2016. The Act deals with the rights and entitlements of persons with disability with special emphasis on increasing accessibility and community participation. Learning disorder and autism spectrum disorders are new entrants to the schedule of disabilities consisting of physical disability, intellectual disability, mental disability, and disability due to chronic medical conditions and multiple disabilities.

INTERFACE OF THE COMMON LAW AND MENTAL HEALTH

Criminal Responsibility

Patients with mental illness stand in the court of law in the same way as any other offender in criminal cases. Two important components required for proving guilty of a crime are "actus reus" (the act was unlawful) and "mens rea" (the mind was guilty). According to Section 84 of the IPC, which is inspired from the famous McNaughton rules, "Nothing is an offence which is done by a person who, at the time of doing it, by reason of unsoundness of mind, is incapable of knowing the nature of the act, or that he is doing what is either wrong or contrary to law".

Civil Responsibility

According to Section 118 of the Indian Evidence Act, 1872, all persons are competent to testify in court unless proven otherwise and mental illness in itself does not make the person incompetent to testify.

The Indian Contract Act, 1872 in Chapter 2, section 12 under exclusions describes a person to be of sound mind for the purpose of making a contract, if, "at the time when he makes it, he is capable of understanding it and of forming a rational judgment as to its effect upon his interest."

No person of unsound mind (as declared by a competent court) can contest an election or exercise the franchise of voting. Soundness of mind is task-specific and situation-specific, falling under the purview of the court of law.

Testamentary Capacity

According to the Indian Succession Act, 1925, "Will" is the legal declaration of the intention of a testator with respect to his property which he desires to be carried into effect after his death.

Testamentary capacity refers to person's full sense and mental sanity to have confirmed and signed the Will after understanding what his assets comprised and what he is doing by making a Will. It is the legal status of executing a Will.

The act of making a Will should be voluntary without any undue influence, fraud or coercion and the testator should have a sound mind with adequate knowledge of the nature of act, extent of property, potential beneficiaries, and the consequences of the decision (Jiloha, 2009).

Psychiatrist in Court

A psychiatrist may be called in court as an expert witness, with special knowledge and experience in a defined field to assess the mental condition and fitness of the person in question. The psychiatric assessment should always be detailed and admission can be advised in case of need of behavioral observation. The psychiatrist should follow a code of conduct and show due respect to the court of law. One should carefully listen to the questions asked, giving a clear and concise report with no medical jargon or moral judgment (Chadda, 2013).

NATIONAL MENTAL HEALTH POLICY

In contrast to legislation, a mental health policy is an organized set of values, principles, and objectives, for improving mental health and reducing the burden of mental disorders (World Health Organization, 2005). It is a blueprint of attaining the set objectives. Ministry of Health and Family Welfare, Government of India launched the National Mental Health Policy of India, "New Pathways New Hope" on October 10, 2014 with the following goals:

- To reduce distress, disability, exclusion, morbidity, and premature mortality associated with mental health problems across lifespan
- To enhance understanding of mental health in country
- To strengthen the leadership in mental health sector at national, state, and district levels.

The policy envisions "to promote mental health and prevent mental illness, to enable recovery, to promote destigmatization and desegregation leading to socioeconomic inclusion of persons affected with mental illness, and to provide accessible, affordable, quality health, and social care within a rights-based framework."

The policy is a progressive and welcome step pertaining to the provision of mental health services. It strengthens the seriousness of mental illnesses, and consolidates the rights-based framework on which further legislation and mental health programs may be built.

CONCLUSION

The interface of law and mental health is intriguing and needs to be studied in detail for a better understanding of the need of legislation in the first place and its effective implementation. With the constant burden of inequality, vulnerability, and stigma being carried by patients with mental illnesses, it becomes important to safeguard their rights in a legislative framework. Legislation has brought all the components of mental health care delivery under its purview to ensure an equality and basic standard of health care provision, expected from a developed society. In addition, mental illnesses bring forth challenges in the common laws of the land which need to be tailored to accommodate the uniqueness of these patients.

REFERENCES

Bhargava R, Sivakumar T, Rozatkar A. Persons with disabilities (equal opportunities, protection of rights and full participation) act 1995. In: Chavan BS, Gupta N, Arun P, Sidana A, Jadhav S (Eds). Community Mental Health in India. New Delhi: Jaypee Brothers Medical Publishers (P) Ltd; 2012. pp. 169-75.

Chadda RK. Forensic evaluations in psychiatry. Indian J Psychiatry. 2013;55(4):393.

Choudhary LN, Narayan M, Deep Shikha. The ongoing process of amendments in MHA-87 and PWD Act-95 and their implications on mental health care. Indian J Psychiatry 2011;53(4):343-50.

Freeman M, Pathare S. WHO Resource Book on Mental Health, Human Rights and Legislation. Geneva, World Health Organization 2005.

Jiloha RC. Mental capacity/testamentary capacity. Clinical Practice Guidelines of the Indian Psychiatric Society. Forensic Psychiatry. 2009;20-34.

Jiloha RC. The Mental Health Act of India. In: Malhotra S, Chakrabarti S (Eds). Developments in Psychiatry in India. India: Springer; 2015. pp. 611-22.

The Narcotic Drugs and Psychotropic Substances (Amendment) Act. Ministry of Law and Justice, Government of India. 2014.

National Mental Health Policy of India: New Pathways, New Hope. New Delhi, Ministry of Health, Government of India. 2014.

National Trust for the Welfare of Persons with Autism, Cerebral Palsy, Mental Retardation and Multiple Disabilities Act (Act 44 of 1999). Ministry of Social Justice and Empowerment, Government of India. 1999.

Sayers J. The World Health Report 2001—Mental health: new understanding, new hope. Bull World Health Organization. 2001;79:1085.

Trivedi JK. Mental Health Act: salient features, objectives, critique and future directions. Indian J Psychiatry. 2009:51:11-9.

World Health Organization. Mental health Care Law: Ten basic principles: With annotations suggesting selected actions to promote their implementation. Geneva: WHO, 1006.

World Health Organization. Mental Health Policy, Plans and Programmes (updated version 2). Geneva, World Health Organization, 2005.

World Health Organization. WHO Mental Health Atlas. Geneva, WHO, 2014.

Chapter 41

Social Impact of Terrorism and Extremism

Debasish Basu, Gagan Hans

SUMMARY

It is abundantly clear that terrorism and extremism in various modalities, magnitude and means are here to stay, and in fact generally on the rise in terms of geographic coverage and frequency. No continent, country, region or society can be said to be immune to these activities any longer. It is also apparent that the very purpose of terrorist acts is to create "terror", not only in the minds of those directly affected by such acts, but more importantly, in the larger society as an overt threat of dire consequences, if the terrorist/extremist demands are not met. Thus, the social impact of terrorism and extremism goes beyond individual psyche (where it can cause several psychiatric disorders and/or psychological sequelae) to the collective psyche or the social mindset. The impact of these acts on society can be economic, psychosocial or existential. These acts set in motion a series of counter-terrorist measures and generate a sense of paranoia in the society, which paradoxically may further fuel the cycle of terrorism in the long run. The whole issue is extremely complex and even controversial.

INTRODUCTION AND SCOPE

Terrorism has emerged as one of the major global challenges in the last few decades. "Terrorism" refers to a broad and very heterogeneous group of offending behaviors. It is difficult, therefore, to make valid and empirically supported generalizations. It can have varied presentations depending on the geographical region of the world that makes studying it as a phenomenon relatively difficult although there is no denying the fact that there are common features observed globally.

The scope of terrorism has increased manifold in the recent years with the adoption of newer methods by the terrorists to escape conventional methods of surveillance with a common goal of inflicting maximum damage to human lives and property. It has been well-established that terrorism is a kind of psychological warfare where primary motive is a creation of a state of panic and chaos in a society through adoption of barbaric and unconventional methods (Kaplan, 1981). Thus, the intention of executing an act of terrorism is to create crippling fear in the minds of individuals in a society (Jones & Fong, 1994).

Terrorism can have an impact on both the individual and the community/nation which may be defined as the personal threat and the national threat respectively. The personal threats are more likely to elicit a greater degree of fear in the mind of an individual rather than the national threats. Terrorists have usually declared a state of war on the government and through the acts of terrorism they demonstrate their capabilities of striking at will and relative impotency of the authorities to safeguard lives of the ordinary citizens. They want to create an atmosphere of helplessness and hopelessness where the assumptions about personal security are invalidated (Trivedi, 2004).

The National Consortium for the Study of Terrorism and Responses to Terrorism, cited by the Global Terrorism Index (2015) has proposed the following criteria for qualifying an event as an act of terrorism related, if two of the following three criteria are met:

1. "The violent act was aimed at attaining a political, economic, religious, or social goal
2. The violent act included evidence of an intention to coerce, intimidate, or convey some other message to a larger audience other than to the immediate victims
3. The violent act was outside the precepts of international humanitarian law".

Krug (2002) in world report on violence and health has defined terrorism as a form of asymmetric warfare in which "an organized group lacking conventional military strength and economic power seeks to attack the weak points inherent in relatively affluent and open societies. The attacks take place with unconventional weapons and tactics and with no regard to military or political codes of conduct."

A common feature of many different forms of terrorism and extremism is that their impact goes (or is intended to go) far beyond individual harm or threat. Rather, the harm and threat is directed to the society at large. As the Prevention of Terrorism Act (POTA, 2002) of India puts it: "Terrorist act produces a prolonged psychological effect on society, disrupts even tempo and tranquility and produces a sense of insecurity in the minds of a section of the society or the whole society".

Hence, the importance of studying and appraising the social impact of terrorism and extremism. In the following sections, after discussing the definitions of some relevant terms, glancing a bird's eye view on the prevalence of terrorism and major terrorist incidents, and briefly visiting the complex issue of psychosocial roots of terrorism, we discuss the main mandate of this chapter. The psychosocial impact of terrorism and extremism is not only on those directly exposed to these acts but also on those large segments of society who are indirectly affected. A short section will examine broad mitigating strategies, and a final section will touch upon the psychosocial impact of counter-terrorist measures as well.

DEFINITIONS: TERRORISM, EXTREMISM, RADICALIZATION, COUNTER-TERRORISM

Defining terrorism has been more difficult in present times than it has ever been in the past. The definition varies from one geographical area to other. Although many definitions have been suggested no definition is complete in the sense of conveying the multiple sub-phenomena associated with it. What has definitely helped flourish terrorism is that it can be used both in the context of violent resistance to the state as well as in the service of the state interests. The United Nations (1999) defines a terrorist act as:

- "Any act intended to cause death or serious bodily injury to a civilian, or to any other person not taking an active part in the hostilities in a situation of armed conflict, when the purpose of such acts, by their very nature or context, is to intimidate a population, or to compel government or an international organization to do or to abstain from doing any act."

- Religious extremism can be defined as "An outright opposition to rational thinking or rigid interpretation of religion that are forced upon others using social or economic coercion, laws, intolerance or violence" (ICAN, 2014). The global rise in the phenomenon of religious extremism and intolerance has provided a fertile breeding ground for terrorism and related activities.
- Home Affairs Committee of the House of Commons, United Kingdom (2012) has defined radicalization as "A process by which ordinary individuals come to sympathize with and support violent protests and terrorism and includes both social and psychological determinants and vulnerabilities that shape otherwise healthy young people to engage with and adopt terrorist ideology". Radicalization can happen because of a multitude of factors, the nature of which suggests a complex interplay of personnel and environmental determinants.
- Counter-terrorism can be loosely defined as "The practice, military tactics, techniques, and strategy that government, military, law enforcement, business, and intelligence agencies use to combat or prevent terrorism. Counter-terrorism strategies include attempts to counter financing of terrorism" (Royal College of Psychiatrists, 2016b).

PREVALENCE OF TERRORISM AND MAJOR TERRORIST INCIDENTS

Barring very few regions of the world, terrorism has a global presence now with cases being reported all over the world almost on daily basis. Though the nature and frequency of terrorist activities differs in the different parts of the world, the common theme is the violent nature of the attacks. However, some terrorist attacks stand out from the rest in context of sheer magnitude and subsequent impact globally, like the September 11, 2001 attack when terrorists hijacked four commercial jets imposing as passengers and subsequently crashed two jets in World Trade Center's twin towers resulting in complete collapse and a death toll of over 3,000 people. Some other major terrorist attacks in the recent times have been the bombing of Air India's airliner in 1985 flying from Canada to India which killed 329 passengers, Beslan School siege in Russia, 2004 resulting in death of 385 people in which majority of victims were school children, 2014 Gamboru Ngala attack by Boko Haram militia in Nigeria killing 336 people, 2016 Karrada bombings in Baghdad killing 341 people, and so on; unfortunately, the list is ever expanding. All these terrorist attacks have shaped the course of our history very significantly and have led to major geopolitical changes by influencing the foreign policies of major military powers of the world.

Similarly, in India there has been a major upsurge of the terrorism-related activities in the last few decades. The Mumbai attack of 2008 killed 173 people while injuring at least 308. It was carried out by Islamic terrorists. The horrific incident drew condemnation from all around the world. Global Terrorism Index (2015) has placed India among top ten countries in the world which are affected by terrorism. Terrorism in India can be broadly categorized into three mutually exclusive groups, all of which have their separate ideology, i.e., communist, Islamist and separatist. Recent years have seen an upscaling of violence in different parts of the country with terrorist attacks becoming more and more deadlier than before. In some areas of Northeast India and Jammu & Kashmir, it has assumed newer dimensions in the recent years. The state of Punjab which was in the grip of major turmoil in 1990s has reverted back to normalcy in recent times. The ongoing insurgency in Jammu & Kashmir continues to have significant psychological effects in the aftermath of violence. The terrorists with affiliations to the communism have also been actively involves in the terrorist activities in central India resulting in significant loss of lives.

PSYCHOSOCIAL ROOTS OF TERRORISM AND EXTREMISM: A BRIEF NOTE

Although there is a large body of work in this area, it is only briefly recapitulated here because the mandate of this chapter is psychosocial sequelae of terrorism rather that its causes and roots. Determining that how people get radicalized to carry out barbaric terrorist acts has been a matter of debate. However, there is a no denying the fact that it results from a complex interplay of a multitude of factors, including extremist religious beliefs, personal susceptibility, unstable family environment, poor educational status, inadequate employment opportunities, sociopolitical turmoil, ongoing war, substance abuse, etc. although it is not uncommon to find exceptions to these factors. Bartocci (2014) observed that there is a very little evidence to support that the people who commit terrorist acts have mental illnesses. Though people, who have psychiatric difficulties with poor coping, may be vulnerable to exploitation and persuasion by extremists, especially at the time of distress when they choose to isolate themselves from mainstream. Sometimes it may be extremely difficult to disentangle political affiliations from delusions/overvalued ideas, even when there is a culturally compatible group holding the same set of beliefs (Bhui, 2016).

This phenomenon may have exceptions, especially as an emerging trend observed in the western countries termed as "lone wolf" terrorists, who may act rather impulsively and erratically like, e.g. knife attacks at a busy marketplace, ploughing a vehicle in a busy street to inflict maximum causalities. Alfaro et al. (2015) have observed that the people indulging in these kinds of terrorist attacks are at high-risk of having a pre-existing mental illness and may act for retribution of perceived insult of their religious beliefs or to apparently avenge death of people in various ongoing wars in different parts of the world. In addition, some vulnerable individuals may be seeking self-identity by becoming a part of the terrorist organizations (Bhui, 2016).

The terrorist organizations have used this modus operandi as a major method of recruitment to their ranks throughout the world and their propaganda is specially designed to target this population on various social media sites on the internet.

PSYCHOSOCIAL IMPACT ON THOSE DIRECTLY OR INDIRECTLY EXPOSED TO TERRORIST OR OTHER EXTREMIST ACTS

Psychiatric

Table 1 lists the psychiatric morbidities, commonly observed in terrorism survivors (Trivedi, 2004; Yehuda & Haymen, 2005):

Table 1: Psychiatric morbidity seen in terrorism survivors

Acute reaction to stress	
Adjustment disorders	• Brief depressive reaction • Prolonged depressive reaction • Mixed anxiety/depressive reaction • Mixed with irritability/anger
Anxiety states	• Generalized anxiety disorder • Mixed anxiety and depressive state • Panic attacks • Dissociative disorder
Depression	
Post-traumatic stress disorder	
Others	• Exacerbation of pre-existing mental illness • Exacerbation of personality traits • Neuropsychiatric effects of concussion • Head injury • Brain damage • Epilepsy • Alcohol and other substance abuse • Enduring personality change

Individual response to terrorist events is highly variable. Grieger (2006) suggests that although the nature of the traumatic event may be an important predictor of the psychological response, there is a significant contribution from the factors like genetic makeup, social contexts, past experiences and future expectations, close proximity to the event, severity of exposure, low levels of social support, previous psychiatric illness, history of trauma, and ongoing negative life events.

Yehuda & Haymen (2005) have made an important observation that there may be important contributions from the neurobiological systems in the development of the psychological effects and the knowledge about the same may be important in the development of preventive strategies. They also reported that two factors which play the most important role in the development of long-term mental illness risk are: (1) Directness and severity of the exposure of an individual, (2) Degree of personal susceptibility.

There have been suggestions regarding a triphasic response (Tyhurst, 1951) following a major trauma. The initial "impact" phase is characterized by a stunning and numbing response by the survivor who may remain preoccupied by the events of the trauma. This is followed by the "recoil" phase where the survivors want to talk about the event and also try to seek some support. This phase gives way to the "post-trauma" phase where the survivor comes to term with what exactly has happened, and how significantly it has affected the life of the individual? It is during this phase that the survivors show a mix of reactions ranging from anger to depression and anxiety.

Grieger (2006) suggests that although in the immediate aftermath of a terrorist incident prevalence of the individuals presenting with psychiatric complaints to the emergency departments may increase significantly, a large proportion of this population will not have a diagnosable psychiatric disorder. The vast majority will have behavioral and emotional changes only. The small percentage of the population with diagnosable conditions will have disorders across a spectrum, with maximum people having acute stress disorder and bereavement. Some individuals will also develop serious conditions like post-traumatic stress disorder and depression. The course of these disorders is also highly variable. Some people will experience remission, while in others the symptoms may continue for a long course, if left untreated. The other heath-related behaviors may also change significantly in the aftermath of a terrorist incident.

The development of acute stress disorder and post-traumatic stress disorder is more likely in individuals with direct exposure to traumatic event with grave threat to life and experiencing extreme fear (Bryant, 2003). Acute stress disorder is a time-limited disorder with a highly variable course and extent of distress. It is likely that maximum number of individuals with acute stress disorder will never seek medical attention. Though initially thought to be important predictor for the development of subsequent post-traumatic stress disorder the evidence for the same is lacking. If there are prominent symptoms of dissociation following a traumatic event, these patients have a significant risk of developing subsequent post-traumatic stress disorder and depression (McFarlane, 2000).

During a traumatic event and subsequent recovery, there may be a significant increase in the use of tobacco, alcohol and other illicit drugs as a means of coping with the emotional turmoil. This leads to increase in criminal activities inherent with substance abuse in the community, resulting in increased rates of injury, assaults and other related behaviors.

Children often are worst affected by terrorism. They may suffer because of the direct exposure to terrorism-related activities or because of the death/disability of parents and caregivers. The manifestations depend on the age of the child as well as the severity and intensity of the exposure. Whereas the behavior manifestations in young children may be in the form of excessive crying, showing clinging behavior or other developmental difficulties, older children may have the symptoms depression or post-traumatic stress disorder, and may develop alcohol, nicotine or other illicit drug dependence (Trivedi, 2004). Some children may show "traumatic play" in which the child reenacts trauma or trauma related themes in play.

Psychological

Psychological reactions to the terrorist events may vary a lot in a given population. In addition to responses to the event, the individuals who have been in proximity of the event, are also likely to suffer from constant fear of a possible repetition of the events of similar nature. The reactions are likely to be influenced by the extent of personal damage suffered, proximity to the event, coping styles and threat perception of the individual.

Terrorist attacks usually instill deep and lasting fear in a society which is targeted. They serve a dual purpose by drawing attention of the media worldwide, and disrupting the social functions and the infrastructure of the targeted societies. It might be apt to draw the conclusion that the terrorism is a psychological warfare and terrorist design attacks to have a maximum impact on target population. All this has an impact on the health-related behaviors of the population. The acute effects may be in the form of anxiety, depression and a sense of feeling vulnerable with resultant paranoia of suspect communities. The chronic effects are seen after the media coverage subsides and are reflected in newer counter-terrorism measures taken by such societies. It becomes apparent that the individuals, who were not directly affected by the primary attack, also start to feel vulnerable with resultant feeling of stress and anxiety.

Social

The changes which occur are not only restricted to the health systems but have an impact on the overall lifestyle of the individuals living in terrorism affected areas. The uncertainties of the daily schedule with regular and unpredictable cycles of violence have a tremendous impact on all the members of the society. When there are security concerns in a society all other work takes a secondary role. The businesses, academic institutions and offices have to adjust their working, taking into consideration the security concerns. Terrorism also negatively impacts the tourism industry and in places, where majority of the population is dependent on tourism for their livelihood, the rates of unemployment may rises sharply further complicating the turmoil.

Terrorism has been one of the most common causes of mass migrations in the recent years. This gives rise to another subgroup of highly vulnerable refugee population caught in the middle of the conflict. The resultant effect is a great deal of psychological distress in these individuals. The over identification of these people as terrorism perpetrators adds to their trauma. The process of radicalization and subsequently carrying out terrorist activities is an outcome of various interplaying factors acting together, which are not limited to any particular ethnicity, religion or culture (Royal College of Psychiatrists, 2016a).

Narco-terrorism: A Special Case of Social Impact

Narco-terrorism refers to use of money raised from illegal drugs trade (within or across the state or national borders) essentially to fund terrorist organizations and activities (Curtis, 2002). Illicit drugs trade (including forced cultivation of poppy and coca plants; production, distribution and sale of drugs) is used only as a means to raise massive funds to fuel terrorism (Bjornehed, 2004). However, the social impact is vast in terms of utilization of huge resources in supply control, generation of a parallel economy and livelihood, and devastating effects on the society of widespread drug use and addictions.

MINIMIZING THE PSYCHOSOCIAL IMPACT OF TERRORISM AND EXTREMISM

Individual Level

The widespread psychological impact of a terrorist attack can result in extreme and dangerous reactions from a minority of the affected population, including rioting, targeting suspected minority groups and creating atmosphere of chaos and panic. Sensational media reporting may make the matters worse in times of crisis (Ayalon & Lahad, 2000).

The scientific literature over the past two decades has given fresh insights about the effects of psychological trauma following a terrorist act, coping mechanisms of the populations, and effective treatments. Yehuda & Haymen (2005) suggest that following the trauma most of the individuals cope well and do not require any professional intervention. A small subgroup of the affected individuals may develop post-traumatic stress disorder, depression and substance use disorders, and for these people the mental health resource utilization rates are likely to be high.

As is universal with mental health disorders, the failure of recognition of the symptoms is a common occurrence. The stigma attached with mental health may further complicate the issue of effective treatment seeking (Greenberg, 2015).

Yehuda (1999, 2002) has concluded that based on our present understanding, it is very difficult to predict who are more likely to develop long-term mental health concerns following the exposure to traumatic events.

There are some symptoms which have been considered as potential markers for subsequent psychopathology like dissociation, intrusive thoughts, hyperarousal and avoidance, but research has failed to prove them to be reliably consistent. Thus, it is important that the individuals exposed to trauma should be provided access to adequate mental health services for early identification and treatment of the disorders.

Aggregate Level

Building resilience of a community is important in fight against terrorism. While we have discussed how terrorism impacts the health behavior of a community, it is also important to remember that another important area of impact is the interaction between various members of the same community. While it is not uncommon for hate crimes and retaliatory attacks to rise sharply against minority groups following a terrorist attack, another equally important area of concern is that some members of these minority groups choose to socialize within their own ethnic and religious groups rather than playing an active role in a larger community. Both these actions are counterproductive for communal harmony and create an atmosphere of hostility, suspicion and increasing paranoia.

McCauley & Moskalenko (2011) have pointed to the fact that the factors which can help prevent radicalization of an individual are very poorly understood. The veil of separation between being religious/nationalist to that of an extremist who can justify violence to achieve objectives is vague and at what point this transformation takes place is difficult to define. No single model can be used for the prevention of radicalization. Mental health issues can play some role in the process of radicalization but there are other factors which are far more important in this entire transformation.

The current understanding of the pathways leading to terrorism is largely based on the reconstructed biographies of people who have been convicted on terrorism charges, It is self-explanatory that there can be a great deal of variation as biographies are essentially unique to each individual (Arena & Arrigo, 2005).

Royal College of Psychiatrists (2016a) suggest that the media should provide a balanced opinion without sensationalizing the facts to maintain calm in the society. The psychiatrists and other professionals with relevant experience can give a balanced view of the situation to the media. The risk factors for developing mental health problems can be discussed on such platforms and people should be encouraged to seek help in case of persistent difficulties.

It has been shown that the "psychological debriefing" or "trauma counseling" has no benefit in the aftermath of a traumatic event and can lead to potential harm to the individuals (National Institute for Health and Care Excellence, 2005).

Planning for emergency situations is important part of the resilience building of the community. The emergency situation has psychological consequences for both the affected people and emergency responders. The planners should adopt evidence-based approaches while preparing the emergency responders to deal with the psychological effects of their work (Greenberg, 2013).

The building of the community resilience is best achieved beforehand of the actual situation. This is best achieved by wider cooperation between all the stakeholders, including the emergency responders and media to deal with a crisis in most efficient way. There must be protocols in place to deal with emergency situations and these must be revised from time to time keeping the threat level to a community in perspective.

PSYCHOSOCIAL IMPACT OF COUNTER-TERRORIST MEASURES

The psychosocial impact of terrorism has a peculiar and unique counterpart: counter-terrorist measures and their own psychosocial impact. Terrorist attacks provoke strong anti-terrorism measures at the government, military, police and importantly, societal levels. In an attempt to identify potential terrorists or extremists, governments often resort to screening individuals on the basis of their racial, ethnic, political or religious identities or characteristics. This is known as "profiling", which is often used at airports, border controls and similar check points.

At a societal level, following a severe terrorist attack such as "9/11", society becomes guarded and suspicious against general members of a particular racial or religious community, and every member of that community is viewed with varying degrees of wariness, hypervigilance, suspicion, and even frank animosity and hatred. These social mindset changes often lead to "hate crimes" targeted against innocent members of that particular community.

Thus, profiling (by the government) and hate crimes (by the public), both are offshoots of counter-terrorism which cause further social impact on the members of the "suspected" community by fostering more defensive behavior, marginalization, stigmatization, and, paradoxically, might actually facilitate radicalization processes especially among the young and underprivileged members of the target communities. Thus, the "cycle of mutual disbelief and violence" is propagated further (Royal College of Psychiatrists, 2016b).

CONCLUSION

It is abundantly clear that terrorism and extremism in various forms, magnitude and means are here to stay, and in fact increasing in terms of geographic coverage and frequency. No continent, country, region or society can be said to be immune to these activities any longer. It is also apparent that the very purpose of terrorist acts is to create "terror", not only in the minds of those directly affected by such acts, but more importantly in the larger society as an overt threat. Thus, the social impact of terrorism and extremism goes beyond individual psyche (where it can cause several psychiatric disorders and/or psychological sequelae), to the collective psyche or the social mindset. These acts set in motion a series of counter-terrorist measures and generate a sense of paranoia in the society, which paradoxically may further fuel the cycle of terrorism in the long run. The whole issue is extremely complex and even controversial.

Further research is needed which can help us understand both the factors contributing to increasing rates of radicalization and extremism in the society as well as the social and psychological impacts on a population in the aftermath of a terrorist attack. There should be a balanced approach between the valid recognition of threat perception to a community and the creation of an atmosphere of undue hostility, fear, suspicion, and paranoia.

REFERENCES

Alfaro GL, Barthelmes RJ, Bartol C, et al. Lone Wolf Terrorism. Georgetown University. 2015.

Arena MP, Arrigo BA. Social psychology, terrorism, and identity: a preliminary re-examination of theory, culture, self, and society. Behav Sci Law. 2005;23(4):485-506.

Ayalon O, Lahad M. Life on the Edge: Coping with War, Terror and Violence. Haifa: Nord Publications; 2000.

Bartocci G. Cultural psychiatry and the study of the bio-psycho-cultural roots of the supernatural: clinical application. World Cult Psychiatry Res Rev. 2014;9:56-64.

Bhui K. Flash, the emperor and policies without evidence: counter-terrorism measures destined for failure and societally divisive. BJ Psych Bull. 2016;40(2):82-84.

Bjornehed E. Narco-terrorism: the merger of the war on drugs and the war on terror. Global Crime. 2004;6:305-24.

Bryant RA. Early predictors of post-traumatic stress disorder. Biol Psychiatry. 2003;53:789-95.

Curtis G. The Nexus among Terrorists, Narcotics Traffickers, Weapons Proliferators, and Organized Crime Networks in Western Europe. Washington, DC: Library of Congress; 2002.

Global Terrorism Index: Measuring and Understanding the Impact of Terrorism. New York: Institute for Economics & Peace; 2015.

Greenberg N. Fostering resilience across the deployment cycle. In: RR Sinclair and TW Britt (Eds). Building Psychological Resilience in Military Personnel: Theory and Practice. Chicago: American Psychological Association; 2013.

Greenberg N, Brooks S, Dunn R. Latest developments in post-traumatic stress disorder: diagnosis and treatment. Br Med Bull. 2015;114:147-55.

Grieger TA. Psychiatric and societal impacts of terrorism. Psychiatric Times. 2006;23(7):24.

Hobfoll SE, Spielberger CD, Breznitz S, et al. War-related stress: addressing the stress of war and other traumatic events. Am Psychol. 1991;46:848-55.

Home Affairs Committee. The Roots of Violent Radicalisation. House of Commons, London, United Kingdom; 2012.

Hunt E, Jones N, Hastings V, et al. TRiM: an organizational response to traumatic events in Cumbria Constabulary. Occupational Medicine. 2013;63:549-55.

ICAN: Extremism as Mainstream: Implications for women, development and security in the MENA/Asia region. International Civil Society Network, USA; 2014. pp. 1-12.

Jones F, Fong Y. Military Psychiatry and Terrorism. Department of the Army, Textbook of Military Medicine Washington DC; 1994. pp. 264-9.

Kaplan A. The psychodynamics of terrorism. In: Alexander Y and Gleason J (Eds). Behavioral and Quantitative Perspectives on Terrorism. New York: Pergamon; 1981. pp. 35-50.

Krug EG. World report on violence and health. World Health Organization, Geneva, Switzerland, 2002.

McCauley C, Moskalenko M. Friction:How Radicalization to Them and Us. London: Oxford University Press; 2011.

McFarlane AC. Posttraumatic stress disorder: a model of the longitudinal course and the role of risk factors. J Clin Psychiatry. 2000;61(suppl 5):15-20.

National Institute for Health and Care Excellence (NICE): Post-Traumatic Stress Disorder: Management. NICE. 2005.

Prevention of Terrorism Act (POTA), 2nd edition. Lucknow: Eastern Book Company; 2002.

Royal college of Psychiatrists. Responding to large scale traumatic events and acts of terrorism. PS03/16; 2016.

Royal College of Psychiatrists. Counter-terrorism and Psychiatry. Position Statement PS04/16; 2016.

Trivedi JK. Terrorism and mental health. Indian J Psychiatry. 2004;46:7-14.

Tyhurst JS. Individual reactions to community disaster: the natural history of psychiatric phenomena. Am J Psychiatry. 1951;107:764-69.

United Nations: International Convention for the Suppression of the Financing of Terrorism. Adopted by the General Assembly of the United Nations in Resolution 54/109 of 9 December 1999. United Nations, 1999.

Yehuda R. Risk Factors for Posttraumatic Stress Disorder. Progress in Psychiatry Series. Washington, DC: American Psychiatric Association; 1999.

Yehuda R. Post-traumatic stress disorder. New England Journal of Medicine. 2002;346:108-14.

Yehuda R, Haymen SE. The impact of terrorism on brain and behaviour: What we know and what we need to know. Neuropsychopharmacology. 2005;30:1773-80.

Chapter 42

Mass Media, Information Technology, and Mental Health

Vinay Kumar, Koushik Sinha Deb, Rishi Gupta

SUMMARY

Media and information technology form the interface through which we reach the world outside the immediate grasp of our five senses. Mass media therefore is the prime cultivator of our perceptions, influencing our thinking, attitudes, and behavior. The depiction of "madness" and the "mad" in mass media significantly affect the society's view of these disorders and their sufferers. As the mentally ill are often depicted as unstable, violent, odd or comical, there is a general increase in stigma related to mental illness, especially in those people who are avid consumers of mass media. Negative depiction of mental health professionals and mental health treatments often leads to reduced utilization of these services by those who need them the most. Social media use itself can also negatively affect mental health through precipitation of depression, anxiety, online-bullying and through exposure to inappropriate content. Despite the pitfalls, responsible use of information technology can result in great benefits. Virtual and augmented reality can be used to develop newer techniques of therapy in delusions, autism, and attention deficit hyperactivity disorder (ADHD). The enmeshment of modern life in technology has made it a very powerful tool that needs to be used carefully, lest it becomes the healthcare problem itself.

INTRODUCTION

Life in the 21st century is intimately intertwined with various forms of mass and social media, and it is difficult to imagine a life completely untouched by these sources of information and influence. Mass media refers to all sources of publicly delivered information and entertainment, and its history can be traced back to the early days of civilization when dramas were performed in various cultures, and heralds bore the word of the king to the corners of the empire. Modern and truly massive mass media spread with the invention of the printing press by Johannes Gutenberg in 1453 (Assmann, 2012), and since then has ramified into myriads of forms ranging from print media (newspapers, magazines, journals), electronic media (radio, television, movies) and finally to the internet (blog, vlog, Rich Site Summary—RSS, and mobile apps). In addition to being the primary source of knowledge regarding the world which is outside the immediate reach of our five senses, mass media is also credited as the prime cultivator of perceptions, influencing our thinking, attitudes, and behavior (Wahl, 1992).

The advent of the internet in mid-1960s resulted in democratization of content creation and information delivery, and freed mass media from the perception of being the mouthpiece

Table 1: Characteristics and differences between mass media and social media

Characteristics	Mass media	Social media
Communication type	One way and one-to-many	Two way and one-to-one
Consumer participation	Passive, targets isolated consumers	Active, connects consumers
Information	Controlled, censored, content-driven	Uncontrolled, uncensored, conversation-driven,
Information delivery	Transient with limited number of targeted channels	Continuous with unlimited number of channels
Investment	Requires significant financial investment	Requires social investment
Credibility	Varies, dependent on the perception of the source	Varies, dependent on the perception of the source

of the minority elite. Over time, websites and applications which promote the formation of an alternative online community, through user conversations, dialogues and opinions developed, and came to be collectively known as Social Networking Sites (SNSs). Such sites currently involve dedicated online communities, forums, photograph sharing websites, video sharing websites, online weblogs (blogs), dating services, and instant chat and messaging platforms. Transparency, democracy, anonymity, and ease of access have propelled social media as the primary channel of information for a large proportion of the population. Mass media and social media differ in fundamental ways of information delivery which are detailed in **Table 1**.

Mass and social media, in their universal outreach, can be significant resources for mental health information and service delivery. Unfortunately, they are also often implicated as perpetrators of mental health-related stigma or as causes of mental distress and disorder due to dysfunctional use. This chapter analyzes the interface between media influence and mental health, and looks into possible ways in which information technology can be used as a tool to improve mental health.

MASS MEDIA AND MENTAL HEALTH

Literature and media have depicted mental health and illness in various forms since antiquity. The analysis of even William Shakespeare's (1564–1616) work shows his curious fascination with madness, provides a fairly accurate description of various mental ailments which will currently fall under the categories of depression, psychosis, and obsessive compulsive disorder **(Table 2)** (Andreasen, 1976; Ottilingam, 2007).

With the advent of movies and television, the focus shifted to the portrayal of the mentally ill in these new formats of information and entertainment. As early as in 1960s, social scientists reported the perils of stereotype creation by skewed mass media portrayal of people with mental illness, similar to other marginalized populations of women, minorities and the elderly (Wahl & Lefkowits, 1989). Mental illness, even in those early days stood out as a common instrument for plot development, recorded in over 18% of movies (between 1930 and 1959) (Gerbner, 1961), 10% of prime time serials (Turow & Coe, 1985), and in more than 47% of

Table 2: Depiction of mental illness in the work of William Shakespeare

Play/Sonnet (Year)	Character	Current equivalent diagnosis
The Merchant of Venice (1600)	Antonio (main protagonist)	Depression
Hamlet (1603)	Hamlet	Bipolar disorder
King Lear (1608)	King Lear	Depression/Dementia
Macbeth (1611)	Lady Macbeth	Schizophrenia/PTSD
Othello (1622)	Othello	Morbid jealousy (Othello syndrome)

PTSD, post-traumatic stress disorder.

Table 3: Theories on media and mass perception*

Theory	Principle component	Example
Cultivation theory	Repeated exposure to constant and regular messages on television will "reiterate, confirm, and nourish values" and modify perceptions of reality to conform to those presented on television	People living in the world of television might see the real world more in terms of the pictures and values presented in the virtual world
Social learning theory	New behaviors are acquired by observing and imitating others	People and specially children imbibe behaviors as well as social conventions and rules of conduct with mentally ill persons while watching mass media portrayals

*Modified from (Stout et al., 2004).

children's television programming (Wilson et al., 2000a). Rather than fulfilling the expected role of media as a "mediator" between the scientific knowledge and general public, analysis of the media representation of mental illness showed that the "media image" was pulling public ideas away from expert views in the direction of "bizarre, sordid, fearful, or frivolous" portrayals of the subject (Gerbner & Tannenbaum, 1960).

These deviated representations affected viewers, and media consumption was found to influence viewers' attitudes and knowledge regarding mental disorders (Kimmerle & Cress, 2013). People who watched crime related shows on television remained more afraid of being victim to violent crimes (Gerbner et al., 1978), and patients' attitudes toward health care providers (favorable vs. unfavorable) could be mapped to their television watching habits (Morgan & Shanahan, 2010). Subsequent work on communication research has brought forth two theories which might explain such effect **(Table 3)** (Stout et al., 2004). While the "cultivation theory" helps us understand how media representation over time might create stigma for mental illness, Bandura's now famous "social learning theory" highlights the generation of discriminative and distancing behavior toward person with mental disorders.

Media Depiction of the Mentally Ill

The media depiction of mentally ill persons has often been stereotypical, stigmatizing and factually incorrect (Miller, 2007). Multiple studies report that in media representations, common symptoms of mental illnesses are glossed over, leaving in only the most "appealing" ones (Smith, 2015a). For example, in most television shows and movies, schizophrenia patients are depicted as having either elaborated visual or auditory hallucinations, or sometimes even dissociative identity disorder (a result of a concrete translation of the word). Rare disorders, such as gender identity disorder, and anterograde amnesia, are depicted as occurring much more frequently than they actually do, and often in a more melodramatic manner than in reality. Frequently, in a bid to increase the impact of the content, the more negative and bizarre aspects of mental illnesses are overemphasized, editing out the harrowing experience for both the patient and his caregivers. The mentally ill are often depicted as violent, strange and unpredictable, while their distress is rarely highlighted. The extent of violence attributed to the mentally ill in media far exceeds than what it is in real life. Of all the patients with mental illness, less than 3% exhibit violent behavior, even though the media depicts this number to be almost ten times as much (Diefenbach, 1997; Diefenbach & West, 2007) (Fazel et al., 2009).

A 2006 literature review by Pirkis et al. (2006) included additional analysis of filming techniques used to indicate the ominousness of characters with mental illness. Cinematic tropes, such as the close-up shots, individual point of view, discordant music, atmospheric lighting, and stark and dim settings were more frequently used in scenes depicting persons with mental illness. Characters with mental illness are often given unattractive features, like "rotting teeth or unruly hair" (Wilson et al., 2000). Hyler and colleagues (1991) in a similar content analysis categorized the stereotypes of negative portrayals of the mentally ill in media and movies into eight subtypes **(Table 4)**.

Even children's television programming suffered from such wrong portrayal. Wilson et al. (2000) monitored of all children's TV program in New Zealand for over a week and reported that out of 128 episodes monitored, 46% referred to mental illness, mostly (80%) as cartoons (Wilson et al., 2000b). "Crazy", "mad", "nuts", "bananas", and "loons" were the common vocabulary used to describe mentally ill characters, and none of them were shown to have any positive traits. Most of these characters acted in an evil, aggressive, or irrational manner and were feared by the "good" protagonist as well as by the viewer. Another study by Lawson and Fouts (2004) examined the depiction of mental illness in Disney movies as they are considered to be "timeless classics" viewed by several generations of children. Of the 34 films examined, reference to mental disorders was made in 85% of films which was significantly greater than children's real life exposure. Portrayals were often overtly negative and patients were often "taken away" from society in "loony vans" (Lawson & Fouts, 2004). As children are more impressionable than adults and spend a significant amount of time watching television, these depictions leave a deep and lasting impact generating fear and stigma (Wahl, 2003).

Depiction of Mental Illness

Very few studies have looked into the portrayal of specific categories of mental disorders like schizophrenia or obsessive compulsive disorder (OCD). Wahl (1995) reviewed the Reader's Guide of all even-numbered years between 1964 and 1992 for references to schizophrenia and found only 9.1% of the articles referring to the disorder. Further, most of articles were published in popular science magazines with focused clientele, rather than in magazines of

Table 4: Negative stereotypes of mentally ill persons in media*

S. No.	Stereotype	Description	Examples
1.	The homicidal maniac	The most Common stereotype, unpredictably violent, prone to gruesome and grotesque atrocities	The Maniac Cook (1909), Psycho (1960), The Exorcist (1973)
2.	The rebellious free spirit	Eccentric, odd, or different characters who are often mislabeled as mentally ill, and inappropriately treated	One Flew Over the Cuckoo's Nest (1975), Dumbo (1941), Beauty and the Beast (1992)
3.	The enlightened	Fun loving, pacifist or wise, intellectual patients who cannot be understood by others	King of Hearts (1968), Good Will Hunting (1997)
4.	The female seductress	Females are depicted as nymphomaniacs with seductive powers that can destroy men	Dressed to Kill (1980), Basic Instinct (1992)
5.	The narcissistic parasite	Depicted as "overprivileged, self-obsessed, and overconcerned with their trivial problems"	Lovesick (1983)
6.	The zoo specimen	Most derogatory portrayal where persons are dehumanized with prominent mannerism and posturing akin to animals in a zoo	The Snake Pit (1948)
7.	The simpleton	Often children in children's program, the character lack comprehension and provides comic relief	There's Something About Mary (1998), Rain Man (1988)
8	The victim	Patients are often victim to crime or exploitation, unresponsive to therapy and non-contributing to society	Shutter Island (2010), Perfect Blue (1997)

*Modified from Hyler and colleagues (1991) and Pirkis et al. (2006).

general interest. In a more recent study, (Owen, 2012) did a similar content analysis of 41 movies depicting 42 characters with schizophrenia and found that the interpretations of the illness were often overtly negative and violent. Wahl (2000) also conducted a similar review in 2000 looking into the references and description of OCD in popular magazines from 1983 to 1997. For OCD, although the description was far more accurate compared to the representation in movies and television, only few of the articles under the target heading were on the subject. Most articles were about obsessed fans stalking celebrities. Depictions of body image ideal in media have also been extensively researched as a cause of various eating disorders, including anorexia, bulimia and orthorexia (Grabe et al., 2008; López-Guimerà et al., 2010). Studies report a definite temporal correlation between exposure to western media and new case findings or increase in prevalence of these disorders in cultures previously unexposed to such values (Becker, 2004; Lee, 2000). The media representations of persons suffering from eating disorders have also been found to be inaccurate and stigmatizing (Spettigue & Henderson, 2004). Almost all movie and television characters suffering from eating disorders are depicted as white and of upper socioeconomic strata, creating a stereotype of eating disorders as a problem of the rich white women, ignoring other patient groups. In various movies, binges were often used as a sign of breakdown or failure to control ones' behavior, often de-medicalizing it and putting the onus on the sufferer (Hogan & Strasburger, 2008).

Substance abuse depiction in movies and media, in contrary, suffers from overt normalization, which minimize the harm caused by drugs. Alcohol and tobacco use often represents the normal "routinized background" in movies and television. Nonproblematic drug use in "foreground" characters is also often depicted as positive attributes, imbibing characters with vitality, vigor, and life. Even problematic drug use (intoxication), when it happens occasionally, either as experimentation or as a corollary to great emotional upheaval, is depicted as normal. Characters having significant drug dependence fall into the stereotypes of being a either a "tragic hero", a "rebellious free spirit", a "demonized addict", or a "comedic user" (Cape, 2003). The portrayal of smoking in movies often moves beyond normalization to romanticize smoking, marking it as a surrogate for manliness, thoughtfulness and power. According to some authors, the glamorized depiction of smoking in the movies of 1980s led to an increased prevalence of smoking in youngsters (Charlesworth & Glantz, 2005) resulting in a national call of assigning ratings to restrict access to movies with smoking (Strasburger & American Academy of Pediatrics. Council on Communications and Media, 2010). A similar analysis from India looking into 44 top grossing Bollywood movies between 2006 and 2008 shows that more than 50% of the youth rated films having depictions of tobacco use (Nazar et al., 2013). More recently, attention has been paid to the media portrayal of other psychoactive substances, apart from alcohol and tobacco. An analysis of the 200 most popular movies of all times reported that in addition to tobacco and alcohol, illicit drug-use was also portrayed in a positive light and without any negative consequences in most movies (Gunasekera et al., 2005). A survey of American teenagers who indulged in risky sexual behavior and drug use found these individuals to spend more time watching television than their non-watching peers, supporting the normalization effect of the media on drug use and high-risk behavior (Klein et al., 1993). Such portrayals have been linked with early initiation, progression to hard drug use and dependence in teens and adolescents (Nunez-Smith et al., 2010).

Finally, suicide depiction in media often lacks the sensitivity required to report such devastating outcome. Suicide and self-harm attempts are untoward consequences of many mental disorders and life stress, a fact that media often overlooks in its eagerness to sensationalize and romanticize the acts. Studies have consistently found significant relationship between suicide portrayals and its impact on the viewers (Gould et al., 2003), and many international organizations including the World Health Organization (World Health Organization, 2017) have come out with guidelines for responsible reporting of suicides **(Table 5)**. Yet, media reporting often turns a blind eye to these guidelines for the sake of sensationalism (Bohanna & Wang, 2012).

Media reporting of suicide can significantly enhance or weaken suicide prevention efforts of the country. Extensive coverage of an event of suicide, the details of the place and process, and reporting suicide as an unexplainable sudden event propagates myths about suicide—that it is unpredictable and unpreventable. The risk is particularly high when the event is reported in persons who are of high social status and can be easily identified with by the vulnerable reader. The copycat effect of subsequent suicides in the vulnerable reader is known as the "Werther effect", after the protagonist of Goethe's novel "The Sorrows of Young Werther", who

Table 5: Responsible media reporting for suicides	
Positive reporting practices (Dos)	*Reporting practices to be avoided (Don'ts)*
Do provide accurate information about where to seek help	Don't place stories about suicide prominently and don't unduly repeat such stories
Do educate the public about the facts of suicide and suicide prevention, without spreading myths	Don't use language which sensationalizes or normalizes suicide, or presents it as a constructive solution to problems
Do report stories of how to cope with life stressors or suicidal thoughts, and how to get help	Don't explicitly describe the method used
Do apply particular caution when reporting celebrity suicides	Don't provide details about the site/location
Do apply caution when interviewing bereaved family or friends	Don't use sensational headlines
Do recognize that media professionals themselves may be affected by stories about suicide	Don't use photographs, video footage or social media links

Modified from World Health Organization (2017). Preventing suicide: A resource for media professionals, update.

commits suicide when faced with the loss of his love (Kim et al., 2013). Conversely, responsible reporting educates the reader about the suicide prevention strategies, provides information about early warning signs of self-harm and may encourage those at risk to seek help rather than to commit the unfortunate act. Scientific literature refers to this protective effect of media reporting as the "Papageno effect", after Mozart's opera "The Magic Flute", where Papageno, who became suicidal after loss of his love, gets reminded of the alternatives and ultimately finds hope and redemption (Niederkrotenthaler et al., 2010).

Depiction of Mental Health Professionals and Psychiatric Treatment

The mental health professionals too are depicted in a manner which is not consistent with real life. They are shown as either incompetent, eccentric and idiotic people, with distinctive mannerisms, or as evil, scheming villains (Schneider, 1987). Often, the therapist is depicted as an attractive female, who accomplishes treatment more by virtue of her positive relationship with the patient, rather than any definite therapy (Gabbard, 2001). Occasionally, the therapist is depicted as all-knowing savior who is completely absorbed in his work, devoting his time in life to nothing else but his profession, and being able to cure mental illnesses by a single brilliant stroke of catharsis. Other times, the therapist is depicted to be an ever-rationalizing person, who puts his/her patients to comfort by superficial psychodynamic explanations of their symptoms. The portrayals often leave the rationality of scientific treatment behind for the benefit of dramatization, thereby altering the perception of the viewer regarding the expectation, settings and method of psychiatric management. The therapist is often seen to treat patients at home, in park, by the sea-side, in a café, but rarely in his office. A 2011 Indian study that analyzed the portrayal of psychiatrists in Bollywood movies for over a decade (2001–2010) found 33 psychiatrists appearing in significant roles in the 26 movies selected. Indian cinema depicted psychiatrists mostly as middle-aged males, who were friendly toward their patients. Unfortunately a significant 42.4% of the characters were clinically incompetent, and 70% of the movie instances made inaccurate diagnoses. Further, ethical boundary violations were very common by movie characters with around 24% of the fictional psychiatrists transgressing nonsexual boundaries, and 15.2% violating both sexual and nonsexual boundaries (Banwari, 2011). Such depictions not only prejudice the viewer's perspective of psychiatrist but also contribute to the stigma associated with mental disorders.

Another area of common misrepresentation in media is that of mental health treatment. As with other aspects of mental health, mass media tends to depict those mental health treatments which create a deeper impact on the viewers. Therefore, pharmacotherapy is rarely depicted in movies while electroconvulsive therapy (ECT) receives an inordinate focus, whenever such a treatment is depicted. Unfortunately, most of the depictions of ECT in even Western cinema have been reported to be inaccurate, with ECT being shown in a negative light in majority of movie depictions (McDonald & Walter, 2001). Portrayals of ECT are similarly distorted and dramatized in Indian cinema, with the procedure mostly serving as a trope for dramatic tension rather than as a treatment modality. In Bollywood movies, ECT is frequently used as a punitive measure, and is usually delivered by force without consent, without much premedication, using nonstandard ECT devices, and with the purpose to either punish a mentally ill patient, erase their identity, or create insanity where there was none (Andrade et al., 2010). Amongst other psychiatric treatments, psychotherapy often finds a place in the methods shown, albeit in a distorted and unrealistic manner. Psychotherapy is often used as an exposition tool to explore the mental world and agony of the "hero" rather than as a principled treatment process. Dynamic discussions therefore remain the director's favorite method of therapy, while magical emotional catharsis is depicted as a favored way of cure. An exploration of 400 movies for psychiatric treatments by Gabbard in 2001 found that none of the movies depicted treatment by way of medications (Gabbard, 2001). On few occasions when psychiatric medications were indeed administered in movies, they were shown to have the purpose of sedating the patients, or caused cognitive impairment and severe adverse effects. Even in movies that did have a favorable outlook toward psychiatric disorders, psychiatric medications were generally portrayed as a form of treatment which the protagonist had to "escape," or perish (Owen, 2012).

Stigma and Role of Mass Media

For many, mass media is often the primary source of knowledge regarding the symptoms and effects of mental illnesses. Misrepresentations in mass media therefore misinform viewers and often decrease rather than increasing understanding (Stuart, 2013). Indeed, knowledge regarding schizophrenia and OCD has been reported to reduce proportionally with the increase in television watching hours and knowledge gained regarding schizophrenia has been more if people watched a documentary, rather than if they watched a fictional movie, even though the content presented in both were the same (Kimmerle & Cress, 2013). The general perception of mentally ill persons as unpredictably violent can also be traced back to such depictions in mass media. In a study, two-fifths of a sample of general population believed mental illness to be associated with violence and attributed this knowledge to what they saw on television (Philo et al., 1994). The stigma perpetuated by media not only touches the general population but also affects patients themselves as a form of self-stigma (Smith, 2015b). Studies have consistently shown "self-stigma" to be associated with late detection, late treatment seeking and early dropout from treatment, often leading to a poorer outcome of mental disorders (Maier et al., 2013). Occasionally, media viewing itself can lead to induction or perpetuation of mental disorders in the general public (Padhy et al., 2014). "Copycat" suicides in vulnerable population, initiation and progression in substance use disorders, and development of eating disorders subsequent to media influenced body image "ideals" represent a few of such disorders (Spettigue & Henderson, 2004). Additionally, excessive and dysfunctional use of the internet by many adolescents and young adults has started finding its way into psychiatric classificatory systems, and thus itself comprises a mental disorder (Gentile et al., 2017).

Fortunately, not all portrayals of mental illness in mass media are negative. Several movies have made an attempt to portray mental illnesses and treatments as they are in real life, without excessive melodrama. The depiction of mentally ill people in a positive light, for example as accomplished scholars, can lead to a reduction in stigma (Nairn & Coverdale, 2005). Mass media, when utilized responsibly, can also help in improving the mental health of the general population (Gabbard & Gabbard, 1999). Mass media can be instrumental in delivering mental health awareness content to the general public (Cheng et al., 2016). The utilization of the mass media by several celebrities to spread awareness regarding different mental illnesses has helped to improve the knowledge and attitudes of people regarding psychiatric disorders in recent times. In India, the demonstration of a short educational film regarding ill effects of tobacco consumptions which has been made mandatory before every movie show, and the complete media ban on tobacco and alcohol products in movies and television have met with partial success (Arora et al., 2008). Suicide prevention helplines, emergency police dial number for women safety and adverts on child safety also help in decreasing the occurrence of major stressors which may lead to later psychiatric disorders.

SOCIAL MEDIA AND MENTAL ILLNESS

According to the International Telecommunication Union, 48% of the 7.4 billion world population currently use the internet. Internet technology adoption has been spearheaded by adolescents and youth, and as of 2017, 70% of the world's youth (15–24 years) have an online connection. For developed countries, an even higher proportion (94%) of young adults have access to the internet, while 67% of youths in developing countries have access to such services (International Telecommunication Union, 2017). Majority of internet use currently occurs on mobile broadband and out of the 830 million young people who are online, 320 million (39%) are exclusively from China and India. The commonest activity, children and adolescents world-over report using the internet for, is to access social media (Messina & Iwasaki, 2011; Pradeep & Sriram, 2016). The social media may comprise of social networking websites, media sharing websites, chat rooms, forums, blogs (a truncation of the term "weblog"), vlogs (video-blogs) and virtual worlds, including virtual gaming worlds, virtual reality and mixed reality interfaces. The vastness, variety and omnipresence of such online social media underscore its tremendous potential to affect the attitudes and behaviors of its users.

The virtual self-representation in the online world is considered a necessary step in formation of self-identity in adolescents (Villani et al., 2016). Adolescents' self-esteem has been shown to correlate directly with the type of feedback that they receive from their peers on these social networking websites, with positive feedback leading to better self-esteem, and a negative feedback reducing self-esteem (Valkenburg et al., 2006). The ability to present only their "best" self might be a contributor to social media attraction, as a study found that self-esteem was better when people viewed their online profile than when they viewed a mirror (Gonzales & Hancock, 2011). In fact, social updates and friends on SNSs have been shown to be significantly proportional to the adolescent's self-esteem. The "online self" becomes so ingrained in the lives of some children that when forced to delete their online account, children have committed suicide (Sivashanker, 2013). In adolescent girls, time spent in social networking websites significantly related to internalization of the slim body image, weight surveillance, and drive for thinness (Tiggemann & Slater, 2013). Some studies have shown that spending as little as 3 hours on these websites each week leads to increased depressive symptoms and decreased social support in users (Kraut et al., 1998). The association between the use of social networking websites and depression has been so consistent, the term "Facebook Depression" (O'Keeffe et al., 2011) has been coined to refer to its occurrence.

The fact that social networking websites represent a space, where children and adolescents interact with each other frequently and publicly, similar to a neighborhood or a school, has resulted in the phenomenon of cyberbullying (Runions & Bak, 2015). In contrast to traditional bullying which was previously limited by time, contact and situation, cyber-bullying penetrates into the victims' very personal space, right inside their homes (Modecki et al., 2014). The internet's ability to maintain anonymity and distance, and its lack of monitoring and repercussions promote and protect bullies. Also, the fact that the perpetrators cannot directly see the extent of the trauma that is being inflicted, makes them more likely not to limit their actions in the absence of this empathic feedback. Victims of online bullying face the risk of depression (Mota et al., 2015), and when severe enough, can result in suicide (Bauman et al., 2013). In India too, a survey carried out by Intel titled "Teens, Tweens, and Technology 2015" reported that almost 30% children surveyed experienced being bullied online, 50% reported bullying someone online at least once, and 65% reported witnessing online cruelty (McAfee Internet Security, 2015). A direct relationship between the time spent on social networking websites and the risk of being victim of bullying (Kwan & Skoric, 2013) has been reported and depression has been shown to mediate this link between online harassment and suicide, particularly in women (Smith et al., 2014).

A few applications and websites have taken another step forward, and made suicide the central theme of the social network, wherein completing the "tasks" in the social list culminates in the user committing suicide. Though counter-intuitive, an alarmingly large number of children have fallen victim to such social tasks with the "blue-whale" game making headlines in recent times. However, the blue whale is only one of the many such human experiments that get conducted in the sinister "dark web" of the internet. The dark web refers to the section of the internet which is not visible directly in search engines, and need to be accessed directly by entering the exact web address (Pergolizzi et al., 2017). Because of its undocumented nature, the dark web is essentially untraceable and is therefore host to many illegal activities, including sale of illicit drugs, child pornographic content, and groups which promote distressing activities as public torture, murder, or suicide. Such content, when accessed by susceptible population such as children, can have a profound impact on their mental health.

The use of social media has also been associated with anxiety and compulsive behavior (McCord et al., 2014). People of all ages have been shown to become anxious when not allowed to check their social networking pages, with this anxiety being demonstrated more by the younger generation than the older (Rosen et al., 2013). The phenomenon, called FOMO (Fear Of Missing Out) in "tech"-parlance, has been postulated to be due to the "Zeigarnik" effect (Perry & Singh, 2016). While face to face conversations have distinct start and end points, conversation on social media can continue in interrupted bursts indefinitely. Zeigarnik effect refers to the human desire for closure, thereby making users overtly attentive with unfinished conversations over the internet. A similar phenomenon termed as the "phantom vibration syndrome," entails the constant checking of one's smartphone because of feeling that it has vibrated (Rosenberger, 2015). Social media communications also suffer from the risk of disclosing personal details to unknown individuals, of getting incorrect advice, or being presented with too much information, more than what can be processed by a single person in a meaningful manner (Kuss & Griffiths, 2017). Internet advices may deter people from visiting a healthcare profession, delaying diagnosis and management, occasionally with catastrophic results.

Despite these negative effects, social media when used in moderation, can help adolescents develop essential social skills, provide them with a virtual platform, where they can experiment with values, morals, gender and identity before going out in the real world, and can give them a larger exposure to the world, culture, and ethos (Lemma, 2010). Social media additionally can be used to deliver mental health information to the general public, patients and mental health professionals (Moorhead et al., 2013), and forums can be used to answer questions regarding mental health. Social forums also help patients to connect with other sufferers of similar ailments and foster creation of user groups (Prescott et al., 2017). Such user groups have been shown to improve coping, resource generation and resource sharing by patients and their care providers (Naslund et al., 2016). The cost of delivering information over social media is minimal, and the content can be delivered in very less time, in formats not possible previously in print. The traditional view of social media's perceived lack of credibility and quality control gets neutralized by its transparency and self-censorship through the opposing comments of other participants. Indeed, in regimes of government censorship and business marketing, many users trust social media reports more in comparison to official channels of information (McMullan, 2006).

The myriad ramifications of social media and its intimate involvement in every facet of modern life makes it difficult to quantify its effect on mental health in unidimensional positive and negative outcome measures. The internet and social media therefore have often been considered as a "cultural tool" by sociologists (Greenfield & Yan, 2006), and like other cultural tools (automobiles, firearms, etc.), their use and outcome often depends on the user and the mode of use rather than on the intrinsic nature of the tool itself.

Information Technology and Recent Advances in Psychiatry

Technology for information processing has moved far beyond the computers into mobile and wearable devices, opening newer possibilities of detection, diagnosis and management of mental disorders. The CATEGO program (Wing et al., 2012) developed for the diagnosis of symptoms of schizophrenia in the International Pilot Study Of Schizophrenia (IPSS) was one of the first computer based systems developed for diagnosing mental disorders (Helzer et al., 1981). Subsequently, most established diagnostic instruments, including the Composite International Diagnostic Interview (CIDI) (World Health Organization, 2001), Mini International Neuropsychiatric Interview (MINI) (Sheehan et al., 2010) and Primary Care Evaluation of Mental Disorders (PRIME-MD) (Kobak et al., 1997) have been ported for automated measurement to computer systems. Several similar tools have been developed for substance use disorders, viz: Addiction Severity Index – Multimedia Version (ASI-MV), the Drinker's Check-up, and the Behavioral Self-Control Program for Windows (Hester & Miller, 2006) and for eating disorder diagnosis, viz: Eating Disorder Diagnostic Algorithm (EDDA) (Thiels & Deb, 2014). However, upcoming measurement systems for psychiatric diagnosis aspire to move beyond these static algorithms to measure mental state continuously and at the native location of the subjects using principles of "ecological momentary assessment"(Myin-Germeys et al., 2016). Initial deployment of the concept in mood detection applications based on mobile platforms shows promising decrease in recurrence rate of mood episodes and hospital visits in patients suffering from recurrent mood disorders (Faurholt-Jepsen et al., 2014).

Service delivery through tele-psychiatry has been reported to be highly efficacious in treating all age-groups, from children and adolescents, up to the geriatric population (Myers et al., 2006; Tang et al., 2001). The cost limitation of tele-psychiatry has resulted in development of multiple alternative cost effective solutions of online and computer based treatment. Computer and internet based psychotherapy modules have been developed for depression and anxiety (Spek et al., 2007), PTSD (Spence et al., 2011), social phobia (Carlbring et al., 2009), and irritable bowel syndrome (Ljótsson et al., 2010). Most such internet delivered therapies have been shown to be effective as well as cost-saving (Ebert et al., 2015). With increasing processing power and access to virtual reality, innovative new therapies are now being developed which were previously impossible. Avatar therapy for refractory auditory hallucinations, where patients create and interact with virtual avatars who take the role of persecutors, represents one such new area (Craig et al., 2017). Virtual and augmented reality training in phantom limb syndrome (Dunn et al., 2017), as well as in post stroke rehabilitation (Laver et al., 2017) open completely new areas of work. Several such virtual and game world interaction show promise for ADHD and autistic spectrum disorders, and herald the way for novel therapy techniques in psychiatry.

CONCLUSION

Ever since the advent of information technology, the human race has made progress at an unimaginable pace, changing life and lifestyle over the course of mere decades. However, the comforts of technology has also led to a more sedentary lifestyle, disruption of the normal circadian rhythm, and easier misrepresentation of facts. Where on the one hand, technology has made possible the delivery of important healthcare messages to a large number of people in a cost effective manner, it has also introduced several health issues which need addressing themselves. Mass media and information technology therefore remain akin to a double-edged sword—one that can win great achievements, but that also needs to be used with extreme care.

REFERENCES

Andrade C, Shah N, Venkatesh BK. The depiction of electroconvulsive therapy in Hindi cinema. J ECT. 2010;26:16-22.

Andreasen NJ. The artist as scientist. Psychiatric diagnosis in Shakespeare's tragedies. JAMA. 1976;235:1868-72.

Arora M, Reddy KS, Stigler MH, et al. Associations between tobacco marketing and use among urban youth in India. Am J Health Behav. 2008;32:283-94.

Assmann A. The printing press and the internet: from a culture of memory to a culture of attention. In: Gentz N, Kramer S (Eds). Globalization, Cultural Identities, and Media Representations. New York: SUNY Press; 2012. p. 11.

Banwari GH. Portrayal of psychiatrists in Hindi movies released in the first decade of the 21st century. Asian J Psychiatry. 2011;4:210-3.

Bauman S, Toomey RB, Walker JL. Associations among bullying, cyberbullying, and suicide in high school students. J Adolesc. 2013;36:341-50.

Becker AE. Television, disordered eating, and young women in Fiji: negotiating body image and identity during rapid social change. Cult Med Psychiatry. 2004;28:533-59.

Bohanna I, Wang X. Media guidelines for the responsible reporting of suicide: a review of effectiveness. Crisis. 2012;33:190-8.

Cape GS. Addiction, stigma and movies. Acta Psychiatr Scand. 2003;107:163-9.

Carlbring P, Nordgren LB, Furmark T, et al. Long-term outcome of Internet-delivered cognitive-behavioural therapy for social phobia: a 30-month follow-up. Behav Res Ther. 2009;47:848-50.

Charlesworth A, Glantz SA. Smoking in the movies increases adolescent smoking: a review. Pediatrics. 2005;116:1516-28.

Cheng J, Benassi P, de Oliveira C, et al. Impact of a mass media mental health campaign on psychiatric emergency department visits. Can J Public Health. 2016;107:e303-11.

Craig TK, Rus-Calafell M, Ward T, et al. AVATAR therapy for auditory verbal hallucinations in people with psychosis: a single-blind, randomised controlled trial. Lancet Psychiatry. 2018;5(1):31-40.

Diefenbach DL. The portrayal of mental illness on prime-time television. J Community Psychol. 1997;25:289-302.

Diefenbach DL, West MD. Television and attitudes toward mental health issues: Cultivation analysis and the third-person effect. J Community Psychol. 2007;35:181-95.

Dunn J, Yeo E, Moghaddampour P, et al. Virtual and augmented reality in the treatment of phantom limb pain: a literature review. NeuroRehabilitation. 2017;40:595-601.

Ebert DD, Zarski AC, Christensen H, et al. Internet and computer-based cognitive behavioral therapy for anxiety and depression in youth: a meta-analysis of randomized controlled outcome trials. PLoS One. 2015;10:e0119895.

Faurholt-Jepsen M, Frost M, Vinberg M, et al. Smartphone data as objective measures of bipolar disorder symptoms. Psychiatry Res. 2014;217:124-7.

Fazel S, Gulati G, Linsell L, et al. Schizophrenia and violence: systematic review and meta-analysis. PLoS Med. 2009;6:e1000120.

Gabbard G. Psychotherapy in Hollywood cinema. Australasian Psychiatry. 2001;9(4):365-9.

Gabbard G, Gabbard K. Psychiatry and the Cinema. Washington DC, American Psychiatric Press; 1999.

Gentile DA, Bailey K, Bavelier D, et al. Internet gaming disorder in children and adolescents. Pediatrics. 2017;140:S81-5.

Gerbner G. Psychology, psychiatry, and mental illness in the mass media: a study of trends, 1900–1959. Mental Hygiene. 1961;45:89-93.

Gerbner G, Gross L, Jackson-Beeck M, et al. Cultural indicators: violence profile no. 9. J Commun. 1978;28:176-207.

Gerbner G, Tannenbaum PH. Regulation of mental illness content in motion pictures and television. Int Commun Gazette. 1960;6:365-85.

Gonzales AL, Hancock JT. Mirror, mirror on my Facebook wall: effects of exposure to Facebook on self-esteem. Cyberpsychol Behav Soc Netw. 2011;14:79-83.

Gould M, Jamieson P, Romer D. Media contagion and suicide among the young. Am Behav Sci. 2003;46:1269-84.

Grabe S, Ward LM, Hyde JS. The role of the media in body image concerns among women: a meta-analysis of experimental and correlational studies. Psychol Bull. 2008;134:460-76.

Greenfield P, Yan Z. Children, adolescents, and the internet: a new field of inquiry in developmental psychology. Dev Psychol. 2006;42:391-4.

Gunasekera H, Chapman S, Campbell S. Sex and drugs in popular movies: an analysis of the top 200 films. J R Soc Med. 2005;98:464-70.

Helzer JE, Brockington IF, Kendell RE. Predictive validity of DSM-III and Feighner definitions of schizophrenia. A comparison with research diagnosis criteria and CATEGO. Arch Gen Psychiatry. 1981;38:791-7.

Hester RK, Miller JH. Computer-based tools for diagnosis and treatment of alcohol problems. Alcohol Res Health. 2006;29:36-40.

Hogan MJ, Strasburger VC. Body image, eating disorders, and the media. Adolesc Med State Art Rev. 2008;19:521-46.

Kim JH, Park EC, Nam JM, et al. The Werther effect of two celebrity suicides: an entertainer and a politician. PLoS One. 2013;8:e84876.

Kimmerle J, Cress U. The effects of television and film exposure on knowledge about and attitudes toward mental disorders. J Community Psychol. 2013;41:931-43.

Klein JD, Brown JD, Childers KW, et al. Adolescents' risky behavior and mass media use. Pediatrics. 1993;92:24-31.

Kobak KA, Taylor LH, Dottl SL, et al. A computer-administered telephone interview to identify mental disorders. JAMA. 1997;278:905-10.

Kraut R, Patterson M, Lundmark V, et al. Internet paradox: a social technology that reduces social involvement and psychological well-being? Am Psychol. 1998;53(9):1017-31.

Kuss DJ, Griffiths MD. Social networking sites and addiction: ten lessons learned. Int J Environ Res Public Health. 2017;14(3). pii: E311.

Kwan GC, Skoric MM. Facebook bullying: an extension of battles in school. Comput Hum Behav. 2013;29:16-25.

Laver KE, Lange B, George S, et al. Virtual reality for stroke rehabilitation. Cochrane Database Syst Rev. 2017;11:CD008349.

Lawson A, Fouts G. Mental illness in Disney animated films. Can J Psychiatry. 2004;49:310-4.

Lee S. Eating disorders are becoming more common in the East too. BMJ. 2000;321:1023.

Lemma A. An order of pure decision: growing up in a virtual world and the adolescent's experience of being-in-a-body. J Am Psychoanal Assoc. 2010;58:691-714.

Ljótsson B, Falk L, Vesterlund AW, et al. Internet-delivered exposure and mindfulness based therapy for irritable bowel syndrome: a randomized controlled trial. Behav Res Ther. 2010;48:531-9.

López-Guimerà G, Levine MP, Sánchez-Carracedo D, et al. Influence of mass media on body image and eating disordered attitudes and behaviors in females: a review of effects and processes. Media Psychol. 2010;13:387-416.

Maier JA, Gentile DA, Vogel DL, et al. Media influences on self-stigma of seeking psychological services: the importance of media portrayals and person perception. Psychol Pop Media Cult. 2013;3:239-56.

McAfee Internet Security, 2015. Teens, 'tweens, and technology Data Sheet, Reading Today; 2015.

McCord B, Rodebaugh TL, Levinson CA. Facebook: social uses and anxiety. Comput Hum Behav. 2014;34:23-7.

McDonald A, Walter G. The portrayal of ECT in American movies. J ECT. 2001;17:264-74.

McMullan M. Patients using the Internet to obtain health information: how this affects the patient-health professional relationship. Patient Educ Couns. 2006;63:24-8.

Messina E, Iwasaki Y. Internet use and self-injurious behaviors among adolescents and young adults: an interdisciplinary literature review and implications for health professionals. Cyberpsychol Behav Soc Netw. 2011;14(3):161-8.

Miller G. Mental health and the mass media: room for improvement. Lancet. 2007;370(9592):1015-6.

Modecki KL, Minchin J, Harbaugh AG, et al. Bullying prevalence across contexts: a meta-analysis measuring cyber and traditional bullying. J Adolesc Health Off Publ Soc Adolesc Med. 2014;55: 602-11.

Moorhead SA, Hazlett DE, Harrison L, et al. A new dimension of health care: systematic review of the uses, benefits, and limitations of social media for health communication. J Med Internet Res. 2013;15(4):e85.

Morgan M, Shanahan J. The state of cultivation. J Broadcast Electron Media. 2010;54(2):337-55.

Bottino SM, Bottino CM, Regina CG, et al. Cyberbullying and adolescent mental health: systematic review. Cad Saude Publica. 2015;31:463-75.

Myers K, Valentine J, Morganthaler R, et al. Telepsychiatry with incarcerated youth. J Adolesc Health. 2006;38:643-8.

Myin-Germeys I, Klippel A, Steinhart H, et al. Ecological momentary interventions in psychiatry. Curr Opin Psychiatry. 2016;29:258-63.

Nairn RG, Coverdale JH. People never see us living well: an appraisal of the personal stories about mental illness in a prospective print media sample. Aust N Z J Psychiatry. 2005;39:281-7.

Naslund JA, Aschbrenner KA, Marsch LA, et al. The future of mental health care: peer-to-peer support and social media. Epidemiol Psychiatr Sci. 2016;25:113-22.

Nazar GP, Gupta VK, Millett C, et al. Tobacco imagery in Bollywood films: 2006-2008. Heart Asia. 2013;5:44-6.

Niederkrotenthaler T, Voracek M, Herberth A, et al. Role of media reports in completed and prevented suicide: Werther v. Papageno effects. Br J Psychiatry. 2010;197:234-43.

Nunez-Smith M, Wolf E, Huang HM, et al. Media exposure and tobacco, illicit drugs, and alcohol use among children and adolescents: a systematic review. Subst Abuse. 2010;31:174-92.

O'Keeffe GS, Clarke-Pearson K, Council on Communications and Media. The impact of social media on children, adolescents, and families. Pediatrics. 2011;127:800-4.

Ottilingam S. The psychiatry of King Lear. Indian J Psychiatry. 2007;49:52-5.

Owen PR. Portrayals of schizophrenia by entertainment media: a content analysis of contemporary movies. Psychiatr Serv. 2012;63:655-9.

Padhy S, Khatana S, Sarkar S. Media and mental illness: relevance to India. J Postgrad Med. 2014;60: 163-70.

Pergolizzi JV, LeQuang JA, Taylor R, et al. The "Darknet": the new street for street drugs. J Clin Pharm Ther. 2017;42:790-2.

Perry B, Singh S. A virtual reality: Technology's impact on youth mental health. Indian J Soc Psychiatry 2016;32:222-6.

Philo G, Secker J, Platt S, et al. The impact of the mass media on public images of mental illness: media content and audience belief. Health Educ J. 1994;53:271-81.

Pirkis J. Blood RW, Francis C, et al. On-screen portrayals of mental illness: extent, nature, and impacts. J Health Commun. 2006;11:523-41.

Pradeep P, Sriram S. The virtual world of social networking sites: adolescent's use and experiences. Psychol Dev Soc. 2016;28:139-59.

Prescott J, Hanley T, Ujhelyi K. Peer communication in online mental health forums for young people: directional and nondirectional support. JMIR Ment Health. 2017;4:e29.

Preventing suicide: a resource for media professionals, update 2017. Geneva: World Health Organization; 2017

Rosen LD, Whaling K, Rab S, et al. Is Facebook creating "iDisorders"? The link between clinical symptoms of psychiatric disorders and technology use, attitudes and anxiety. Comput Hum Behav. 2013;29:1243-54.

Rosenberger R. An experiential account of phantom vibration syndrome. Comput Hum Behav. 2015;52:124-31.

Runions KC, Bak M. Online moral disengagement, cyberbullying, and cyber-aggression. Cyberpsychol Behav Soc Netw. 2015;18:400-5.

Schneider I. The theory and practice of movie psychiatry. Am J Psychiatry. 1987;144(8):996-1002.

Sheehan D, Sheehan K, Shytle R. Reliability and validity of the Mini International Neuropsychiatric Interview for Children and Adolescents (MINI-KID). J Clin Psychiatry. 2010;71:313-26.

Sivashanker K. Cyberbullying and the digital self. J Am Acad Child Adolesc Psychiatry. 2013;52(2):113-5.

Smith B. Mental illness stigma in the media. Rev J Undergrad Stud Res. 2015a;16.

Smith B. Mental illness stigma in the media. Rev J Undergrad Stud Res. 2015b;16.

Smith PK, Thompson F, Davidson J. Cyber safety for adolescent girls: bullying, harassment, sexting, pornography, and solicitation. Curr Opin Obstet Gynecol. 2014;26:360-5.

Spek V, Cuijpers P, Nyklicek I, et al. Internet-based cognitive behaviour therapy for symptoms of depression and anxiety: a meta-analysis. Psychol Med. 2007;37:319-28.

Spence J, Titov N, Dear B, et al. Randomized controlled trial of Internet-delivered cognitive behavioral therapy for posttraumatic stress disorder. Depress Anxiety. 2011;28:541-50.

Spettigue W, Henderson KA. Eating disorders and the role of the media. Can Child Adolesc Psychiatr Rev. 2004;13:16-9.

Stout PA, Villegas J, Jennings NA. Images of mental illness in the media: identifying gaps in the research. Schizophr Bull. 2004;30:543-61.

Strasburger VC; American Academy of Pediatrics. Council on Communications and Media. Policy statement: children, adolescents, substance abuse, and the media. Pediatrics. 2010;126:791-9.

Stuart H. Media portrayal of mental illness and its treatments: what effect does it have on people with mental illness? CNS Drugs. 2006;20(2):99-106.

Tang WK, Chiu H, Woo J, et al. Telepsychiatry in psychogeriatric service: a pilot study. Int J Geriatr Psychiatry. 2001;16:88-93.

Thiels C, Deb KS. EDDA: an eating disorder diagnostic algorithm according to ICD-11. Eat Weight Disord. 2014;19:111-4.

Tiggemann M, Slater A. NetGirls: the Internet, Facebook, and body image concern in adolescent girls. Int J Eat Disord. 2013;46:630-3.

Turow J, Coe L. Curing television's ills: the portrayal of health care. J Commun. 1985;35:36-51.

Valkenburg PM, Peter J, Schouten AP. Friend networking sites and their relationship to adolescents' well-being and social self-esteem. CyberPsychol Behav. 2006;9:584-90.

Villani D, Gatti E, Triberti S, et al. Exploration of virtual body-representation in adolescence: the role of age and sex in avatar customization. SpringerPlus. 2016;5:740.

Wahl O. Depictions of mental illnesses in children's media. J Ment Health. 2003;12:249-58.

Wahl OF. Obsessive-compulsive disorder in popular magazines. Community Ment Health J. 2000;36:307-12.

Wahl OF. Media Madness: Public Images of Mental Illness. New Brunswick, NJ: Rutgers University Press; 1995.

Wahl OF. Mass media images of mental illness: a review of the literature. J Community Psychol. 1992;20:343-52.

Wahl OF, Lefkowits JY. Impact of a television film on attitudes toward mental illness. Am J Community Psychol. 1989;17:521-8.

World Health Organization Composite International Diagnostic Interview. World Health Organization. 2001.

Wilson C, Nairn R, Coverdale J, et al. How mental illness is portrayed in children's television: a prospective study. Br J Psychiatry. 2000a;176:440-3.

Wilson C, Nairn RA, Coverdale J, et al. How mental illness is portrayed in children's television: a prospective study. Br J Psychiatry. 2000b;176:440-3.

Wing JK, Cooper JE, Sartorius N. Measurement and Classification of Psychiatric Symptoms. Cambridge: Cambridge University Press; 2012.

Chapter 43

Farmers' Suicides in India: Three Decades of Protracted Issue

Prakash Balkrishna Behere, Manik Changoji Bhise, Aniruddh Prakash Behere

SUMMARY

Suicide by farmers has been the topic of talk for over three decades in various public domains. Over 3 lakh farmers have committed suicide in country and phenomenon still continues to affect different parts. It has been attributed to financial, social, and lifestyle changes of farmers. Despite the rise in farm produce, the agriculture sector has been under chronic financial strain in last few decades. With the globalization of markets, cost of doing farm business has increased significantly. Farmers are exposed to competitive seed, fertilizer, and chemical markets, while prices of their produce remain largely controlled by governments under the banner of food items, essential for living. Recently there have been psychological autopsy studies on farmers' suicide which have established the role of psychological factors like mental illness, addictions, and impact of stressful life events in their suicide. So far, there have been inconstancies in preventive strategies. Most of the time has been lost in ex gratia and welfare activities. At this juncture, unless there is concrete prevention policy, this issue will be further protracted.

INTRODUCTION

Farmers' suicides in India have become a protracted issue for over three decades now. Since 1995, over 3 lakh farmers have committed suicide in the country. Initially thought as a regional problem, it has now been reported from most parts of the country. In Maharashtra, with changing environmental and drought situations, farmers from Marathwada and surrounding regions have committed suicide in large numbers. Its cognizance is taken by the National Crime Records Bureau of India, which has created farmers' suicides as a separate category in their report on "accidental deaths and suicide" (National Crime Records Bureau, 2014). Over three decades, much has been said and done about etiology of this issue. States like Karnataka came up with few policies to tackle it. There were loan waivers for farmers by the Union and State Governments, and ex gratia financial help, agricultural implements, livestock, etc. were distributed. Recently, Maharashtra waived off farmers' loans with a rider that loan should be from co-operative banks. Among all this hue and cry, there are silent sufferers, the family members left behind by the victim, who are often neglected (Bhise & Behere, 2016, 2017). Their agony so far is reflected in very few studies from the country. This chapter discusses the problem from a mental health point of view looking into the causation and probable solutions.

BEFORE INCEPTION OF ISSUE IN INDIA

Suicide by farmers has been brought to the light by media reports and some studies in rural areas in the late 1990s. Prior to this, though not known as a separate category in India, studies on farmers across the globe had established their vulnerability for suicide. In the late 1980s, it was observed that the suicide rate amongst Australian farmers was twice as high as the general male population, ranging from 47.7 per 100,000 for male farm managers to 54.6 per 100,000 for agricultural laborers against a rate of 21.1 per 100,000 for general male population (Gun et al., 1996). The most common method for committing suicide was hanging followed by carbon monoxide poisoning. This correlates with literature that method of suicide adopted is usually the one which is lethal and easily available. Another study revealed that in the decade 1988–1997, one farm-related suicide had happened every 4 days. This was far higher than found in rural Australia during the same period (Page & Fragar, 2002). After this, the Australian government took preventive steps like programs to increase the adaptability of farmers to stressors, increased community suicide awareness through targeted programs, access to counseling services and mental health first aid skills, and targeted resilience building and interventions in high-risk areas like drought, etc. Subsequently, during Victorian drought from 2001 to 2007, there was no significant increase in the number of farmers' suicides (Guiney, 2012). During the 1980s, research on mental health of farmers in rest of the world was also accumulating. A study conducted by the Health Department in the UK found that farmers are essentially practical people and like to do things on the go. More than half of the farmers had difficulty maintaining records and keeping up with the myriad of forms, regulations, and legislation pertaining to their profession (Hawton et al., 1998). Almost all were worried about money, and more than a quarter had financial problems. Additionally, a third had physical health issues. Another study from the UK reported that levels of depression and anxiety were higher in farmers than in the general population, with farmers more likely to report that life was not worth living (Eisner et al., 1998).

North America experienced a farming crisis in the 1980s that led to a rise in the number of suicides by farmers. There was a nearly 6-fold elevation in suicide rate in farmers during the period of 1984–1989 in Alabama (USA), compared to people working in public administration (Liu & Waterbor, 1994). Iowa also saw a raised proportional mortality ratio of 1.20 in the same period. Minnesota, North and South Dakota, Montana and Wisconsin saw a suicide rate of 50.1/100,000, which was significantly higher than that of the general population (Pylka & Gunderson, 1992). All these studies were conducted within same decade and indicated the worsening state of farm crisis in North America. This trend continued into next decade. Between 1990 and 1998, in three states Kentucky, South Carolina, and North Carolina, suicide rates for white male farmers were significantly higher than that in the general white male population (Browning et al., 2008). Some proposed factors for this were chronic medical illness, depression, financial crisis, stressful life events, etc.

The fact that the farming sector experiences one of the highest suicide rates than any other profession is in stark contrast to the portrayal of this field having a happy and healthy way of living. Farmers' suicides have been reported across India from Kerala, Karnataka, Uttar Pradesh, Punjab and the Vidarbha region. In view of this, the recommendations of numerous inquiry commissions have been implemented.

In India, the Vidarbha region in Maharashtra was the first to report a volley of farmers' suicides in the 1990s. The fact that suicide rates are high among farmers is apparent from SCRB (State Crime Records Bureau) data. This is troublesome as almost 3.4 million cotton farmers are present in the Vidarbha region (including Washim, Buldana, Nagpur, Akola, Amravati, Gondia, Yavatmal, Chandrapur, Bhandara, Wardha, and Gadchiroli districts) (Behere & Rathod, 2006). Behere and Rathod (2006) further investigated the status of farmers' suicide in this region using psychological autopsy, at the request of the district administration of Wardha. This approach offered insight into the drastic step of suicide committed by farmers.

During the same time frame in India, there were few more studies on suicide from rural areas, where farming is a major occupation. Though these studies did not focus on only farmers, they can be a reflection of what was happening in rural India, where farming is a prime source of living. A study by Banerjee et al. (1990) from 24 Parganas District of West Bengal found that in the year under study (i.e. 1979), a higher proportion of females had committed suicide than males. Pesticide poisoning was the most common method adopted for suicide. Interpersonal issues and quarrels with a spouse were cited as causes for suicide. Another study by Nandi et al. (1979) from West Bengal reported minimal impact of restriction of Endrin, a lethal pesticide, on occurrence of suicide among farmers, and attributed high suicide rates in Daspur police station region to the interpersonal issues, stress due to modern farm practices and chronic incurable disease in victims. Suicide in Punjab farmers was also an intriguing phenomena at that time. Media was reporting indebtedness as the prime cause of suicide by farmers while Punjab, farmers were known for their prosperity. Bhalla et al. (1998) reported that in rural Punjab, young farmers and agriculture laborers with minimal or no education were at higher risk of committing suicide. Most suicide victims had small or marginal land holding. Nearly 70% of the victims were unable to maintain satisfying relationships and had frequent discords with other family members. Compared to the general population, significantly higher proportion of suicide victims had substance abuse and dependence issues. Most (92%) of them were reported to have mental stress at the time of death. Depressive symptoms were present in 54.7%, and irritability and aggression (9.4%), emotional isolation (9.4%), and insomnia (7.5%) were the associated symptoms. Indebtedness was reported in 18% of the cases, much lower than expected from media reports. This study had played a pivotal role in understanding of farmers' suicide, and was a joint effort of social scientists, mental health professionals, and economists. First time in India, it had asserted the role of psychological factors in farmers' suicide. Unfortunately even today, the role of mental health professionals in prevention activities is largely questioned by governments and intellectual circles.

QUEST FOR IDENTIFICATION OF RISK FACTORS

Media has been one of the biggest driving as well as diverting force in the quest for risk factors of suicide by farmers in India. Since the beginning, it has been highlighting indebtedness and economic difficulties as the "only" cause of suicide by farmers. There were some good articles by Sainath (2007) in The Hindu newspaper, which covered different dimensions of the issue and solutions to it. When one looks at the available literature, attempts by scholars from different fields look akin to the story of "the elephant and blind men." There are studies from sociologists, economists, administrative institutions, agricultural scientists, and mental health professionals, which have found evidence in favor of their hypothesis. So far, collaborative efforts by different intellectual circles are lacking. At present, the issue is further complicated by political sensitization and interests of some groups involved. Initially, the economic and the social aspects of this issue were investigated. Field studies were carried out by the Indira Gandhi Institute of Development Research, Mumbai (Mishra, 2006) and the Tata Institute of Social Sciences (2005). Daughter's/sister's marriage, indebtedness, conflict in the family, suicide in the neighborhood or in the family, crop failure, lowering of social status, economic downfall, addiction, and health problems (including problems of mental health) were found to be associated with farmers' suicides. Conversely, findings by the Yashwantrao Chavan Academy of Development Administration, Pune differed from these, even though they studied an almost identical sample (Lochan & Lochan, 2006). Above studies have been criticized for not being able to conceptualize the association between farm crisis and suicides, and did not include a nonsuicidal and nonfarmer control group.

Literature associating suicide by farmers with the agrarian crisis in India is also available. Green revolution has increased the yield of crops, but it came at its own cost. Foodgrain stocks have been surplus for domestic needs for a decade. Scenes of grains getting spoiled in government warehouses are common. For farmers, over the years the government has stopped subsidies on fertilizers and pesticides leading to 800 times rise in the cost of these inputs. Payments to laborers and machines owners have also increased by more than 100-fold. Newer high yielding varieties of crops needed additional fertilizers and more frequent pesticide sprays. These crops also needed more frequent irrigation than traditional crops. Thus, the cost of doing farming has significantly increased the last 30 years. On the other hand, prices of farm produce have increased only 8–10 times in the same period. Thus, over the last three decades, farming has become less viable in terms of earning. Majority of farmers reported that, given a choice, they would quit farming for some other source of earning. This is further compounded by open markets and globalization. Cost of living in the villages has increased significantly. Farmers have to spend significantly more amount of money on education, health and other amenities for the family than in the past. All this is leading to high financial demands on farmers, forcing them to borrow money from multiple sources. Based on their findings on this issue, authors proposed "vicious cycle of indebtedness" which traps farmers **(Figure 1)**. Considering the fact that larger proportions (82% of all farmers interviewed) of suicide and nonsuicide households had debt, and that cost of living and cost of doing farming both increased significantly in recent years, we can say that seeking debt is a common practice in India (Bhise & Behere, 2010). The most common source of debt is commercial banks, which issue "crop loan" to farmers, meant to be spent on agriculture. It is hoped that providing money to spend on agriculture will help in better inputs and ultimately good yields for crops so that these debts are paid back to banks, with good profit to farmers.

This cycle of debt goes on for years without much stress to farmers. But in actual life, the scenario is different. There are so many additional expenses in a farmer's life. A farmer gets trapped into this cycle with mounting amounts of debt when these additional or unexpected expenses come in his way. The most common reasons for these additional expenses that were incurred by suicide victims in our study were family expenses, e.g. health, education, festivals, marriage of sister or daughter, digging well, etc. When these expenses come in the way,

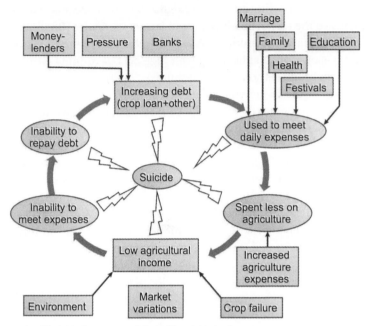

Figure 1: Vicious cycle of indebtedness associated with suicide by farmers.
Source: Bhise and Behere (2010).

crop loans are diverted to meet these financial burdens. This leads to a shortage of finances to run agriculture, leading to decreased inputs on crops. This in association with high costs of pesticides, seeds, and agricultural labor, ultimately leads to low agricultural income. This is compounded by poor rains, crop failures, and fluctuating market prices for agricultural produce. Further, this leads to an inability to repay existing debt as was evident among suicide victims in our study. Current banking policy is that unless previous debts are cleared off, fresh loans can not be obtained. This leads to a feeling of helplessness, as to run farms, many such farmers do not have enough funds in hand. This along with additional expenses that can not be met with by crop loans propels farmers toward private moneylenders, who charge extremely high-interest rates. All these factors lead to severe distress among the farmers. Pressure from moneylenders and banks further adds to the distress among farmers. Once deeply rooted in this cycle, there is no way out. The ego of farmers can break-down at various stages leading to suicide. Thus, though suicide victims had relatively similar amounts of debt as controls, they have other debt characteristics that played a crucial role in pushing them deep into the *vicious cycle of indebtedness* in our study (Bhise & Behere, 2010).

Indebtedness and financial distress in farmers have also been documented in other studies on farmers' suicide. Mishra (2006) had reported similar findings on indebtedness in his case-control study from central India. A study from Kerala reported that both suicide victims and control families reported a very low average annual income (₹ 20,000 to ₹ 45,000). These farmers did not have sufficient resources to rise above certain barrier of income (Xavier et al., 2007). There is complete lack of other allied sources of income for farmers such as dairy, fishery, etc. To meet the ends in the face of inadequate income, farmers have to obtain loans from private moneylenders who extort them with high-interest rates. Other Indian studies have also emphasized the role of indebtedness in farmers' suicides (Bhalla et al., 1998; Behere & Behere, 2008). In a qualitative study from central India, indebtedness was perceived as one of the important reasons for suicide, along with high cost of running farm business and low market price for farm produces (Dongre & Deshmukh, 2010).

The literature on suicide in general and mental illness reveals a strong correlation between the two. Contribution of mental illness to the suicide risk at an individual level is far greater than the impact of social or economic factors (Cavanagh et al., 2003). Psychological autopsy studies across India such as Gururaj et al. (2004) from Bangalore, Chavan et al. (2008) from Chandigarh, Vijayakumar & Rajkumar (1999) from Chennai have reported the presence of diagnosable mental illness in suicide victims. As of now in India, studies on farmers' mental health and suicide are very few. Rather there are some leaders in the field, who have minimized the role of psychological factors. An example quoted by Dr RS Murthy in his oration speech is here: Ms Vandana Shiva, an international environmental activist, said on BBC Hard Talk Show "When 40,000 Indian farmers end their life, it is no more an issue of psychological aberration; it is no more an issue of depression on the part of particular farmer. It has become an economic phenomenon." He went on to say that with complex phenomena like suicide, there is a need to take a multifaceted approach (Murthy, 2012). Sometimes eminent psychiatrists themselves underrate or rather question the involvement of mental health professionals in the prevention of farmers' suicide in India. In a recent editorial in a national journal, it is quoted "there is a certain folly in suggesting mental health professionals" role; can such a professional go from farm to farm each season to offer antidepressants and psychotherapy to farmers, whose families face financial ruin?' Keeping this aside, in recent years, there had been some studies looking at mental health perspective of the issue (Rao et al., 2017). In our study from Wardha district in Vidarbha, Maharashtra, 60% of the farmers' suicide victims had some diagnosable psychiatric illness. Most common were depression (37.7%) and alcohol dependence (10%) followed by other psychiatric illnesses. In addition, 42% had alcohol abuse. In 20% of the cases, victims had expressed suicide ideas to close family members or friends (Bhise & Behere, 2016). A study from Kerala had similarly found a high prevalence of psychiatric illness among farmers who committed suicide. There, alcohol abuse (23.2%) was a commonest psychiatric diagnosis, followed by depression (17.9%). Also, 23.1% of the victims had past history of suicide attempt. However, only 10% had received treatment for past attempt (Xavier et al., 2007). A recent study from Assam correlated farmers' suicide with stressful life events prior to committing suicide. Some of the stressful life events often recognized by the family members were major personal illness or injury, and excessive alcohol or drug use by family members. In few cases, indebtedness was a major stressor. Property or crops damage, death of spouse, and family conflict were other major stressors. Few had experienced the death of a close family member and sexual problems as a stress factor (Thakuria & Mazumder, 2017). Findings from a qualitative study investigating farmers from the Vidarbha region found that stress, family responsibilities, poor financial return, perceived debt, government apathy, high input costs, poor irrigation, pressure to return loans, crop failure, and substance use were major reasons for committing suicide (Dongre & Deshmukh, 2010). Solutions suggested by the participants themselves included support and counseling services, including a monitoring system for the vulnerable, transparent disbursement of relief packages, and capacity building among farmers.

In our study on survivors of farmer's suicide in Wardha district, we found that significantly higher proportion of survivors had psychological distress than controls. Female survivors, spouses and parents of suicide victims had a high risk of distress. Psychological distress was commonly expressed in form of depressive and somatic symptoms (Bhise & Behere, 2016, 2017).

FACTORS RESPONSIBLE FOR NONRESOLUTION OF ISSUE

Crisis mitigation for farmers' suicides in the country so far has failed on multiple occasions. Over the last three decades, the issue stands unresolved indicating that there are some fallacies in approaches so far. Initially, there has been a strong denial of the existence of this crisis. It was termed as mere "media hype" by many. This led to prolonged apathy and distress in the farming sector. Initial descriptions in media were predominantly of suicide due to the financial crisis. In lines with this, in the Union budget of 2008–09, there was debt waiver of farm loans. Though temporarily applauded by many, soon it was realized that this scheme had minimal impact in prevention of farmers' suicides (Jadhav, 2008). Other schemes for farmers like the supply of livestock and farm implements, redistribution of subsequent loans, etc. failed in alleviating this crisis. Another fallacy in initial approach by the government institutions was a focus on ex gratia financial help. Provision of financial help to the bereaved families, though important in itself, did not have effect in the prevention of suicide. Ownership of farm and presence of indebtedness or financial burden were the criteria used to define farmers' suicides, and eligibility to ex gratia help was decided accordingly. This, as found in our study led to nonreceipt of government aid by 55% of the households of the farmers committing suicide. This also to the exclusion of those with any illness (not only psychiatric) or stress due to significant life events prior to suicide, from the category of "farmers" suicide' in government records. Due to the complex interplay of farm and family environment and stressors associated with it, it is difficult to judge whether suicide was due to financial loss or due to other causes. It is time now to break this barrier of "welfare approach" and take systematic steps incorporating social, economic, and psychological measures aimed at strengthening farmers and prevention of farmer's suicides. Educating farmers in the safe use of pesticides is an important prevention strategy, ignored so far. Considering the fact that 60–70% suicide victims used pesticide poisoning as a method of suicide, and also that access to pesticides is need of modern farming, a midway solution on the issue is a must. Sri Lanka has set a very good example by regulating pesticides (Gunnell et al., 2007; Hawton et al., 2009). Over decades, they have reduced suicide rate by almost half of what was in the early 1990s. There was the withdrawal of some highly lethal pesticides from market lethality of most of the pesticides was reduced. This was combined with a mass campaign for safe storage and safe use of pesticides, identification of high-risk individuals and training of primary healthcare workers in management of pesticide poisoning. Few experimental strategies like storage of pesticides in one central place in a village in lockers, provision of lockable boxes for storage of pesticides, etc. were accepted well by local people in Sri Lanka. Similar provisions in India can help reduce deaths from pesticide poisoning (and suicide in general). This along with other psychosocial and economic strategies will go a long way in suicide prevention.

Involvement of mental health professionals in farmers' suicide prevention activities has met with resistance from media, political fronts and farmer groups as well. This is in lines with the stigma associated with mental illness in society. This also indicates that we the mental health professionals, in general, need to work in liaison with society to spread mental health awareness to break the stigma. Another aspect of this barrier is fear of loss of financial benefits if suicide is termed to be due to mental illness. At the policy level, this needs to be handled delicately. As discussed above, irrespective of whether financial crisis is present or not, all suicides by farmers should be categorized as "farmers' suicides", and there should be flexibility in provisions of help to the affected families as per their needs. A system for early identification of farmers with psychological distress and provision of mental health care for those screened will be an important step in reducing suicides.

CONCLUSION

Contrary to the commonly held notion, farmers' suicide is not only a mental health issue but is rather contributed to by several factors including family disputes, alcohol abuse, and depression caused by a poor financial status, grain drain, chronically remaining in debt, high input costs and poor returns, and the practice of government compensation following suicide. The issue thus requires a sensitive handling using a multipronged approach including welfare measures, as well as raising mental health awareness, early detection of risk factors, and creating treatment facilities. The psychosocial risk factors need to be carefully managed by a professional approach involving all the stake holders.

REFERENCES

Banerjee G, Nandi DN, Nandi S, et al. The vulnerability of Indian women to suicide a field-study. Indian J Psychiatry. 1990;32(4):305-8.

Behere PB, Behere AP. Farmers' suicide in Vidarbha region of Maharashtra state: a myth or reality? Indian J Psychiatry. 2008;50:124-7.

Behere PB, Rathod M. Report on Farmers' Suicide in Vidarbha, Wardha. Report submitted to Collectorate Wardha, Government of Maharashtra, India; 2006.

Bhalla GS, Sharma SL, Wig NN, et al. Suicides in rural Punjab. Report submitted to Government of Punjab by Institute for Development and Communication. Himalaya Press; 1998.

Bhise MC, Behere PB. A case-control study of psychological distress in survivors of farmers' suicides in Wardha district in Central India. Indian J Psychiatry. 2016;58(2):147-51.

Bhise MC, Behere PB. Risk factors for farmers' suicides in central rural India: matched case-control psychological autopsy study. Indian J Psychol Med. 2016;38:560-6.

Bhise MC, Behere PB. Psychological autopsy of farmers' suicides. Dissertation submitted to Maharashtra University of Health Sciences, Nashik in partial fulfillment of MD. Psychiatry, 2010.

Browning SR, Westneat SC, McKnight RH. Suicides among farmers in three southeastern states, 1990-1998. J Agric Saf Health. 2008;14(4):461-72.

Cavanagh JT, Carson AJ, Sharpe M, et al. Psychological autopsy studies of suicide: a systematic review. Psychol Med. 2003;33:395-405.

Chavan BS, Singh GP, Kaur J, et al. Psychological autopsy of 101 suicide cases from northwest region of India. Indian J Psychiatry. 2008;50:34-8.

Dongre A, Deshmukh PR. Farmers' suicides in the Vidarbha region of Maharashtra, India: a qualitative exploration of the causes. J Inj Violence Res. 2012;4(1):2-6.

Eisner CS, Neal RD, Scaife B. Depression and anxiety in farmers. Prim Care Psychiatry. 1998;4:101-5.

Guiney R. Farming suicides during the Victorian drought: 2001-2007. Aust J Rural Health. 2012;20:11-5.

Gun RT, Langley AJ, Dundas SJ, et al. The Human Cost of Work: A Review of the Occurrence and Causes of Occupational Injury and Disease in South Australia, 2nd edition. Adelaide: South Australian Health Commission; 1996.

Gunnell D, Fernando R, Hewagama M, et al. The impact of pesticide regulations on suicide in Sri Lanka. Int J Epidemiol. 2007;36(6):1235-42.

Gururaj G, Isaac MK, Subbakrishna DK, et al. Risk factors for completed suicides: a case-control study from Bangalore, India. Inj Control Saf Promot. 2004;11(3):183-91.

Hawton K, Fagg J, Simkin S, et al. Methods used for suicide by farmers in England and Wales: the contribution of availability and its relevance to prevention. Br J Psychiatry. 1998;173:320-4.

Hawton K, Ratnayeke L, Simkin S, et al. Evaluation of acceptability and use of lockable storage devices for pesticides in Sri Lanka that might assist in prevention of self-poisoning. BMC Public Health. 2009;9:69.

Jadhav N. Farmers' Suicide and Debt Waiver: An action plan for agricultural development of Maharashtra. Report submitted to Government of Maharashtra; 2008.

Liu T, Waterbor JW. Comparison of suicide rates among industrial groups. Am J Ind Med. 1994;25(2):197-203.

Lochan M, Lochan R. Farmers' Suicide: Facts and possible policy interventions. Pune, Yashwantrao Chavan Academy of Development Administration; 2006.

Mishra S. Farmers' suicides in Maharashtra. Economic Political Weekly. 2006;41(16):1538-45.

Murthy RS. Farmers suicide: need for mental health interventions. Indian J Soc Psychiatry. 2012;28:26-35.

Nandi DN, Mukherjee SP, Banerjee G, et al. Is suicide preventable by restricting the availability of lethal Agents? A rural survey of West Bengal. Indian J Psychiatry. 1979;21:251-5.

National Crime Records Bureau of India: Accidental Deaths and Suicide in India. Ministry of Home Affairs, Government of India, 2014.

Page AN, Fragar LJ. Suicide in Australian farming, 1988-1997. Aust N Z J Psychiatry. 2002;36:81-5.

Pylka KP, Gunderson PD. An epidemiologic study of suicide among farmers and its clinical implications. Marshfield Clinic Bulletin. 1992;26:29-57.

Rao TS, Gowda MR, Ramachandran K, et al. Prevention of farmer suicides: greater need for state role than for a mental health professional's role. Indian J Psychiatry. 2017;59:3-5.

Sainath P. Farm suicides rising, most intense in four States. The Hindu, November 12, 2007.

Tata Institute of Social Sciences, Rural Campus. Causes of Farmer Suicides in Maharashtra: an enquiry. Final report submitted to the Mumbai High Court, 2005.

Thakuria P, Mazumder A. A study on stressful life events and farmers suicide. Indian J Forensic Med Toxicol. 2017;11(1):70-2.

Vijayakumar L, Rajkumar S. Are risk factors for suicide universal? A case control study in India. Acta Psychiatr Scand. 1999;99:407-11.

Xavier PV, Dinesh N, John AJ, et al. Position paper and action plan on farmers' suicide: presentation to Chief Minister and Health Minister, Kerala. J Psychiatry. 2007;22(1):68-75.

Rural Mental Health

Vimal Kumar Sharma

SUMMARY

This chapter outlines different patterns of distribution of rural population around the world. Rapid rural development and advancement in communication technology have narrowed down the differences in ways of living in rural and urban population. Most populated countries such as China and India still have a sizable rural population. This is true of African subcontinent as well as central parts of Australia.

Contrary to public belief that people living in rural area suffer less from mental illness, epidemiological studies around the world found no difference in mental health morbidity in this population. The prevalence of various mental disorders along with suicide rates in rural population is briefly outlined.

Service provision for mentally ill people living in rural areas remains a major challenge due to multitude of factors. Lack of resources and facilities needed to provide treatment and care to sufferers of mental illness, reluctance of specialist mental health professionals to work for or reach out to this population, reluctance to accept help for mental illness due to cultural belief systems, stigma attached to mental illness and poor affordability for health are some of common barriers in organizing mental health services for rural population.

The last section of the chapter outlines the way forward on how to meet the rural world's mental health needs. Raising awareness of mental illness as well as overcoming unhelpful cultural myths through public health education programs, training frontline health workers in mental health, using modern technology to reach out to this population and improving resources and facilities for the care of people with mental health problems are some of practical ways to address this need.

INTRODUCTION

Rural area is referred to countryside with thinly spread smaller size of population mainly involved with agricultural work. The Indian census, for example, defines rural area with population of less than 5000, density of population no more than 400 per square kilometer, and 25% or more working males working in agricultural sector.

In 1960, two-thirds (66%) of the world's population resided in rural area, which came down to around 46% by 2015. The proportion of population living in rural areas is lower in developed or high income countries like Europe and North America (18–25%), as compared to low and middle income countries (69% and 50% respectively), as per the World Bank data

(World Bank, 2015). It is worth noting that the industrialization and development of countries over the years has led to more and more urban migration and therefore a sizable decline in world's rural population.

Trinidad and Tobago and Burundi top the list, where nearly 90% of people live in rural areas. African subcontinent on the whole holds the highest proportion of rural population; however, based on the overall population of countries such as India and China, the maximum number of people (over one billion) live in rural areas is in these two countries.

The rural population is highest in developing (low income) countries. Poverty, illiteracy and poor birth control are some of the factors responsible for higher rural population in these countries. Most rural communities are still reliant on agriculture as their main occupation.

Mental health services available to rural dwellers are very inadequate. Lack of mental health specialists is often blamed for the poor mental health service provision. However, a number of other factors such as stigma-based views toward mental illness and their cultural beliefs for causes and remedies of mental disorders lead to poor acceptance or even rejection of the recommended ways of treating mental health problems. Mental health service provision to rural communities requires a deeper understanding of their needs, beliefs and attitudes toward mental illness as well as a good deal of knowledge of existing ways and resources, they routinely use in dealing with them.

EPIDEMIOLOGY OF MENTAL DISORDERS IN RURAL POPULATION

Mental disorders are as prevalent in rural population as much as in urban dwellers. The prevalence rate of all mental and behavioral disorders in rural population is around 10–15%. In recent years, the problems of substance misuse and self-harm as well as suicide has gone up in rural population. In a 20-year comparative study in rural India, Nandi et al. (2000) found slight decline of prevalence of mental disorders from 11.7% to 10.5% with biggest decline in cases of hysteria, anxiety and phobic disorders with a similar increase in cases of depression. However, that may not be the case in the recent years. A recent national survey carried out in several states in India by the National Institute of Mental Health and Neurosciences, Bengaluru found that about 10% of rural population suffered from mental disorders as compared to around 14% in urban areas (Gururaj et al., 2016). In another study of rural older adults, Tiwari et al. (2013) found that 24% of this population had mental disorders mainly depression, cognitive impairment and dementia (Tiwari et al., 2013). A raised suicidal rate among rural farmers in India is a well-known fact in recent years (Behere & Behere, 2008). Surprisingly in a recent survey in rural India, Rathod et al. (2017) found alcohol consumption predominantly in men (23%), and nearly half of them had problem drinking (Rathod et al., 2017). In China, on the other hand the mental disorders are relatively less prevalent. Gu et al. (2013) did a systematic review where prevalence of major depressive disorder was estimated to be around 2% in rural population (Gu et al., 2013).

Psychiatric morbidity in rural African subcontinent is on the other hand higher. In a study carried out in nineties in a South African village, Rumble et al. found over 27% population experiencing mental health problems (Rumble et al., 1996). In another recent study in Western Kenya, 45% of people had life time prevalence of mental illness (Kwobah et al., 2017). In a study in rural agricultural population of Western Kenya, 10.8% of people had common mental disorders, mainly anxiety and depression (Jenkins et al., 2012).

In the developed countries such as USA and Australia, the prevalence rates of mental illness in rural population is the same (around 20%) as in their urban counter parts, yet the services available to rural population for their mental disorders are poor (Gramm et al., 2010). There are more suicides among rural population. In a meta-analysis of prevalence studies of mental disorders in the developed countries on the other hand, Peen et al. found that urbanization raised prevalence rate of mental disorders urban dwellers compared to rural ones (Peen et al., 2010).

As there is increase in the longevity of the rural population in last 10 years along with societal changes, the rural population is at a higher risk of developing mental health population.

MENTAL HEALTH SERVICE PROVISION AND ITS CHALLENGES

Mental health services to rural population are scarcely available throughout the world. This is particularly a bigger problem in low and middle income countries. Kumar (2012) highlighted a huge treatment gap, poor resources and lack of government's attention on mental health of rural India. There are significant challenges to provide acceptable level of mental health services to rural population. Some of them are outlined in the following section (Kumar, 2012).

Low Priority Given to Mental Health by Authorities

Mental health generally receives lower priority in the overall health spending despite the fact that mental health leads to significant morbidity in rural population. This is even worse for rural communities especially of low and middle income countries, where a large proportion (over half) of people live in rural areas (Monteiro et al., 2014). Lack of governments' sustainable initiatives and programs on rural mental health lead to poor distribution of mental health related resources and somewhat demoralization in health workers who are keen to provide services for mentally ill people.

Poor Resources and Accessibility

The number of mental health professionals working in rural areas is fewer even in high income countries. The situation is even worse for low-middle income and low income countries. The World Mental Health Atlas reveals that whereas high income countries spend around $57 per capita on mental health, the figures for low to middle income countries are below $2 per person per year, most of which is spent on in-patient facilities (World Health Organization, 2015). Rural communities of low-middle countries are therefore left with hardly any mental health resource. The number of psychiatrists in high income countries is significantly more compared to in low-middle income countries, with some places having just one or two psychiatrist for the whole country, and mainly in the cities.

As outlined above, rural population has no local mental health facilities. It becomes inconvenient and expensive for the individuals living in rural community to travel to cities to seek help for mental illness. The situation is no better in high income countries where primary care physicians have little knowledge and skills to manage mental health problems, and rural communities have scarce specialist resources (Gramm et al., 2010).

Poor Acceptability of Services

Rural communities still have their cultural beliefs and misconceptions toward behavior resulting from mental illness as being considered to be caused by supernatural causes or bad spirits (Ngui et al., 2010). Poor literacy largely plays an important part in such deeply held beliefs. They often seek help from faith-healers. People with mental illness are stigmatized, believing they are being possessed by evil spirits (Mohit, 2001). As a result, they avoid seeking help from mental health specialists even if that help is made available.

Inadequate Mental Health Knowledge and Skills amongst Health Workers

Health workers and primary care doctors serving rural communities are not skilled to identify and manage mental disorders (Sharma & Copeland, 2009). Inadequate training on mental health is well-recognized by the WHO and considered as an important reason for treatment gap for mental disorders (World Health Organization, 2010, 2016).

WAY FORWARD TO MEET THE MENTAL HEALTH NEEDS OF RURAL POPULATION

A proper planning of the mental health services for people living in rural areas needs a multi-facet approach. Some authors have outlined that community mental health services should take account of socio-economic context, individual and population-based preventative approach, open and easy access, team-based approach, long term and sustainable approach, and the cost-effectiveness of the services provided (Thornicroft et al., 2016). The services should focus on strengths and aspirations of people with a focus on recovery and fulfillment, should strengthen from family to communities to organizations' support, and should apply evidence-based interventions with genuine involvement of people (Jacobson & Greenley, 2001). Mental Health Action Plan (2013–2020) expects majority of countries to fulfill its objectives of (1) Effective leadership and good governance in providing community focused mental health services, (2) Comprehensive integrated and responsive mental health and social care in the communities, (3) Implement mental health promotion and prevention strategies, and (4) Develop and strengthen integrated information systems to gather evidence and carry out applied research in collaboration with academic institutes. These objectives have to be taken into consideration in service organization (World Health Organization, 2013).

Involving Communities

A broad understanding of rural communities' mental health needs is only possible by approaching people, families and key community leaders to find out what they understand about mental health problems. This knowledge would be valuable to develop appropriate public educational programs for mental health. Community involvement in organizing health services is a widely recommended essential approach (Thornicroft et al., 2016; World Health

Organization, 2013). User involvement is well-advanced in the western world and has made a real impact on effective service development (Simpson & House, 2002).

Public Education about Mental Health

Mental health must be everyone's business. Teachers at school, employers at work place, police, families, friends and relatives in their social interactions often notice change in people's behavior, performance, etc. Having some understanding through mental health public education that mental ill health may be attributable to the change of behavior, can prompt them to get right help at earliest opportunity.

There should therefore be a public mental health education program as a part of government's initiative. Advancing technology now available to rural people and media, including social media could be used for this purpose. Public health education program should also address the issue of stigma and discrimination, and misconceptions associated with mental disorders. A simple message should be effectively conveyed to people that mental illness is a health issue, and people with timely and right care, and treatment can fully recover.

Skilling Health Workers in Mental Health—Training and Education

Mental Health Gap Action Programme (mhGAP) by WHO highlighted that in low and middle income countries, around 80% of all people with mental disorders do not receive adequate treatment for their mental health conditions (World Health Organization, 2016). This proportion is even higher for rural communities in low income countries which form nearly one-third of the world's population. As a result, training of frontline health workers in mental health, so that they can identify, diagnose and manage mental health problems of rural people themselves as far as possible, is only the answer. Hence, mhGAP provided intervention guidelines (mhGAP-IG, World Health Organization, 2016) for health workers to learn to identify and manage priority conditions such as depression, psychosis, bipolar disorder, epilepsy, childhood developmental and behavioral disorders, dementia, substance misuse, self-harm, and other emotionally and medically unexplained complaints. Another progress has been the development of program to reduce treatment gap for mental disorders (PRIME— **Pr**ogramme for **I**mproving **M**ental health car**E**) for low and middle income countries and a detailed evaluation process (Lund et al., 2012, 2016; World Health Organization, 2016). The program incorporates the mhGAP-IG for up-skilling health workers. The PRIME package targeted community level (frontline workers), health care facility level (health center) and organizational level (district health administration). Initial PRIME field trials in five countries, Ethiopia, India, Nepal, South Africa and Uganda have shown some promising findings (Fekadu et al., 2016; Jordans et al., 2016; Kigozi et al., 2016; Petersen et al., 2016; Shidhaye et al., 2016). Three of the five trials (India, Nepal & Ethiopia) included mostly rural population. These studies identified various challenges of integrating mental health in primary care level. A sufficient length of mental health training, ongoing support from specialist, and making medicines and other resources available at primary care level are some of them. It is also important to find out about primary care workers' attitudes toward mental illness. Ma et al. (2015) discovered that many primary care workers had negative views of mental illness in rural China.

Mental health assessment tools for primary care have been developed like Global Mental Health Assessment Tool (GMHAT) (Sharma & Copeland, 2009; Sharma, 2015). The primary care version—GMHAT/PC is a semi-structured, computer-assisted clinical assessment tool, designed to help health workers in making quick, convenient and comprehensive standardized mental health assessments in both primary and general health care. The assessment program consists of various screens. Initially program gives details on how to use the tool and how to rate the symptoms. The first two screens assess details about present, past, personal and social history, which also includes history of epilepsy, trauma and learning disorder. Subsequent screens assess mental status in a quick yet comprehensive manner. The initial questions are for screening major symptom complexes, which if answered positively lead on to additional questions. The symptom areas screened by the tool include worries, anxiety, panic attacks, concentration, low mood, mania, psychosis, suicidal risk, sleep, appetite, obsessive-compulsive symptoms, hypochondriasis, memory impairment, disorientation, substance misuse, personality, etc. It is now widely being used and has also been translated into different languages including Hindi, Arabic, English and Spanish (Krishna et al., 2009; Sharma et al., 2004, 2008, 2010, 2013; Tejada et al., 2016). The questions have been arranged in clinical order. A training program of 2–3 days was also developed by the GMHAT team for frontline workers to provide knowledge and skills to help them identify, diagnose and manage mental disorders at primary care level. The findings of field trials are promising and detailed in a book recently published by Indian Psychiatric Society (Behere et al., 2017). GMHAT/PC may prove to be very useful clinical tool for frontline health workers in association with mhGAP-IG.

Treatment and Specialist's Support to be Made Available at Rural Community Level

All recent PRIME field studies' findings highlighted that poor supply of medicines particularly in rural areas caused problems in treating people with mental illness (Lund et al., 2016). A need of ongoing support from mental health specialists was also considered necessary. These matters require a strong commitment at a higher governmental level. While the practitioners who provide general health care can serve the rural population for their mental health needs, the mental health specialists may help the practitioners in management of mental health problems by training, educating and supporting them.

Technology Support—in Detecting and Treating Mental Health Problems

People from low-income countries are also able to afford technology like mobile phones and tablets. The mobile network is now available in the remote areas of these countries. It is therefore necessary to explore the ways to reach out to people living in rural and remote areas using smart phones and computers. Health workers following training may use tools such as GMHAT/PC that is now available in android app and can easily be used for mental health assessment using android phone.

Advancement of tele-medicine is very promising. People from remote areas can easily communicate with specialists from any part of the world (Rathod et al., 2017). The governments should invest in technology to maximize the health care benefits for rural and remote population.

CONCLUSION

In the 21st century, it is heart-breaking to see the neglect of people with severe mental illness in some rural communities. Patients' human rights are often ignored and they are treated without much respect or dignity (Ngui et al., 2010). It is important that in organizing and planning mental health services for the rural communities, patients' human rights issues are duly considered, and health workers are trained in treating patients with mental illness and their relatives with respect and dignity. Mental health sufferers' rights should also be protected by appropriate legal framework. In a recent Lancet communication, Patel et al. (2016) highlighted that despite high level initiatives taken by Lancet in 2007 with a follow-up in 2012 and by the WHO in its mental health action plan 2013–2020, people with mental illness are still deprived to receive evidence-based treatment (Patel et al., 2008, 2016; World Health Organization, 2013).

REFERENCES

Behere P, Behere A. Farmers' suicide in Vidarbha region of Maharashtra state: a myth or reality? Indian J Psychiatry. 2008;50(2):124-7.

Behere P, Sharma V, Kumar V, et al. Mental Health Training for Health Professional: Global Mental Health Assessment Tool (GMHAT). Indian Psychiatric Society; 2017.

Fekadu A, Hanlon C, Medhin G, et al. Development of a scalable mental healthcare plan for a rural district in Ethiopia. Br J Psychiatry. 2016;208(s56):s4-12.

Gramm L, Stone S, Pittman S. Mental health and mental disorders—a rural challenge: a literature review. Rural Healthy People. 2010;1:97-114.

Gu L, Xie J, Long J, et al. Epidemiology of major depressive disorder in Mainland China: a systematic review. PLoS One. 2013;8(6):e65356.

Gururaj G, Varghese M, Benegal V, et al. National Mental Health Survey of India, 2015-16: Summary. Bengaluru, National Institute of Mental Health and Neuro Sciences; 2016.

Jacobson N, Greenley D. What is recovery? A conceptual model and explication. Psychiatr Serv. 2001;52(4):482-5.

Jenkins R, Njenga F, Okonji M, et al. Prevalence of common mental disorders in a rural district of Kenya, and socio-demographic risk factors. Int J Environ Res Public Health. 2012;9(5):1810-9.

Jordans MJ, Luitel NP, Pokhrel P, et al. Development and pilot testing of a mental healthcare plan in Nepal. Br J Psychiatry. 2016;208(s56):s21-8.

Kigozi FN, Kizza D, Nakku J, et al. Development of a district mental healthcare plan in Uganda. Br J Psychiatry. 2016;208(s56):s40-6.

Krishna M, Lepping P, Sharma VK, et al. Epidemiological and clincial use of GMHAT-PC (Global Mental Health assessment tool—primary care) in cardiac patients. Clin Pract Epidemiol Ment Health. 2009;5:7.

Kumar A. Mental health services in rural India: challenges and prospects. Health. 2012;3(12):757-61.

Kwobah E, Epstein S, Mwangi A, et al. Prevalence of psychiatric morbidity in a community sample in Western Kenya. BMC Psychiatry. 2017;17(1):30.

Lund C, Tomlinson M, De Silva M, et al. PRIME: a programme to reduce the treatment gap for mental disorders in five low- and middle-income countries. PLoS Med. 2012;9(12):e1001359.

Lund C, Tomlinson M, Patel V. Integration of mental health into primary care in low- and middle-income countries: the PRIME mental healthcare plans. Br J Psychiatry. 2016;208(s56):s1-3.

Ma Z, Huang H, Chen Q, et al. Mental health services in rural China: a qualitative study of primary health care providers. BioMed Res Int. 2015;2015:1-6.

Mohit A. Mental health and psychiatry in the Middle East: historical development. East Mediterr Health J. 2001;7:336-47.

Monteiro NM, Ndiaye Y, Blanas D, et al. Policy perspectives and attitudes towards mental health treatment in rural Senegal. Int J Ment Health Syst. 2014;8(1):9.

Nandi D. Psychiatric morbidity of a rural Indian community: changes over a 20-year interval. Br J Psychiatry. 2000;176(4):351-6.

Ngui EM, Khasakhala L, Ndetei D, et al. Mental disorders, health inequalities and ethics: a global perspective. Int Rev Psychiatry. 2010;22(3):235-44.

Patel V, Garrison P, de Jesus Mari J, et al. The Lancet's series on global mental health: 1 year on. Lancet. 2008;372(9646):1354-7.

Patel V, Saxena S, Frankish H, et al. Sustainable development and global mental health—a Lancet Commission. Lancet. 2016;19(387):1143-5.

Peen J, Schoevers R, Beekman AT, et al. The current status of urban-rural differences in psychiatric disorders. Acta Psychiat Scand. 2010;121(2):84-93.

Petersen I, Fairall L, Bhana A, et al. Integrating mental health into chronic care in South Africa: the development of a district mental healthcare plan. Br J Psychiatry. 2016;208(s56):s29-39.

Rathod S, Pinninti N, Irfan M, et al. Mental health service provision in low- and middle-income countries. Health Serv Insights. 2017;10:1178632917694350.

Rumble S, Swartz L, Parry C, et al. Prevalence of psychiatric morbidity in the adult population of a rural South African village. psychol Med. 1996;26(5):997-1007.

Sharma V. Psychiatry in primary health care: Indian perspectives. Developments in Psychiatry in India. New Delhi: Springer India; 2015. pp. 439-47.

Sharma V, Copeland J. Detecting mental disorders in primary care. Ment Health Fam Med. 2009;6(1):11-3.

Sharma V, Durrani S, Sawa M, et al. Arabic version of the Global Mental Health Assessment Tool—Primary Care version (GMHAT/PC): a validity and feasibility study. East Mediterr Health J. 2013;19(11):905-8.

Sharma V, Jagawat S, Midha A, et al. The Global Mental Health Assessment Tool-validation in Hindi: a validity and feasibility study. Indian J Psychiatry. 2010;52(4):316-9.

Sharma V, Lepping P, Cummins AG, et al. The Global Mental Health Assessment Tool—Primary Care Version (GMHAT/PC). Development, reliability and validity. World Psychiatry. 2004;3(2):115-9.

Shidhaye R, Shrivastava S, Murhar V, et al. Development and piloting of a plan for integrating mental health in primary care in Sehore district, Madhya Pradesh, India. Br J Psychiatry. 2016;208(s56):s13-20.

Simpson EL, House AO. Involving users in the delivery and evaluation of mental health services: systematic review. BMJ. 2002;325(7375):1265.

Tejada P, Jaramillo LE, García J, et al. The Global Mental Health Assessment Tool Primary Care and General Health Setting Version (GMHAT/PC)–Spanish version: a validity and feasibility study. Eur J Psychiat. 2016;30(3):195-204.

Thornicroft G, Deb T, Henderson C. Community mental health care worldwide: current status and further developments. World Psychiatry. 2016;15(3):276-86.

Tiwari SC, Srivastava G, Tripathi RK, et al. Prevalence of psychiatric morbidity amongst the community dwelling rural older adults in northern India. Indian J Med Res. 2013;138(4):504-14.

World Bank. The World Bank Annual Report 2015, Washington DC, World Bank, 2015.

World Health Organization. Mental Health Gap Action Programme (mhGAP) Intervention Guide for mental, neurological and substance use disorders in non-specialized health settings. 2010.

World Health Organization. Mental Health Action Plan 2013-2020. 2013.

World Health Organization. Mental health Atlas Geneva: WHO; 2014.

World Health Organization. Mental Health Gap Action Programme (mhGAP) Intervention Guide for mental, neurological and substance use disorders in non-specialized health settings. Geneva: WHO; 2016.

Chapter 45

Urban Mental Health

Nitin Gupta, Shiva Prakash Srinivasan

SUMMARY

Urbanization is becoming a ubiquitous phenomenon. Most of the movement from rural to urban areas is happening in the developing nations which already have large populations. This has led to many unintended consequences including sociological changes, financial and economic changes, climacteric changes and health changes. Mental health has been one aspect that has been gradually receiving more attention. Mental health problems have varied across cultures and time and space. This review will attempt to coalesce the extant literature on various aspects of mental health in urban settings. We will explore the effects of urbanization on mental health across various age groups, service care provision in urban settings and finally discuss some role of the mental health professionals in policymaking in making healthier cities.

INTRODUCTION

Urbanization is a well-recognized and ubiquitous phenomenon. Urbanization which is the increase in the number of cities and urban population, is not only a demographic movement, but also includes social, economic and psychological changes that accompany this movement. There is growth in industry and development in other aspects that is associated with the increase in urbanization. This is especially true in developing nations where nearly 3/4ths of the world's population is concentrated. This mass migration of persons from rural to urban areas has had many unintended consequences including effect on the social, economic, environmental and health-related aspects. As per the UN report 2016 (United Nations, 2016), 24 of the 31 megacities in the world are in the developing nations. Of these 24 megacities, 5 are in India. The urban areas also house more than half of the entire population in the world now. These megacities are a melting pot of various cultures leading to issues of acculturation both for the service providers as well as the individuals. In a nation as vast and diverse as India, the differences are more pronounced.

EPIDEMIOLOGY

The Census of India, 2011, defines urban areas as all places within a municipality, corporation, cantonment board or notified town area committee (referred to as statutory town). Census also notifies areas to be urban, if it has a population of more than 5,000; at least 75% of the male population is engaging in non-agricultural pursuits, and has a population density of at least 400 person per sq. km. (referred to as census town). Urban areas are classified as Mega cities when the population exceeds 10 million, Million plus cities when population exceeds one million but less than 10 million, and class I cities when the population is less than a million but more than 100,000. As against 5,161 urban areas in 2001, census 2011 shows 7,935 urban areas which is an increase of 54% in the number of towns. As of 2011, 377 million people live in urban areas of the country and urban dwellers comprise 31.16% of the total population against 27.8% in 2001. The census also recognizes that for the first time since Independence, the absolute increase in population is higher in urban areas rather than rural areas. This massive growth in urban areas was attributed to migration, natural increase and inclusion of new areas under the title "urban". It is estimated that 80% of urban increase in population in the next two decades will occur in developing nations.

A meta-analysis of various epidemiological studies (Reddy & Chandrashekar, 1998) done in India revealed a dramatic urban slant to the prevalence of mental health problems with a prevalence of 80.6 per 1,000 population in urban areas as compared to 48.9 per 1,000 population in rural areas. The only diagnoses that were made more frequently in rural areas were epilepsy and hysteria. The study noted that stress-related disorders including neurotic depression, anxiety, and obsessions contributed to the difference between the urban and rural population. In a related analysis done 2 years later, Ganguli (2000) found that the psychiatric morbidity among industrial workers in North India was two and a half times more than the other urban population and up to five times more than the rural population. The most recent and exhaustive study on epidemiology of psychiatric disorders, National Mental Health Survey of 2015–16 shows that mental disorders are more prevalent in urban region. The survey estimates that the life time prevalence of psychiatric disorders was 13.7% for the country, with the corresponding numbers for rural, urban non-metro and urban metro (million plus city) being 12.3%, 12.8%, and 19.3%, respectively. Current prevalence of psychiatric disorders (except nicotine use disorder) in individuals over 18 years at national level was 10.6%, the corresponding numbers for rural, urban non-metro and urban metro being 9.6%, 9.7%, and 14.7%, respectively. Further, across various diagnostic categories, prevalence of schizophrenia and related psychosis, mood disorders and neurotic and stress-related disorders, was nearly 2–3 times more in urban metros.

This pattern of urban rural differentiation in the prevalence of mental health problems has been noted for child mental health problems too. In a meta-analysis of epidemiological studies of the epidemiology of child mental health problems (Malhotra & Patra, 2014), in spite of the methodological differences, the prevalence of child mental health problems in the community ranged from 0.8 to 29.4% in the urban sample and 1.3–2.73% in the rural sample. In the school samples, the prevalence in urban areas ranged from 6.33 to 45.6% in urban areas and 4.6–33.3% in rural areas. The meta-analysis also suggested that there are approximately 29 million children in need of mental health services.

As per the Indian census 2011 (Census of India, 2011), the elderly constitute 8.1% of the urban population as compared to 7.9% of the rural population. While there are no detailed studies comparing the differences in the urban rural prevalence of mental health problems in the elderly, barring a few studies, a detailed review (Varghese & Patel, 2004), found a consistently high prevalence of mental health problems in geriatric age group, ranging from 33.3 to 61%. Dementia prevalence ranged from 1.6 to 2.44% in persons older than 65 years.

HEALTHCARE PROVISION

The WHO Mental Health Atlas program (World Health Organization, 2011) profiled mental health care systems in the member countries. Estimates for India include 0.329 mental health outpatient facilities per 100,000 population, 0.0823 psychiatric beds per 100,000 population in general hospitals and 1.469 beds per 100,000 population in mental hospitals. The human resources details paint a more dismal picture. As of 2011, there were only 0.301 psychiatrists per 100,000 population in India. Psychologists and social workers were 0.047 per 100,000 population and 0.033 per 100,000 population, respectively. This represents a serious dearth of both infrastructure and human resources for mental health care in India. With a growing population in urban areas, this service gap would keep expanding.

This service gap was studied in detail in a landmark study (Desai et al., 2004) which employed both qualitative and quantitative methods of evaluation. The study was conducted in three major cities of India (Chennai, Delhi, and Lucknow) and provided nearly consistent results. The research design involved mapping exercises with estimation of service loads, in-depth interviews, key informant interviews and focused group discussions. The primary results indicated an uneven availability of mental health services even in the urban areas with the government sector catering to half to two-thirds of the service load, the private sector caring for one-third to half and only a small portion being catered by the NGO sector. The human resource deficit in the studied urban areas for psychiatrists ranged from 22 to 60%, psychologists from 78 to 97%, social workers from 69 to 94% and psychiatric nurses from 45 to 76%. Chennai fared the worst in the manpower sector but still had more beds per 10,000 population than the other sites (2.5 as compared to 0.5 in Delhi and 2.0 in Lucknow). Even in the presence of such different services, the relative mental health service gap was calculated in each of the cities with a consideration of the average prevalence of mental health problems at 10%. The gap ranged from 82% in Lucknow to 96% in Chennai with Delhi at 92%.

The study also attempted to see the barriers to availing mental health services and found that financial problems, social stigma, and lack of awareness featured as the top three perceived reasons according to providers. The community also identified financial problems, lack of awareness of services and illnesses, and social stigma as barriers to seeking help. They also identified a lack of trust on government mental hospitals regarding the care provided and the hygiene conditions in such places as specific barriers to going to the government sector for care. Overall the study concluded that while the National Mental Health Programme (NMHP) and the District Mental Health Programme (DMHP) target the rural population, it is possible to erroneously assume that the urban areas have good coverage for mental health services. Given the rapid urbanization of the population in India across all age groups, it is imperative to rethink the method of delivery of care for persons with mental health problems.

MECHANISMS OF EFFECT OF URBANIZATION ON MENTAL HEALTH

The health of individuals in urban areas may be affected by multiple factors. One of the common causes is the increase in persons moving to urban areas, which requires a growth in infrastructure. However, infrastructure growth often does not keep up pace with population growth. This in turn may increase the risk of poverty and exposure to environmental adversities including overcrowding, unhealthy living situations and poverty. Poverty in itself has a multidimensional relationship with mental illnesses (Patel & Kleinman, 2003). Srivastava (2009) link identifies multiple studies that links lower socioeconomic status to alcoholism in men, increased risk of intimate-partner violence and depression in women, and so on.

At a more micro level Wandersman and Nation (1998) evaluated the effects of neighborhood characteristics on mental health and identified that socioeconomic status, racial and ethnic composition, and residential patterns are related to mental health problems, mediated by the processes of social organization, psychological stresses, and subcultural influences. The review based its findings on the available literature on the effects of childhood maltreatment, juvenile delinquency, juvenile violence, and high school dropout rates being linked to neighborhoods with a number of families in poverty, level of cultural heterogeneity, number of divorced adults, and female headed households. Regarding childhood maltreatment, the effect was mediated by weak neighborhood ties, few internal resources and stressful day to day interactions. Significant associations were noticed between neighborhood physical and social incivilities and an increase in risk of crime, juvenile delinquency, anxiety, depression, and somatic symptoms.

EFFECTS OF MAKING STRUCTURAL CHANGES IN URBAN PLANNING ON MENTAL HEALTH

The role of urban planning on health has been an age-old concept finding its roots in the formation of the Health of Towns Association in the UK in 1844. This has been recognized by the WHO in the introduction of the "healthy cities" concept (Awofeso, 2003). The concept is based on the public health objective of reducing the inequalities in social conditions and thus health among the growing urban populations the world over. It identifies the difficulties faced by the poor in urban areas including life- threatening living and working conditions as a potential area for interventions that will not be economically burdensome.

Various aspects of child development are affected by the design of the building. A detailed review (Williams & Williams, 2017) in an architectural journal identifies urban designs, that increase access to daily physical activities lasting 60 minutes, promote healthy weight, prevention of weight-related chronic diseases, improved behaviors, self-esteem, and academic performance. This includes both indoor and outdoor environments, such as access to staircases, play areas for climbing, balancing, jumping, pushing and pulling, and so on. The review also finds that quiet indoor environments, that reduce the rumbles less than that of a loud whisper, support the needs of children with learning disabilities. The individuals in the field of architecture have also been able to identify design principles for creating inclusive urban designs for persons with dementia (Pani, 2016). These include the communal and the private environments being familiar, accessible, legible, distinctive, safe, and comfortable. There are also recommendations for development of intergenerational spaces that are both therapeutic for the children as well as the elderly.

NATIONAL URBAN HEALTH MISSION

Government of India with the objective of addressing the health care needs of the urban poor (slum-dwellers, marginalized groups like rickshaw pullers, street vendors, homeless people and others), launched National Urban Health Mission (NUHM) as a sub-mission under the National Health Mission. NUHM intends to provide essential primary health care services in urban slums and to reduce the out-of-pocket expenditure of such individuals. It also envisages collaborating with Ministries of Urban Development, Housing and Poverty Alleviation, Women and Child Development and Human Resources Development to deal with wider determinants of health like drinking water, sanitation, school education, etc. Although all national health programs are to be implemented under NUHM, there is a heavy thrust on vector borne diseases, reproductive, maternal, newborn, child and adolescent services while mental health issues and indeed all non-communicable illnesses take back seat (NUHM framework document). The NUHM proposes to make available mental health services at community health center, but currently there is negligible intervention at primary level and minimal outreach activities. In effect, those with mental illness continue to seek mental health services at government-run tertiary centers or private practitioners, both of which focus on acute treatment with little role in preventive or rehabilitative services. The National Mental Health Survey 2015–16, has shown that mental disorders in urban metro area is more than metro non-urban areas. So the need is high in this region but somehow it is not yet in priority area of policymakers. Mental health services are better in urban than rural counterparts but urban areas certainly are not necessarily providing acceptable standards of care and future is not much promising either.

CONCLUSION

Urban mental health as described above has been an issue that has not got sufficient attention. This might be due to the fragmented approach to addressing the various issues related to health in urban settings. There is a clear deficit in the human resources but, that is not all. There also appears to be a lack of coordination between various stakeholders involved in the care of individuals in the urban areas (Desai et al., 2004; Patel et al., 2007). The mental health policy as of now through the DMHP and NMHP targets the rural population without necessarily considering the unique needs of the urban population. There is evidence to show that major policy changes such as increased taxes on alcohol and related substances may have a significant effect in reduction of its use.

Working toward improving the mental health care delivery system, the ancillary medical personnel are not used appropriately. There is sufficient evidence for the role of trained community health workers providing group and individual counseling sessions for women in urban slum areas having a positive effect on their physical and psychological health. The other contributors to the development of an appropriate mental health care system include the mental health professionals themselves. There is a dire need to improve mental health care in the primary care system by means of education of the primary care physicians in the care of persons with common mental disorders. This need can be met by a better consultation-liaison model and also by direct education of the general practitioners in the care of such individuals.

REFERENCES

Awofeso N. The healthy cities approach—reflections on a framework for improving global health. Bull World Health Organ. 2003;81(3):222-3.

Census India 2011. Office of the Registrar General & Census Commissioner, India Ministry of Home Affairs, Government of India 2011.

Desai NG, Tiwari SC, Nambi S, et al. Urban mental health services in India: how complete or incomplete? Indian J Psychiatry. 2004;46(3):195-212.

Ganguli HC. Epidemiological findings on prevalence of mental disorders in India. Indian J Psychiatry. 2000;42(1):14-20.

Malhotra S, Patra BN. Prevalence of child and adolescent psychiatric disorders in India: a systematic review and meta-analysis. Child Adolesc Psychiatry Ment Health. 2014;8:22.

Pani B. Improving the lives of people with dementia through urban design. J Urban Design Mental Health. 2016;1:1-12.

Patel V, Araya R, Chatterjee S, et al. Treatment and prevention of mental disorders in low-income and middle-income countries. Lancet. 2007;370(9591):991-1005.

Patel V, Kleinman A. Poverty and common mental disorders in developing countries. Bull World Health Organ. 2003;81(8):609-15.

Reddy VM, Chandrashekar CR. Prevalence of mental and behavioural disorders in India: a meta-analysis. Indian J Psychiatry. 1998;40(2):149-57.

Srivastava K. Urbanization and mental health. Ind Psychiatry J. 2009;18(2):75-6.

United Nations, Department of Economic and Social Affairs, Population Division. The World's Cities in 2016 – Data Booklet (ST/ESA/ SER.A/392), United Nations. 2016.

Varghese M, Patel V. The graying of India: mental health perspective. In: Agarwaal SP, Goel DS, Ichhpujani RL, Salhan RN, Shrivatsava S (Eds). Mental Health: An Indian Perspective 1946-2003. New Delhi: Directorate General of Health Services, Ministry of Health and Family Welfare; 2004. pp. 240-8.

Wandersman A, Nation M. Urban neighborhoods and mental health. Psychological contributions to understanding toxicity, resilience, and interventions. Am Psychol. 1998;53(6):647-56.

World Health Organization. WHO Mental Health Atlas 2011. Geneva, World Health Organization, 2011 - India. [online] Available from http://www.who.int/mental_health/evidence/atlas/profiles/ind_mh_profile.pdf. [Accessed January, 2018].

Williams L, Williams Q. Spatial designs to enhance early development and well-being in urban environments. J Urban Design Mental Health. 2017;2:8.

Chapter 46

Globalization, Market Economy, and Mental Health

R Srinivasa Murthy

SUMMARY

Social psychiatry has seen a change in its focus, outlook, and prominence over period of time. The emergence of globalization and focus on the individual for the last half a decade has now given space to critical evaluation of the impact of globalization and market economy on the common man. Globalization has effects on mental health in varied ways. The current chapter examines the development of globalization in the last few decades. Subsequently the effect of globalization and market economy on mental health is discussed, especially with regards to the newer understandings in mental health. Various issues related to globalization like rising inequity, rapid urbanization, loneliness, refugees, farmer suicides, climatic changes, industrial disasters, and child trauma are discussed. Finally the possible ways of developing a healthy approach to globalization are considered in this chapter.

INTRODUCTION

Social psychiatry during the last 100 years has seen many ups and downs. The large scale epidemiological studies of the early part of the 20th century emphasized the role of social factors in the prevalence of mental disorders. In the middle of the 20th century, the heyday of social psychiatry, there was recognition of the importance of social institutions like family and community for social cohesion beyond the individual level characteristics and actions. However, social psychiatry, so apparently promising in the optimistic context of postwar America in the 1950s and 1960s, saw its influence and status decline within American psychiatry in the late 1960s and 1970s (Blazer & Kinghorn, 2015).

The emergence of globalization and focus on the individual was a phenomenon of the last 50 years. The wheel has turned full circle, and currently globalization and market economy are seen as the enemies of the common man. These days it is common to read articles/books in the lay press titled, "capitalism, is there no alternative" (Fisher, 2008); "the great affluence fallacy" (Brooks, 2016); "globalisation: the rise and fall of an idea that swept the world" (Saval, 2017); "No, is not enough" (Klein, 2017).

It is significant to note that there were expressions of the negative impact of globalization on health even during the peak of the globalization movement (Walt, 1998; Woodward, 2001; Feachem, 2001; Lee, 2001; Miranda & Yamin, 2002; Benatar, 2005, 2011; Fisher, 2008; Piketty, 2014) and these have become coon in recent times (Friedman, 2016; Brooks, 2016; Mason, 2016;

Garten, 2016; Saval, 2017; Klein, 2017). There are many manifestations of the distrust and unhappiness among the general public as manifested by the events of recent times in both developed and developing countries. Some of these are the violent protests in Hamburg at the time of the G-20 meeting in July 2017, the Brexit vote and the hung parliament in the June 2017, UK election, the growing epidemic of opioid addiction in West Virginia attributed to large inequalities, the increasing rates of depression in the population in the economically rich countries, the rise of the right wing politics in countries like India, the farmers suicides in India, the refugee crisis in Europe, and the acute awareness of the damage to the planet by climate change.

As a result globalization and market economy, at one time considered a progressive development, is coming under scrutiny. The overall feeling is one of being in a new situation of loosing the past and not knowing what is there to replace the same, as expressed by Schwartz (2000).

"The burden of our civilization is not merely, as many suppose, that the product of industry is ill-distributed, or its conduct tyrannical, or its operation interrupted by embittered disagreements. It is that industry itself has come to hold a position of exclusive predominance among human interests, which no single interest, and least of all the provision of the material means of existence, is fit to occupy."

The current chapter addresses this topic by examining (i) the development of globalization in the last few decades, (ii) the effect of globalization and market economy in terms of the mental health impact, (iii) place the impact of globalization against what is known about mental health (especially what is the new understanding of mental health), and (iv) consider ways of developing a healthy approach to the globalization.

GLOBALIZATION

Globalization has been part of human history. What is special about globalization of the last few decades is the rapidity of the pace, and the extent of loss of boundaries and a degree of homogenization of living conditions.

The likely impact of globalization was recognized in the early phase itself. For example, Woodward et al. (2001) noted that globalization is one of the key challenges facing health policymakers and public health practitioners. They called for attention to the economic benefits of globalization to be translated into health benefits; need to be aware of the potential adverse effects of globalization on population level health-influences like tobacco marketing; international rules need should take full account of the effects on the healthcare systems and health related sectors. They concluded:

"it is important to monitor the effects of globalization and health, and to ensure that the results of such monitoring are fed effectively into the decision making processes at the national and international levels".

Huynen et al. (2005) recognizing that globalization is causing profound and complex changes in the very nature of our society, presented a conceptual framework to understand the health impacts of globalization, providing a "think-model" and a "basis for the development of future scenarios on health." Similar caution and concerns have been voiced by a number of health professionals (Walt, 1998; Woodward et al., 2001; Feachem, 2001; Lee, 2001;

Miranda & Yamin, 2002; Benatar, 2005, 2011; Fisher, 2008; Piketty, 2014; Friedman, 2016; Mason, 2016; Garten, 2016; Saval, 2017).

Lyon Declaration of 2011 presents the linkage of globalization and mental health as follows: "Globalization results from a continued process of increasing human, information and commercial exchanges across physical and political frontiers. Cultural exchanges have grown markedly since the mid-1980s with the information and communication technologies revolution to the point of creating a "world-wide village" where everyone is "a neighbor". These technologies have expanded the volume and pace of interactions; hence the emergence of a global awareness which includes demands for enhanced governance and better transparency. A global citizenship is emerging that supports solidarity: this is a hazardous but vital challenge to take up although there is a risk it may be ineffectual". Further, "The market is deemed to be rational and the state is to keep its intervention to a minimum. The underlying ideology is that individual initiative drives the success or failure of the nation's economy. In this ideology, there are two significant disconnections: explicitly the economic sphere from the political one, and the financial sphere from the economic one. As a result, there is no concern about environmental and social consequences. Today, hyperfinance rules the world and uncontrolled greed is the engine of growth". One of the effects of globalization and market economy is the concept of "precarity". The word precarity is most of the time used in its negative sense as a synonym of uncertainty, risk of catastrophe, poverty, etc. The state of precarity is both antagonistic and complementary to individual autonomy. Like for autonomy, dependency has to be respected. It is true from infancy to old age. Illness, trauma, and other states of debility increase the level of precarity, which simply and positively means: the absolute need of the others, to live. From this standpoint, one might speak of a "healthy precarity" defined as the social support that is needed at every stage of life, in a shared and reciprocal fashion. Beyond the useful concept of vulnerability, that of precarity has the valuable merit, in this individualistic era, to include the other, in its own definition.

Mental health implications of globalization comes from the recognition, "the conditions which keep and favor reliable human bonds constitute the foundation of a healthy precarity; they concern every person responsible on a social, economic, and political level. These conditions, implying justice and equity, strengthen the personal feeling of mastering a future in which everyone can take part. Neglecting these conditions is as harmful to the individual and to society as those concerning attacks against freedom and security. It does violence to the human person....Social, economic, and political contexts are prone to massively switch human bonds to unreliability and mistrust, leading to a negative precarity, with psychosocial effects prejudicial to mental health. These negative effects are focused on the loss of confidence in oneself, in one's family, in others and in the future. These effects could be described in various ways, for instance termed as depression, withdrawal, individualistic atomization, social paranoia, along with a fading of any future project but a catastrophic one". Recognizing the importance the Lyon declaration called for, "there is no global public space able to objectivize measure and qualify negative psychosocial effects of globalization. We propose to establish a perennial international network, initiated at the congress of the five continents. The objective is to demand a vital human ecology from the economical and political decision-makers who should take into account what is favorable and unfavorable to social bonds in governance principles, laws and regulations. To achieve this, we propose to create an International Observatory on Globalization and Human Ecology which will be the vector for research, exchanges and recommendations on precarity and suffering connected to the alienating effects of world "financiarisation" and "merchandisation".

IMPACTS OF GLOBALIZATION RELEVANT TO MENTAL HEALTH

The relationship between globalization and mental health has been recognized for over two decades. Different investigators have focused on varied aspects. For example, Timimi (2005) observed:

"Children's behavior is influenced by child rearing philosophies and cultural socialization processes. Globalization is imposing Western culture and views of mental health around the world with the assumption that they are superior to those in non-Western cultures. Although there are numerous examples of problematic child rearing beliefs in non-Western cultures (such as female circumcision), many practices are effective and should be preserved".

Bhugra and Mastrogianni (2004) recognized the breaking down of the cultural boundaries and changes in idioms of distress and pathways to care. They called for training packages that could enhance clinicians' cultural competency in multicultural settings.

Clark (2014a,b,c,d) in a series of four articles pointed to the dangers of medicalization of mental health. The other danger of movement of highly trained professionals from low- and middle-income countries (LMICs) to richer countries is depriving the needed professional services to populations of LMICs.

The most recent review of mental health, the Lancet—WPA Future of Psychiatry, summarizes the challenges as follows:

"A large body of evidence shows the importance of social determinants for mental disorders. Societal factors such as social inequality, crime, poverty, poor housing, adverse upbringing conditions, poor education, unemployment, and social isolation are related to increased rates of mental disorders. The relevance of some social determinants varies across the world. Examples are substantial urbanisation in LMICs; increasing social isolation in high-income countries; the changing flow of refugees in some regions; and different levels of economic instability, civil unrest, and inequality between rich and poor people. Most of these social determinants influence physical health problems too, but they can be seen as particularly relevant to psychiatry" (Bhugra et al., 2017).

There is growing evidence of the impact of globalization resulting in income inequality, urbanization, disasters, migration/refugees, climate change, loneliness, etc. The next section considers the evidence of these effects of globalization.

Inequality and Mental Health

Globalization increases inequalities in the population. Richer and stronger groups of populations are the beneficiaries of globalization (Stringhini et al., 2017). Wilkinson and Pickett (2010, 2017) have been examining this area. In their 2017 review, they conclude:

"For the last 40 years, research evidence has been accumulating that societies with larger income differences between the rich and poor tend to have worse health and higher homicide rates...taken together, the hundreds of research papers on these effects of inequality suggest that the relationships meet the epidemiological criteria for causality...mental illness is the most recent addition to this list of effects of greater inequality". Ribeiro et al. (2017) in a meta-analysis of research in this area report greater inequality is associated with higher rates of anxiety and depression, though there is heterogenicity among the studies. They call for inclusion of income inequality in the public health agenda. It is salient to note that Wilkinson and Pickett (2010) present international research studies showing associations with drug abuse, teenage pregnancies, violence, imprisonment, and quality of life (QoL). These reports raise the possibility of reduction of inequality as a contributor to population wellbeing.

Urbanization and Slums

During the last century, the migration of the populations living in urban areas has shown a massive shift. This is not only in terms of numbers but significantly populations are moving from isolated, integrated, and supportive communities to anonymous social units, with significant mental health effects. In most developing countries, over 10% of the population living in urban areas live in slums. The mental health impact of living in slums is getting greater attention. Urbanization affects mental health through the influence of increased stressors and factors such as an overcrowded and polluted environment, high levels of violence, access to illicit drugs, and reduced social support. For example, low-paid urban workers often live in crowded spaces with poor basic sanitation, food supplies, and shelter, as well as, few, if any, basic governmental and social support services (Bhugra et al., 2017).

Loneliness

Loneliness is gaining attention as an important factor for mental ill health. A number of longitudinal studies indicate that loneliness precedes depression, sleep difficulties, high blood pressure, physical inactivity, functional decline, cognitive impairment, and increased mortality. Physical and mental health components of QoL are significantly reduced by loneliness. Severe loneliness is associated with reduced patient satisfaction (Musich et al., 2015). A wide range of group and individual-based interventions have been developed to address social isolation. A recent meta-analysis reported that 80% of participatory interventions produced beneficial effects (Dickens et al., 2011). In a longitudinal study, researchers from Harvard and Peking universities analyzed 12 years' worth of data from men and women aged 65 years or older and found that loneliness and depressive symptoms appeared to be related risk factors of worsening cognition (Rubin, 2017).

Farmers Suicide

The problem of increasing rates of farmers suicides has been linked with the larger economic changes like opening of the economy to foreign investment, globalization, and related developments. In developing countries like India, there are three dimensions to the end result, namely, the agricultural dimension, the economic dimension, and the psychosocial dimension. Agricultural dimension has included the monsoon and the market; limited irrigation-rainfed agriculture is very risky; after spending so much on cash crops, the farmers find that the returns are lower than the cost—for cotton, the cost per quintal is ₹ 2585, while the support price is ₹ 1760; lack of crop insurance; low support price; high-cost intensive farming; shift to cash crops by large groups of farmers with increase in production and fall in prices; repeated crop failures; small land holdings; and use of Bt Cotton. Economic dimension has included decrease plan outlay in the Five-year plans—fall from 14.9% in the First plan to 5.2% in the Tenth plan; high interest charged by moneylenders; limited loans available from the banks; harsh measures used to recover loan money; and loans taken for social needs like marriages and education. The psychosocial dimension includes the loss of cohesive communities, loss of social supports, increasing inequalities, generation gap and raising individualism with an aspirational young generation (Srinivasa Murthy, 2012).

Climate Change

Climate change and its impact on populations is a part of everyday news. We are witness to unprecedented disasters. It is significant that the health concerns are reflected by a number of professional groups. The 2015 Lancet Commission on Health and Climate Change has been formed to map out the impacts of climate change, and the necessary policy responses, in order to ensure the highest attainable standards of health for populations worldwide. This Commission is multidisciplinary and international in nature, with strong collaboration between academic centers in Europe and China.

The central finding from the Commission's work is that tackling climate change could be the greatest global health opportunity of the 21st century. The key messages from the Commission are summarized below, accompanied by ten underlying recommendations to accelerate action in the next 5 years.

One of the recommendation (No. 4) emphasizes lifestyles and mental health as follows:

Encourage a transition to cities that support and promote lifestyles that are healthy for the individual and for the planet. Steps to achieve this include development of a highly energy efficient building stock; ease of low-cost active transportation; and increased access to green spaces. Such measures improve adaptive capacity, whilst also reducing urban pollution, greenhouse gas emissions, and rates of cardiovascular disease, cancer, obesity, diabetes, mental illness, and respiratory disease.

The American College of Physicians, the American Academy of Pediatrics, and nine other medical societies have joined forces to raise public awareness and action against the harmful effects of climate change on the health of Americans (Medscape, 2017).

The report, *Medical Alert! Climate Change is Harming Our Health*, outlines three specific types of harms from climate change: Direct harms, such as injuries and deaths due to increasingly violent weather, asthma, and other lung diseases that are exacerbated by extremely hot weather, wildfires, and longer allergy seasons. The spread of disease through insects that carry infections such as Lyme disease, Zika virus, or West Nile virus and through contaminated food and water. The effects on mental health resulting from the damage climate change can do to society, such as increasing depression and anxiety. In a new position statement, the American Psychological Association (APA) focuses on the profound impact of climate change on mental health, which may include the development or exacerbation of mental illnesses such as anxiety, depression, post-traumatic stress disorder (PTSD), or substance abuse. "Those with mental health disorders are disproportionately impacted by the consequences of climate change. APA recognizes and commits to support and collaborate with patients, communities, and other health care organizations engaged in efforts to mitigate the adverse health and mental health effects of climate change," the APA statement said.

Exposure to disasters results in mental health consequences, some chronic. Children, the elderly, people with pre-existing mental illness, the economically disadvantaged, and first responders are at higher risk for distress and other adverse mental health consequences from climate- or weather-related disasters. Communities that rely on the natural environment for sustenance and livelihood, as well as populations living in areas most susceptible to specific climate change events, are at increased risk for adverse mental health outcomes. Just the threat of climate change can cause some people to experience adverse mental health outcomes, and media and popular representations of climate change can influence stress responses and mental well-being. Extreme heat can put people with mental illness at higher risk for poor physical and mental health; and individuals with existing anxiety or depression or PTSD could see a worsening of symptoms. Individuals may develop these disorders as a result of the stress of the event. Distress reactions may also occur in the form of risky behaviors, such as increased alcohol or drug use and for many individuals, just the thought of climate change is enough to produce severe anxiety and/or depression, and perhaps a sense of hopelessness. For others, it gives rise to a strong denial reaction.

As part of the future mental health scenarios, climate change as a cause and an area for intervention will be in focus of a wide range of professionals and policymakers.

Industrial Disasters

The Bhopal gas disaster in 1984 is an example of the negative impact of uncontrolled industrialization in developing countries. The mental health impact on Bhopal even after three decades of the disaster is a continuing challenge. The inadequacy of the response to mitigate the impact is another dimension of disasters (Srinivasa Murthy, 2014). A review of 105 major industrial incidents (1971–2010) report workers in industrializing countries continue to face far greater levels of hazard exposure than those of developed countries (Beck, 2016). Unfortunately, the industrializing countries have limited capacity to care for the mental health impact of the disasters (Christodoulou et al., 2016; Srinivasa Murthy, 2014a, 2016).

Refugees

Migration of populations have been part of human history. However, in the recent past, especially in the last few years, migrations are occurring in response to conflicts, political instability, economic crisis, and the populations moving are treated as "unwelcome" in most countries. Menatl health of the refugees is compromised (Refugees Study Centre, 2014, 2017).

The stresses of forced emigration—physical, social, and psychological—have taxed all societal systems. These stresses stem not only from factors directly related to migration or living in refugee camps, but also from living under the authority of individuals with, most often, a different culture, language, and traditions (Bhugra et al., 2017).

Refugees could be at excess risk of psychiatric morbidity because of forced migration, traumatic events and resettlement in unfamiliar environments. Being a refugee and asylum seeker, both directly and indirectly, can be stressful and disturbing, and such experiences are closely related to suicide and self-harm. Prevalence of suicidal behavior among refugees is reported to range from 3.4 to 34% (Vijayakumar, 2016).

Another practice that has mental health impact on children is the separation of children from parents. MacKenzie et al. (2017) point out that harming children by separating them from their parents unnecessarily is unsound practice from the perspective of developmental and mental health science. Doing so simply to send a warning to other families is also immoral (MacKenzie et al., 2017).

There is widespread recognition for development and implementation of psychosocial-mental health interventions to address the needs of refugees (Krausz & Choi, 2017)

CHILD TRAUMA

Child neglect and abuse is gaining recognition as public health priority. Adverse conditions in early life are associated with higher risk of mental disorders. The evidence of the long-lasting effects of "child neglect and abuse" are increased rates of mental disorders. Physically abused, emotionally abused, and neglected individuals have a higher risk, 2–3 times, of developing depressive disorders than nonabused individuals. Children with a history of bullying, 40–50 years later, had an increased risk for depression and suicidal thoughts and were likely to have lack of social relationships, lower educational levels and also more likely to be unemployed and earning less. Other significant associations with childhood adversities are occurrence of first-onset and recurrent mania, fatigue syndromes, adult violent offending, and criminality. There is growing evidence of the mediation of the effects of child neglect and abuse as biologically based with associated changes at the level of stress response, changes in brain structures, inflammatory response and neurocognitive functions (Srinivasa Murthy, 2014b).

DISCUSSION

This section will bring together some of the dominant themes to present a road map for future.

It is needless to say that we are going through a period of intense stress at all levels from the individual to the environment. This is expressed differently by different thinkers. Few of these are captured below to reflect the situation humanity is in at this historical point of time.

There is growing understanding of the social origins of mental disorders and need for social interventions, in addition to individual interventions. Rebuilding communities will be an agenda of the coming times (McKnight & Block, 2012; Yarlagadda et al., 2014; Bianchi et al., 2017; Hamber & Gallagher, 2015; Junger, 2016; Giacco, 2017).

The challenge of change is reflected in an ancient Basuto proverb "if a man does away with his traditional way of living and throws away his good customs, he had better first make certain that he has something of value to replace them".

Pankaj Misra's (2017) recent book, "Age of Anger" makes two important points, to describe the current social situation and individuals. He places the current situation against the developments after enlightenment and the failed goal of equality. He makes two important observations, relevant to social psychiatry—amoral individualism and ressentiment. He summarizes, current social situation of individualism and impact on the individual as follows:

"Many of these shocks of modernity were once absorbed by inherited social structures of family and community, and the state's welfare cushions. Today's individuals are directly exposed to them in an age of accelerating competition on uneven playing fields, when it is easy to feel that there is no such thing as either society or state, and that there is only a war of all against all".

He ends the book with a conclusion of being in a, period of endless transition. He calls for, "the need for some truly transformative thinking, about the self and the world."

Brooks (2016) points to the paradox of the needs of individual and community: "In the great American tradition, millennials would like to have their cake and eat it, too." A few years ago, Macklemore and Ryan Lewis came out with a song called "Can't Hold Us," which contained the couplet: "We came here to live life like nobody was watching/I got my city right behind me, if I fall, they got me." In the first line they want complete autonomy; in the second, complete community.

The other theme is the growing need for a caring community: "We are discovering that it takes a village to do more than raise a child. It is the key to a satisfying life. It turns out we need our neighbors and a community to be healthy, produce jobs, protect the land, and care for the elderly and those on the margin" (McKnight & Block, 2012).

Rethinking of Development

One of the urgent need is to rethink development from the human perspective. For too long, society has been driven by productivity as a goal by itself, irrespective of the impact on the individuals. There are some initial attempts at rethink in terms of replacing gross national product with gross national happiness and similar thoughts. In this direction, social psychiatry, has an important role, in outlining the human needs and sources of human satisfactions (Yarlagadda et al., 2014, Blazer & Kinghorn, 2015; White et al., 2017; Bhugra et al., 2017).

Rethinking of Mental Health

The turn of the 20th century brought individualism to the forefront of mental health, an important break from the dominant role played by religion till that time. The gains of the focus of individual has been many. However, as reviewed earlier, there is need to reset the clock to have a harmony between the individualism and community life. In this effort, social psychiatry, with roots in the societal forces has much to offer.

Empowering of the individuals and families is need of the times. This is challenging as noted by Imhasly-Gandhy (2017), a psychotherapist from India:

"As clinicians and researchers we are most close to individuals and families and the challenge. The transformation of ideals, which have persisted for generations, cannot be changed in the span of a generation by rational arguments. Nevertheless, as psychologists, we can help change the individuals who have suffered and have transformed themselves and in turn influence others, leading to the formation of a critical mass. This broadening of consciousness through discussions and debates has an influence on the unconscious of others at large...we need to have the courage to deal with these issues and not transmit our entire unattended baggage to our future generations".

Rebuilding of Communities

Although the causes of mental disorders are complex and multiple, solutions have to be local and rooted in local practices and institutions. Traditionally, crisis situations were solved by elders in the family, community leaders, and religious leaders. There is a need to rebuild community life through common cultural, social, and recreational activities to provide opportunities for group commitment to values and norms of behavior (McKnight & Block, 2012). In addition, small homogeneous communities can build places for people to meet, play, and resolve their growth-related problems. Religious centers like temples, gurdwaras, churches, and mosques can play a vital part by responding to the needs of the younger generation.

Research

There is an urgent need for monitor(ing) the effects of globalization and health, and to ensure that the results of such monitoring are fed effectively into the decision-making processes at the national and international levels (Bhugra et al., 2017). This need is greater in the LMICs.

There is need to understand the impact of many effects of globalization and market economy at the level of individuals, families, communities, and state levels. Equally important is to develop interventions to address the impact at all levels both on the short- and long-term perspectives. It is best to avoid in these efforts to look the different components of society as competing or contrasting points but as complimentary. Such a harmony of the needs of the individual with that of the processes of globalization would be an important contribution of the field as well as adaptation of ideas and practices to the local cultures and communities (Nath, 2017).

The mental health group of Future of Psychiatry (Bhugra et al., 2017), recognizing that psychiatry in the first quarter of the 21st century is at the cusp of major changes, identifies the scope as follows:

"Increased emphasis on social interventions and engagement with societal expectations might be an important area for psychiatry's development. This could encompass advocacy for the rights of individuals living with mental illnesses, political involvement concerning the social risk factors for mental illness, and, on a smaller scale, work with families and local social networks and communities. Psychiatrists should therefore possess communication skills and knowledge of the social sciences as well as the basic biological sciences".

CONCLUSION

The challenges and opportunities of current situation is best presented by the Global Risk Report (2017) as follows:

"The 12th edition of The Global Risks Report is published at a time when deep-rooted social and economic trends are manifesting themselves increasingly disruptively across the world. Persistent inequality, particularly in the context of comparative global economic weakness, risks undermining the legitimacy of market capitalism. At the same time, deepening social and cultural polarization risks impairing national decision-making processes and obstructing vital global collaboration. Technology continues to offer us the hope of solutions to many of the problems we face. But the pace of technological change is also having unsettling effects: these range from disrupting labor markets through automation to exacerbating political divisions by encouraging the creation of rigid communities of like-minded citizens. *We need to become better at managing technological change, and we need to do it quickly. Above all, we must redouble our efforts to protect and strengthen our systems of global collaboration.(emphasis added).* Nowhere is this more urgent than in relation to the environment, where important strides have been made in the past year but where much more remains to be done. This is a febrile time for the world. We face important risks, but have also opportunities to take stock and to work together to find new solutions to our shared problems. More than ever, this is a time for all stakeholders to recognize the role they can play by exercising responsible and responsive leadership on global risks".

Social psychiatrists, with their recognition that mental health of individuals are largely social in origin, are eminently placed to contribute to the future mental health of humanity.

REFERENCES

American Psychological Association. Psychology and Global Climate Change: Addressing a Multi-faceted Phenomenon and Set of Challenges. Washington, APA, 2009.

Beck M. The risk implications of globalisations: an exploratory analysis of 105 major industrial incidents (1971-2010). Int J Environ Res Public Health 2016;13(3).pii: E309.

Benatar SR. Moral imagination: the missing component of global health. PLoS Med. 2005;2:e400.

Benatar SR, Gill S,Bakker I, et al. Global health and the global economic crisis. Am J Public Health. 2011;101(4):646-53.

Bhugra D, Mastrogianni A. Globalisation and mental disorders. Br J Psychiatry. 2004;184:10-20.

Bhugra D,Tasman A, Pathare S, et al. The WPA-Lancet Psychiatry Commission on the Future of Psychiatry Lancet Psychiatry. 2017;4(10):775-818.

Bianchi R, Schonfeld IS, Laurent E, et al. Burnout or depression: both individual and social issue. Lancet. 2017;390(10091):230.

Brooks D. The great affluence fallacy, New York Times, August 9, 2016.

Blazer GD, Kinghorn W. Positive social psychiatry. In: Jeste DV, Palmer BW (Eds). Positive Psychiatry—A Clinical Handbook. Washington: APA Press; 2015.

Christodoulou GN, Mezzich JE, Christodoulou NG, et al. Disasters-Mental Health Context and Responses. New Castle upon Tyne: Cambridge Scholars Publishing; 2016.

Clark J a Medicalisation of global health 1: has the global health agenda become too medicalized? Glob Health Action. 2014;7:23998.

Clark J b Medicalisation of global health 2: the medicalization of global mental health. Glob Health Action. 2014;7:24000.

Clark J c Medicalisation of global health 3: the medicalization of the non-communicable diseases agenda Glob Health Action. 2014;7:24002.

Clark J d Medicalisation of global health 4: the universal health coverage campaign and the medicalization of global health. Glob Health Action. 2014;7:24004.

Climate Change a Major Mental Health Threat, Experts Warn— Medscape - May 12, 2017.

Dickens AP, Richards SH, Greaves CJ, et al. Interventions targeting social isolation in older people: a systematic review. BMC Public Health. 2011;11:647.

Feachem RGA. Globalisation is good for your health, mostly. Br Med J. 2001;323(7311):504-6.

Fisher M. Capitalist Realism: Is There no Alternative? Winchester: OBooks; 2008.

Friedman TL. Thank You for Being Late: An Optimist's Guide to Thriving in the Age of Accelerations. London: Penguin; 2016.

Furos J, Sundaram S. Globalisation and mental health: The Lyon declaration. Asian J Psychiatry. 2012;5:283-5

Garten JE. From Silk to Silicon: The Story of Globalization. New York: Harper; 2016.

Giacco D, Amering M, Bird V, et al. Scenarios for the future of mental health care: a social perspective. Lancet Psychiatry. 2017;4(3):257-60.

Global Risk Report, 2017, 12th edition. Geneva: World Economic Forum; 2017.

Hamber B, Gallagher E. Psychosocial Perspectives on Peacebuilding. London: Springer; 2015.

Huynen MM, Martens P, Helderink HB, et al. The health impacts of globalization: a conceptual framework. Global Health. 2005;1:14.

Imhasly-Gandhy R. Eros, love and the process of individuation in Indian society, In: Nath R (Ed). Healing Room: Harper Element; 2017.

Junger S. Tribe-on Homecoming and Belonging. New York: Twelve; 2016.

Klein N. This Changes Everything. London: Penguin Random House; 2015.

Klein N. No, is Not Enough. London: Penguin Random House; 2017.

Krausz RM, Choi F. Psychiatry's response to mass traumatization and the global refugee crisis. Lancet Psychiatry. 2017;4(1):18-20.

Lee K. A dialogue of the deaf? The health impacts of globalization. J Epidemiol Community Health. 2001;55(9):619.

Lyon declaration: When Globalisation drives us mad towards an ecology of social bonds. Lyon, Conference of the Five Continents, 2011.

Mason P. Postcapitalism: A Guide to our Future. London: Penguin Random House; 2016.

MacKenzie MJ, Bosk E, Zeanah CH. Separating families at the border — consequences for children's health and well-being. NEJM, 2017: 376:2314-5.

McKnight J, Block P. The Abundant Community-awakening of the Power of Families and Neighbourhoods. 2012. Berrett Koehler Publisher Inc, California, USA.

Miranda JJ, Yamin AE. Where is the real debate on globalization? J Epidemiol Commun Health. 2002;56:719.

Misra P. Age of Anger—A History of the Present. New Delhi: Juggernaut; 2017.

Musich S, Wang SS, Hawkins K, et al. The impact of loneliness on quality of life and patient satisfaction among older, sicker adults. Gerontol Geriatr Med. 2015:1-9.

Nath R. Healing Room-The Need for Psychotherapy, Harper Element, 2017.

Piketty T. Capital in the Twenty First Century. Cambridge: Harvard University; 2014.

Refugees Study Centre: Faith and Responses to Displacement. Forced Migration Review. 2014;48.

Refugees Study Centre: Shelter in Displacement. Forced Migration Review 2017;55.

Ribeiro WS, Bauer A, Andrade MCR, et al. Income inequality and mental illness-related morbidity and resilience: a systematic review and meta-analysis. Lancet Psychiatry. 2017;4(7):554-62.

Rubin R. Loneliness might be a killer, but what's the best way to protect against it? JAMA. 2017 318(19):1853-1855.

Saval N. Globalisation: the rise and fall of an idea that swept the world. The Guardian. 2017.

Schwartz B. The Cost of Living: How Market Freedom Erodes the Best Things in Life. New York: Norton; 2000.

Srinivasa Murthy R. Farmers suicide: need for mental health interventions. Indian J Soc Psychiatry. 2012;28:26-35.

Srinivasa Murthy, R. Impact of child neglect and abuse on adult mental health. Institutionalised Children Explorations and Beyond. 2014b;1:150-62.

Srinivasa Murthy R. Mental health of survivors of 1984 Bhopal disaster: A continuing challenge. Ind Psychiatry J. 2014a;23(2):86-93.

Srinivasa Murthy R. Conflict situations and mental health care in developing countries. In: Christodoulou GN, Mezzich JE, Christodoulou NG (Eds). Disasters-Mental Health Context and Responses. New Castle upon Tyne: Cambridge Scholars Publishing. 2016. pp. 153-72.

Stringhini S, Carmeli C, Jokela M, et al. Socioeconomic status and the 25X25 risk factors as determinants of premature mortality: a multicohort study and meta-analysis of 1.7 million men and women. Lancet. 2017;389(10075):1229-37.

The Medical Society Consortium on Climate and Health: Medical alert! Climate change is harming our health. Fairfax, Center for Climate Change Communication, 2017.

Timimi S. Effect of globalization on children's mental health. BMJ. 2015;331:37-9.

Vijayakumar L.Suicide among refugees-a mockery of humanity. Crisis. 2016;37(1):1-4.

Walt G. Globalisation of international health, Lancet. 1998;351(9100):434-7.

White RG, Jain S, DMR Orr, et al. The Palgrave Handbook of Sociocultural Perspectives on Global Mental Health. London: Palmgrave-Macmillan; 2017.

Wilkinson R, Pickett K. The Spirit Level—Why Greater Equality Makes Societies Stronger. New York: Bloomsbury; 2010.

Woodward D, Drager N, Beaglehole R, et al. Globalisation and health: a framework for analysis and action. Bull World Health Organ. 2001;79(9):875-81.

Wilkinson R, Pickett K. Inequality and mental illness. Lancet Psychiatry. 2017;4:512-3.

Yarlagadda S, Maugham D, Lingwood S, et al. Sustainable psychiatry in the UK. Psychiatr Bull. 2014;38:285-90.

Index

Page numbers followed by *b* refer to box, *f* refer to figure, *fc* refer to flowchart, and *t* refer to table.